THERAPEUTIC PHARMACOLOGY

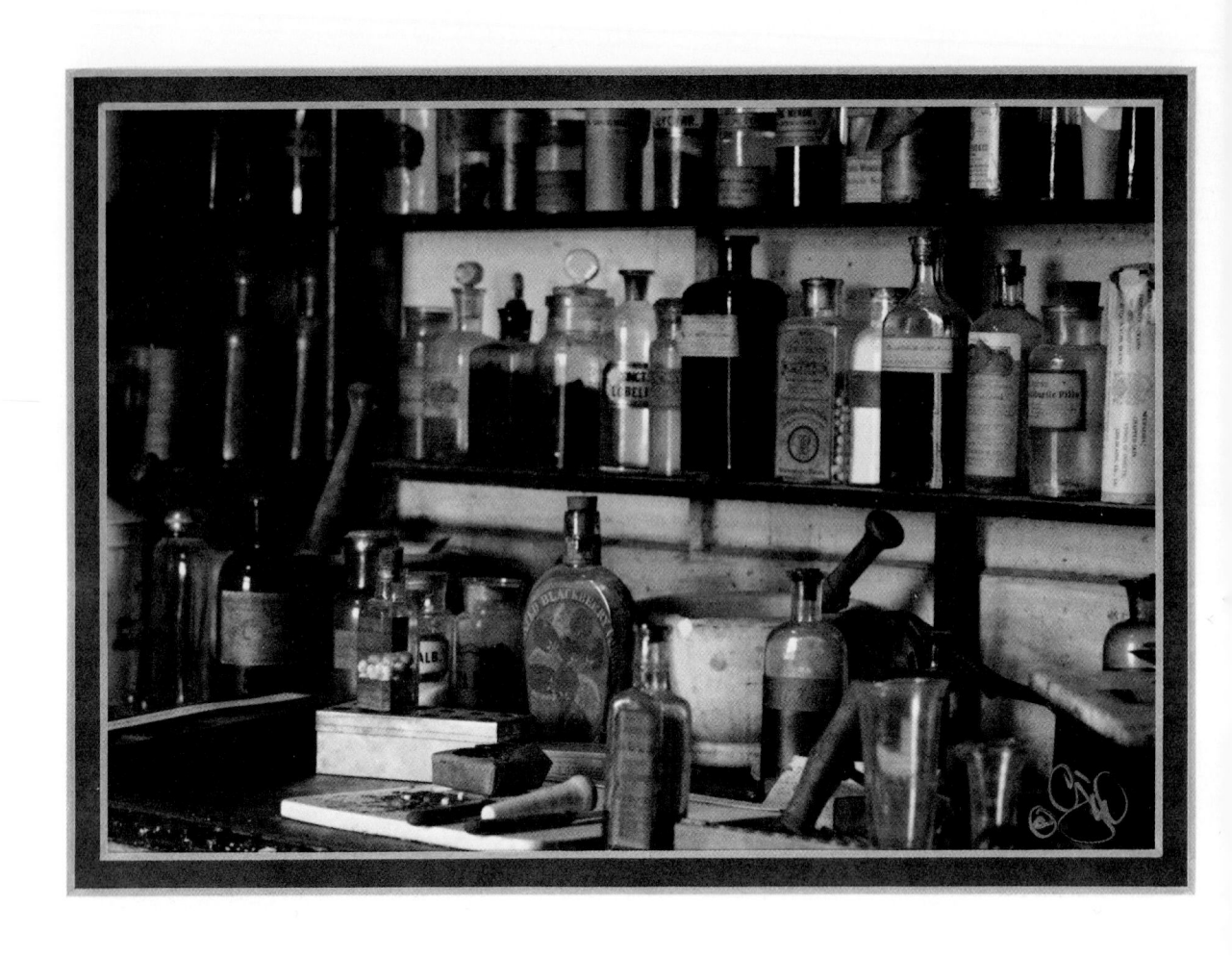

THERAPEUTIC PHARMACOLOGY

Glenn D. Appelt, Ph.D., R.Ph., F.A.C.A.
Professor of Pharmacology
School of Pharmacy
University of Colorado
Boulder, Colorado

Jennifer McNew Appelt, M.A., M.A.C.E.
Lecturer, English Department
University of Colorado, Boulder, Colorado

Formerly Director of Continuing Education
University of Kentucky, College of Pharmacy
Lexington, Kentucky

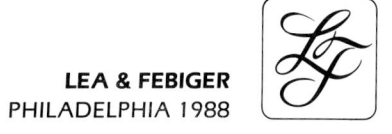

LEA & FEBIGER
PHILADELPHIA 1988

Lea & Febiger
600 Washington Square
Philadelphia, PA 19106-4198
U.S.A.
(215) 922-1330

Library of Congress Cataloging-in-Publication Data

Appelt, Glenn D.
  Therapeutic pharmacology.

  Includes bibliographies and index.
  1. Pharmacology. 2. Chemotherapy. I. Appelt,
Jennifer McNew. II. Title. [DNLM: 1. Drug Therapy.
2. Pharmacology, Clinical. QV 38 A646t]
RM300.A64 1988   615.5'8   87-21351
ISBN 0-8121-1115-X

Cover and frontispiece photograph by permission of Cynthia Davis, Denver, CO. © Cynthia Davis 1983.

Copyright © 1988 by Lea & Febiger. Copyright under the International Copyright Union. All Rights Reserved. This book is protected by copyright. *No part of it may be reproduced in any manner or by any means without written permission from the publisher.*

PRINTED IN THE UNITED STATES OF AMERICA

Print number: 5   4   3   2   1

To our many students
from whom we have learned so much and
to our very special student, Christy,
who makes all our efforts worthwhile

PREFACE

Therapeutic Pharmacology was written to provide health professionals with a clear understanding of the use of drugs from a clinical standpoint. To this end, the book is organized by organ systems, and each of the ten chapters presents anatomy and physiology, pathophysiology, disorders affecting the organ system, therapeutics, and significant drug interactions. We believe the organ system organization is a strong, practical, and necessary approach that provides integrated knowledge regarding the uses of drug therapy in clinical medicine. This focus also enables health care practitioners to communicate effectively with patients and peers.

Use of the organ system approach permits a unified and sequential consideration of healthy and functional organ processes, disorders affecting the system, pathologic changes that occur in disease, and specific drug treatments used to correct or manage the disorder/disease. Regarding the latter, the concise, practical descriptions of drug therapies interface basic pharmacology (mechanism of action, drug interactions) with applied pharmacology (clinical indications, adverse effects/precautions, drug interactions).

Considering that health professionals' clinical contacts are ordinarily with sick people who have one or more diseased organ systems, we believe that prior knowledge of what constitutes a nondiseased, functional system will better allow the student to fully understand the severity or benign nature of afflictions. Additionally, most patients do not first inquire about specific drug classes (e.g., the anticholinergics) but rather they express immediate concern about their illness symptoms or noticeable dysfunctions of particular organ systems. Consequently, we feel the use of the organ system approach prepares the student to both effectively respond to initial patient complaints and to monitor logical drug treatment regimens based upon the organ system(s) affected.

We also believe that an understanding of the disease processes involved in illness and the drugs utilized in therapy will foster more effective interprofessional communication and will optimize comprehensive health care team approaches. The organ system focus, which circumvents strict pharmacologic classifications of, for example, antibiotics, diuretics, and antineoplastics, allows the health professional student to concentrate upon the pharmacology and therapeutics of individual organ systems in a rational progression—from wellness, to illness, to therapeutics.

Use of learning objectives at the beginning of each chapter and a self-assessment examination at the end enhances *Therapeutic Pharmacology*'s value as a teaching textbook. The objectives, which also serve as a type of chapter outline, and the examinations, which describe a variety of clinical situations health practitioners encounter daily, serve as practical learning devices for the student and as discussion topics for classroom use. Although the clinical situations carry a pharmacy orientation, they are easily adaptable to all practice environments.

Of interest to those using the book primarily as a reference text are the suggested readings and the drug tables included in each chapter. The readings represent publications from a variety of sources: scientific and professional journals, annual reviews of pharmacology, textbooks, literature from pharmaceutical companies, and even articles from the lay press. By presenting a cross section of relevant information, we hope to encourage our readers to expand their reference base. The drug tables, which list the therapeutic agents available at this writing, include the drug's international generic name, trade names of products presently marketed in the United States, and recommended daily dosage ranges. Although we exerted the utmost care in preparing the drug tables, we strongly urge our readers to refer to the manufacturers' product literature regarding specific dosage/administration guidelines and recommended clinical indications.

As is the case with all authors, without the help of many others we would have been unable to complete this book. We are especially indebted to Lea & Febiger for all their support and able assistance, and so we thank George H. Mundorff, Executive Editor, Pharmacy, for believing in us from the beginning; Dorothy A. DiRienzi and Thomas J. Colaiezzi for guiding us through all the production phases; and John F. Spahr and John F. Spahr, Jr., for being such fine gentlemen. We also gratefully acknowledge the support of the administration of the University of Colorado for granting a sabbatical leave, which allowed us the time needed to finish our book. We were most fortunate to have the help of David Stirts, an excellent artist with the University of Colorado Academic Media Services, who prepared our illustrations. We appreciate the kindness of two Lea & Febiger authors, Emmanuel Stein and James Crouch, for the use of illustrations from their publications. And lastly, we express our deep appreciation to our parents, who not only kept us in school long ago, but also taught us the value of perseverance and patience.

Boulder, Colorado

Glenn D. Appelt
Jennifer McNew Appelt

CONTENTS

1

CENTRAL NERVOUS SYSTEM — 1
- Chapter Objectives — 1
- Introduction — 2
- Anatomy and Physiology of the Central Nervous System — 3
  - The Brain and the Spinal Cord ● Subcortical Brain Regions ● Ascending Reticular Activating System ● Limbic System ● Hypothalamus ● Medial Forebrain Bundle ● Periventricular System ● Spinal Cord
- Neurotransmission in the Central Nervous System — 9
  - CNS Neurons ● Noradrenergic Pathways ● Dopaminergic Pathways ● Serotonergic Pathways ● Cholinergic Pathways ● GABA-ergic Pathways ● Glycine Pathways
- Disorders of the Central Nervous System — 12
  - Pain Disorders ● Sleep Disturbances ● Sleep-Wake Disorders ● Disorders that Occur Only During Sleep ● Insomnia ● Seizures ● Affective Disorders ● Psychoneurosis ● Organic Brain Psychosis ● Schizophrenia ● Attention Deficit Disorder ● Alzheimer's Disease ● Parkinsonism ● Infections
- Therapeutic Applications of Drugs Affecting the Central Nervous System — 24
  - General Anesthetics ● Local Anesthetics ● Sedatives and Hypnotics ● Anticonvulsant Drugs ● Narcotic Analgesics ● Narcotic Analgesic Antagonists ● CNS Stimulants ● Psychotherapeutic Drugs ● Anticonvulsant Drugs ● Antiparkinsonism Drugs ● Anti-infectives
- Drug Interactions — 79
- Summary — 83
- Suggested Readings — 84
- Chapter Examination — 84

2

AUTONOMIC NERVOUS SYSTEM — 89
- Chapter Objectives — 89
- Introduction — 90

ix

Anatomy and Physiology of the Autonomic Nervous System	91
Parasympathetic Division ● Sympathetic Division ● Characteristics of the Autonomic Nervous System	
Drug Action on ANS Neurotransmission	95
Cholinergic Transmission ● Acetylcholine Receptor ● Nicotinic Acetylcholine Receptor ● Muscarinic Acetylcholine Receptor ● Adrenergic Transmission ● Adrenergic Receptors ● Alpha-adrenergic Receptors ● Beta-adrenergic Receptors	
Disorders Treated with Autonomic Drugs	105
Diseases Treated with Cholinergic Drugs ● Diseases Treated with Cholinergic Blocking Drugs ● Diseases Treated with Adrenergic Drugs ● Diseases Treated with Adrenergic Blocking Drugs	
Autonomic Drugs	111
Cholinergic Drugs ● Anticholinesterase Drugs ● Muscarinic Receptor Blocking Drugs ● Drugs Blocking Nicotinic Receptors ● Synthetic Ganglionic Blocking Drugs ● Drugs Blocking Nicotinic Receptors at the Neuromuscular Junction ● Adrenergic Drugs ● Adrenergic Blocking Drugs ● Drugs that Block Adrenergic Neurons ● Drugs that Reduce Central Adrenergic Outflow ● Drugs that Inhibit Monoamine Oxidase ● Drugs that Inhibit Catecholamine Synthesis	
Drug Interactions	144
Summary	146
Suggested Readings	146
Chapter Examination	147

3

CARDIOVASCULAR SYSTEM	149
Chapter Objectives	149
Introduction	150
Anatomy and Physiology of the Heart and Blood Vessels	150
Heart ● Blood Vessels	
Diseases of the Heart and Blood Vessels	160
Arrhythmias ● Congestive Heart Failure ● Coronary Artery Disease ● Hypertension ● Infections	
Drugs Used in the Treatment of Cardiovascular Disease	169
Cardiac Arrhythmias ● Congestive Heart Failure ● Coronary Artery Disease ● Hypertension ● Anti-infectives	
Drug Interactions	200
Summary	204
Suggested Readings	205
Chapter Examination	206

4

CIRCULATORY/RETICULOENDOTHELIAL SYSTEM	209
Chapter Objectives	209
Introduction	210

CONTENTS **xi**

Anatomy and Physiology of the Circulatory/Reticuloendothelial System   **211**
   Blood ● Lymphatic System ● Blood-forming Organs
Diseases Involving the Blood Elements and Clotting Mechanisms   **221**
   Erythrocyte Disorders ● Leukocyte Disorders ● Acquired Immune Deficiency Syndrome (AIDS) ● Hemorrhagic Disorders ● Hyperlipoproteinemias
Drugs Affecting the Circulatory/Reticuloendothelial System   **228**
   Drugs Used in the Treatment of the Anemias ● Drugs Altering Blood Coagulation ● Drugs Used to Treat Hyperlipidemias ● Drugs Used in the Chemotherapy of Hematologic Malignancies
Drug Interactions   **252**
Summary   **255**
Suggested Readings   **256**
Chapter Examination   **256**

5

RENAL SYSTEM   **259**
   Chapter Objectives   **259**
   Introduction   **260**
   Anatomy and Physiology of the Kidney   **263**
     Blood Circuit ● Tubular Urine Circuit ● Factors Influencing Diuresis
   Functions of the Kidney   **268**
     Excretion of Waste ● Acid-Base Balance ● Water Balance ● Electrolyte Balance ● Renin Secretion
   Diseases Treated with Diuretic Drugs   **271**
     Edematous Conditions ● Nonedematous Conditions
   Disorders Treated with Uricosuric Drugs   **274**
     Gout
   Drugs Affecting the Renal System   **274**
     Diuretic Drugs ● Urocosuric Drugs
   Special Aspects of Electrolyte Patterns Seen in Diuretic Therapy   **281**
     Hypokalemia ● Hyperkalemia ● Hyponatremia ● Hyperchloremia
   Factors Involved in the Clinical Selection of a Suitable Diuretic   **282**
   Drug Interactions   **283**
   Summary   **285**
   Suggested Readings   **286**
   Chapter Examination   **286**

6

ENDOCRINE SYSTEM   **289**
   Chapter Objectives   **289**
   Introduction   **290**
   Anatomy and Physiology of the Endocrine System   **293**
     Pituitary Gland ● Thyroid Gland ● Parathyroid Glands ● Adrenal Glands ● Gonads ● Pancreas
   Special Aspects of Endocrine Glands   **302**

Dysfunction of the Endocrine Glands ... 304
  Anterior Pituitary Gland ● Posterior Pituitary Gland ● Thyroid Gland ● Parathyroid Glands ● Adrenal Glands ● Gonads ● Pancreas
Drugs Affecting the Endocrine System ... 309
  Anterior Pituitary Hormones ● Posterior Pituitary Preparations ● Thyroid Gland Preparations ● Antithyroid Drugs ● Thyroid Parafollicular C Cell Hormone ● Parathyroid Gland Preparations ● Adrenal Gland Preparations ● Sex Hormone Preparations ● Pancreatic Preparations
Drug Interactions ... 328
Summary ... 330
Suggested Readings ... 331
Chapter Examination ... 331

7

RESPIRATORY SYSTEM ... 335
Chapter Objectives ... 335
Introduction ... 336
Anatomy and Physiology of the Respiratory System ... 336
Disorders of the Respiratory System ... 340
  Allergy ● Diseases/Disorders of the Nose, Throat, and Ear ● Chronic Obstructive Pulmonary Disease ● Bacterial/Viral Infectious Diseases of the Lower Respiratory Tract ● Infectious Fungal Disease ● Pulmonary Tumors
Drugs Used in Respiratory Disorders and Infections ... 347
  Antihistamines; H_1 Receptor Blockers ● Antibacterial Drugs ● Antibacterial Drugs that Affect Cell Wall Synthesis ● Antibacterial Drugs that Affect Protein Synthesis ● Antibacterial Drugs that Act Primarily as Antimetabolites ● Antimicrobial Drugs that Alter Plasma Membrane Permeability
Drugs Used in Respiratory Tract Obstruction ... 366
  Bronchodilators ● Anticholinergic, Antimuscarinic Bronchodilator Drugs ● Mucolytic Drugs ● Corticosteroids ● Nasal Decongestants ● Antitussives
Drugs Used in Lung Carcinoma ... 370
Drug Interactions ... 370
Summary ... 372
Suggested Readings ... 372
Chapter Examination ... 373

8

DIGESTIVE/GASTROINTESTINAL SYSTEM ... 375
Chapter Objectives ... 375
Introduction ... 376
Anatomy and Physiology of the Digestive/Gastrointestinal System ... 376
  Mouth and Esophagus ● Stomach ● Small Intestine ● Colon ● Additional Organs Vital to Digestion

Disorders of the Digestive/Gastrointestinal System	382
Disorders of the Mouth/Salivary Glands ● Esophageal Disorders ● Stomach Disorders ● Intestinal Disorders ● Liver Disorders ● Gallbladder Disorders ● Pancreatic Disorders	
Drugs Used in the Treatment of Digestive/Gastrointestinal System Disorders	389
Drugs Used in the Treatment of Peptic Ulcer ● Laxatives ● Digestive Aids ● Antidiarrheals ● Miscellaneous Gastrointestinal Drugs ● Antihemorrhoid Preparations ● Antiemetics ● Antibiotics/Anti-infections Used in Gastrointestinal Infections ● Antineoplastics ● Anthelmintics	
Drug Interactions	410
Summary	411
Suggested Readings	411
Chapter Examination	411

9

REPRODUCTIVE/GENITOURINARY SYSTEM	415
Chapter Objectives	415
Introduction	416
Anatomy and Physiology of the Reproductive/Genitourinary System	416
Female Genital System ● Male Genital System ● Renal/Urinary Excretion System	
Diseases and Disorders of the Genitourinary System	419
Venereal Infections ● Nonvenereal Infections ● Carcinomas of the Female Reproductive System ● Carcinomas of the Male Reproductive System ● Carcinoma of the Urinary Bladder	
Drugs Used in the Treatment of Genitourinary Diseases and Infections	423
Drugs Used to Treat Infections ● Drugs that Affect Uterine Musculature ● Antineoplastic Drugs	
Drug Interactions	435
Summary	435
Suggested Readings	436
Chapter Examination	436

10

INTEGUMENTARY/CONNECTIVE TISSUE SYSTEM	439
Chapter Objectives	439
Introduction	440
Anatomy and Physiology of the Integumentary/Connective Tissue System	440
Connective Tissue ● Functions of the Skin ● Sweat Glands ● Skin Appendages	
Diseases and Disorders of the Integumentary/Connective Tissue System	442
Skin Infections ● Skin Infestations ● Miscellaneous Skin Disorders ● Skin Cancers ● Disorders of the Joints and Connective Tissues	

Drugs Used in the Treatment of Integumentary/Connective Tissue
   Disorders	**446**
   Drugs Used to Treat Skin Diseases ● Drugs Used to Treat Diseases of
   the Joints and Connective Tissues
Drug Interactions	**456**
Summary	**457**
Suggested Readings	**457**
Chapter Examination	**458**

# APPENDICES	**461**

Appendix A. Ocular Anti-inflammatives and Anti-infectives	**461**
Appendix B. Fluid-electrolyte and Nutritional Replenishers	**462**
Appendix C. Vitamins	**463**
Appendix D. Immunologic Agents	**464**
Appendix E. Radiopaque Agents and Radiographic Adjuncts	**464**
Appendix F. Immunosuppressive Drugs	**465**

# INDEX	**467**

chapter 1

CENTRAL NERVOUS SYSTEM

CHAPTER OBJECTIVES

After studying this chapter, you should be able to:
1. Name the major anatomic divisions of the human brain.
2. Describe the physiologic functions associated with each brain division.
3. Discuss neurochemical transmission in the central nervous system (CNS).
4. List several chemicals that are designated as CNS neurotransmitters.
5. Discuss the significance of the central monoamine systems.
6. Discuss several theories regarding the mechanism of action of anesthetics.
7. List several volatile general anesthetics and describe the pharmacologic characteristics of at least two of these drugs.
8. Describe the toxicity associated with halothane, nitrous oxide, and ketamine.
9. Explain the use of local anesthetics in surgical procedures.
10. Discuss the characteristics of NREM and REM sleep.
11. Name two examples of barbiturates considered as: ultra-short acting; short acting; intermediate acting; long acting.
12. List several therapeutic uses of barbiturates.
13. Discuss the treatment of acute barbiturate intoxication and chronic barbiturate abuse.
14. List several non-barbiturate sedative-hypnotics and give at least two possible advantages of these drugs over barbiturates.
15. Discuss the use of sedative-hypnotics in the treatment of pain.
16. Discuss the characteristics of several forms of seizures.
17. Name at least two drugs of choice in the treatment of petit mal seizures; grand mal seizures; psychomotor-grand mal mixed seizures; Jacksonian seizures.
18. Name several adverse effects that occur with hydantoin anticonvulsants; succinimide derivatives; and phenacemide.
19. Comment on phenobarbital-phenytoin combination therapy in the control of grand mal seizures.
20. Discuss the pharmacologic activity and therapeutic indication for carbamazepine; valproic acid; and acetazolamide.
21. Discuss factors associated with drug selection and dosage adjustment in the control of seizures.
22. List the major naturally occurring opium alkaloids and designate whether the individual alkaloid is a phenanthrene or benzylisoquinoline type.
23. Name three pharmacologic properties of morphine sulfate not related to central nervous system depression.
24. Describe the treatment of acute opiate overdose.
25. Compare the pharmacologic properties of meperidine HCl to morphine sulfate.

26. Discuss the pharmacologic properties of methadone and explain its selection for use in heroin withdrawal treatment programs.
27. Describe the opiate withdrawal syndrome and compare it to withdrawal from barbiturates.
28. Discuss several interactions of the opiates with other drugs.
29. Describe the effect of methylxanthines on phosphodiesterase activity and adenosine receptors.
30. Describe the effects of caffeine on the myocardium; blood vessels; gastric secretion; and bronchiolar muscles.
31. Outline several proposed mechanisms of action for amphetamine activity.
32. Evaluate d-amphetamine, methylphenidate, phenteramine, and phenmetrazine in modern therapeutics and list valid clinical indications for these drugs.
33. Describe criteria that link neurotransmitters to behavioral change.
34. Discuss at least two theories relating to the biochemical causation of schizophrenia.
35. Considering the different chemical divisions of the phenothiazine derivatives, differentiate the likelihood of common adverse effects that occur in each division.
36. State the site(s) in the CNS affected by the phenothiazines to produce hypotension; to cause hypothermia; to elicit an antiemetic effect; and to induce neurologic adverse effects.
37. List and explain several therapeutic interactions that occur with the phenothiazine derivatives.
38. Discuss at least two theories concerning the antipsychotic mechanism of action of the phenothiazine derivatives.
39. Explain the clinical indications and therapeutic expectations of the tricyclic antidepressants (TCADs).
40. Describe two theories regarding the mechanism of action of imipramine.
41. Discuss the major limitations of the monoamine oxidase inhibitors (MAOIs) in the treatment of depression.
42. List the main pharmacologic properties of lithium carbonate.
43. State the proposed sites of action that are involved in skeletal muscle relaxation produced by diazepam and meprobamate.
44. Discuss the possibility of the development of physical dependence on the benzodiazapine group of antianxiety drugs.
45. Name several side effects that are common to the propanediol group of tranquilizers.
46. Discuss the possible significance of diazepam-induced depression of limbic system activity as compared to chlorpromazine-induced activation in this region.
47. Discuss the etiology of parkinsonism, emphasizing cholinergic-dopaminergic mechanisms.
48. Describe a proposed mechanism of action for levodopa; amantadine; biperidin; trihexyphenidyl; and bromocryptine mesylate.
49. Explain the possibility of clinical improvement with levodopa in reserpine-induced parkinsonism as compared to the lack of benefit in chlorpromazine-induced parkinsonism.
50. State the effect of the following drugs on the clinical activity of levodopa: pyridoxine; chlorpromazine; haloperidol; and carbidopa.

INTRODUCTION

The central nervous system (CNS) consists of the brain and spinal cord; the latter's primary function is the transport of information to and from the brain (Figure 1.1). Sensory nerve fibers enter the CNS and carry information previously coded at peripheral sites. To illustrate, sensory fibers transmit the type, intensity, and location of a sensation into the spinal cord and brain where interpretation of the information occurs. The human brain, resembling a sophisticated computer, has an unequaled capacity for both the integration and storage of incoming information. This process involves decoding, rerouting, and interacting with prior information to permit translation by the brain into appropriate reaction by the individual.

The CNS, as with the autonomic nervous system (ANS), is superimposed upon all other organ systems for the purpose of coordinating their diverse functions (Figure 1.2). Thus, the total organism achieves an integrated and smoother activation of all processes. Only recently explored at a molecular level, the brain is the root of consciousness, a phenomenon that is basic to life. Besides consciousness, functions such as behavior, memory, recognition, and learning are all based in the brain. Abstract reasoning and creative thought, characteristic feats of man's ability as a living organism, are formulated in the brain.

In 1981, Sperry received the Nobel Prize in Medicine for discovering that the left side of the brain relates to reason, logic, measurement, and speech, and the brain's right side dominates creativity, inspiration, and feelings. Synchronization of man's two brains (left and right sides or hemispheres) apparently increases and heightens awareness in the individual. Although research in this area of brain function is in its beginning stage, biofeedback techniques for anxiety control and related problems indicate the strong interrelationship of the brain with the ANS.

The human brain, weighing about 1.4 Kg and protected by the bony cranium, contains more than 11 billion interconnecting neurons. These neurons form before birth and are irreplaceable if injured or destroyed. Although estimates indicate that adults lose about 10,000 neurons daily, a 100 year old should still have 97% of the total number of neurons present at birth.

The pharmacologic thrust toward understanding the biochemical and molecular mechanisms of drug action on the brain is one of modern medicine's most exciting challenges. Extensive research efforts continually yield information about chemical agents that may effectively treat mental illnesses that are refractory to other therapy.

ANATOMY AND PHYSIOLOGY OF THE CENTRAL NERVOUS SYSTEM

Knowledge of the anatomic characteristics of the brain and the spinal cord and the physiologic functions of each region enhances one's

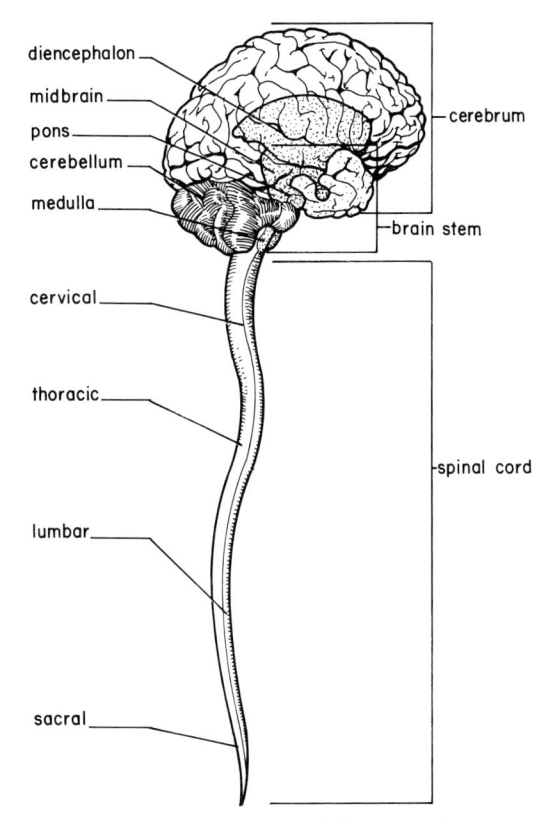

Fig. 1.1 General anatomy of the central nervous system. (From Crouch, J.E.: Essential Human Anatomy. Philadelphia, Lea & Febiger, 1982.)

understanding of drug action on the central nervous system.

THE BRAIN AND THE SPINAL CORD

The brain is enclosed in a protective bony shell called the cranium; this bony covering (skull) resists moderate blows. If viewed from the top without the bony skull, the brain looks like a huge, soft, pinkish-gray walnut, complete with a wrinkled surface and division into two halves or hemispheres. These wrinkles or infoldings greatly increase the surface area of the cerebral cortex and are quite uniform in normal brains. Thus, they serve as guides or landmarks in determining specific functional areas of the brain for speech, vision, and hearing. A deep vertical fissure divides the brain into left and right hemispheres; other infoldings separate individual lobes in each hemisphere.

4 THERAPEUTIC PHARMACOLOGY

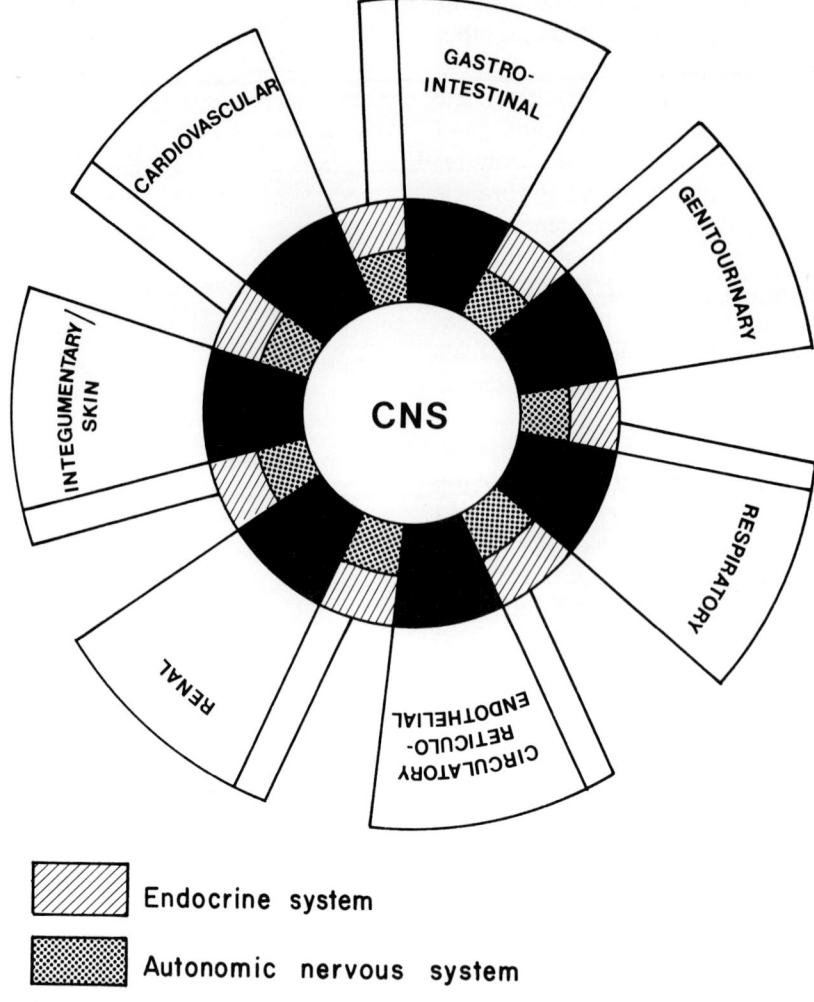

Fig. 1.2 Central nervous system as core influence.

Divided into three subunits based upon embryologic considerations, the brain develops at the cranial end of the neural tube, forming the forebrain, hindbrain, and the midbrain. The spinal cord forms from the rest of the neural tube.

The forebrain develops into the two cerebral hemispheres, the thalamus and the hypothalamus. The hindbrain evolves into the medulla, pons, and cerebellum. Located between the pons and the thalamus, the midbrain structurally remains essentially unaltered from the neural tube. The cavity of the neural tube designates the ventricular system in the formed brain.

The thalamus and hypothalamus (diencephalon) form the upper part of the brain stem. Subthalamic nuclei lie between the dorsolateral aspect of the hypothalamus and the dorsal thalamus. These nuclei functionally relate to the extrapyramidal motor system.

The cerebral cortex, the basal ganglia or striatum, and the limbic system (including the olfactory bulbs, septal nuclei, amygdala, and hippocampus) comprise the telencephalon. The major sulci divide the telencephalon into frontal, parietal, temporal, and occipital lobes.

The hindbrain and midbrain (lower brain stem) are sites of outflow for all cranial nerves except the olfactory nerves and the optic nerves. The cranial nerves are either somatic (as represented by those linking to facial muscles) or autonomic (as noted in the parasympathetic vagus nerves). Additionally, the cranial nerves serve somatosensory, visceral, and special senses, such as taste, hearing, and vestibular functions.

Located on the top surface of the lower brain stem, the cerebellum, meaning "little brain," has two hemispheres and a central connecting structure. The cerebellum, containing the centers for muscle coordination, equilibrium, and muscle tone, receives information from the spinal cord and from vestibular afferents for posture maintenance. Thus, this structure is instrumental in maintaining motor function and control. Proprioceptive input, equilibrium, and modulation of voluntary motor movements are also under cerebellar control.

Three supporting membranes that minimize shocks and jolts to the head are the meninges. These membranes suspend the brain and spinal cord in a liquid medium of cerebrospinal fluid. The dura mater ("tough mother") is the tough outer membrane that adheres to the skull and the spinal cord through fat pads. The delicate inner membrane, called the pia mater ("tender mother"), adheres to the brain and contains blood vessels. A web-like membrane, the arachnoid, holds the dura mater and pia mater together.

The brain's outer rind is a grayish layer of nerve cells about 0.3 cm thick. This "gray matter" contains neurons that distribute nerve impulses across selected synapses. The white tissue ("white matter") that lies underneath the gray matter conducts impulses along nerve fibers.

Known as the cerebral cortex, the gray matter analyzes incoming sensory information and initiates voluntary motor behavior. Centers for speech, sensation, and movement are located in the cerebral cortex; thus, this part of the brain is responsible for the special uniqueness of the human mind and constitutes one of the most complex structures in nature.

The cerebral cortex weighs about 454 g and contains dendrites and axon terminals (synapses) of 9 billion neurons. Supporting cells and blood vessels comprise the remainder of the cerebral cortex. The major structure in the human CNS, the cerebral cortex substantially evolved from lower animals and occupies a higher percentage of space in the human brain. The folds and wrinkles in the brain, plus the fact that the cortex practically covers other parts of the brain, indicate expansion of the brain within the skull.

The cerebral cortex is functionally divided into receiving areas, output areas, and association areas. Sensory neurons from the primary senses supply the receiving areas. Found in the same general region of the brain, receptors in these receiving areas respond to a particular sensory stimulus. Output areas of the cerebral cortex supply neuraxons to subcortical regions of the brain and carry impulse traffic to glands and muscles. The association cortex does not directly receive or directly supply neurons; rather, it functions in assimilation and control of complex behavior.

The distribution of thalamocortical projection neurons determines the major separation of functions in different areas of the cerebral cortex. In addition to areas of the primary sensory cortex that receive visual, auditory, and somatosensory information from subcortical thalamic sites, secondary sensory areas are not linked by specific thalamic projections. The prefrontal cortical region or "association" cortex, highly developed in man, connects by association fibers with the occipital and temporal cortex.

Located in the frontal regions of the brain, motor areas of the cerebral cortex initiate impulses when decisions signal behavioral response. Some of the motor cortex neurons extend their axons downward through the cerebral peduncles and pyramids of the medulla oblongata. These neuraxons pass to the lower brainstem and finally to the upper spinal cord where they are designated as corticospinal fibers. These pathways are vital in initiating voluntary muscle movement. Because of their passage through pyramidal cells, these classical avenues are called pyramidal tracts. The extrapyramidal system consists of motor neuraxon pathways that do not intercept the pyramidal cells but connect with the basal ganglia, the thalamus, and the cerebellum to modulate motor function. As noted later, extrapyramidal side effects are common with certain classes of CNS drugs, especially the phenothiazine tranquilizers.

The striatum (basal ganglia) is divided into the neostriatum (caudate nucleus and putamen) and the paleostriatum (globus pallidus). The group of nuclei that form the basal ganglia comprise a secondary motor system. The basal ganglia modulate the nonvoluntary, nonconscious adjustments of muscles concerned with posture and muscle tone. Parkinsonism, a disease characterized by muscle rigidity, tremors, a "pill-rolling" movement of the fingers, and a decrease in facial expression, results from abnormalities in this brain region.

SUBCORTICAL BRAIN REGIONS

Certain of the brain's subcortical areas, responsible for many necessary integrating functions, are prime targets for psychotropic drug action. Three of these sites (the ascending reticular activating system, the limbic system, and the hypothalamus) comprise the anatomic substrate for human emotion.

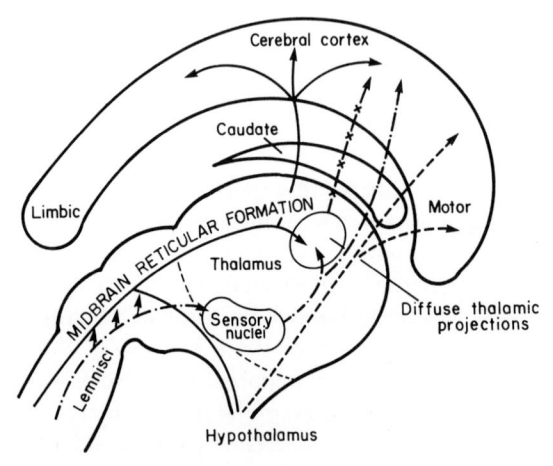

Fig. 1.3 Reticular formation. (Modified from Science, 127:59, 1958.)

ASCENDING RETICULAR ACTIVATING SYSTEM (ARAS)

The ascending reticular activating system (ARAS) is a diffuse collection of neuron cell bodies and neuron fibers in the central brain stem (Figure 1.3). The ARAS receives impulses through collaterals that are branches of sensory neurons, which transverse the classical lemniscal pathways. Sensory input results in direct transmission of impulses to the appropriate area of the cortex and channeling of impulses through the ARAS. Both paths are essential for an individual's awareness of any sensory stimulus. Unless the cortex is aroused by the ARAS before recognition of information, activation of the cortex is impossible. The ARAS is multisynaptic and distributes axons throughout the brain. The mutisynaptic nature renders the ARAS susceptible to drug influence.

The reticular core is the fundamental center of integration in the brain since other centers can't function in its absence. It extends from the mid-medulla oblongata upwards through the pontine and midbrain tegmentum.

Impulse output from the ARAS rises higher into the thalamus and the cortex to determine the arousal state of the CNS. One of the primary functions of the ARAS is control of the brain's arousal level. Accordingly, the ARAS receives and relays input from all sensory modalities. Stimulation that results from the impulse traffic on these pathways is transmitted to the cerebral cortex. The ARAS initiates impulses to the cerebral cortex, thus preparing it for receipt of further information via sensory pathways. Activation of the cerebral cortex by the ARAS produces an alert and behaviorally aroused state with an enhanced awareness of environmental stimuli.

The ARAS' role as a selective sieve or screening system for sensory input explains adaptation by the ARAS to an individual milieu. For example, an individual born and reared in a rural environ with its accompanying serene and quiet ambience often experiences difficulty sleeping in a city apartment that is located on a busy freeway. After a few nights, this person usually adapts to the car noises as his ARAS selectively blocks the nonthreatening arousal of the cortex. The inhibition of cortical arousal, however, is not generalized to include all sensory input as smoke (a potentially dangerous and unusual sensory input) immediately wakes this individual.

LIMBIC SYSTEM

Functionally implicated in modulating emotional behavior, the limbic system represents temporal lobe structures that include the fornix, hippocampus, anterior thalamus, hypothalamic nuclei, the mammillary bodies, amygdala, and septal nuclei (Figure 1.4). Although the differences between the ARAS and the limbic system were once easily contrasted, these differences are now less apparent due to increases in functional knowledge of the brain. Rich in interneurons, the limbic system unites with the ARAS and the thalamus. Whereas the thalamus is the region through which emotional stimuli enter consciousness, the limbic system is regarded as the seat of emotion.

The term rhinencephalon, "nose brain," has long denoted the limbic system, especially in lower animals. Although smell and emotional response are closely related in man, the implication that the limbic system's function is limited to olfactory stimuli is inaccurate. Because the limbic system evidently dominates visceral activities, the term "visceral brain" is a more accurate descriptor. For example, a phrase like "you make me sick to my stomach" represents a spontaneous emotional reaction that doesn't logically stem from an intellectual evaluation of a given situation. Rather, the actual anatomic source of this emotional response is the limbic system, not the stomach. Thus, stress, the psychogenic component in many total disease profiles, contributes to organic disease, such as ulcers or hypertension.

HYPOTHALAMUS

The thalamus and hypothalamus are often termed the diencephalon (Figure 1.5). The thalamus, a relay center to and from the cerebral cortex, acts as a center for unlocalized sensations, either agreeable or disagreeable. The hypothalamus, one of the oldest areas of the brain, functions as the central regulator of the ANS. Information from the body that is relevant for maintenance of the organism is integrated into appropriate responses. Each cerebral hemi-

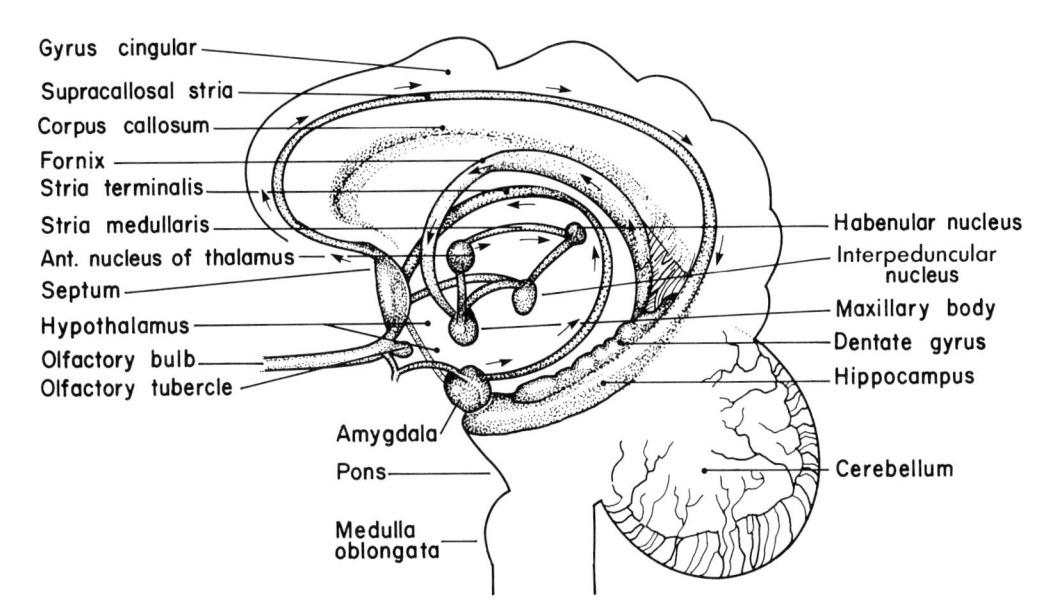

Fig. 1.4 Limbic system. (Modified from Neuropsychopharmacology: A Series from Roche Laboratories. Nutley, NJ, Hoffmann-La Roche, 1976.)

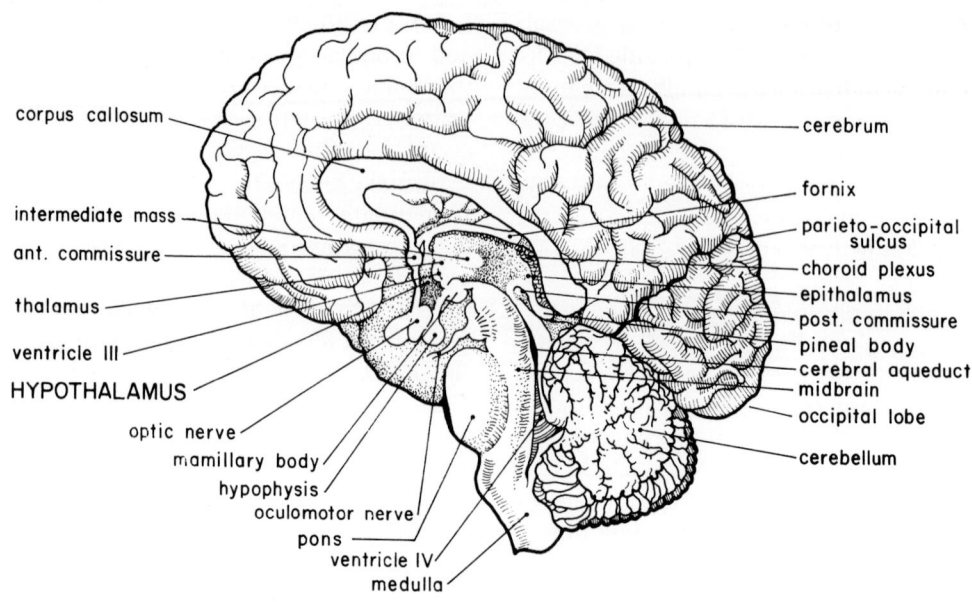

Fig. 1.5 Hypothalamus. (Modified from Crouch, J.E.: Essential Human Anatomy. Philadelphia, Lea & Febiger, 1982).

sphere contains one of a pair of identical hypothalamic nuclei. These nuclei, consisting of groups of dendrites (receiving projections of neurons), perform specific functions. Hypothalamic osmoreceptors, for instance, monitor the blood to insure a normal range of blood osmolarity. Hypo-osmotic or hyperosmotic conditions activate hypothalmic neurons that stimulate compensatory hormone mechanisms. The interface of the hypothalamus with the endocrine system adjusts and maintains homeostasis.

Hypothalamic nuclei monitor blood levels of various chemicals and release substances that the bloodstream delivers to target structures. For example, hypothalamic releasing factors stimulate the anterior pituitary gland to secrete hormones, such as corticotropin and thyrotropin. The hypothalamus also contains cell bodies of a neurosecretory pathway to the posterior pituitary gland, which connect to this gland via the infundibulum.

Other neuroregulatory processes attributed to hypothalamic regions include temperature regulation ("thermostat"), appetite control ("appestat"), and water intake ("osmostat"). Because the hypothalamus has a rich blood supply, drugs that enter the bloodstream reach the hypothalamus in high concentrations. Consequently, many central acting drugs initially alter autonomic function before having any effect on consciousness.

MEDIAL FOREBRAIN BUNDLE (MFB)

A group of neuraxons rimming the perimeter of the hypothalamus comprise the medial forebrain bundle (MFB). As indicated by experiments of electrical stimulation, this part of the brain is the physiologic substrate for pleasure and reward. Other studies implicate abnormal MFB function in episodes of psychotic behavior; mood alterations (as in depression) involve changes in electrical activity of this brain region.

PERIVENTRICULAR (PV) SYSTEM

The cerebral ventricles exist as four cavities within the brain and consist of two lateral ventricles (one in each cerebral hemisphere) and singular third and fourth ventricles. The periventricular (PV) system is a collection of fibers concerned with punishment or aversion responses in the individual. In contrast to the medial forebrain bundle (MFB), the PV system constitutes a negative area since activation results in discomfort. Current data suggest that the PV system may functionally relate to the MFB, and that activation of the MFB depresses the PV system, producing a cerebral activation process.

SPINAL CORD

Whereas the brain develops at the cranial end of the developing neural tube, the spinal cord constitutes the remainder of this tube. Bony vertebrae of the spinal cord enclose the meninges, cerebral spinal fluid (CSF), and the spinal nerves. The spinal cord, which carries information to and from the brain, is the elongated portion of the CNS that extends down the back from the base of the brain to the sacral vertebrae.

NEUROTRANSMISSION IN THE CNS

The brain contains a number of distinct nerve systems that directly or indirectly influence many physiologic functions. Each of these systems is characterized by a specific neurochemical transmitter responsible for impulse transmission at central synapses or central terminal receptor sites. The proper balance and functioning of these neurotransmitters play a vital role in governing states of consciousness and in modulating emotional experience and behavior.

CNS NEURONS

The general features of "typical" human central neurons resemble the model established for peripheral neurons (see Chapter 2). The central neuron model consists of the cell body, including dendrites that emanate from this structure and a nucleus contained within it; and the axon that transports enzymes, vesicles, and precursors from the cell body to the third major structural component—the nerve terminal (Figure 1.6). The latter is the site of neurotransmitter synthesis and storage.

Neurotransmitter synthesis, release, degradation, and reuptake all occur at the nerve terminal (Chapter 2). The terminal contains specialized vesicles or granules that are involved in the uptake, storage, and release of neurotransmitters. Mitochondria, present in the terminal, provide the metabolic energy required for these processes. Degradation enzymes, such as monoamine oxidase, are also contained in the mitochondria.

The depolarization of the nerve terminal membrane by an action potential is accompanied by changes in Na^+, K^+, and Ca^{++} flux. Fusion of the neurotransmitter storage vesicle to the terminal membrane is the initial process in neurotransmitter release; exocytosis of the vesicle contents into the synaptic cleft follows. The neurotransmitter then diffuses into close proximity of postsynaptic receptors where interaction initiates biochemical events that ultimately result in a specific physiologic response.

Monoamine systems in the brain are vital to a number of physiologic functions. Three main monoamine systems are critical for the regulation of a variety of behavioral responses including affective reaction, arousal, cognition, aggression, and sexual drive. The neurotransmitter operant in synaptic events designates these amine systems as noradrenergic (NE), dopaminergic (DA), and serotonergic (5-HT).

Although similar structurally, the monoaminergic neurons differ primarily in the enzymes present to synthesize the respective neurotransmitter. After forming in the cell body, enzymes required for neurotransmitter synthesis travel by axoplasmic flow to the nerve terminals. These nerve terminals consist of numerous branches that contain swellings called varicosities.

Within the varicosities are vesicles that hold the neurotransmitter. The vesicles actively take up amines in the cytoplasm by a process requiring adenosine triphosphate (ATP) and magnesium (Mg). The storage vesicles of norepinephrine neurons contain dopamine-beta-hydroxylase, the enzyme that mediates

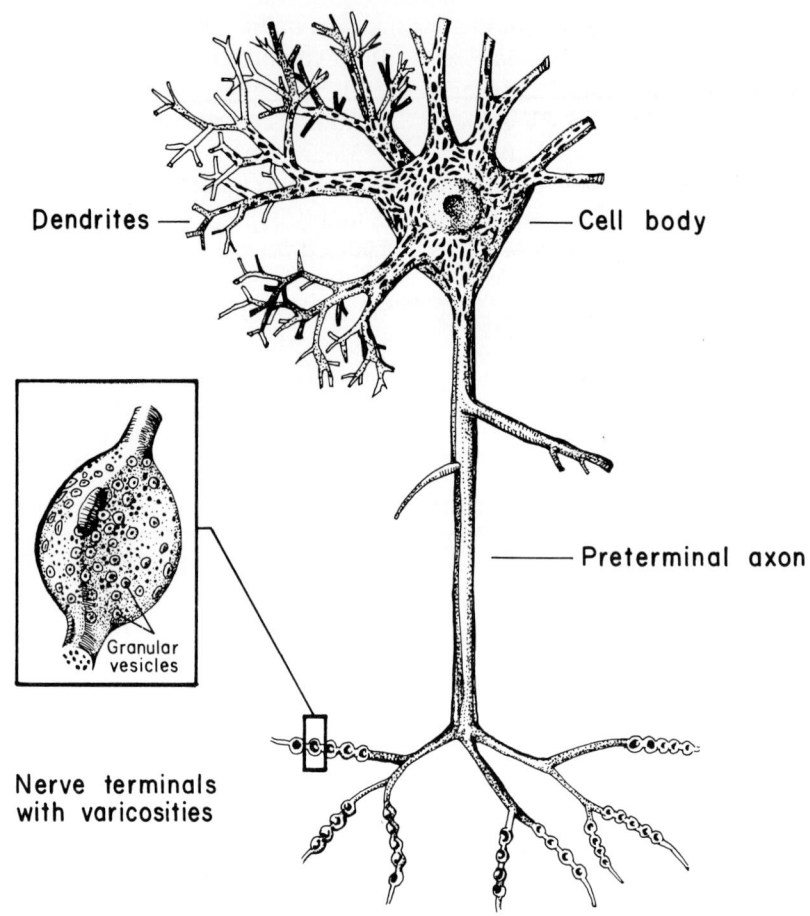

Fig. 1.6 Schematic representation of neuron, showing the cell body, preterminal axon, and nerve endings with varicosities. (Modified from Neuropsychopharmacology: A Series from Roche Laboratories. Nutley, NJ, Hoffmann-La Roche, 1976.)

the synthesis of norepinephrine from dopamine.

NORADRENERGIC (NE, NOREPINEPHRINE, NA) PATHWAYS

The major proportion of NE neurons have their cell bodies in the brain stem. Ascending and descending noradrenergic tracts (Figure 1.7) contain fibers that innervate various regions of the CNS. Noradrenergic neurons are found predominantly at the medullary and pontine levels of the brain stem. Descending fibers originate in the medulla oblongata and terminate in the gray matter at the top of the spinal cord.

A dorsal and ventral bundle divide the ascending noradrenergic neurons. The dorsal bundle contains neurons in or near the locus ceruleus (pons), and the ventral bundle originates from ventral and lateral cell groups in the medulla oblongata and pons. Ascending neurons arise from cell bodies in the medulla oblongata (reticular formation) and pons, and they enter the medial forebrain bundle (MFB). Ascending tracts carry these fibers to the hypothalamus, stria terminalis, the preoptic area, septal area, amygdaloid cortex, cingulate gyrus, and neocortex.

Noradrenergic neurons from the medulla oblongata and pons also innervate the cerebellum.

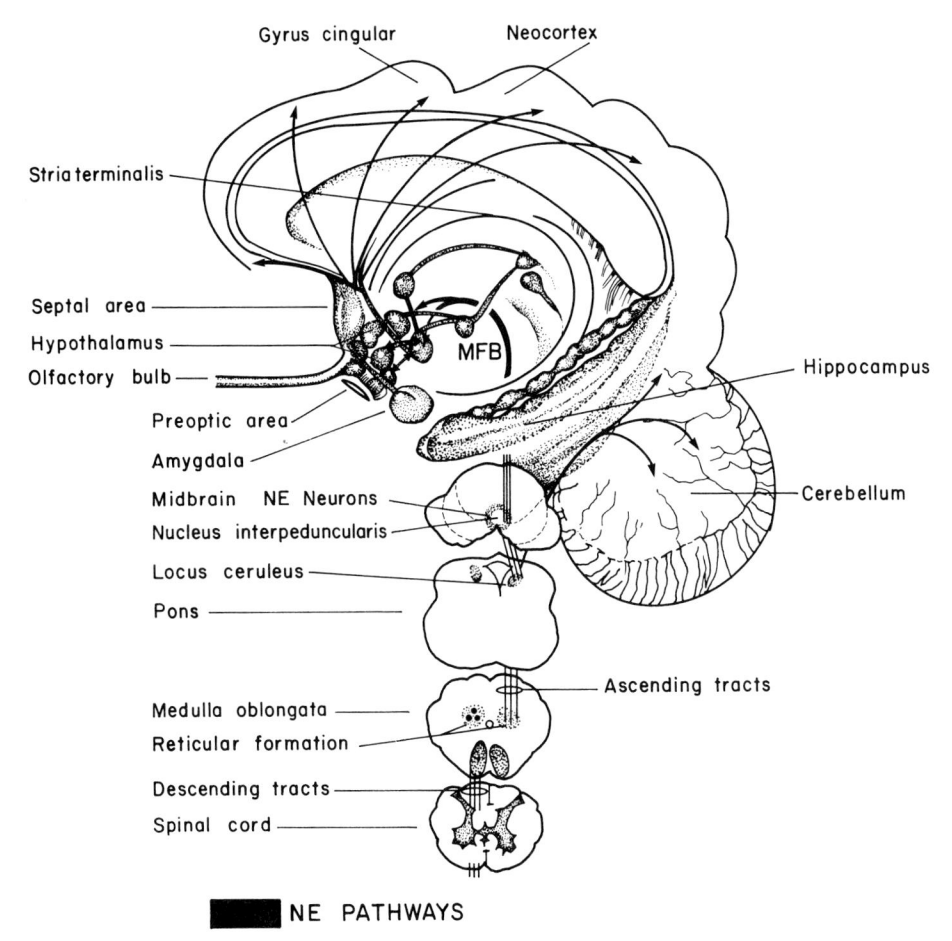

Fig. 1.7 Norepinephrine pathways. *(Modified from Neuropsychopharmacology: A Series from Roche Laboratories. Nutley, NJ, Hoffmann-La Roche, 1976.)*

DOPAMINERGIC (DA, DOPAMINE) PATHWAYS

The nigrostriatal tract, a DA pathway (Figure 1.8), arises from cell bodies in the substantia nigra. These fibers terminate on tiny interneurons in the caudate nucleus and putamen. The mesolimbic system is the second major grouping of dopaminergic fibers. These cell bodies are located in the midbrain just caudal and medial to the substantia nigra. The mesolimbic pathway enters the MFB where the fibers project to various structures of the limbic system and terminate anterior to the caudate nucleus in the nucleus accumbens, olfactory tubercule, and red nucleus of the stria terminalis (the limbic striatum).

A final major DA pathway involves neurons that have cell bodies in the arcuate and anterior periventricular nuclei. These fibers terminate in the median eminence of the hypothalamus and function in the regulation of gonadotropin secretion.

SEROTONERGIC (5-HT, 5-HYDROXYTRYPTAMINE) PATHWAYS

The distribution of serotonergic pathways (Figure 1.9) in the CNS resembles noradrenergic tracts. The neuraxons of the descending tracts

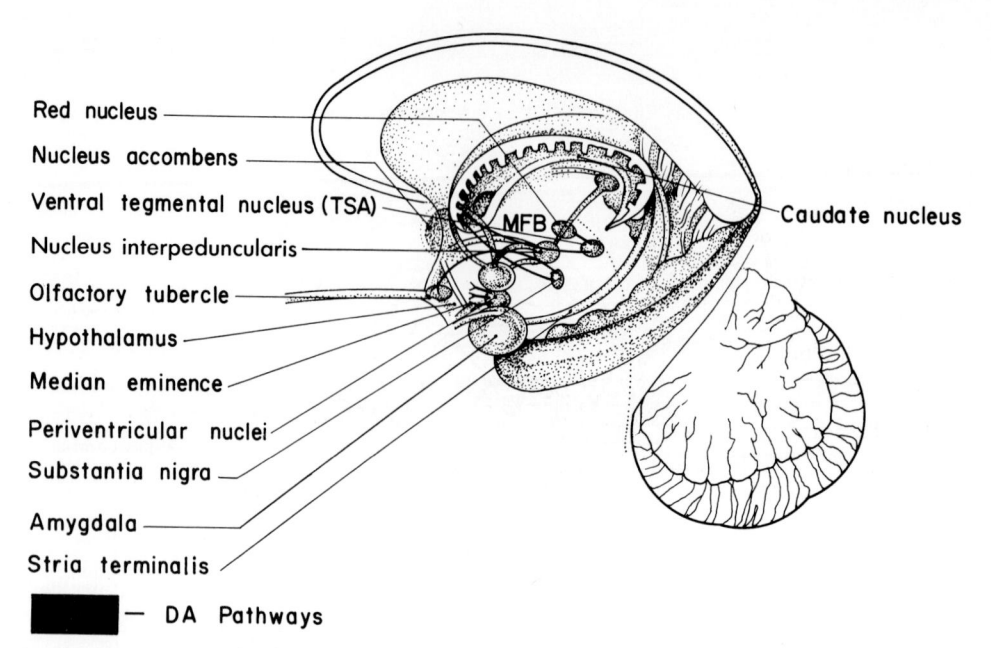

Fig. 1.8 Dopaminergic pathways. (Modified from Neuropsychopharmacology: A Series from Roche Laboratories. Nutley, NJ, Hoffmann-La Roche, 1976.)

project caudally to the spinal cord. Cell bodies in these descending tracts are found in the lower raphe nuclei of the pons.

Ascending fibers rise rostrally from the median and dorsal raphe nuclei and travel together with noradrenergic fibers to the hypothalamus, limbic forebrain, neostriatum, paleostriatum, and neocortex. Additional synaptic connections of serotonergic fibers are made with tryptaminergic cells in the brain stem.

CHOLINERGIC (AC, ACETYLCHOLINE) PATHWAYS

Spinal motorneuron collaterals to the Renshaw cells in the spinal cord are cholinergic. In the brain, significant cholinergic involvement appears in the diffuse projection from the brain stem tegmentum to the neocortex, the striatum, and the hippocampus.

Identified cholinergic pathways (Figure 1.10) originate in the medial septal nucleus and terminate in the hippocampus. The ascending reticular formation and auditory and visual primary afferent fibers also contain cholinergic neurons.

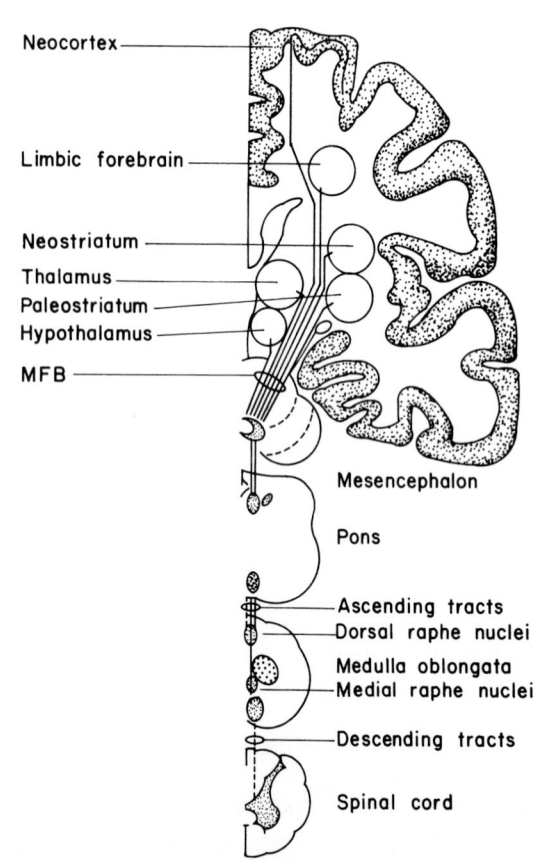

Fig. 1.9 Serotonergic pathways. (Modified from Neuropsychopharmacology: A Series from Roche Laboratories. Nutley, NJ, Hoffmann-La Roche, 1976.)

CENTRAL NERVOUS SYSTEM

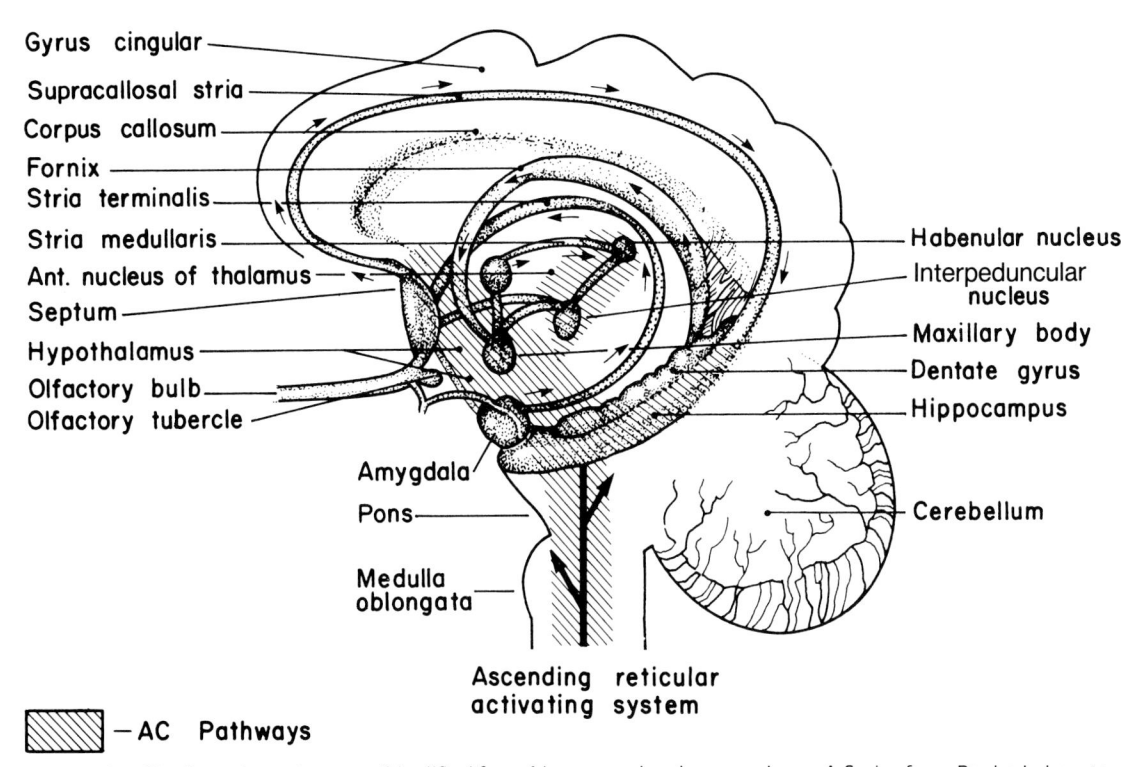

Fig. 1.10 Cholinergic pathways. (Modified from Neuropsychopharmacology: A Series from Roche Laboratories. Nutley, NJ, Hoffmann-La Roche, 1976.)

GABA-ERGIC (GAMMA-AMINOBUTYRATE, GABA) PATHWAYS

Considerable evidence indicates that the amino acid GABA functions as a neurotransmitter at all levels of the CNS. GABA receptors are located at various sites on the central neuron, including somadendritic receptors, presynaptic terminal receptors (GABA$_A$ and GABA$_B$), and terminal autoreceptors.

GLYCINE PATHWAYS

Glycine, an inhibitory amino acid and neurotransmitter, is more prominent in the spinal cord than in the brain. Its role as a neurotransmitter is currently under investigation, as are other amino acids, especially glutamic acid and tryptophan.

DISORDERS OF THE CENTRAL NERVOUS SYSTEM

Central nervous system disorders that are amenable to drug therapy include pain, various sleep disturbances, epilepsy, affective disorders (i.e., depression, mania, neuroses, schizophrenia, organic psychoses), attention deficit disorder (ADD), Alzheimer's disease, parkinsonism, and certain infections.

PAIN DISORDERS

Pain, either acute or chronic, is a composite subjective experience characterized by unpleasant perceptions and emotions, as well as by related autonomic, psychologic, and behavioral responses. Acute pain usually has an important physiologic function. As a protective mechanism for the body, pain occurs as a warning of current or impending tissue damage and causes the individual to quickly remove the pain's source. Thus, reactions to pain (e.g., removing a bothersome splinter or moving away from intense heat) are only natural. Acute pain also functions as a symptom of disease, for example, often prompting people to seek dental assistance for a tooth abscess or medical attention for kidney stones passing down the ureter.

Chronic pain, however, is without any apparent physiologic function and lasts for months or even years beyond a usual course of acute disease. Chronic pain sufferers often encounter severe emotional, physical, economic, and social stresses. Resembling a stuck fire alarm, chronic pain no longer serves a purpose but does not end. The chronic pain of carcinoma or backache of uncertain cause are both persistent and nagging. By becoming the focus of the patient's existence, such painful maladies force other facets of the patient's life into a subordinate position.

Nerve endings sensitive to pain (nociceptors), touch and pressure (mechanoreceptors), and heat (thermoreceptors) are widely distributed in tissues. A physical stimulus compresses or stretches sensitive tissue, whereas chemicals act directly on sensitive nerve endings to cause pain. The pathogenesis of pain sometimes involves inflammation, ulceration, distension, anoxia, or spasm.

The polypeptide bradykinin is a primary endogenous pain-causing chemical that acts in concert with prostaglandins to initiate pain impulses in nerve fibers. Prostaglandins are endogenous hormone-like acidic compounds derived from long-chain polyunsaturated fatty acids (Chapters 9 and 10). Prostaglandins were first found in semen and supposedly were formed in the prostate gland; they are actually ubiquitous compounds that are synthesized in almost all mammalian cells (except erythrocytes) and vitally relate to several physiologic actions.

Damage to cells results in the activation of an enzyme, phospholipase A_2, that initiates a cascade of reactions culminating in the hyperalgesic process. Phospholipase A_2 converts cell membrane phospholipids to prostaglandin precursors (such as arachidonic acid), as well as stimulating the release of a number of chemicals, including bradykinin and histamine.

Arachidonic acid, through the action of the enzyme cyclo-oxygenase, is converted to unstable cyclic endoperoxides; these are further metabolized to stable prostaglandins. Prostaglandins sensitize the nociceptor nerve fiber endings to bradykinin and histamine, generating electrochemical impulses along the pain fiber.

Small unmyelinated C fibers and the delta group of A fibers in afferent neurons carry pain signals from the receptors. C fiber impulse traffic, transmitted slowly on C fibers (0.5 to 2 m/sec), results in burning, aching pain. Delta A fibers conduct pain impulses rapidly (3 to 20 m/sec) and produce sharp, pricking pain. Both C and delta A fibers are widespread in the skin, periosteum, arterial walls, joint surfaces, and the falx cerebelli and tentorium cerebelli in the cranial cavity. Thus, the sudden trauma of a painful stimulus precipitates a "double" pain sensation that is first characterized by a fast pricking pain sensation and then is shortly followed by a burning pain sensation. The pricking pain alerts the individual to the damaging influence and ordinarily results in removal of the painful stimulus. The slow burning sensation, on the other hand, becomes more painful over a period of time and produces the extensive awareness and suffering associated with pain.

Pain fibers (both A and C) enter the spinal cord through the dorsal roots and terminate on neurons in the dorsal horns of the gray matter (substantia gelatinosa). At this junction, the pain impulses pass through one or more short-fibered neurons and then travel via the long fibers that cross to the opposite side of the cord and upward to the brain in the spinothalamic and spinoreticular tracts.

As the pain pathways pass into the brain, they separate into two separate pathways. Whereas small delta A fibers comprise the sharp pain pathway, the burning pain pathway consists almost exclusively of the slow type C fibers. While delta A fibers terminate in the thalamus and in the somatic sensory cortex, the C fibers end in the brainstem reticular formation and thalamus, thus allowing pain impulse

CENTRAL NERVOUS SYSTEM

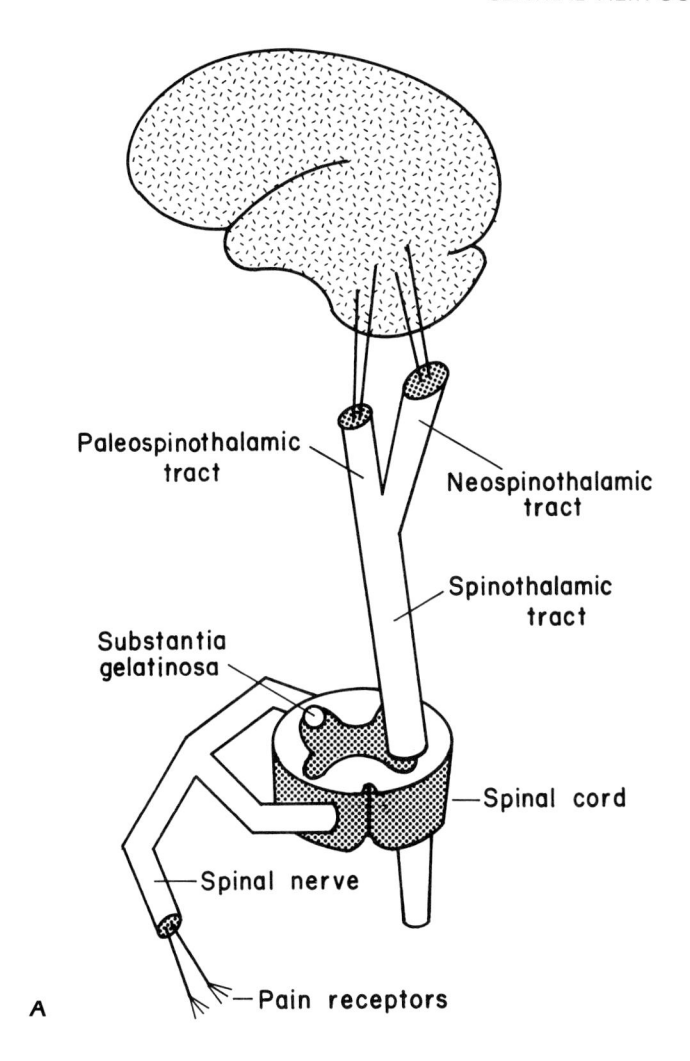

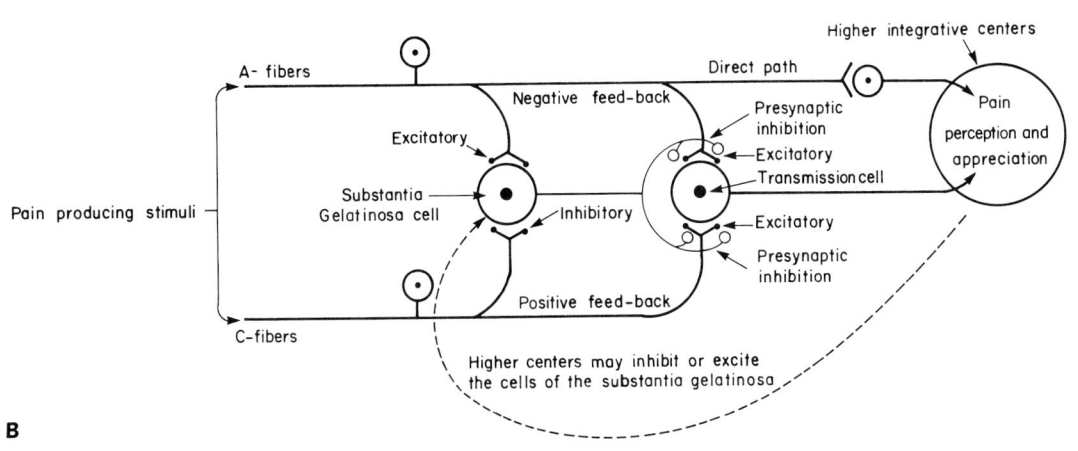

Fig. 1.11 Gate theory of pain. (A modified with permission from Drug Topics, Medical Economics Co., February 7, 1983; B modified from Bowman, W.C., and Rand, M.J.: Textbook of Pharmacology, 2nd Ed. Oxford, Blackwell Scientific Publications, 1980.)

transmission to all areas of the brain. By relaying burning and aching signals, the C fibers have a potent effect on the CNS. Their function causes responses such as arousal from sleep, creation of a sense of anxiety and urgency, and promotion of defense and aversion reactions — all responses designed to rid the person of a painful stimulus.

Although people possess essentially equal thresholds for pain, their degree of reaction or tolerance to pain varies. Pain causes both reflex motor activity and psychic reactions (including anguish, anxiety, crying, depression, nausea, and excessive muscular excitability).

The Gate Control Theory represents an anatomic model for pain perception (Figures 1.11A and 1.11B). A neural pathway, designated as the spinal gate, exists in the substantia gelatinosa and receives pain nerve fibers from the periphery. The relative amounts of activity in the large and small fibers control the spinal gate. Whereas activity in the large fibers inhibits pain impulses (similar to closing a gate), small fiber activity opens the spinal gate with resultant stimulation of neuron transmission and continued propagation of the pain signal. Descending control systems influence the gate operation, in addition to these peripheral afferent cues. The brain evidently initiates an inhibitory response by closing the spinal gate.

Two types of non-pain signals reduce the degree of pain impulse transmission through the spinal cord. The first is stimulation of large sensory fibers from peripheral mechanoreceptors and/or thermoreceptors (e.g., massage and heat). The second type of non-pain influence involves corticofugal (away from the cerebral cortex) signals that descend down the spinal cord. Pain suppression may last for an hour or more after these signals cease. One hypothesis indicates that these two non-pain signals terminate in the substantia gelatinosa (where chemicals known as enkephalins are released) and act on receptors to close the spinal gate. The inhibitory fibers terminate on the pain neuraxons prior to their synapse with the neurons of the substantia gelatinosa, hence, the designation "presynaptic inhibition."

Enkephalins, present in the CNS, are endogenous opiate-like neurotransmitters that apparently mediate the integration of sensory information regarding pain and emotional behavior. Neurons that release enkephalins form synapses on the terminals of excitatory central neurons (Figure 1.12). Enkephalins released from the inhibitory neurons bind to opiate receptors on excitatory nerve terminals. The enkephalin-receptor binding increases the sodium ion conductance across the excitatory terminal membrane and partially depolarizes it. Consequently, when a nerve impulse reaches the terminal, the net depolarization decreases because of the prior partial depolarization of the terminal membrane.

A corresponding reduction in the amount of excitatory neurotransmitter, such as acetylcholine, released is consistent with inhibition of excitatory neuron activity. Thus, while enkephalin action is initially excitatory, the resultant effect on pain signal transition is inhibitory.

Stereospecific saturable enkephalin receptors are distributed along the C fiber pathway; significant sites of receptor population include the substantia gelatinosa, the ARAS, and brain areas that mediate emotional behavior and emotional response to pain (e.g., the limbic system). Theoretically, a release of the enkephalins with subsequent receptor activation at these sites could reduce the individual's reaction to pain.

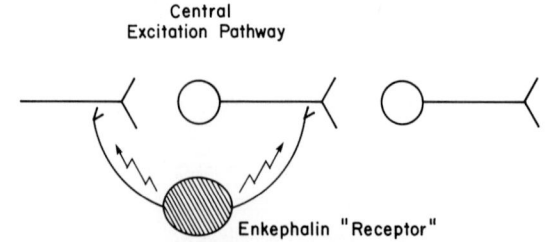

Fig. 1.12 Enkephalin impact on excitatory neuron.

SLEEP DISTURBANCES

Insomnia, or an inability to sleep, is one of the most common complaints patients report to physicians; in fact, an estimated 1 in 5 patients who see a doctor voice this problem. Although people spend approximately ⅓ of their lives in

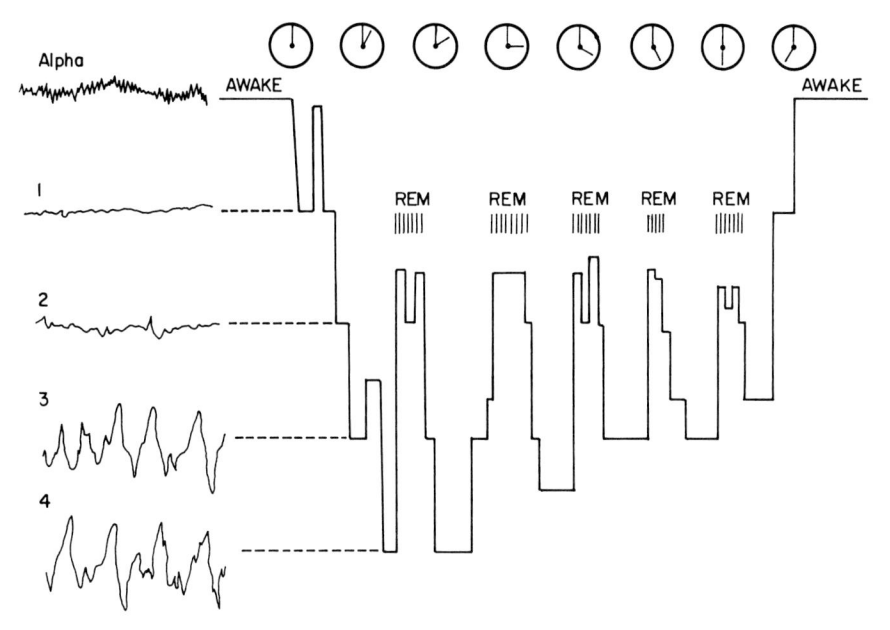

Fig. 1.13 EEG sleep waves; the stages of sleep as indicated by the cortical EEG (on the left). REM sleep is the deepest form of sleep, yet the cortical EEG approaches that of wakefulness. (From Bowman, W.C., and Rand, M.J.: Textbook of Pharmacology, 2nd Ed. Oxford, Blackwell Scientific Publications, 1980.)

sleep, the physiologic basis of sleep and its transitions with wakefulness remain a mystery.

The physiologic substrate for the maintenance of an "awake" cerebral cortex and conversely for the transition to an "asleep" cerebral cortex is the ascending reticular activating system (ARAS). The ARAS is a diffuse collection of neuron cell bodies and neuron fibers in the central brain stem. Output from the ARAS ascends higher into the brain to the thalamus and cortex to determine the state of sensory arousal. Input to the ARAS occurs from all sensory modalities and this arousal results from greater sensory neuron traffic. Cerebral cortical influence executes modulation of ARAS activity.

Investigations in sleep research record sleep stages with encephalograms (EEGs), electrooculograms (EOGs) from each eye, and electromyograms (EMGs), generally of the mentalis or submentalis (chin) muscles.

Taken from the surface of the skull, the EEG indicates the electrical potential of neurons on or near the surface (cortex) of the brain. This test indicates four rhythms in humans whose eyes are closed (Figure 1.13). Alpha waves of 8 to 13 cycles per second (cps) indicate the alpha rhythm, the predominant rhythm in relaxed adults. The beta rhythm, seen in drowsy adults, is the predominant rhythm observed in young children. In this rhythm, the cps value is greater than 13. Theta (at 4 to 7 cps) and delta (at less than 4 cps) are the two other rhythms the EEG notes. Of these, the delta rhythm is normal only in the sleeping adult and child.

The EMG records the muscle activity in chin muscles, and the EOG measures electrical activity (DC) around the eyes. These recordings help determine the several sleep stages.

Two states recognized are NREM (nonrapid eye movement) and REM (rapid eye movement) sleep. The NREM state, divided into four stages, represents slow wave sleep.

Stage 1, a brief transitional stage between wakefulness and lower sleep stages, is characterized by a low-voltage, mixed frequency EEG that is relatively slower than that found in wakefulness. Also occurring in Stage 1 are slow, rolling eye movements and a decreased muscle tone (as compared to wakefulness). Perceived differently from person to person, Stage 1 sleep is variously described as wakefulness, drowsiness, and sleep.

Stage 2 sleep shows an EEG similar to that of Stage 1, but it contains sleep "spindles" and "K-complexes," particular waveforms that are characteristic of Stage 2. Generally, muscle tone is lower than in Stage 1.

The Stage 3 EEG shows a slower frequency and increased amplitude, indicating the formation of delta waves. Since this high-amplitude, slow activity continues into Stage 4, these stages are referred to as delta sleep.

Stage 4 sleep has the slowest frequency and highest amplitude with the "deepest" sleep occurring in this stage. The major EEG difference in Stage 3 and Stage 4 is the percentage of delta waves per unit of recording.

Rapid eye movements characterize REM sleep, also called paradoxical, aroused, or desynchronized sleep. The REM sleep EEG is similar to that of Stage 1 NREM sleep and looks like an awakened brain. Dreaming also occurs during REM sleep.

The typical sleep cycle involves a quick passage through Stages 1 and 2 and then a moderate period of time (1 to 2 hours) in delta sleep, Stages 3 and 4. Approximately 90 minutes after sleep onset, the patient enters the first REM period that lasts several minutes. This cycle is repeated four to five times during the night. As the nocturnal sleep period proceeds, delta sleep consumes less time and the REM episodes lengthen and intensify. The final REM period in a "normal" sleep cycle usually lasts from 30 to 60 minutes. When deprived of REM sleep, most individuals become anxious and irritable; also, when allowed uninterrupted sleep, they show REM rebound.

SLEEP-WAKE DISORDERS

Estimates indicate that serious sleep problems occur in between 12 and 15% of today's population.

DISORDERS OF EXCESSIVE SLEEPINESS

Sleep Apnea. Occurring when airflow ceases through a person's nostrils and mouth for more than 10 seconds, sleep apnea may result from either some airway obstruction or abnormality of the breathing apparatus. Treatment of this form of apnea usually involves surgery or procedures such as a tracheostomy. Central sleep apnea, on the other hand, results from brain damage or depressant drug intoxication.

Narcolepsy. Narcolepsy is a condition characterized by an uncontrollable desire for sleep or by sudden episodes of sleep at various time intervals. Cataplexy is often associated with attacks of narcolepsy, as are higher than normal incidences of behavioral problems. Narcoleptic patients' EEGs indicate an abnormal sleep pattern at the onset of sleep. Four main symptoms of narcolepsy are sleep attacks, catalepsy, sleep paralysis upon awakening, and hypnagogic hallucinations.

DISORDERS THAT OCCUR ONLY DURING SLEEP

Sleepwalking and nocturnal enuresis occur most often in children.

PARASOMNIAS

Sleepwalking (somnambulism) occurs during Stages 3 and 4 REM sleep, a situation considered normal in children. Similarly, children experience sleep terror (pavor nocturnus) during the same stages of REM sleep. This condition differs from nightmares and, as in somnambulism, usually ceases as children mature.

Sleep-related nocturnal enuresis, characterized by a brief arousal from Stages 3 and 4 sleep, is another condition most children outgrow by puberty.

INSOMNIA

Insomnia, a disorder of initiating and maintaining sleep, is defined as abnormal wakefulness or the inability to sleep. Insomniacs sleep less than they feel is necessary for their optimum daytime functioning. Difficulty in falling asleep, an inability to remain asleep, abbreviated sleep with premature awakening, or often a combination of these problems characterize insomniacs' complaints.

Psychologic causes of insomnia include worry, excitement, or anxiety. Insomnia often coexists with psychiatric disturbances, such as schizophrenia or affective disorders. Other causes of insomnia include disruption of circadian rhythms (for example, jet lag), sleeping in a strange environment, or a temporary disrupting situation, such as grief. Since insomnia is often a secondary problem to a behavioral disorder, short-term upset, or organic problem, alleviation or correction of the primary disorder usually improves insomniac states.

SEIZURES

Epilepsy is characterized by the occurrence of sudden and transitory periods of abnormal motor, sensory, autonomic, or psychic dysfunction. Epileptic seizures are usually correlated with abnormal and excessive discharges in the brain as evidenced by changes in the encephalogram (EEG).

Convulsions, common in many cases of epilepsy, indicate generalized motor involvement. Neuron defects frequently cause the involuntary paroxysms of muscle contractions. The origin of convulsive seizures is a focal area in the brain that has been predisposed to abnormal neuron firing. The abnormal focus may be either functional (as in a site close to a tumor) or of unclear biochemical or organic origin.

An epileptic seizure results when random excitatory discharges from the focal region spread to other neurons in the motor cortex. Studies relate this spread of excitation to blood sugar levels, blood pH, osmotic pressure, electrolyte profile, and endocrine influence. Other research implicates stress (mental or physical), fatigue, and nutritional status in promoting the aberrant spread that forms an aggregate of excited neurons. Involvement of motor pathways leads to skeletal muscle contractions. Motor involvement is either generalized as in grand mal and myoclonic seizures or is partial as in simple motor (Jacksonian) and temporal lobe (limbic) seizures.

Unconsciousness and tonic-clonic convulsions characterize grand mal seizures. An aura (visual, auditory, epigastric, or psychic) usually precedes the unconsciousness. After the person becomes unconscious, initial convulsions explosively force air out of the lungs, resulting in the epileptic "cry." Generalized motor tonic-clonic seizures follow this eerie, birdlike scream.

Opisthotonus characterizes the tonic component of the seizure. In other words, the person is forced into an arched position when the violent spasm of all body musculature pulls his back muscles. This back arching causes convexity in the ventral body region. In clonic seizures, alternate contraction and relaxation of all muscles occur. Postseizure depression of motor and sensory function makes the person sleep for several hours.

Petit mal, a form of generalized seizure, does not involve motor dysfunction. Termed absence seizures, these attacks cause the patient to lose mental consciousness of his surroundings and sometimes to simply stare off into space. This type of seizure, occurring as frequently as several hundred a day, is most common in the prepubertal years.

Myoclonic attacks are generalized seizures that are characterized by rhythmic body jerks without loss of consciousness.

Focal or partial seizures, defined as aberrant motor or psychomotor activity, result from a local discrete spread of excitation that does not become generalized. Jacksonian epilepsy or simple motor seizures often follow physical injury to a brain region, such as in post-auto accident patients. Convulsions in Jacksonian seizures are often confined to a single limb or muscle group (Jacksonian motor epilepsy) or to specific and localized sensory disturbance (Jacksonian sensory epilepsy); other limited signs and symptoms depend upon the particular cortical area that produces the abnormal discharge.

Psychomotor seizures are partial attacks that apparently involve the temporal lobe and limbic structures. Simple sensory changes in the visual, auditory, olfactory, and autonomic functions are usually the only outward sign of these seizures.

Possible origins of seizure foci include congenital defects, head trauma, hypoxia at birth, inflammatory vascular changes of unknown cause or following disease, tumors, and brain abscess. Also, studies implicate biochemical lesions in epileptic seizures. One theory states that a reduction in inhibitory components of neuron circuits causes paroxysmal discharges in primary epileptic foci. Gamma-aminobutyric acid (GABA) is a neurotransmitter of inhibitory neuron systems in the CNS. Convulsant drugs that induce epileptiform discharge patterns in central neurons also inhibit GABA function. Conversely, compounds that increase GABA influence often reduce seizure activity. Ongoing studies concern detection of differences between biochemical patterns in epileptiform cerebral cortex and nonepileptiform tissue.

AFFECTIVE DISORDERS

Affective disorders range from benign conditions that are not associated with marked disability to debilitating diseases that prevent the individual from functioning in society.

DEPRESSION

The affective (pertaining to a feeling or mental state) disorder, depression, is a multifaceted syndrome characterized by changes in mood, activity, behavior, sleep, and neuroendocrine functions, including sexual activity. Since these functions are mediated by biogenic amine neurotransmitters, a logical hypothesis implicates biochemical errors in the CNS as causes of depression.

Changes in neurotransmitter systems have long been associated with behavioral pathology. A problem in this approach is assigning chronologic order to the events (i.e., determining if the biochemical change elicits a behavioral aberration or if the behavioral aberration results in a biochemical shift). No unequivocal, reproducible demonstration of a specific biochemical change causing clinical depression has emerged. Even so, the observation that drugs which alter brain biogenic amine metabolism are beneficial in certain depression states supports a biochemical theory of depression.

Not a single disease entity, depression occurs in a variety of forms. Temporary mood state changes, such as in grief states, differ from the persistent malignant syndrome that characterizes clinical endogenous depression. Also, depression may occur as a secondary disease in other psychiatric or medical disorders, including cardiovascular disease and cancer. Involutional melancholia, psychotic depression reaction, and unipolar or bipolar depression are other forms of clinical depression. Unipolar depression is characterized by only depression, whereas bipolar depression contains a patient history of mania together with depression. Criteria established for this differentiation are useful in achieving the best treatment protocol for each patient.

Disturbances of sleep patterns are common to depressed patients, i.e., they experience markedly short Stage 4 sleep. Anxiety and depression, two distinct syndromes, also coexist in most depressed patients.

The "catecholamine hypothesis of depression," one of several biochemical theories of depression etiology, relates clinical depression to depleted stores of catecholamines. According to this theory, low norepinephrine concentration in critical brain regions causes clinical depression. Serotonin levels in the brain are also related to affective disease, such as depression. The "indoleamine hypothesis," another depression etiology theory, correlates low brain serotonin concentration with depression. An interfacing of these two hypotheses represents an alternative approach to understanding the causes of depression.

Biochemical-behavioral correlation studies boldly link discrete physiologic aberration with mental state. Some affective disorders apparently result primarily from biochemical or genetic defects with little impact from environmental factors. However, in other instances, strong adverse environmental influences may induce biochemical changes that precipitate behavioral toxicity. Another possibility is that the biochemical changes induced in behavioral toxicity have no significant role in causing the mental illness, but rather, they are the end-result of behavior on physiologic processes.

Regardless of the implications of any biochemical change, a beneficial diagnostic "spin-off" accrues. Blood catecholamine levels and urine catecholamine metabolite profiles, for example, may become important diagnostic tools in determining the nature and/or severity of the affective disorder. When combined with diagnostic psychologic and behavioral criteria, this information offers an opportunity for more definitive and successful chemotherapeutic intervention in the treatment regimen.

Biochemical theories of depression do not necessarily involve changes in a single brain neurotransmitter or neurosystem. To illustrate, mania and depression apparently reflect an altered balance between two or more neurosystems in the brain. Such an "imbalance hypothesis," involving cholinergic, catecholaminergic, and indoleaminergic interactions, more realistically reflects the complexity of the clinical disease.

Depression is either exogenous or endogenous in nature. Exogenous depression follows an external stress-inducing stimulus or series of traumatic events. Usually amenable to drug therapy, this form of depression rarely lasts longer than a few months. Endogenous depression is a more insidious condition since no precipitating occurrences are readily identified as causative factors. These patients lose interest in external surroundings for no apparent reason and withdraw from social interaction. Although some menopausal women experience endogenous depression concurrently with significant hormone changes, no cause-effect relationship implicates endocrine imbalance in endogenous depression.

MANIA

Biologic hypotheses of mania are similar to those set forth for depression. In depression, a functional deficit of neurotransmitter monoamines occurs at central synapses; conversely, a functional excess of these amines possibly exists in mania. A modified indoleamine hypothesis proposes a decrease in serotonin (5-HT) in both depression and mania, with the greater deficit occurring in depression.

PSYCHONEUROSIS (NEUROSIS)

According to Freud, anxiety is the central and basic problem in psychoneurosis. Doubtless, anxiety is an important component in psychoneurotic reactions, particularly in acute attacks. However, other primarily subjective symptoms include restlessness, irritability, hyperexcitability, psychologic rigidity, and fatigue. Psychoneurosis is also often accompanied by objective symptoms, such as breathlessness, increased muscular tension, sweating, trembling, and insomnia.

ORGANIC BRAIN PSYCHOSIS

Organic brain psychosis, a mental disease related to a discernible organic lesion or toxic reaction, is usually produced by a chemical toxin (e.g., lead poisoning) or by physical damage to a brain region.

SCHIZOPHRENIA

Schizophrenia is a functional psychosis best described as a group of symptoms with certain common features. Functional psychoses are those major mental disorders that have no known specific causative factor. The schizophrenias and affective disorders comprise the overwhelming majority of the cases of functional psychoses. Major disturbances in thought content, bizarre behavior, a regression in intellectual functioning, inappropriate affective expression, and frequent hallucinations and delusions characterize schizophrenia symptomatology.

The age of onset of schizophrenia is usually from adolescence to early adult life. Exceptions include paranoid schizophrenia, which ordinarily appears after the age of 30, and childhood schizophrenia.

The classic description of the primary symptoms of schizophrenia, as described by Bleuler, includes the four A's: association, affect, ambivalence, and autism. Changes in association are manifest as illogical, tangential, irrelevant, or inappropriate ideas or responses. Loss of logical association and thought organization result in interruption of one idea with others.

Affect, an expression of mood or emotion, is oftentimes rigid, indifferent, and inappropriate. For example, a patient may express indifference toward serious life events or may even laugh at a situation where concern or worry are usual appropriate responses.

Ambivalence in the schizophrenic patient makes decision making or dealing with coexistent positive and negative feelings extremely difficult. For example, when asked if ambivalence exists, the patient may reply, "Well, yes and no."

Autism, the excessive focusing on internal feelings, results in an inability to relate to other people. A detachment from reality coexists with a lack of emphasis on the individual's external life.

Besides these four primary symptoms, accessory symptoms are also important in schizophrenia diagnosis. Hallucinations, usually auditory, are common and the perceived voices may be either threatening or pleasurable. Also noted are delusions that often involve persecution. Catatonia, or related phenomena, and memory disturbances complete the list of accessory symptoms that are useful in schizophrenia diagnosis. Of additional interest is the absence of any physical changes consistently present in schizophrenia.

Several subtypes of schizophrenia are described clinically; of these, the undifferentiated and paranoid forms are the most common. Characterized by a thought disorder, undifferentiated schizophrenia does not distinctly show the symptomatology described for the simple hebephrenic, catatonic, or paranoid subtypes. Paranoid schizophrenia represents a patient profile in which more clear-cut delusions and auditory hallucinations are present. Also, intellectual function, except for delusional perception, usually remains intact.

Epidemiologic evidence indicates that schizophrenia occurs most frequently in the lowest social classes of urban populations. The conditions of life in this environment may somehow aid and abet the schizophrenic disease process. Some reasons for this social-schizophrenia correlation include the likelihood of a highly stressful environment in that social milieu, inadequate stress-coping techniques because of a lack of money, fewer institutional resources for stress prevention, and a psyche-draining lifestyle that reduces the individual's emotional resources for stress management.

Increased and prolonged psychosocial stress may "overactivate" hypothalamic nuclei, resulting in an exaggerated release of polypeptide-releasing hormones. These hypothalamic "releasing-hormones" stimulate the anterior pituitary gland to secrete hormones, including corticotropin (ACTH). Activation of the adrenal gland represents a characteristic endocrine response to stress. Thus, a prolonged stress reaction, occurring in a noxious psychosocial environ, could overburden neuron pathways in the brain to precipitate mental disease in much the same manner as stress contributes to organic disorders in psychosomatic disease.

Several studies indicate that extensive abnormalities in the interaction of families precede the onset of schizophrenia. A pattern of dominant mother and submissive father characterizes the marital profile common to parents of schizophrenics. Noted within the preschizophrenic family are communication problems, which are variously described as unclear, blurred, misunderstood, wandering, vague, and subtly contradictory. These disturbances precede development of the disease and apparently affect the development of a child's perceptual functions, essential for the child's determination of reality and his relation to it. These psychosocial conditions impair the capacity of the preschizophrenic individual to cope with and resolve the problems of living. Life condition stresses thus develop and expand to activate the schizophrenic process in a genetically predisposed person.

Recent studies indicate that brain biochemical differences reflect the genetic predisposition that exists in schizophrenia. A provocative biochemical theory of schizophrenia focuses on dopamine, a CNS catecholamine neurotransmitter. If dopamine is present in excessive amounts, abnormal motor and mood states occur that resemble schizophrenia. A significant brain research finding is that the activity of dopamine-beta-hydroxylase, the enzyme that converts dopamine (DA) to norepinephrine (NE), is significantly reduced in schizophrenia. This is consistent with the theory that the norepinephrine-mediated reward system is impaired in schizophrenia. The lack (genetically-induced) of dopamine-beta-hydroxylase permits dopamine to accumulate and presumably function in an expanded and perhaps aberrant role as a neurotransmitter or neuromodulator. Although studies such as those that show the brain of postmortem schizophrenics contains less dopamine-beta-hydroxylase are suggestive, dopamine's precise role in the etiology of schizophrenia is still undetermined.

Another biochemical theory of schizophrenia involves the formation of endogenous psychotogens. This hypothesis, in its simplest form, holds that schizophrenia results from an aberrant metabolic pathway that forms an endogenous hallucinogen. Schizophrenic patients may possess more active alternate metabolic pathways that convert endogenous chemicals to psychotogens. Examples of these proposed endogenous psychotogens include methylated derivatives of the neurotransmitters serotonin (5-HT) and dopamine (DA).

ATTENTION DEFICIT DISORDER (ADD)

The "hyperactive" or "hyperkinetic" label is an outdated description of a childhood syndrome that is more accurately characterized by a deficit in attention. Thus, attention deficit disorder (ADD) in children is a more appropriate term. Although the pathogenesis of the disease is unknown, proposed unsubstantiated causes include food additives, encephalitis early in life, difficult birthing, and maturation lag.

The ADD child has a poor attention span, distractability, emotional lability, aggressiveness, and hyperactivity. This syndrome apparently affects approximately 3% of schoolage children (most are usually elementary schoolage); also, boys are more frequently diagnosed as having ADD than are girls. These children are not necessarily more active than normal children, but they are unable to remain still for any period of time.

Minor neurologic problems or EEG abnormalities occur in ADD cases. A history of difficult birth, early injury, or infection may also contribute to the disorder. Spontaneous remission sometimes occurs in cases just prior to the teenage years. Both ADD diagnosis and treatment effectiveness are difficult to determine. Untreated cases apparently have higher delinquency rates and such patients may develop schizophrenia or other psychiatric disorders.

ALZHEIMER'S DISEASE

Alzheimer's disease is the most common form of dementia. Senile dementia of the Alzheimer type accounts for 50 to 60% of all cases of dementia. The incidence of Alzheimer's disease is age-related and occurs most frequently in the elderly. The incidence of severe, nonreversible dementia rises from about 1% in those between 65 and 70 years of age to about 15% in those over 85. Current estimates indicate that between 2 and 4 million people in the United States are affected with Alzheimer's disease. A progressive deterioration of personality and intelligence that eventually leads to the individual's inability to function independently characterizes this disease.

Genetic factors are a contributing factor in the etiology of Alzheimer's disease. The genetic influence apparently results from a simple autosomal dominant characteristic. Although Alzheimer's disease appears frequently in individuals with Down's or trisomy 21 syndrome, attempts at elucidating abnormalities in chromosome 21 have been unsuccessful. Nongenetic factors also implicated but not yet substantiated in the disease onset include viral infection.

Three major pathophysiologic features of Alzheimer's disease are neuron atrophy, increased numbers of amyloid plaques and neurofibrillary tangles, and deficient acetylcholine neurotransmitter activity (as measured by reduced choline acetyltransferase activity). These histologic changes are quantitative rather than qualitative; other findings such as inconsistent degrees of deficiency in the CNS suggest that there are subgroups of Alzheimer's disease patients.

Pronounced cognitive impairment is the most obvious symptom initially identified with the development of Alzheimer's disease. Memory loss, reduced ability to concentrate, and poor learning skills lead to changes in the more subtle forms of mental activity, such as reasoning and judgment. Patients with Alzheimer's disease often exhibit aggressive behavior, inappropriate sexual behavior, paranoid delusions, depression, or emotional lability. The further advancement of the disease often leads to the individual's inability to function independently, rendering the patient helpless and submissive. Thus, the management of Alzheimer's disease involves psychologic and social measures, as well as pharmacotherapeutic intervention.

PARKINSONISM (PARALYSIS AGITANS)

Parkinsonism is clinically characterized by tremor, rigidity, and akinesia. Over 150 years ago in an essay entitled "Essay on the Shaking Palsy," Dr. James Parkinson described the syndrome associated with parkinsonism. Involuntary tremor (mainly in the hands and ankles) often involves a "pill rolling" movement of the thumb and index finger. Rigidity of muscles results from an impairment of CNS inhibitory mechanisms, and akinesia (actually evidenced as hypokinesia) occurs along with muscle weakness.

A characteristic body posture ensues with the head usually flexed on the chest, the body bowed, and the arms, wrists, and knees bent. The patient's center of gravity is forward and by walking on the forepart of his feet, the patient takes almost running short steps to prevent falling face forward to the ground. A blank, staring appearance results from reduced facial movements. Patients also have difficulty in swallowing and chewing and their speech is monotonous and slurred. As fine hand tremor makes writing difficult, improvement in patient writing often gauges the effectiveness of antiparkinsonism drugs.

The basal ganglia contain high concentrations of acetylcholine and dopamine. Dopaminergic and cholinergic neuron systems are mutually antagonistic in the striatum and substantia nigra and these opposing neurochemical pathways influence extrapyramidal control of skeletal muscle activity.

Parkinsonism theory states that the dopaminergic neuron system is deficient, thereby releasing the cholinergic neuron system to produce a central cholinergic predominance. Abnormal control of muscle activity occurs and clinical symptoms of parkinsonism become apparent.

Eighty percent of the dopamine found in the human brain is concentrated in the basal ganglia. Only 10% of the normal amount of dopamine in this brain region is noted in parkinsonism patients.

Controversy exists as to whether the tyrosine hydroxylase deficiency common in parkinsonism results from the disease or is a potential cause of the illness. Tyrosine hydroxylase, an enzyme that converts tyrosine to levodopa, is a presynaptic enzyme expected to be in low levels when degeneration of neurons occurs. Thus, its deficiency in the substantia nigra and corpus striatum of parkinsonism patients may be the result of the disease, rather than its cause.

INFECTIONS (MENINGITIS, ENCEPHALITIS)

Life-threatening infections of the CNS may develop either by spread of the micro-organism from adjacent infectious foci or by septicemic invasion. Bacterial meningitis is usually caused by Hemophilus influenzae, Neisseria meningitides, and Streptococcus pneumoniae infections. Meningitis due to Mycobacterium tuberculosis and fungal meningitis and encephalitides also occur clinically.

Antibiotic treatment is required that maintains a blood level resulting in CSF concentrations well above the minimal inhibitory concentration for the causative organism. Early disease diagnosis is essential and constant patient monitoring is necessary.

THERAPEUTIC APPLICATIONS OF DRUGS AFFECTING THE CENTRAL NERVOUS SYSTEM

Besides treating CNS diseases, drugs affecting sleep and pain response are also valuable in producing surgical anesthesia. Thus, these drugs allow for the correction of physical disease, mainly in areas unrelated to the CNS.

GENERAL ANESTHETICS

A goal of surgical anesthesia is abolition of the patient's perceptions and reactions to pain. General anesthesia is induced by the administration of gases or volatile liquids (see Table 1.1) through the respiratory tract or by the intravenous administration of ultra-short acting barbiturates, such as thiopental. Surgical anesthesia is also achieved through local, regional, or conduction anesthesia by applying drugs directly to nerves or nerve roots. This type of selective blockade reduces the centripetal (impulses to the brain) conduction of pain signals from only a particular region of the body.

The importance of controlling the dosage of an anesthetic, thereby regulating the depth of anesthesia, requires a "flow sheet" of signs and symptoms that reflect the degree of anesthesia. A conventional scale utilizes the physiologic effects produced by classical volatile anesthetics (such as diethyl ether). In present medical practices, the presence of other drugs masks or otherwise affects many of the suggested observations. Nevertheless, the definitions and descriptions of the various stages of anesthesia remain valuable in delineating the pharmacologic effects of anesthetic drugs. Figure 1.14 designates the stages of anesthesia: Stage 1: Analgesia; Stage 2: Excitement; Stage 3: Surgical Anesthesia; and Stage 4: Medullary Paralysis.

Depression of the higher brain centers and the beginning of disinhibitory behavior characterize Stage 1 (Analgesia). Although conscious, the Stage 1 patient "feels no pain" and is sometimes euphoric. The intensity of the analgesia that occurs with nitrous oxide permits certain minor procedures, e.g., dental extractions. Patients in Stage 1 anesthesia often report dreams, fantasies, and a variable degree of amnesia.

Stage 2 (Excitement) presents with more marked disinhibition as a result of the release of lower brain centers from the inhibitory influence of cerebral cortical centers. In this stage, the patient loses consciousness and becomes excited. Struggling, shouting, and drunken-like behavior also occur.

Stages 1 and 2 represent the induction period. The degree of excitement depends upon several factors including the dose and type of preanesthetic medication, the particular general anesthetic agent, the intensity of external sensory stimulation, and the patient's personality set.

After Stage 2, the responses of the patient are reflex. The onset of a regular pattern of respiration indicates entrance into Stage 3 (Surgical

Table 1.1 GENERAL ANESTHETICS

Available products	Trade names
Inhalation Anesthetics:	
Cyclopropane	—
Enflurane	Ethrane
Ethylene	—
Halothane	Fluothane; Halothane
Isoflurane	Forane
Methoxyflurane	Penthrane
Nitrous oxide	—
Intravenous Anesthetics:	
Etomidate	Amidate
Ketamine	Ketalar; Ketaject
Methohexital sodium	Brevital sodium
Thiamylal sodium	Surital
Thiopental sodium	Pentothal

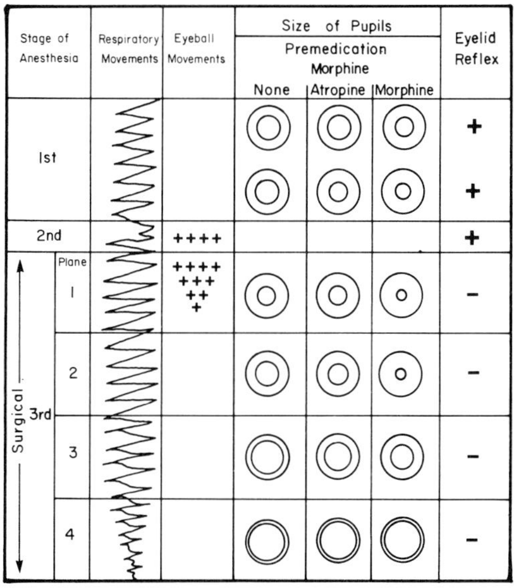

Fig. 1.14 Stages of anesthesia. (From Modell, W., Schild, H.O., and Wilson, A.: Applied Pharmacology. Philadelphia, W.B. Saunders Co., 1976.)

Anesthesia). This physiologic sign is important since other responses, such as pupillary size and blood pressure, are affected by excitation and preanesthetic medication. Along with regular and full respiration, blood pressure readings and responses to surgical stimuli are practical guides to the anesthesia depth.

Four planes divide Stage 3. In planes i. and ii., respiration continues with full and regular movements and eye movements disappear. CNS depression continues in a descending manner to the thoracic portion of the spinal cord where the intercostal muscles become paralyzed because their innervation originates from the thoracic cord. The diaphragm, innervated by the phrenic nerve from the cervical cord, becomes paralyzed after the activity ascends to the neck level cord. Whereas incomplete intercostal paralysis characterizes plane iii., complete intercostal paralysis indicates the beginning of plane iv.

In Stage 4 (Medullary Depression), respiration ceases, the blood pressure falls to dangerous levels, tachycardia occurs, and the pupils maximally dilate. Unless measures are taken to reverse the anesthetic depressant activity, death intervenes.

Muscle relaxation is a major determinant in the relative ease of exposure of deep structures during surgery. Surgical procedures not requiring extensive skeletal muscle relaxation are usually performed during plane ii. of Stage 3, but the common intra-abdominal operations require plane iii. The adjunctive use of skeletal muscle relaxants allows surgery in a lighter plane. A curariform drug, for instance, permits surgery in plane ii. of Stage 3, rather than in plane iii.

VOLATILE ANESTHETICS

Volatile anesthetics, which are absorbed and excreted rapidly through the lungs, readily control the depth of anesthesia. Also, the emergence phase is usually brief following their administration.

Halothane. A nonflammable, nonirritating general anesthetic, halothane represents the first of a series of newer halogenated hydrocarbon anesthetics that gained popularity in modern medicine.

Mechanism of Action. Halothane has significant depressant effects on central synapses in the ascending reticular activiating system (ARAS) and the higher cortical centers. Although the biochemical mechanisms of anesthetic action are unclear, they may involve physico-chemical alterations in cerebral neurons. Clathrate formation of water molecules in neuraxon "pores" is a mechanism proposed for the inhibition of CNS function. The relative lipid-solubility (as well as the surfactant properties) correlates well with their potency.

The lipid matrix of central neuron membranes is the apparent primary site of action of anesthetics. Also, hydrophobic regions of membrane-bound proteins may bind anesthetics, which alters neuron activity. Thus, the loss of sensation and consciousness, characteristic of halothane anesthesia, is evidently due to physical changes in the neuraxon or terminal membrane nature.

In addition to the anesthetic's site of action in the brain, the substantia gelatinosa of the spinal cord (where depression of the gate-control system for impulses occurs) is also a site of general anesthetic activity.

Clinical Indications. Halothane produces profound anesthesia without oxygen deprivation. Since halothane is not a potent analgesic, nitrous oxide is ordinarily used for inducing and maintaining halothane anesthesia. Halothane produces bronchiolar dilation, and the drug is sometimes used as an anesthetic for asthma patients.

Adverse Effects/Precautions. Halothane anesthesia reduces myocardial contractility and cardiac output. Arterial hypotension and a decrease in peripheral resistance also represent cardiovascular depression. Because halothane sensitizes the myocardium to catecholamines, cardiac arrhythmias may occur. Endogenous epinephrine release that results from insufficient anesthesia or inadequate ventilation probably contributes to this problem.

Repeated use of halothane may cause liver damage. Characterized by high mortality rates, halothane-induced hepatitis represents a hypersensitivity reaction and occurs in about 1 in 1,000 to 10,000 exposures to the drug; the incidence increases with repeated exposures.

Halothane induction, in rare instances, triggers an unusual and sometimes fatal hypermetabolic reaction in the skeletal muscle of susceptible patients. Rapid elevation in body temperature and increases in oxygen consumption and carbon dioxide production characterize this condition, which is termed "malignant hyperthermia."

Methoxyflurane. Methoxyflurane, a potent nonflammable anesthetic, has significant volatile analgesic properties.

Mechanism of Action. Methoxyflurane's depressant effects on synapses in the ARAS induce anesthesia. As with higher doses of halothane, methoxyflurane's effects extend to other CNS areas and result in respiratory and vasomotor center depression.

Clinical Indications. The combination of methoxyflurane with nitrous oxide in oxygen and thiopental allows for fast anesthesia induction and permits sufficient analgesia at the later anesthesia planes. Potential kidney toxicity limits the drug's use for deep or prolonged anesthesia.

Adverse Effects/Precautions. Because of its high fat solubility and lipoid tissue affinity, methoxyflurane remains in the body for extended periods. Methoxyflurane's main disadvantage is that liberation of nephrotoxic fluoride ions results from the drug's long stay in the body. Thus, high-output renal failure, progressing to total renal failure, sometimes results. This renal toxicity has caused curtailment of the use of methoxyflurane. Malignant hyperthermia may also occur with methoxyflurane.

Enflurane. Enflurane, a potent nonflammable anesthetic, has properties similar to those of halothane.

Mechanism of Action. The sites and mechanisms of action of enflurane are the same as those proposed for halothane.

Clinical Indications. Enflurane is a widely used general anesthetic.

Adverse Effects/Precautions. Patients should be screened for evidence of prior seizure disorders because of enflurane's association with seizure activity. Also, respiratory and circulatory depression may occur in deep enflurane anesthesia. As with all halogenated hydrocarbon anesthetics, malignant hyperthermia is possible.

Isoflurane. A nonflammable volatile anesthetic, isoflurane resembles enflurane and offers smooth and rapid induction into and emergence from surgical anesthesia.

Mechanism of Action. The brain ARAS is the primary site of isoflurane anesthetic action. The physico-chemical mechanisms of isoflurane action are similar to those indicated for halothane.

Clinical Indications. Introduced for clinical use in 1981, isoflurane achieved wide acceptance as a general anesthetic agent. Isoflurane allows rapid anesthesia adjustment and maintains stable cardiac output during surgery.

Adverse Effects/Precautions. Isoflurane produces progressive respiratory depression and hypotension. No reports of renal or hepatic toxicity following isoflurane therapy have been made. Malignant hyperthermia may occur.

Nitrous Oxide (Laughing Gas). Nitrous oxide, a colorless anesthetic gas, has neither a significant odor nor taste.

Mechanism of Action. Nitrous oxide depresses the higher cortical centers and the ARAS. Although it possesses appreciable analgesic activity, nitrous oxide is too weak for general anesthesia use except as an induction agent or if hyperbaric conditions are achieved.

Clinical Indications. Combination of nitrous oxide with hypnotics, analgesics, or muscle relaxants achieves satisfactory surgical anesthesia due to nitrous oxide's lack of potency. Other clinical uses for nitrous oxide include selected dental procedures and as an induction agent for more powerful anesthetics, such as halothane.

Adverse Effects/Precautions. Nitrous oxide lowers methionine synthetase levels and thus reduces vitamin B_{12} synthesis. Although this effect is not significant with nitrous oxide use as an anesthetic, reports indicate a neurologic syndrome related to vitamin B_{12} deficiency following nitrous oxide use over long periods, as in substance abuse cases.

INTRAVENOUS ANESTHETICS

Intravenous anesthetics include the thiobarbiturates, ketamine, and etomidate.

Thiopental. The sulfur analog of pentobarbital, thiopental is a potent ultra-short acting thiobarbiturate.

Mechanism of Action. Pronounced lipid solubility of thiopental results in rapid passage into the brain. Ease of penetration of the blood brain barrier produces an almost immediate onset of action. The biochemical mechanism of barbiturate (thiopental) central depressant activity apparently relates to activation of receptors that exist as a component of a supramolecular complex, which also contains a GABA recognition site, a benzodiazepine affinity site, and a chloride ionophore. Facilitation of GABA-ergic inhibition may relate to decreases in GABA's rate of dissociation from its receptor. The lipophilic qualities of the thiobarbiturate molecule may also alter physico-chemical properties of the central neuron membranes. Thiopental produces hypnosis and anesthesia without analgesia.

Redistribution of thiopental to other lipid-rich sites in the body results in the ultra-short duration of thiopental central depression. Plasma levels of thiopental decrease rapidly following redistribution of the drug from the brain lipids first to heavily perfused organs, then to skeletal muscle, and finally to fatty tissue. Additionally, catabolism of thiopental is a factor in terminating CNS effects.

Clinical Indications. Used as an intravenous anesthetic, thiopental speeds the induction period.

Adverse Effects/Precautions. Thiopental use should be avoided as an intravenous anesthetic in shock or bronchial asthma patients, as well as in those with intermittent porphyria. Thiopental anesthesia, although rapid, is not as easily controlled as volatile anesthesia agents. Consequently, thiopental administration necessitates careful monitoring of anesthesia stages.

Ketamine. Ketamine, a phencyclidine (PCP) derivative, produces dissociative anesthesia.

Mechanism of Action. The biochemical mechanism whereby ketamine produces anesthesia is unclear. The rapid onset of the drug's anesthetic action usually produces surgical anesthesia within 30 seconds and lasts for 5 to 10 minutes.

Clinical Indications. Ketamine rapidly induces analgesia and amnesia. Used as the sole anesthetic agent in diagnostic and surgical procedures not requiring skeletal muscle relaxation, ketamine also serves as an inductive agent for other general anesthetics. A supplement for low-potency agents, such as nitrous oxide, ketamine is given both intramuscularly and intravenously. Since this drug frequently produces psychic problems in adults, ketamine's use is ordinarily limited to superficial procedures in infants and children.

Adverse Effects/Precautions. Ketamine stimulates the sympathetic nervous system, increasing blood pressure. Intracranial pressure increases with ketamine.

Approximately 12% of the patients who receive this drug experience emergence psychic difficulties. These reactions (including terrifying dreams and extensive reality distortion) are lowest in the young (15 years or less) and the elderly (over 65). A reduced dosage of ketamine and addition of intravenous diazepam to the regimen lowers the incidence of psychologic manifestations during emergence.

Etomidate. Etomidate, an imidazole congener, is used as an intravenous hypnotic drug in anesthesia induction.

Mechanism of Action. Although etomidate has no analgesic properties, it possesses significant hypnotic activity. The intravenous administration of etomidate has limited effects on cardiac output and peripheral or pulmonary circulation. Rapid biotransformation of etomidate by the liver and kidneys results in an extremely brief duration of action.

Clinical Indications. Employed for anesthesia induction, etomidate is also used to supplement a weak anesthetic, such as nitrous oxide in oxygen. Another of its clinical applications is in short gynecologic procedures, e.g., dilation and curettage.

Adverse Effects/Precautions. About 1 in 5 etomidate users note transient venous pain. A venous irritant effect (perhaps leading to thrombophlebitis) may result from the vehicle propylene glycol that solubilizes etomidate.

Some patients also experience adrenal steroid depletion following etomidate therapy. Another adverse effect is transient involuntary muscle contractions (usually myoclonic jerkings) that occur in about 1 in 3 patients.

ADDITIONAL INTRAVENOUS ANESTHETICS

Methohexital and thiamylal, both thiobarbiturates, have uses similar to those of thiopental and intravenous anesthetics.

A combination product of fentanyl (a narcotic analgesic) and droperidol (a major tranquilizer) is used in surgical procedures as an anesthetic premedication, an anesthetic induction agent, or as an adjunct in the maintenance of general or regional anesthesia. General quiescence, reduced motor activity, and marked analgesia characterize the combined effect (called neuroleptanalgesia) of fentanyl and droperidol. Loss of consciousness does not occur with this drug combination, which is usually administered by intramuscular injection. The clinician should consider the pharmacologic properties of each of the drugs in this combination because of their specialized differences.

LOCAL ANESTHETICS

Local anesthetics (see also Chapter 10) are either of the ester or amide type. By interfering with nerve conduction, local anesthetics produce a reversible loss of sensation in a particular region of the body. Certain local anesthetics (such as tetracaine and dibucaine) are administered into the subarachnoid or intrathecal space and thus are considered as spinal anesthetics which act on the CNS to achieve their pharmacologic effect. Lidocaine, prilocaine, and mepivacaine are used for epidural and caudal anesthesia in certain surgical and medical procedures.

Mechanism of Action. Local anesthetics interfere with the rate of the depolarization phase of the nerve action potential. Consequently, neurons do not adequately depolarize and the nerve action potential is inhibited. Local anesthetics apparently compete with Ca^{++} for a site in the membrane that opens the Na^+ channel in "fast" depolarization.

Clinical Indications. When injected into the spinal cord or adjacent areas, selected local anesthetics produce regional anesthesia for medical and surgical procedures.

Adverse Effects/Precautions. Unlike amide-type local anesthetics, ester-type anesthetics may produce allergic reactions as evidenced by rashes or bronchospasm. CNS stimulation followed by depression and peripheral cardiovascular collapse are serious adverse reactions to systemic local anesthetic administration.

Table 1.2 SEDATIVE-HYPNOTICS

Available products	Trade names	Daily dosage range
Barbiturate type:		
Amobarbital	Amytal	30–200 mg
Amobarbital sodium	Amytal sodium	65–200 mg
Aprobarbital	Alurate	40–160 mg
Butabarbital sodium	Butabarbital sodium; Butasol sodium	60–120 mg
Mephobarbital	Mebaral	150–200 mg
Pentobarbital sodium	Nembutal sodium	60–100 mg
Phenobarbital	Luminal; others	30–100 mg
Secobarbital	Seconal	40–100 mg
Talbutal	Lotusate	120 mg
Nonbarbiturate Type:		
Acetylcarbromal	Paxarel; Sedamyl	500–1000 mg
Chloral hydrate	Noctec	250–2000 mg
Ethchlorvynol	Placidyl	100–1000 mg
Ethinamate	Valmid	500–1000 mg
Flurazepam HCl	Dalmane	15–30 mg
Glutethimide	Doriden; Glutethimide	125–1000 mg
Methyprylon	Noludar	50–400 mg
Paraldehyde	Paral	5–30 ml
Propiomazine HCl	Largon	10–30 mg
Scopolamine HBr	Scopolamine HBr	0.3–0.6 mg
Temazepam	Restoril	30 mg
Triazolam	Halcion	0.25–0.5 mg
Triclofos sodium	Triclos	1500 mg

SEDATIVES AND HYPNOTICS

Although the words "sedative and hypnotic" have no exact scientific definitions, they are still commonly used medical terms. A sedative calms the patient without producing unconsciousness and sleep. Thus, a sedative predisposes a patient to sleep by reducing anxiety and mental stress. A hynoptic, on the other hand, produces a greater degree of CNS depression and actually induces sleep. Depending upon the dosage, the same drug often acts as either a sedative or as a hypnotic (Table 1.2).

The barbiturates, a class of synthetic drugs, produce varying degrees of CNS depression. In this manner, low doses of oxybarbiturates are used as sedatives; higher doses of the same drugs produce a hypnotic effect or sleep; and certain thiobarbiturates are used as anesthetic agents. Thus, a choice of the appropriate barbiturate produces a degree of CNS depression that ranges from mild sedation to a deep stage of anesthesia.

The nonbarbiturate sedative-hypnotics are from several different chemical classes, including benzodiazepine derivatives, and resemble the barbiturates by their ability to reduce anxiety and nervous tension, as well as to induce sleep.

BENZODIAZEPINE DERIVATIVES

Benzodiazepine derivatives are presently one of the most widely used drug classes in modern medicine. Various individual members of the benzodiazepine group are used as antianxiety drugs, central skeletal muscle relaxants, anticonvulsants, and sedative-hypnotics. Certain benzodiazepines, such as flurazepam and nitrazepam, are popular sedative-hypnotic drugs.

Several reasons account for the replacement of the classical sedative-hypnotics, e.g., barbiturates, by the benzodiazepine derivatives. Depression of respiration, a critical consideration in overdose cases, is not as marked with the benzodiazepines. As selective depressants of the CNS, the benzodiazepines do not follow the barbiturate sequence of increasing dosage to produce hypnosis and then anesthesia. Stupor occurs with high benzodiazepine doses, but true anesthseia is not produced. This selectivity is an advantage since even in large doses coma rarely occurs. CNS depressants, such as alcohol, greatly enhance respiratory depression, and the benzodiazepine-alcohol drug interaction is often fatal. Additionally, the benzodiazepines are central skeletal muscle relaxants.

The benzodiazepines may owe many of their pharmacologic effects to activation of receptors that influence GABA function in the CNS. The receptor-effector mechanism activated by the benzodiazepines requires a similar interaction by GABA with its affinity site. The benzodiazepine action is detectable only when GABA-ergic neurons are active or when exogenous GABA is applied to neurons. The benzodiazepine receptor is part of a supramolecular complex that contains the receptors for GABA and benzodiazepines and the GABA receptor-modulated chloride channel.

Chronic use of high doses of benzodiazepines may result in psychic and physical dependence. Abrupt withdrawal of the benzodiazepine in dependent individuals results in CNS excitation, possibly evidenced by convulsions.

Flurazepam. Flurazepam was the first benzodiazepine compound used specifically as a hypnotic drug.

Mechanism of Action. Flurazepam activates receptors that function in concert with GABA receptors to open chloride ion channels (Figure 1.15). An inhibitory effect on central neurons then results.

Clinical Indications. Flurazepam is useful in insomnia cases that are characterized by difficulty in falling asleep and by frequent awakenings and/or early morning awakening. Effectiveness usually remains for about a month after continuous therapy.

Adverse Effects/Precautions. Dizziness, drowsiness, and lightheadedness frequently occur, especially in the elderly. Hazardous tasks undertaken on the day following flurazepam use as a hypnotic require caution. Use of alcohol with flurazepam should be avoided due to the combination's additive effect.

Temazepam. Although most effective in maintaining sleep, temazepam also induces sleep efficiently.

Mechanism of Action. Temazepam interacts with a supramolecular complex that contains the receptors for benzodiazepines, GABA, and the GABA receptor-modulated chloride channel. Temazepam, unlike flurazepam, does not have a major active metabolite. Pharmacologic effects are thus attributed to the unchanged parent compound, temazepam. Since the mean terminal half-life of temazepam is about 10 hours, undesirable "hangover" effects the next day and accumulation of the drug (used on a once daily basis) are unlikely.

Clinical Indications. Temazepam is useful as a hypnotic in treating insomnia.

Adverse Effects/Precautions. Drowsiness, dizziness, and lethargy are the most frequent side effects noted with temazepam.

Triazolam. Triazolam is an effective benzodiazepine hypnotic for short-term use in insomnia.

Mechanism of Action. Triazolam interacts with a supramolecular complex containing the receptors for benzodiazepines, GABA, and the GABA receptor-modulated chloride channel.

Clinical Indications. Triazolam use is the same as that of temazepam.

Adverse Effects/Precautions. Withdrawal of triazolam consistently produces rebound insomnia.

BARBITURATES

Barbiturates, derivatives of barbituric acid, are frequently prescribed sedative-hypnotics. Barbituric acid is synthesized from the reaction of malonic acid and urea (Figure 1.16). The first

32 THERAPEUTIC PHARMACOLOGY

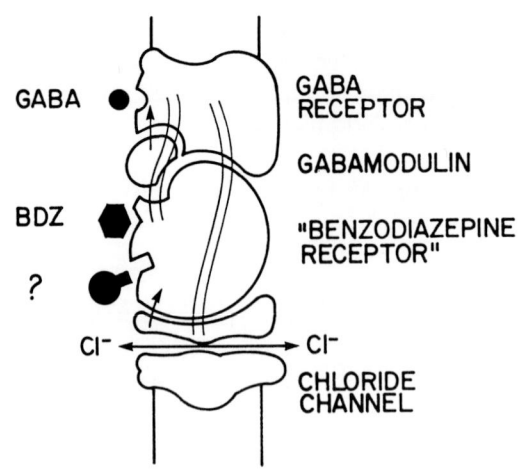

Fig. 1.15 Benzodiazepine receptor. (From Usdin, E., et al.: Pharmacology of Benzodiazepines. Deerfield Beach, FL, Verlag chemie, 1983.)

Fig. 1.16 Barbiturate synthesis and substitution on ring.

clinically available barbiturates, barbital and phenobarbital, were introduced shortly before World War I, circa 1916.

Although barbituric acid does not possess sedative-hypnotic activity per se, replacement of alkyl or aryl groups for hydrogen atoms at position-5 (Figure 1.16) results in sedative-hypnotic activity. This activity also occurs if two ethyl groups replace hydrogen atoms at position-5 (barbital). Increasing the chain length of the alkyl group usually increases hypnotic potency, speeds the onset of action, and decreases the duration of action. There is an upper limit to these generalizations; for example, when the total number of carbon atoms in the alkyl chain reaches eight, the drug becomes extremely toxic.

Aryl substitution, such as the presence of a phenyl group in phenobarbital, imparts antiseizure properties to the drug molecule. Also, replacement of the oxygen at position-2 (Figure 1.16) forms the thiobarbiturates, such as thiopental, which are valuable ultra-short acting intravenous anesthetics. Amobarbital, pentobarbital, phenobarbital, and secobarbital are barbiturates that find wide use as sedative-hypnotics.

The onset of action of the barbiturates depends upon the degree of absorption and the lipid solubility. Sodium salts of the barbiturates are well absorbed orally and are often used clinically. Lipid solubility is an important factor in the onset of barbiturate activity. Thus, amobarbital (with ethyl and isoamyl substitution at position-5) has a more rapid onset than barbital (with two substituted ethyl groups) because of amobarbital's greater lipid solubility.

Blood flow significantly determines the onset of action of a highly lipid soluble barbiturate. Since the brain is a vessel-rich and greatly perfused structure, high CNS concentrations of a lipid soluble barbiturate occur within seconds after intravenous administration. Redistribution of highly lipid-soluble barbiturates to the peripheral muscle-fat compartment terminates the CNS depression of ultra-short acting barbiturates, such as thiopental.

Biotransformation and renal excretion of barbiturates also determine the drug's duration of action. Barbital, for instance, is not metabolized; since its duration of action singularly depends upon renal excretion, the drug is a long acting barbiturate. Barbiturates with an intermediate action are biotransformed by the liver to inactive metabolites that are then excreted in the urine.

The degree of plasma protein-binding by a barbiturate influences the drug's potency and duration of action. Binding to plasma proteins protects the barbiturate from biotransformation, as well as preventing its renal elimination.

An unusual metabolic effect of the barbiturates is their capacity to induce hepatic enzyme synthesis of enzymatic systems which are responsible for their own biotransformation. Their increased metabolism after repeated doses could explain tolerance to barbiturate action.

Psychic and physical dependence may develop with barbiturate use. Abrupt withdrawal of the barbiturate in dependent individuals results in anxiety, irritability, insomnia, tremors, and, in severe cases, life-threatening convulsions. Therefore, careful medical supervision, on an in-patient basis, involving slow withdrawal of the barbiturate over a period of 1 to 2 weeks is recommended.

Acute barbiturate overdose depresses the respiratory center and decreases its responsiveness to carbon dioxide. Supportive measures to maintain respiration and blood pressure and to promote drug excretion are treatment goals.

Barbiturates are not primary analgesics, but they apparently modify an individual's reaction to pain. Certain barbiturates, such as phenobarbital and metharbital, possess anticonvulsant activity.

Barbiturates' ability to activate GABA-ergic pathways resembles benzodiazepine activity. Barbiturates, however, do not interact with benzodiazepine binding sites; rather, they enhance GABA binding to receptors adjacent to chloride channels in the neuron membrane. Thus, the depressant activity of barbiturates relates to their interaction with a membrane-bound supramolecular complex composed of GABA-ergic receptors, chloride ionophores, and benzodiazepine affinity sites (Figure 1.17). Activation opens the chloride ion channel, which causes neuron membrane depolarization.

Pentobarbital. A short-acting barbiturate, pentobarbital is used for both daytime and nocturnal sedation.

Mechanism of Action. Barbiturates depress pathways in the ascending reticular activating system (ARAS). Additionally, the neuron activity of structures in the limbic system decreases. Pentobarbital potentiates the inhibitory effects of GABA-ergic mechanisms in the CNS by an enhancement of GABA receptor binding.

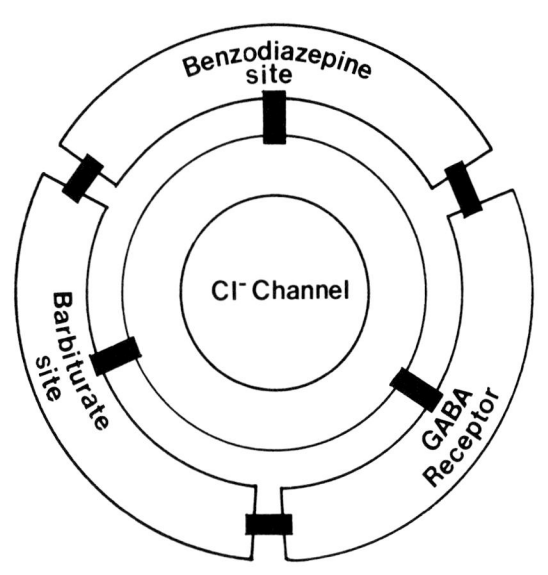

Fig. 1.17 Macromolecular (GABA-BDZ) complex with barbiturate receptor site. (From Study, R.E., and Barker, J.L.: Cellular mechanisms of benzodiazepine action. JAMA, 247:2148, 1982.)

Clinical Indications. Pentobarbital is used as a sedative-hypnotic for the short-term management of insomnia. Tolerance develops to the drug's depressant effects after two weeks.

Adverse Effects/Precautions. CNS effects, such as somnolence, residual sedation ("hangover effect"), and lethargy represent an extension of the drug's primary pharmacologic activity. Paradoxical excitement may occur in susceptible patients. Since psychic and physical dependence to pentobarbital may occur, administration beyond 14 days is not recommended.

Possible hypersensitivity reactions include morbilliform rash, fever, angioneurotic edema, and urticaria. Patients with concurrent asthma or observable allergy signs are more susceptible to these reactions.

Secobarbital. Secobarbital, a short acting barbiturate, is used as a sedative-hypnotic.

Mechanism of Action. Secobarbital inhibits conduction in the ARAS. The molecular mechanism probably involves accentuation of GABA-ergic mechanisms.

Clinical Indications. A short acting barbiturate, like secobarbital, is used as a sedative hypnotic. Administration for longer than 14 days is not recommended. Prolonged, uninterrupted use of secobarbital (even in therapeutic doses) may result in psychic and physical dependence.

Adverse Effects/Precautions. One percent of patients report somnolence, an extension of the drug's pharmacologic effect. Other adverse effects resemble those noted for pentobarbital.

Amobarbital. An intermediate acting drug, amobarbital is used for its sedative and hypnotic action.

Mechanism of Action. Amobarbital depresses the ARAS and interacts with an affinity site on a supramolecular complex that contains a GABA-ergic receptor, a benzodiazepine receptor site, and a chloride ionophore. Activation opens the chloride ion channel in close proximity to the supramolecular receptor complex.

Clinical Indications. Amobarbital is used as a sedative-hypnotic for daytime sedation, nocturnal hypnosis, and preanesthetic medication.

Adverse Effects/Precautions. Idiosyncratic reactions, such as excitement or pain, may occur. Some patients, especially those with asthma, urticaria, or angioneurotic edema, may experience hypersensitivity to amobarbital. Since amobarbital, as all barbiturates, may be habit-forming, the possibility of drug abuse and dependence is a valid concern.

Aprobarbital. Aprobarbital is an intermediate acting sedative-hypnotic barbiturate.

Mechanism of Action. The mechanism and site of action of aprobarbital are the same as those of amobarbital.

Clinical Indications. Aprobarbital is used for sedation and sleep induction on a short-term basis. Since effectiveness is not evident after about two weeks of therapy, drug-free intervals of a week or more should elapse before initiating retreatment for persistent insomnia.

Adverse Effects/Precautions. Aprobarbital has the same types of adverse effects and precautions as those indicated for amobarbital.

Butabarbital. Butabarbital, an intermediate acting barbiturate, is used as a sedative-hypnotic.

Mechanism of Action. The proposed mechanism and site of action are the same as those of amobarbital.

Clinical Indications. Butabarbital is used as a sedative for the treatment of anxiety-tension states. This drug is also an effective hypnotic for inducing and maintaining sleep for short-term management of insomnia.

Adverse Effects/Precautions. Butabarbital's adverse effects and precautions are like those of amobarbital.

Talbutal. Talbutal is an intermediate acting barbiturate.

Mechanism of Action. In therapeutic doses, talbutal depresses the ARAS in the thalamic region of the brain. This activity interferes with nerve impulse conduction to the cortex. The depressant effect relates to an interaction with a supramolecular complex that contains a barbiturate receptor, a chloride ionophore, a benzodiazepine receptor, and a GABA-ergic activation site.

Clinical Indications. Talbutal is used as a hypnotic for the short-term treatment of insomnia.

Adverse Effects/Precautions. Since the adverse effects that occur with talbutal resemble those noted for amobarbital, similar precautions and warnings apply.

Phenobarbital. Phenobarbital, a long acting barbiturate, has sedative-hypnotic and anticonvulsant properties.

Mechanism of Action. The basis of the sedative-hypnotic action is a depressant effect on the ARAS. The molecular mechanism involved is the activation of a barbiturate affinity site located on or near a supramolecular complex that is composed of a chloride ionophore, a benzodiazepine receptor, and a GABA-ergic activation site.

Clinical Indications. Phenobarbital is used both for the short-term treatment of insomnia and as a preanesthetic sedative. It is also widely used as an anticonvulsant.

Adverse Effects/Precautions. The long action of phenobarbital more likely produces next day or residual sedation "hangover" than either the short or intermediate acting barbiturates. Hypersensitivity reactions (such as morbilliform rash, angioneurotic edema, and fever) may occur.

As with all the sedative-hypnotic barbiturates, an oral dose of from 10 to 12 times the therapeutic dose (about 1 g) produces serious poisoning in an adult. Death from respiratory depression commonly occurs after ingestion of more than 2 g of phenobarbital. Concurrent ingestion of alcohol greatly enhances CNS depression of barbiturates.

Mephobarbital. Mephobarbital, a long acting barbiturate, is used as a sedative. This drug also has anticonvulsant properties.

Mechanism of Action. The proposed mechanism and site of action for sedative activity are the same as those of phenobarbital.

Clinical Indications. Mephobarbital is useful as a sedative for the treatment of anxiety, tension, and apprehension. Also, mephobarbital is employed extensively as an anticonvulsant.

Adverse Effects/Precautions. The adverse effects noted with mephobarbital are similar to those of other long acting barbiturates, such as phenobarbital.

MISCELLANEOUS SEDATIVES AND HYPNOTICS

This drug class contains some of the first agents used as sedative-hypnotics, e.g., chloral hydrate and paraldehyde. Drugs that have a similar pharmacologic profile to the barbiturates are also included in this classification.

Chloral Hydrate. Chloral hydrate is an effective hypnotic drug for the treatment of insomnia.

Mechanism of Action. Chloral hydrate is converted in vivo to trichloroethanol, a compound that possesses significant hypnotic activity. This metabolite probably accounts for the pharmacologic activity. In therapeutic doses, chloral hydrate does not significantly depress respiration or the cough reflex.

Clinical Indications. Chloral hydrate is used for nocturnal sedation and as a preoperative sedative.

Adverse Effects/Precautions. Disorientation, sometimes manifested by somnambulism, occasionally occurs in some patients.

Paraldehyde. Paraldehyde, a colorless, bitter liquid which has an intense unpleasant aroma, is occasionally used as a sedative-hypnotic.

Mechanism of Action. In therapeutic doses, paraldehyde produces a nonspecific reversible depression of the CNS. The mechanisms of the hypnotic action of paraldehyde are unknown.

Clinical Indications. Paraldehyde is used as a sedative-hypnotic or to quiet patients with delirium tremens (DTs); however, safer and more effective drugs are usually used in such situations. Taking paraldehyde with food or mixing it with milk or iced fruit juice usually counteracts the taste.

Adverse Effects/Precautions. Prolonged use may result in a drug dependence syndrome that resembles alcoholism. Since hepatitis has been observed with continued use, patients with liver dysfunction may be more susceptible to the action of paraldehyde. Nerve damage, resulting from parenteral administration of this drug, occurs when paraldehyde is injected too close to nerve trunks.

Paraldehyde decomposes upon exposure to air and should not be used if it has either a brownish color or a strong vinegary odor. Plastic containers must be avoided for paraldehyde preparations.

Glutethimide. Glutethimide, a piperidine derivative, is useful as a hypnotic drug.

Mechanism of Action. Glutethimide produces a dose-dependent CNS depression that is similar to the barbiturates; its exact mechanism of CNS depressant action is unknown. The drug shows a pronounced anticholinergic activity, as evidenced by dry mouth, dilated pupils, and inhibition of intestinal motility. Glutethimide suppresses REM sleep and is associated with REM rebound.

Clinical Indications. Glutethimide is used for the short-term (up to 1 week) management of insomnia.

Adverse Effects/Precautions. The most common adverse reactions occur after prolonged use and include osteomalacia and generalized skin rash. Although glutethimide was introduced as a drug less likely to produce the physical dependence associated with the barbiturates, both physical and psychologic dependence on glutethimide occur with prolonged use. Thus, careful evaluation and monitoring of patients receiving glutethimide is necessary.

Methyprylon. Methyprylon, a piperidine derivative, is employed as a hypnotic drug.

Mechanism of Action. Methyprylon produces a CNS depressant action similar to that of the barbiturates. The precise mechanism of methyprylon activity is unknown. Methyprylon suppresses REM sleep and is associated with REM rebound following discontinuation of the drug.

Clinical Indications. Methyprylon is useful in the short-term (up to 1 week) management of insomnia.

Adverse Effects/Precautions. Adverse reactions include dizziness, gastrointestinal upset, headache, and skin rash. Paradoxical excitement may occur with methyprylon, as does the possibility of physical and psychologic dependence.

Ethchlorvynol. Ethchlorvynol is a tertiary alcohol that possesses sedative-hypnotic, anticonvulsant, and muscle relaxant properties.

Mechanism of Action. Ethchlorvynol elicits a dose-dependent CNS depression similar to that of the barbiturates. Although its mechanism of action is unclear, the drug produces EEG patterns that resemble those produced by the barbiturates.

Clinical Indications. Ethchlorvynol is useful in the short-term (up to 1 week) treatment of insomnia.

Adverse Effects/Precautions. Gastrointestinal upset accompanied by nausea and vomiting occur with ethchlorvynol. Other adverse reactions include dizziness, hypotension, and skin rashes. Paradoxical excitement is also sometimes observed. As with the barbiturates, ethchlorvynol use should be avoided in patients who have severe pain, unless analgesics are employed for pain relief.

Since some dosage forms of ethchlorvynol contain tartrazine, patients who are allergy-prone (such as those with bronchial asthma) should use tartrazine-containing drugs cautiously.

Ethinamate. Ethinamate is a carbamate-type nonbarbiturate hypnotic.

Mechanism of Action. A nonselective CNS depressant, ethinamate acts similarly to the barbiturates. However, the exact mechanism of action is unclear.

Clinical Indications. The main therapeutic application of ethinamate is as a short acting hypnotic in the management of insomnia. Ethinamate is not recommended for prolonged use because its effectiveness lessens after about 1 week and its potential for abuse.

Adverse Effects/Precautions. Although adverse reactions are uncommon with ethinamate, they include mild gastrointestinal upset, skin rashes, and paradoxical excitement. Thrombocytopenic purpura and fever are rare occurrences following ethinamate therapy.

ANTICONVULSANT DRUGS

The four major classes of anticonvulsant drugs are the barbiturates, hydantoins, succinimides, and oxazolidinediones (Figure 1.18; Table 1.3). Additionally, several miscellaneous drugs of diverse chemical structure are employed in the management of seizure states. The 6-membered pyrimidine barbiturate ring resembles the 5-membered hydantoin structure by having a nitrogen atom in position-1 of both aromatic rings. The succinimides have a carbon atom at position-1 and the oxazolidinediones contain an oxygen atom at this position. Thus, structural similarity exists in four of the major anticonvulsant groups. The 5-position in the core ring of each of these classes is the prime focus of substitution with various alkyl and aromatic groups. A combination of aromatic and aliphatic groups (for example, phenobarbital, phenyl-ethyl), two aromatic groups (such as phenytoin, 2 phenyls), or two aliphatic groups (for example, ethosuximide, methyl-ethyl) illustrate this substitution. N-methylation is another structural change seen in these groups. N-demethylation ordinarily occurs rapidly in vivo so that a methylated barbiturate is immediately biotransformed to its nonmethylated derivative, such as mephobarbital to phenobarbital.

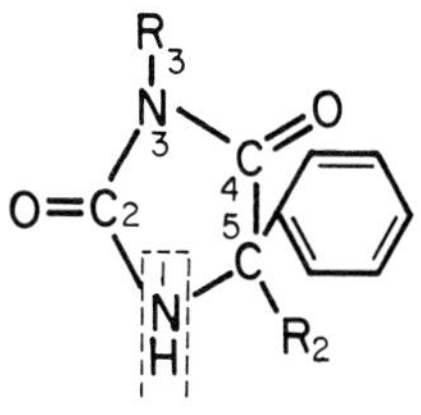

Hydantoin derivatives

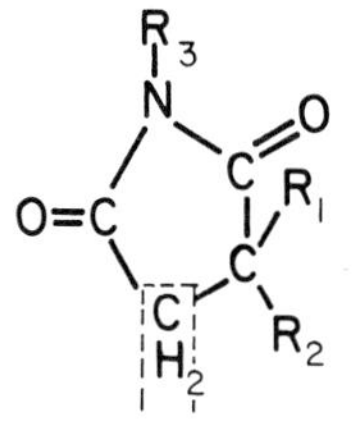

Succinimides

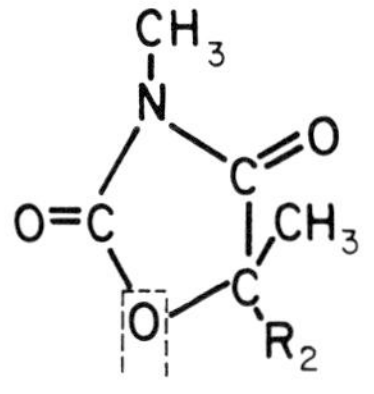

Oxazolidinediones

Fig. 1.18 SAR-Anticonvulsants.

Table 1.3 ANTICONVULSANT DRUGS

Available products	Trade names	Daily dosage range
Acetazolamide	Diamox	250 mg-1 gm
Carbamazepine	Tegretol	200–1200 mg
Clonazepam	Klonopin	Children: 20 mg; Adults: 1.5 mg initially—no more than 20 mg daily maintenance
Diazepam	Valium	5–30 mg
Ethosuximide	Zarontin	750 mg-1.5 g
Ethotoin	Peganone	1–3 g
Mephenytoin	Mesantoin	100–400 mg
Mephobarbital	Mebaral	400–600 mg
Metharbital	Gemonil	100–300 mg
Methsuximide	Celontin	600 mg-1.2 g
Paramethadione	Paradione	600 mg-1.8 g
Phenacemide	Phenurone	1–2 g
Phenobarbital	Luminal	100–300 mg
Phensuximide	Milontin	500 mg-1.2 g
Phenytoin	Dilantin	100–400 mg
Primidone	Mysoline; Myidone	250–750 mg
Trimethadione	Tridione	900 mg-2.1 g
Valproic acid	Depakene; Depakote	60 mg/kg

The drugs most frequently used in the control of tonic-clonic seizures (grand mal) are phenobarbital and phenytoin. Clinicians usually initiate therapy of almost all types of epilepsy with phenobarbital because of its relative safety and broad spectrum of anticonvulsant activity. Although phenobarbital may cause drowsiness, it rarely produces the more limiting adverse effects that the other anticonvulsants cause. Phenytoin, another first drug option in epilepsy therapy, lacks the sedative component of phenobarbital and offers seizure protection in three out of four patients with grand mal epilepsy.

The succinimides are generally considered the drugs of choice for long-term treatment of absence seizures (petit mal). Ethosuximide, used in therapy initiation, combines a relative lack of adverse reactions with a broad spectrum of effectiveness against all forms of absence seizures. Treatment of mixed seizures (absence and tonic-clonic) involves adding phenobarbital or phenytoin to the therapy regimen. Although ethosuximide benefits almost all patients to some degree, the drug controls seizures in 3 out of 4 petit mal patients. Alternate drugs for nonresponsive patients include trimethadione and paradione.

Miscellaneous anticonvulsant drugs (i.e., valproic acid, carbamazepine, acetazolamide, and primidone) are also clinically valuable. One or more of these drugs combined with standard anticonvulsants often offer full seizure protection for refractory patients. Phenacemide, the most toxic of the anticonvulsants, is limited to psychomotor seizures in patients who are completely resistant to other anticonvulsants.

BARBITURATES

Certain barbiturates possess significant anticonvulsant activity in addition to their sedative and hypnotic action.

Phenobarbital. Phenobarbital is the most widely used anticonvulsant barbiturate.

Mechanism of Action. Phenobarbital, an anticonvulsant, is given in doses that are not markedly sedative. The long duration of sustained effect level may also contribute to the drug's value as an anticonvulsant.

A proposed anticonvulsant mechanism for phenobarbital is its general depressant or stabilizing action on excitable cell membranes. Phenobarbital reduces repetitious firing in isolated axons that are exposed to calcium ion and magnesium ion deficient solutions. Thus, membrane stabilization possibly represents an important component in the antiepileptic activity of phenobarbital.

Experimentally, phenobarbital increases the content of the inhibitory neurotransmitter gamma-aminobutyric acid (GABA) in the CNS, especially if the GABA content is abnormally low. Another proposal is that a barbiturate affinity site exists on the CNS supramolecular complex, which contains the benzodiazepine receptor, GABA recognition site, and chloride ionophore. Activation by phenobarbital of the barbiturate receptor enhances GABA receptor binding, thereby inducing a coupling of the receptor-effector reactions that opens neuron membrane chloride ion pores. This interaction results in effects on neuron activity, possibly altering membrane stability characteristics.

Phenobarbital reduces the spread of aberrant impulses over the motor cortex. The dampening of the excitation wave by the "phenyl blanket" is probably a more critical factor in the antiepileptic action of phenobarbital than is inhibition of abnormal neuron firing.

Clinical Indications. Alone or in combination with other anticonvulsants, phenobarbital is indicated in the treatment of all forms of epilepsy. Other uses are in long-term management of generalized tonic-clonic and cortical focal seizures. Phenobarbital is also valuable in the emergency control of acute convulsive states associated with status epilepticus, eclampsia, meningitis, tetanus, and toxic reactions to strychnine or local anesthetics.

Adverse Effects/Precautions. The main adverse effects are sleepiness, depression, headache, slurred speech, visual disturbances, allergic skin reactions, blood dyscrasias, neonatal hemorrhagic disease, and vitamin D deficiency.

Mephobarbital. Mephobarbital (chemically N-methylphenobarbital) is used as an anticonvulsant.

Mechanism of Action. Mephobarbital is biotransformed to phenobarbital, probably accounting for the drug's anticonvulsant action. Chronic oral administration has led to the accumulation of phenobarbital but not mephobarbital. Upon the oral administration of mephobarbital, plasma levels of phenobarbital are higher than mephobarbital itself. Mephobarbital's mechanisms of action are the same as those proposed for phenobarbital.

Clinical Indications. Mephobarbital is used, alone or in combination with other anticonvulsants, in the treatment of tonic-clonic seizures (grand mal) and absence seizures (petit mal).

Adverse Effects/Precautions. The adverse reactions associated with mephobarbital anticonvulsant therapy resemble those of phenobarbital and include effects related to sedation and disinhibition. Specific reactions are drowsiness, dizziness, ataxia, diplopia, and personality changes.

Metharbital. Metharbital is a long-acting anticonvulsant barbiturate that is biotransformed to barbital. Chemically, the phenyl group on carbon position-5 in mephobarbital is replaced by an ethyl group.

Mechanism of Action. Metharbital's bioconversion by demethylation to barbital explains this drug's mechanism of action. Barbital probably acts as an anticonvulsant by mechanisms similar to those of phenobarbital.

Clinical Indications. Metharbital is employed in the management of tonic-clonic seizures (grand mal), absence seizures (petit mal), myoclonic seizures, and mixed seizures.

Adverse Effects/Precautions. Adverse effects observed with metharbital resemble those of phenobarbital and mephobarbital.

HYDANTOINS

The hydantoins are ureides that are chemically related to the barbiturates. These 5-member ring compounds are condensation products of urea and acetic acid, as compared to urea and malonic acid in the case of barbiturates.

Phenytoin (Diphenylhydantoin). Phenytoin is the most commonly used hydantoin anticonvulsant.

Mechanism of Action. Phenytoin prevents the spread of abnormal electrical activity throughout the cerebral cortical neurons. The stabilization of the cortical neurons possibly relates to alterations in sodium flux through membrane pores. One proposal is that the anticonvulsant activity of phenytoin results from the drug's capacity to extrude intracellular brain sodium and thus suppresses the excitation wave spread.

Explanations for membrane stabilization include a reduction of post-tetanic potentiation, prolonged refractory period, elevation of synaptic threshold, and augmentation of inhibitory chemicals, such as GABA.

Clinical Indications. Phenytoin, alone or in combination with phenobarbital, is used in the management of grand mal epilepsy, symptomatic convulsions, and psychomotor seizures. Phenytoin may aggravate petit mal epilepsy.

Phenytoin sometimes relieves trigeminal neuralgia and atypical face pain. The drug is also valuable as an antiarrhythmic drug in specified clinical situations.

Adverse Effects/Precautions. Common side effects are ataxia, nystagmus, and slurred speech. Tremors, nervousness, drowsiness, and fatigue are other adverse reactions.

Hyperplasia of the gums, occurring in about 1 in 5 patients, is more common and severe in younger patients. The irritating alkaline nature of the commercially used sodium salt of phenytoin may cause the nausea and epigastric pain sometimes reported after oral administration of the drug. An allergic rash, often mistaken for measles, and infectious mononucleosis occurs occasionally (in 2 to 10% of the patients on phenytoin therapy).

Hirsutism of the extremities in young females is another reported adverse effect. Rare toxic reactions include toxic psychosis, hepatitis, and a systemic lupus erythematosus-like syndrome.

Because phenytoin therapy results in lower calcium serum levels, some patients have developed rickets after many years of phenytoin treatment. This effect possibly results from a more rapid activation of vitamin D due to the hepatic enzyme induction of phenytoin.

Mephenytoin. Mephenytoin has anticonvulsant properties similar to those of phenytoin.

Mechanism of Action. Mephenytoin apparently inhibits convulsant processes through the same mechanisms as phenytoin.

Clinical Indications. Mephenytoin is indicated for those patients refractory to less toxic anticonvulsants. The drug's value is in the treatment of resistant cases of tonic-clonic seizures (grand mal), psychomotor seizures, focal seizures, and Jacksonian seizures.

Adverse Effects/Precautions. Mephenytoin is more toxic than phenytoin. Rash, neutropenia, and drowsiness are commonly reported side effects. Also, pantocytopenia, aplastic anemia, and hepatic damage occur more frequently with mephenytoin than with phenytoin.

Ethotoin. Ethotoin is an orally effective antiepileptic hydantoin derivative.

Mechanism of Action. Ethotoin, like phenytoin, apparently stabilizes excitable neuron membranes and prevents the spread of seizure activity, rather than abolishing the focus of seizure discharges.

Clinical Indications. Ethotoin is useful in the treatment of tonic-clonic (grand mal) seizures and psychomotor seizures.

Adverse Effects/Precautions. Ethotoin produces less gingival hyperplasia and hirsutism than does phenytoin. However, reported side effects of ethotoin include diarrhea, blood dyscrasias, and dose-related drowsiness and sedation. Ethotoin is contraindicated in patients who have hepatic abnormalities or hematologic disorders.

SUCCINIMIDES

Succinimides have generally replaced other anticonvulsants as drugs of choice in the treatment of petit mal epilepsy.

Ethosuximide. Ethosuximide is the most commonly employed succinimide derivative in the treatment of petit mal seizures.

Mechanism of Action. Succinimide derivatives, such as ethosuximide, selectively block pentylenetetrazol-induced seizures in mice (a screening technique frequently used to test for effective drugs in petit mal seizures). Ethosuximide suppresses the paroxysmal 3 cycle-per-second spike and wave associated with the loss of consciousness that occurs in absence seizures (petit mal).

Ethosuximide depresses the motor cortex and elevates the CNS threshold to convulsive stimuli. Effects on glucose transport and a decrease in tricarboxylic acid cycle substrates may explain the drug's anticonvulsant activity.

Clinical Indications. Ethosuximide is valuable in treating petit mal seizures.

Adverse Effects/Precautions. Side effects include gastrointestinal irritation, drowsiness, depression, headache, and skin rashes. Caution is advised with dosage increases or decreases, as well as with the addition or elimination of other medications. Abrupt withdrawal of anticonvulsant medication may precipitate seizures. When used alone in mixed types of epilepsy, ethosuximide, like the other succinimides, may increase the frequency of grand mal seizures in some patients.

Methsuximide. A succinimide derivative, methsuximide is used in the treatment of absence seizures that are refractory to other medication.

Mechanism of Action. Methsuximide, like ethosuximide, increases the seizure threshold and reduces the paroxysmal spike and wave pattern that characterizes petit mal seizure.

Clinical Indications. Methsuximide is indicated for petit mal epilepsy that is refractory to other drugs.

Adverse Effects/Precautions. Drowsiness, ataxia, and dizziness are commonly reported side effects. Chronic methsuximide administration is indicated by an accumulation of inactive metabolites.

Phensuximide. Phensuximide, a succinimide derivative, is employed in the treatment of petit mal epilepsy.

Mechanism of Action. As with the other succinimides, phensuximide suppresses the paroxysmal cortical spike-wave sequence noted in absence seizures. Elevation of the seizure threshold and depressant effects on the motor cortex contribute to the anticonvulsant activity.

Clinical Indications. Phensuximide is indicated in the treatment of petit mal seizures.

Adverse Effects/Precautions. Drowsiness, ataxia, and dizziness are frequently reported side effects. Symptoms related to gastrointestinal irritation (i.e., nausea, cramps, and anorexia) are also common. A harmless urine discoloration (to a pink, red, or red-brown) may occur with this drug. Cautious phensuximide use is advised in patients with acute intermittent porphyria.

OXAZOLIDINEDIONES

Due to their serious side effects and potential for producing fetal malformations, the oxazolidinediones find limited use as anticonvulsants.

Trimethadione. Trimethadione is employed in the control of petit mal seizures.

Mechanism of Action. The oxazolidinediones, such as trimethadione, suppress the abnormal paroxysmal 3 cycle-per-second spike and wave EEG pattern common to petit mal. Trimethadione apparently raises the threshold for cortical seizures, decreases the projection of focal seizure activity, and reduces repetitive spinal cord transmission. The cortical excitation wave spread is not reduced with trimethadione.

Trimethadione prevents or reduces seizure activity that various chemicals (including pentylenetetrazol, thujone, picrotoxin, and strychnine) induce. Unlike phenobarbital and phenytoin, trimethadione does not modify the maximal seizure patterns in patients receiving electroconvulsive therapy.

Clinical Indications. Trimethadione is indicated for the control of absence (petit mal) seizures that are refractory to other anticonvulsant medication.

Adverse Effects/Precautions. The most persistent side effect is a reversible visual disturbance described as the "glare phenomenon." Occurring early in therapy, this distinct reaction makes outdoor objects in bright light appear as though they're covered with snow.

Blood dyscrasias are serious adverse reactions noted with trimethadione. Eighty percent of the patients receiving trimethadione show a usually nonthreatening neutropenia that should be distinguished from agranulocytosis. Fatal aplastic anemia, thrombocytopenia, and leukopenia are other blood abnormalities that have occurred with trimethadione use. Caution is advised in using this drug in acute intermittent porphyria patients.

A systemic lupus erythymatosus-like syndrome is another complication of trimethadione therapy. Also, a myasthenia gravis-like syndrome may occur with long-term use of trimethadione. This drug may also potentiate allergic reactions (for example, morbilliform rash). Since trimethadione may produce fetal malformations and serious side effects, the drug's use is limited to petit mal seizures that are unresponsive to less toxic anticonvulsant therapy.

Paramethadione. Paramethadione is an alternate to trimethadione in the treatment of selected cases of absence (petit mal) seizures.

Mechanism of Action. Paramethadione's proposed mechanism of action is similar to trimethadione's. However, the drugs differ in that paramethadione's sedative effect is greater than that of trimethadione.

Clinical Indications. Paramethadione is often effective in the control of absence seizures that are refractory to other anticonvulsants. Paramethadione is apparently less toxic and less effective than trimethadione.

Adverse Effects/Precautions. Although the adverse effects of paramethadione and trimethadione are essentially the same, reports of serious toxic reactions are fewer with paramethadione.

MISCELLANEOUS ANTICONVULSANTS

Several miscellaneous anticonvulsants of diverse chemical structure and pharmacologic profile are available for clinical use.

Valproic Acid and Derivatives. Valproic acid and its derivatives, sodium valproate and divalproex sodium, are anticonvulsants that are mainly used in the treatment of absence seizures.

Mechanism of Action. Valproic acid probably owes its anticonvulsant activity to the elevation of GABA levels in the CNS.

Clinical Indications. Used alone or with other anticonvulsants, valproic acid is employed in the treatment of petit mal and complex absence seizures. It is also used as adjunctive therapy in patients who have multiple seizure types that include absence seizures as a component of the pathologic condition.

Adverse Effects/Precautions. Nausea, vomiting, and indigestion are common side effects reported in the initial stages of valproic acid therapy. These reactions usually disappear upon continued treatment. In addition to the sedative effects of valproic acid, CNS reactions include ataxia, nystagmus, dizziness, and incoordination.

Elevations of serum transaminases (SGOT and SGPT) and lactic dehydrogenase (LDH) occur frequently and are apparently dose-related. These results probably reflect potentially serious hepatatoxicity, as patients taking valproic acid have died from hepatic failure.

Carbamazepine. Carbamazepine primarily treats refractory seizure disorders.

Mechanism of Action. Carbamazepine offers anticonvulsant protection in both chemically and electrically-induced seizures in animals. The drug's exact mechanism of action is unknown. Carbamazepine's effects resemble those of phenytoin, as evidenced by a reduction of posttetanic potentiation.

Clinical Indications. Carbamazepine is employed in the management of refractory seizure disorders including partial seizures with complex symptomatology, generalized tonic-clonic seizure (grand mal), and mixed seizure patterns. This drug is ineffective in absence seizures (petit mal), myoclonic spasms, or predominant unilateral seizures.

Adverse Effects/Precautions. Potentially fatal blood dyscrasias, including aplastic anemia, thrombocytopenia, and leukopenia, have occurred following carbamazepine therapy. Frequently reported adverse reactions are drowsiness, incoordination, nausea, vomiting, and confusion. Abrupt discontinuation of carbamazepine after its effective anticonvulsant use may result in seizures or status epilepticus.

Clonazepam. Clonazepam, a benzodiazepine, has significant anticonvulsant activity.

Mechanism of Action. Clonazepam antagonizes pentylenetetrazol and electrically-induced seizures in mice. Additionally, clonazepam blocks seizures induced by photic stimulation in susceptible baboons. In addition to suppressing the spike and wave EEG pattern of absence seizures, clonazepam also decreases the frequency, amplitude, duration, and spread of discharge in minor motor seizures.

Clinical Indications. Clonazepam is useful alone or as an adjunct in the treatment of the Lennox-Gastaut syndrome (petit mal variant), akinetic, and myoclonic seizures. This drug also may control absence seizures that are refractory to other anticonvulsants.

Adverse Effects/Precautions. Frequently reported side reactions include drowsiness (50% of patients) and ataxia (30% of patients). Neurologic side effects include abnormal eye movements, nystagmus, vertigo, and choreiform movements. Clonazepam may increase or precipitate the incidence of the onset of generalized tonic-clonic (grand mal) seizures; this situation may necessitate adding other anticonvulsants or increasing their dosage. As with all benzodiazepines, withdrawal symptoms may occur after abrupt discontinuation of long-term, high dose clonazepam therapy.

Acetazolamide. A carbonic anhydrase inhibitor, acetazolamide is used as an adjunctive drug in selected seizure disorders.

Mechanism of Action. Inhibition of carbonic anhydrase in the CNS apparently blocks abnormal, paroxysmal, excessive neuron discharge. Beneficial effects may relate directly to carbonic anhydrase inhibition or to the acidosis acetazolamide therapy produces.

Clinical Indications. As an adjunctive drug, acetazolamide is used to control petit mal seizures in children. Adjunctive acetazolamide therapy is also useful in certain cases of both childhood and adult tonic-clonic seizures and mixed seizure patterns.

Adverse Effects/Precautions. Adverse reactions include paresthesias, anorexia, polyuria, and occasionally drowsiness and confusion. These side effects (during short-term therapy) are minimal.

Primidone. Since primidone is 2-desoxyphenobarbital and chemically not a malonylurea derivative, it is not a true barbiturate.

Mechanism of Action. Primidone has anticonvulsant activity on its own, but it is also biotransformed to phenobarbital and phenylethylmalonamide (PEMA), both active anticonvulsants. Primidone elevates electroshock or chemoshock thresholds and alters seizure patterns in experimental animals.

Clinical Indications. Alone or in combination with other anticonvulsants, primidone is indicated for the control of grand mal, psychomotor, or focal epileptic seizures. This drug may also control tonic-clonic (grand mal) seizures that are refractory to other anticonvulsants.

Adverse Effects/Precautions. Ataxia and vertigo are frequently reported early side effects. Dizziness and sedation are sometimes severe at the beginning of primidone therapy.

Phenacemide. An open-chain monoureide, phenacemide is the most toxic of all anticonvulsants.

Mechanism of Action. Phenacemide elevates the threshold for minimal electroshock convulsions and abolishes the tonic phase of maximal electroshock seizures in experimental animals. This drug also antagonizes chemoshock (pentylenetetrazol-induced) in animals.

Clinical Indications. Phenacemide is used to control severe epilepsy, particularly mixed forms of psychomotor seizures that are refractory to other drugs.

Adverse Effects/Precautions. Personality changes occur in 1 in 5 patients who receive phenacemide. Reports of fatal hepatitis necessitate liver function tests before and during phenacemide therapy. Blood dyscrasias (including fatal aplastic anemia) also limit phenacemide use.

NARCOTIC ANALGESICS (TABLE 1.4)

Analgesics are classified according to both their ability to relieve pain and their capacity to cause tolerance and physical dependence. The nar-

Table 1.4 NARCOTIC ANALGESICS AND NARCOTIC ANTAGONISTS

Available products	Trade names	Daily dosage range
Narcotic analgesics:		
Alphaprodine HCl	Nisentil	0.4–0.6 mg/kg, IV
Butorphanol	Stadol	2 mg, IM
Codeine phosphate and sulfate	Codeine sulfate; Codeine phosphate	15–60 mg q.i.d., orally, IM, IV, or SC
Fentanyl	Sublimaze	0.05–0.1 mg, IM
Hydromorphone HCL	Dilaudid	2–4 mg
Levorphanol tartrate	Levo-Dromoran	2 mg
Meperidine HCl	Demerol	50–150 mg, IM
Methadone HCl	Dolophine HCl	2.5–10 mg, IM
Morphine	Morphine sulfate; Roxanol	10–30 mg q.i.d.
Nalbuphine HCl	Nubain	10 mg/70 kg, SC, IM, or IV
Oxycodone HCl	Oxycodone HCl	5–10 mg
Oxymorphone HCl	Numorphan	0.5 mg initially, IV
Pentazocine HCL	Talwin	30–50 mg
Propoxyphene HCl	Darvon	65 mg q. 4 hrs as needed
Propoxyphene napsylate	Darvon-N	100 mg q. 4 hrs as needed
Non-narcotic (phenothiazine) analgesic:		
Methotrimeprazine	Levoprome	10–20 mg IM q. 4–6 hrs as needed
Narcotic Antagonists:		
Levallorphan tartrate	Lorfan	1 mg IV
Naloxone HCl	Narcan	0.4–2 mg IV

cotic analgesics act mainly on the CNS, whereas non-narcotic analgesics (e.g., aspirin and acetaminophen) have significant peripheral activity in relieving and controlling pain.

The potent narcotic analgesics include "opiates," a term designating alkaloids obtained from the opium poppy. Morphine and codeine represent these naturally occurring opiate analgesics. Semisynthetic opiate-like drugs are molecular modifications of the natural alkaloids and include hydromorphone and oxycodone. Synthetic narcotic analgesics (such as meperidine and methadone) contain essential structural characteristics of the opiates and semisynthetic opiate-like narcotic analgesics that are necessary for their pain relieving properties.

The narcotic analgesics reduce pain perception by elevating the pain threshold. Continuous moderate to severe dull pain that originates in the smooth muscles of the internal hollow organs is especially amenable to narcotic analgesics. Additionally, the reaction to pain is modified by reducing the unpleasant emotional responses associated with pain. Even though sharp pain (like that which follows a fracture) is felt, narcotic analgesics significantly alter the reaction to the sensation; thus, the patient does not appear to mind the pain. This instance illustrates a characteristic effect of the narcotic analgesics. Finally, somnifacient (sleep-producing) activity, even in the presence of trauma associated with severe pain, is another important effect of narcotic analgesics. Sleep is a "natural antidote" for pain and is generally desired for achieving analgesia. However, situations that require the patient to remain ambulatory and active are exceptions to this effect.

Narcotic analgesics, including the opiates and opiate-like drugs, act on the CNS to relieve pain. In contrast to the newer psychoactive drugs that are used in psychoses and neuroses, the opiates are among the oldest drugs discovered by man.

Opium is the dried milky exudate from the incised unripe seed capsule of Papaver somniferum, the opium poppy. Opium ordinarily contains from 9 to 14% morphine, although samples containing 20% have been reported. Morphine is the most prominent alkaloid (both quantitatively and pharmacologically) contained in opium.

The earliest record of the medicinal use of Papaver somniferum was in Sumaria, dating from the fourth milleneum B.C. In the seventh century B.C., Assyrian tablets describe the method of collecting opium, a procedure employed today. After incision with a knife, the seed capsule is left for the sap to ooze out; the dried exudate is then scraped from the incision wounds.

Opium contains two series of alkaloids: the phenathrene series to which morphine belongs and the benzylquinoline series, represented by papaverine (Figure 1.19). Morphine (from Morpheus, the Greek god of dreams) was isolated as a pure alkaloid in 1805 by the German pharmacist, Serturner. Prior to the 1930s, certain structural modifications of morphine were attempted to both improve morphine as an analgesic and to reduce the alkaloid's addictive liability. These efforts included synthesis of dihydromorphinone (a potent analgesic still used in medicine) and diacetylmorphine (heroin) that was briefly promoted as a potent nonaddictive analgesic.

Evidence indicates that saturable stereospecific opiate receptors exist in the CNS. The opiate receptors are apparently of different types and represent affinity sites not only for exogenous chemicals (opiates such as morphine) but also for endogenous opiate-like molecules, e.g., endorphins and enkephalins.

An early receptor hypothesis, first presented in 1954 and later expanded in the 1970s, recognized the commonality in morphine and similar analgesics of a tertiary nitrogen that can be protonated at physiologic pH. According to this theory, the resultant positive charge, imparted to the molecule, becomes available for interaction with a postulated anionic receptor site.

The phenolic hydroxyl group in the phenanthrene nucleus is the second essential pharmacophore proposed as necessary for analgesic activity. As the phenolic hydroxyl and protonated nitrogen cannot occupy the same flat surface of the receptor, an indentation or cavity in the receptor allows a close fit by accommodating carbon-15 and carbon-16 of the morphine molecule. The morphine molecule must be-

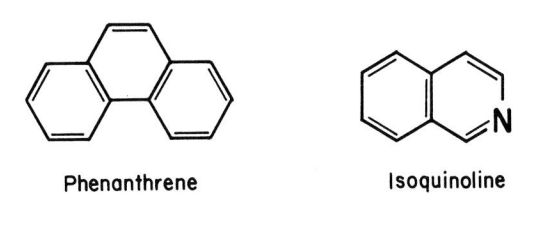

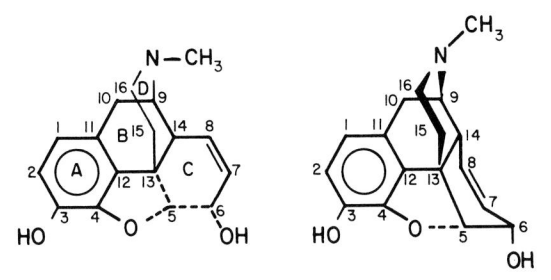

Fig. 1.19 Phenanthrene and Isoquinoline nuclei; Morphine structure.

come oriented in a stereospecific manner for interaction with the opiate receptor. The C-ring is in the "boat" configuration and projects into the plane of the paper, whereas the D-ring (containing the carbon-15 and carbon-16 segment) is in the "chair" position and projects upward to slip into the groove or cavity of the receptor substance. A basic chemical similarity exists in the narcotic analgesics in that gamma-phenyl-N-methyl-piperidine exists as a common structural feature. The "chair" representation of the piperidine moiety best illustrates the outward projection to fill the opiate receptor indentation attachment point. Thus, a three point attachment results from the nitrogen attaching to the anionic site, the aromatic ring binding to a flat complementary affinity site, and the aliphatic (C_{15}-C_{16}) group fitting into the receptor cavity (Figure 1.20).

The flexible receptor may assume different configurations, especially after interacting with agonist molecules. Another proposal indicates the possible existence of receptor binding sites, other than the anionic affinity focus, at multiple locations on the same or different receptors. Thus, a modified multiple binding site concept explains the analgesic activity of chemically dissimilar drugs, such as fentanyl and methotrimeprazine.

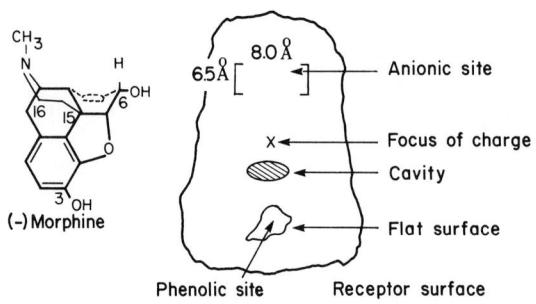

Fig. 1.20 Beckett-Casy opiate receptor -- relationship to morphine. (Modified from Gringauz, A.: Drugs. How They Act and Why. St. Louis, C.V. Mosby, 1978.)

Multiple opiate receptors exist in the CNS. Naturally occurring opiate-like molecules (termed "endorphins" and "enkephalins") function in at least two major opiate peptide systems in the brain. The endorphins and enkephalins serve as either neurotransmitters or hormone-like chemicals (or as both).

The endogenous opiates have a variety of relative affinities for the different receptors. One endogenous opiate system involves beta-endorphin and associates with long neuraxons that interconnect the hypothalamus, the limbic system, and the medial thalamus. Medial thalamic nuclei mediate poorly localized and emotionally-influenced deep pain. Morphine and other opiates are highly valuable in alleviating pain that originates in the viscera or arises from severe injuries, burns, or neoplasms. Opiate receptor density is greater in the medial thalamus than in surrounding thalamic areas.

The second opiate peptide system involves the enkephalins which are found in short neuraxons located throughout the CNS. Evidently these short neuraxons are primarily modulator neurons, whereas the longer neuraxons mediate the emotional and euphoric components of opiate activity. The limbic system (particularly the amygdala) contains a high concentration of opiate receptors. The euphoric effects possibly relate to activation of these limbic system receptors, although analgesic action is unlikely at this site.

Studies of opiate binding to specific sites in the brain and other organs resulted in the subclassification of multiple opiate receptors. Substantial evidence indicates that four major categories of opiate receptors exist: mu, kappa, delta, and sigma. Subtypes of each of these receptors are also proposed.

Morphine-like drugs act primarily on receptors associated with analgesia; i.e., mu and kappa receptors. Associated with sigma receptors are dysphoria or psychomimetic effects; a high concentration and localization of these receptors occurs in the limbic system. Delta receptors are apparently involved in changes in affective behavior. Morphine and related opiate agonists act primarily to activate mu, kappa, and probably delta receptors. While the mu receptors may mediate supraspinal analgesia, respiratory depression, euphoria, and physical dependence, the kappa receptors are associated with spinal analgesia, miosis, and sedation. Lastly, the sigma receptors evidently relate to dysphoria, hallucinations, and respiratory and vasomotor stimulation.

Besides not affecting the sensitivity of sensory receptors associated with pain, morphine and related opiate analgesics also do not modify conduction along afferent impulses in neuraxons. In addition to elevating the pain threshold, these analgesics significantly alter the subjective reaction to pain, probably due to effects on the limbic system.

Alteration of the phenanthrene molecule of morphine results in the synthesis of important semisynthetic alkaloids. For instance, in dihydromorphinone, a ketone oxygen replaces the alcohol hydroxyl, and removal of the double bond produces a potent analgesic. On the other hand, replacing the methyl group on the nitrogen with an alkyl group produces a specific potent morphine antagonist, n-allylnormorphine.

Besides their analgesic action, the narcotic analgesics have other central and peripheral effects. The opiates, opiate-like semisynthetics, and synthetic narcotic analgesics vary in their degree to produce these other actions, although they all share most of these properties to the same extent. The nucleus tractus solitarii and related nuclei concerned with vagal reflexes contain a high concentration of opiate receptors. These high receptor density areas may participate in the cough reflex, gastric secretion, and orthostatic hypotension, thereby correlating receptor activation with physiologic responses other than analgesia.

Although not usually significant when an analgesic is indicated, depression of the medullary cough center is important in therapeutic applications of codeine as an antitussive. Stimulation of the chemoreceptive trigger zone of the medullary vomiting center is ordinarily an undesirable property of narcotic analgesics.

The constipating reaction that results from gastrointestinal effects of narcotic analgesics is usually considered a "side effect," although diarrhea responds to various opiate compounds, such as paregoric (camphorated tincture of opium).

Cardiovascular effects of narcotic analgesics are insignificant in comparison to their activity on the CNS. As the sedating effect of the narcotic analgesics may indirectly reduce cardiac work, morphine therapeutically benefits acute myocardial infarction.

Endogenous opiate binding sites (i.e., mu receptors) are found on afferent terminal neuraxons within the substantia gelatinosa of the spinal cord and in the spinal nucleus of the trigeminal nerve. Narcotic analgesics apparently inhibit neurotransmitter release, such as acetylcholine and substance P that mediate transmission of pain impulses. Stimulated by pain fibers, enkephalinergic neurons may mediate the effect of descending medullary analgesic pathways. Serotonin and norepinephrine are other central neurotransmitters probably released from sensitive afferent nerves in response to noxious stimuli, including pain and associated reactions.

Involvement of serotonin in the development of tolerance to morphine is hypothesized. The synthesis of serotonin increases greatly as tolerance develops, although the accumulation of this neurotransmitter does not occur. Related findings show that reduction in brain serotonin increases sensitivity to painful stimuli and decreases the analgesic potency of morphine.

Norepinephrine and dopamine synthesis, release, and turnover increase in the CNS after morphine administration. Narcotic analgesics inhibit acetylcholine release from neurons and increase total brain levels of this neurotransmitter. Thus, neurotransmitter metabolism interfaces with opiate receptor activation in many physiologic responses to morphine and other narcotic analgesics.

Finally, studies with protein synthesis inhibitors suggest that specific central neuron metabolic alterations characterize tolerance and development of physical dependence, but not the analgesic response. The importance of these biochemical changes and their role in narcotic analgesic activity remain conjectural.

NATURALLY OCCURRING OPIATES

Morphine and codeine are two opiates which find extensive clinical application.

Morphine. Morphine, a naturally occurring phenanthrene alkaloid found in Papaver somniferum, is the prototype of the narcotic analgesics.

Mechanism of Action. Morphine activates the same receptors as the endogenous opiate-like peptides (enkephalins and endorphins). The morphine-receptor binding alters the central release of neurotransmitters from afferent nerves which are sensitive to noxious stimuli. In high doses, morphine raises the threshold to a number of painful stimuli, including heat, electric currents, heavy pressure, thermal radiation, or ischemia. The reactive component of pain (such as suffering, fear, and anxiety) is important in extended pain.

In therapeutic doses, morphine increases the patient's capacity to tolerate pain in that they can still feel the pain, but it is not bothersome. Thus, although morphine apparently acts initially on neural systems responsible for the affective responses to pain, it also reduces the intensity of specific pain sensation by elevating the pain threshold.

Morphine produces a feeling of tranquility and euphoria in patients suffering from pain. However, in pain-free conditions, the individual's response is sometimes an increase in anxiety. When administered as an analgesic, morphine increases tone and decreases peristalis of the gastrointestinal tract, producing an undesirable constipating side effect.

Morphine depresses the medullary respiratory center, even in normal therapeutic doses. Death from acute morphine poisoning results from severe depression of the respiration that occurs when the chemoreceptive medullary respiratory nuclei become insensitive to the pCO_2 and hydrogen ion (H^+) concentration. In morphine overdose, the main stimulus to the respiratory center becomes hypoxia; in acute morphine poisoning, a periodic type of breathing, termed "Cheyne-Stokes respiration," often occurs. Periods of no breathing (apnea), followed by a brief period of rapid respiration, result from anoxia stimulation on the brain stem respiratory centers. After removal of the anoxia stimulus (by respiration), apnea again intercedes until anoxia induces breathing. Thus, periods of fluctuating respiration that alternate with apnea form the clinical picture of Cheyne-Stokes respiration. Inhibition of respiratory drive makes morphine useful in relieving difficult and labored breathing (dyspnea) in acute left ventricular failure or pulmonary edema. The struggle to breathe aggravates the basic cardiac condition and, thus, morphine alleviates this difficulty.

Morphine directly depresses the cough center in the medulla. This action is unrelated to morphine's analgesic or respiratory depressant action.

Morphine depresses the responsiveness of alpha-adrenergic receptors in the cardiovascular system, reducing arterial resistance and venous tone. If the hemodynamic effects become excessive, blood pooling and hypotension occur, especially if the person stands or hypovolemia is present.

Tolerance and physical dependence develop rapidly with morphine use and psychologic dependence usually precedes the resultant physiologic alterations. The drug's abuse potential limits morphine's extensive therapeutic application.

By stimulating the oculomotor nucleus in the midbrain, morphine causes the pupils to constrict. Activating this pupilloconstrictor center increases the impulse traffic along the oculomotor nerve (III) pathway to the circular iris musculature, causing active pupil constriction. Persons who are physically dependent upon morphine do not develop tolerance to the pinpoint pupils.

Clinical Indications. Morphine relieves moderate to severe pain and is also used as a preanesthetic medication. Other clinical indications for the drug include acute pulmonary edema and left ventricular failure.

Adverse Effects/Precautions. Since morphine stimulates the chemoreceptor trigger zone which surrounds the vomiting center in the medulla, nausea and vomiting commonly occur. Lightheadedness, dizziness, sedation, and sweating are frequent side reactions which are especially prominent in ambulatory patients not experiencing pain. As morphine has a marked constipatory effect, anthraquinone laxatives are sometimes administered concurrently to counteract the narcotic-induced constipation. Morphine produces biliary tract spasm, thereby increasing intrabiliary pressure.

The bronchoconstrictor action of morphine aggravates bronchial asthma. Extreme caution is necessary with morphine use in patients who have acute asthma, chronic obstructive pulmonary disease (COPD), or cor pulmonale. The respiratory drive decrease, induced by morphine's depression of the pCO_2 stimulation of the medullary respiratory center, may contribute to apnea or respiratory failure. Major hazards of morphine administration include respiratory depression, apnea, and to a lesser degree, respiratory failure.

Respiratory depressant effects of morphine and its capacity to increase intracranial pressure present an extreme danger in patients who have head injury, a brain tumor, other intracranial lesions, or pre-existing elevated intracranial pressure. Additionally, morphine may obscure the clinical course of head injury patients.

Rapid intravenous injection of morphine increases the incidence of adverse reactions, including respiratory depression, hypotension, apnea, circulatory collapse, and cardiac arrest.

Codeine. Codeine, a naturally occurring phenanthrene alkaloid, is found in Papaver somniferum. Chemically, codeine is methylmorphine, and most of the commercially available codeine is made by methylating the phenolic hydroxyl on the phenanthrene nucleus.

Mechanism of Action. Codeine activates opiate receptors in the CNS and at other organ sites. Codeine has a lesser effect than morphine on cerebral receptors. "Muzzling" the C_3 hydroxyl group on the morphine molecule produces some profound changes in pharmacologic activity. Since codeine does not ordinarily produce euphoria, dependence potential is low with this drug. Also, as an analgesic, codeine in therapeutic doses is far less potent than morphine. Codeine possesses significant antitussive and antidiarrheal activity. An important advantage of codeine over morphine is its effectiveness after oral administration.

Clinical Indications. Codeine, often in combination with other nonopiate analgesics, is widely used to relieve mild to moderate pain. Codeine is also valuable as an antitussive as its effect on the cough center essentially equals that of morphine, yet its activity on higher brain centers is only about 1/20 that of morphine.

Adverse Effects/Precautions. In usual analgesic or antitussive doses, there is a low incidence of adverse reactions. Commonly reported side effects include dizziness, sedation, nausea, constipation, and dry mouth. Susceptible patients report excitement and vertigo following moderate doses. Codeine produces little sedation and the stimulant component of its action, unopposed by a depressant action, may produce excitement. Toxic doses have caused seizures in children.

Codeine is much less potent as a respiratory depressant and also has a lesser effect on the gastrointestinal tract than does morphine. The potential danger of respiratory depression accounts for codeine's cautious use in patients who have head injuries and intracranial lesions.

SEMISYNTHETIC OPIATE-LIKE ANALGESICS

The extension of the planar structure of morphine to a three-dimensional model led to the development of potent semisynthetic and synthetic opiate-like analgesics. Several semisynthetic compounds are clinically suitable as morphine and codeine substitutes.

Hydromorphone (Dihydromorphine). Hydromorphone, a variation of the morphine molecule, is formed by substituting a ketone for the hydroxy at position-C_6 and eliminating the double bond between position-C_7 and position-C_8. Introduced into medicine in 1926, hydromorphone is the second oldest semisynthetic derivative of morphine (the oldest is heroin).

Mechanism of Action. Hydromorphone activates opiate receptors in the CNS.

Clinical Indications. Hydromorphone relieves moderate to severe pain. As an analgesic, hydromorphone is approximately five times more potent than morphine. Hydromorphone's onset of action is faster and its duration of action is briefer than morphine's. Another comparison is that hydromorphone is somewhat more sedative and less euphoriant than morphine.

Adverse Effects/Precautions. Although the adverse effects and precautions for hydromorphone resemble those of morphine, it is less nauseating and constipating.

Oxymorphone. Oxymorphone is created from morphine by substituting a ketone for the hydroxyl at position-C_6, eliminating the double bond between position-C_7 and position-C_8, and adding a hydroxy group at position-C_{14}.

Mechanism of Action. Oxymorphone activates opiate receptors in the CNS.

Clinical Indications. About ten times as potent as morphine in analgesic action, oxymorphone relieves moderate to severe pain. The drug causes more nausea and vomiting than does morphine.

Adverse Effects/Precautions. The adverse effects and precautions for oxymorphone are similar to those of morphine and occur more frequently. Oxymorphone's respiratory depressant activity is pronounced.

Hydrocodone (Dihydrocodeinone). Hydrocodone resembles codeine in the same manner that hydromorphone relates to morphine.

Mechanism of Action. Hydrocodone activates opiate receptors in the CNS and neural elements of the gastrointestinal tract.

Clinical Indications. Hydrocodone is effective in the relief of moderate to severe pain and as an antitussive drug. Used in a variety of combination antitussive and analgesic-antipyretic mixtures, hydrocodone is more potent and has a greater potential for physical dependence than codeine.

Adverse Effects/Precautions. The adverse effects and precautions of hydrocodone resemble those of codeine.

Oxycodone. Structurally similar to hydrocodone, oxycodone differs by having a hydroxy group on position-C_{14} of the phenanthrene nucleus.

Mechanism of Action. Oxycodone stimulates opiate receptors in the CNS.

Clinical Indications. Oxycodone is used in the treatment of moderate to severe pain. The drug is administered parenterally for preoperative medication, anesthesia support, obstetrical analgesia, and anxiety relief in patients with dyspnea associated with acute left ventricular failure and pulmonary edema.

Adverse Effects/Precautions. The adverse effects and precautions of oxycodone resemble those of codeine.

SYNTHETIC NARCOTIC ANALGESICS

Morphinans, phenylpiperidine derivatives, and benzomorphone derivatives represent synthetic drugs that have opiate-like properties.

Levorphanol. Levorphanol is the morphinan analog of morphine formed by elimination of the phenanthrene oxygen bridge which produces a tetracyclic configuration instead of a pentacyclic structure.

Mechanism of Action. Levorphanol activates opiate receptors in the CNS.

Clinical Indications. Levorphanol effectively relieves moderate to severe pain and is used preoperatively to allay apprehension, provide extended analgesia, reduce thiopental requirements, and shorten recovery time. Levorphanol produces less nausea and vomiting than does morphine.

Adverse Effects/Precautions. The adverse effects and precautions of levorphanol resemble those of morphine.

Meperidine. A phenylpiperidine derivative, meperidine was discovered in the search for atropine-like drugs. Meperidine was the first entirely synthetic narcotic analgesic employed clinically.

Mechanism of Action. Meperidine binds primarily to opiate receptors in the CNS. This drug produces less smooth muscle spasm, constipation, and depression of the medullary cough center than equianalgesic doses of morphine. Consequently, meperidine is not clinically useful in treating cough or diarrhea. Meperidine and/or its metabolites apparently interact more strongly with kappa opiate receptors than does morphine.

Clinical Indications. Used both orally and by injection, meperidine relieves moderate to severe pain. Parenteral meperidine is employed for preoperative medication, anesthesia support, and obstetrical analgesia.

Adverse Effects/Precautions. The toxic effects of meperidine resemble atropine and include mydriasis, dry mouth, tachycardia, and excitement. Toxic doses may produce delirium and hallucinations and meperidine use can result in the development of tolerance and physical dependence.

Alphaprodine. A short acting narcotic analgesic, alphaprodine resembles meperidine structurally and pharmacologically.

Mechanism of Action. Alphaprodine activates opiate receptors in the CNS and the gastrointestinal tract.

Clinical Indications. Alphaprodine is used in the treatment of moderate to severe pain. Its analgesic action is prompt and of short duration.

Adverse Effects/Precautions. The side effects and precautions of alphaprodine resemble those reported for meperidine.

Fentanyl. Fentanyl, a phenylpiperidine narcotic analgesic, is used primarily in anesthesia.

Mechanism of Action. Fentanyl activates opiate receptors (primarily the mu receptor) in the CNS.

Clinical Indications. Fentanyl is indicated for analgesic action of short duration before and during anesthesia and is also used in the immediate postoperative period as needed. Another of its applications is as an anesthetic agent with oxygen in selected high risk patients, such as those undergoing open heart surgery or complicated neurologic procedures.

Adverse Effects/Precautions. The adverse effects and precautions noted with meperidine also apply to fentanyl.

Methadone. Methadone, an orally effective synthetic narcotic analgesic, has a prolonged duration of action.

Mechanism of Action. Methadone primarily activates mu opiate receptors in the CNS. Steric factors force orientation of the methadone molecule into a pseudopiperidine ring configuration that interfaces with opiate receptors. The l-isomer of methadone is more potent than the d-isomer as an analgesic. The emetic and constipating actions of methadone are less than those of morphine.

Clinical Indications. Methadone, which relieves severe pain, finds extensive clinical application in narcotic detoxification and in maintenance programs for treating narcotic analgesic dependence syndrome. Methadone substitutes well for most other opiates and is effectively absorbed from the gastrointestinal tract. The drug's long duration of action permits once or twice a day dosage, still another advantage in maintenance programs.

Adverse Effects/Precautions. The adverse effects and precautions for methadone resemble those cited for morphine. Tolerance and physical dependence occur with methadone, but the withdrawal syndrome is less severe than that observed with morphine.

Propoxyphene. A central acting narcotic analgesic, propoxyphene structurally resembles methadone.

Mechanism of Action. Propoxyphene binds to opiate receptors in the CNS. The d-isomer of propoxyphene is the active analgesic moiety. Estimates indicate that 90 to 120 mg of propoxyphene has the analgesic equivalence of 60 mg of codeine. Combinations of propoxyphene and aspirin are widely employed because they afford a higher level of analgesia than either drug given alone.

Clinical Indications. Propoxyphene effectively relieves mild to moderate pain.

Adverse Effects/Precautions. Dizziness, sedation, nausea, and vomiting are the most frequent side effects reported with propoxyphene use. Propoxyphene products in excessive dosage, either alone or in combination with alcohol or other CNS depressants, cause many drug-related deaths. Thus, caution is necessary in using propoxyphene in patients who have a history of CNS drug misuse.

Pentazocine. Pentazocine, a benzomorphone analgesic, has weak narcotic antagonist activity and a low abuse potential.

Mechanism of Action. Pentazocine primarily interacts with kappa and sigma opiate receptors in the CNS. A narcotic antagonist activity is evident because pentazocine precipitates an abstinence syndrome in narcotic-dependent patients. The analgesic and depressant effects of pentazocine result primarily from the l-isomer.

Clinical Indications. Pentazocine relieves moderate to severe pain. Parenteral pentazocine is used for preoperative or preanesthetic medication and as a supplement to surgical anesthesia.

Adverse Effects/Precautions. Common adverse effects are nausea, dizziness or lightheadedness, vomiting, and euphoria. Mood alterations and acute CNS manifestations have also occurred with pentazocine use.

Pentazocine is available in combination with naloxone to counteract the nausea that usually accompanies pentazocine therapy. This combination product is intended for oral use only since severe, potentially lethal reactions (including pulmonary emboli, vascular occlusion, ulceration and abscesses, and withdrawal symptoms in narcotic-dependent individuals) have occurred from injection of the naloxone-pentazocine product.

Severe sclerosis of the skin, subcutaneous tissues, and underlying muscle may occur at pentazocine injection sites. Also, respiratory depressant effects of pentazocine present an exaggerated clinical problem if head injury or increased intracranial pressure exist. Intravenous pentazocine is possibly dangerous in myocardial infarction patients, necessitating cautious administration.

Butorphanol. Butorphanol, a morphinan congener, has both narcotic agonist and narcotic antagonist properties.

Mechanism of Action. Butorphanol interacts primarily with kappa and mu opiate receptors in the CNS. As with pentazocine, butorphanol in analgesic doses increases pulmonary arterial pressure and cardiac work.

Clinical Indications. Butorphanol effectively treats moderate to severe pain. It is also employed for preoperative or preanesthetic medication, balanced anesthesia supplementation, and postpartum pain relief.

Adverse Effects/Precautions. Frequent adverse reactions are sedation, sweating, nausea, vertigo, and lethargy. Narcotic-dependent individuals do not exhibit a withdrawal syndrome following acute or chronic butorphanol use, nor does the drug suppress narcotic withdrawal.

Nalbuphine. Nalbuphine, a narcotic analgesic, has narcotic antagonist activity. Nalbuphine is structurally related to oxymorphine and the narcotic antagonist, naloxone.

Mechanism of Action. Nalbuphine activates kappa opiate receptors in the CNS. Blockade of mu receptors apparently mediates the narcotic antagonist activity. Unlike pentazocine and butorphanol, nalbuphine does not significantly affect pulmonary artery pressure or cardiac work.

Clinical Indications. Nalbuphine relieves moderate to severe pain and is beneficial for preoperative analgesia, as a supplement to surgical anesthesia, and for obstetrical analgesia during labor.

Adverse Effects/Precautions. Sedation occurs in about 1 in 3 patients. Less frequent adverse effects include a sweaty, clammy feeling; nausea and vomiting; dizziness and vertigo; dry mouth; and headache. As with pentazocine, nalbuphine has low abuse potential. Abrupt withdrawal of nalbuphine has promoted narcotic withdrawal symptoms.

NARCOTIC ANALGESIC ANTAGONISTS

Naloxone has replaced nalorphine in the treatment of opiate-induced toxicity. Levallorphan, which has narcotic agonist properties, also reverses narcotic-induced respiration.

Naloxone. Naloxone is a specific pharmacologic antidote for narcotic analgesic overdose.

Mechanism of Action. Naloxone is a competitive antagonist at mu, delta, kappa, and sigma opiate receptors. In higher doses than required for pure agonists, naloxone reverses psychotomimetic and dysphoric effects of the agonist-antagonists, such as pentazocine. Antagonism of respiratory depression is often followed by an "overshoot" phenomenon in which the respiratory rate exceeds the pre-overdose rate.

Clinical Indications. Naloxone is used as an antidote in the treatment of known or suspected narcotic overdose. The intravenous route is preferable in emergency situations.

Adverse Effects/Precautions. Since the duration of respiratory depressant action of the narcotic analgesic overdose often exceeds that of the naloxone activity, repetition of the naloxone doses is sometimes necessary.

MISCELLANEOUS NEWER NARCOTIC AGONIST/ANTAGONISTS

Several of these agents are in clinical testing and may be released for general use.

Dezocine. Dezocine, a mixed agonist/antagonist opiate-like agent, has analgesic activity. Clinical studies show that dezocine is equipotent (or slightly more potent) than morphine in producing analgesia and respiratory depression. Dezocine apparently has a more rapid onset and shorter duration of action than morphine and may have less abuse potential than the morphine-like agonists.

Naltrexone (Trexan). Naltrexone is available for oral use in opiate-dependence maintenance programs.

Nalmefene. A structural analog of naltrexone, nalmefene is an orally effective narcotic antagonist that is used in opiate-dependence maintenance programs.

CENTRAL NERVOUS SYSTEM STIMULANTS (TABLE 1.5)

Numerous natural and synthetic drugs that stimulate the CNS are clinically useful. These CNS drugs increase sensory awareness by activating neuron processes or by blocking inhibitory pathways in the CNS. Some CNS stimulants extend their excitation to the motor cortex, which results in hyperactivity, tremors, and, in some cases, convulsions. The degree of CNS activation results from interaction of excitatory and inhibitory pathways. Interference with inhibitory pathways releases excitatory influences with the predominance of excitatory neuron pathways.

CNS stimulants often lack target cell specificity, a limitation to their clinical efficacy. Thus,

Table 1.5 CENTRAL NERVOUS SYSTEM STIMULANTS

Available products	Trade names	Daily dosage range
Cortical stimulants:		
Caffeine	various	100–200 mg q. 4 hrs as needed
Dextroamphetamine sulfate	Dexedrine	5 mg q. 4–6 hrs
Methamphetamine HCl	Desoxyn; Methampex	20–25 mg
Methylphenidate HCl	Ritalin	10 mg b.i.d. or t.i.d.
Pemoline	Cylert	37.5–75 mg once daily
Medullary Stimulants:		
Doxapram HCl	Dopram	0.5–1.5 mg/kg, IV
Nikethamide	Coramine	1 ml of a 25% solution, IV or IM

the dose of CNS stimulant (such as an amphetamine) necessary for increasing sensory awareness by acting at subcortical and cortical sites approaches the dose that activates CNS motor centers, resulting in hyperactivity and perhaps tremor. In addition, undesirable peripheral activity often occurs with administration of doses that are required to achieve the desired CNS action. For instance, amphetamines have adrenergic agonist activity to stimulate peripheral alpha- and beta-adrenergic receptors. The resultant effects on the cardiovascular system complicate the clinical picture with undesirable side reactions. Finally, the misuse-abuse potential of some CNS stimulants is great. Tolerance, accompanied by psychological and physical dependence, characterize amphetamine use.

CNS stimulants are classified according to their primary central site of action. Thus, therapeutic doses of cortical stimulants (e.g., dextroamphetamine, cocaine, and caffeine) act mainly on the cerebral cortex or on structures that alter cortical function. Medullary stimulants, also called "brain stem stimulants" and represented by nikethimide and doxapram, reverse sedative-hypnotic-induced medullary depression.

CORTICAL STIMULANTS

Cortical stimulants increase alertness and generally induce a heightened awareness of the surroundings. Higher doses produce hyperactivity, autonomic effects on the heart, and muscle tremor.

Amphetamines. Amphetamines have very limited therapeutic application in modern medicine. Dextroamphetamine has a more pronounced effect on the CNS than the l-isomer; however, the drug has lost much of its clinical impact since falling into disfavor as an appetite suppressant. Until 1970, its prescription uses covered numerous conditions, including depression, fatigue, and long-term weight reduction. At that time, the U.S. Food and Drug Administration restricted the legal use of amphetamines (including dextroamphetamine) to the treatment of narcolepsy, hyperkinetic behavior, and short-term weight reduction programs.

Dextroamphetamine (d-Amphetamine). First marketed in 1945 as an appetite suppressant, dextroamphetamine will be discussed as the amphetamine prototype.

Mechanism of Action. This drug's CNS stimulant effects probably result from a biochemical arousal of the ARAS that spreads to all parts of the brain, producing arousal, alertness, and hypersensitivity. Dextroamphetamine also stimulates the reward system, i.e., the medial forebrain bundle (MFB) which produces a sense of well-being. This drug acts as a sympathomimetic by stimulating norepinephrine release from presynaptic granules and causes spontaneous release of norepinephrine from presynaptic neurons. By blocking the presynaptic reuptake of norepinephrine and dopamine, dextroamphetamine enhances the effect of these neurotransmitters on postsynaptic receptors. Dextroamphetamine acts as an appetite suppressant by stimulating hypothalamic nuclei related to satiety, resulting in a feeling of fullness.

The conversion of dextroamphetamine to p-hydroxynorephedrine (a false neurotransmitter) apparently explains dextroamphetamine tolerance. The relatively weak effect of p-hydroxynorephedrine on postsynaptic receptors necessitates higher amounts of dextroamphetamine to both block neurotransmitter reuptake and to produce the anticipated effect.

Clinical Indications. Dextroamphetamine is used as an analeptic in the treatment of narcolepsy and in the management of attention deficit disorder (ADD).

Adverse Effects/Precautions. Excessive central nervous stimulation may occur and cardiovascular responses, including tachycardia and hypertension, are common sympathomimetic effects. Psychologic tolerance develops to the central effects of amphetamines. Toxic psychosis, resembling paranoid schizophrenia, may follow large and repeated doses of dextroamphetamine or its chemical relatives.

Methylxanthines. Caffeine, theophylline, and theobromine are members of the methylxanthine series of naturally occurring alkaloid stimulants, the oldest stimulants known to man (Figure 1.21). Caffeine has pronounced CNS stimulant activity, but theophylline also produces significant CNS stimulation. Caffeine is clinically utilized for its CNS stimulation, whereas in the case of theophylline, the excitation is a side reaction occurring with the drug's use as a bronchodilator. The methylxanthines are also used as diuretics.

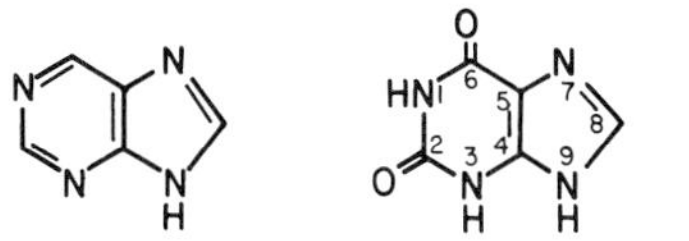

(Caffeine is 1,3,7-trimethylxanthine; theobromine, 3,7-dimethylxanthine; and theophylline, 1,3-dimethylxanthine)

Fig. 1.21 Caffeine — Methylxanthines.

Caffeine (1,3,7 Trimethylxanthine). Caffeine is found in many beverages, over-the-counter stimulants, combination products for pain, and cough/cold preparations. Of the beverages, coffee is the major source of caffeine in the diet of many Americans. Caffeine exerts pharmacologic effects (wakefulness, restlessness, and mental alertness) on the CNS; larger doses produce respiratory stimulation.

Caffeine also affects the cardiovascular system by stimulating the heart and sometimes increasing cardiac output. Increased coronary blood flow also results, probably due to increased myocardial energy requirements. Caffeine dilates some blood vessels, but it constricts cerebral vessels.

Mechanism of Action. Caffeine's mechanism of action as a CNS stimulant is unknown; however, caffeine may act as a stimulant by inhibiting adenosine action in the brain. By activating receptors on presynaptic neurons, adenosine inhibits neurotransmitter release, a probable result of the reduction of calcium ion influx associated with a neuron action potential. Caffeine blocks adenosine receptors in the CNS, thus antagonizing the depressant actions of adenosine and enhancing central neuron firing.

Caffeine apparently induces vasoconstriction of intracranial and extracranial arteries in migraine attacks by antagonizing adenosine-induced vasodilation and by inhibiting norepinephrine release, respectively.

Caffeine inhibits phosphodiesterase, thereby reducing the inactivation of cyclic AMP. The increase in the intracellular concentration of cyclic AMP that occurs at selected sites probably explains caffeine's effects on bronchiolar smooth muscle and the myocardium.

Clinical Indications. Caffeine is used orally as an aid for wakefulness and restoration of mental alertness. Parenterally, caffeine and sodium benzoate (to improve caffeine solubility) is used as an analeptic and diuretic. Caffeine is added to migraine products to increase the oral and rectal absorption of ergotamine, which thereby enhances its action. Caffeine also directly contributes to arterial vasoconstriction.

Adverse Effects/Precautions. Insomnia, restlessness, and nervousness are frequent adverse reactions to caffeine. A caffeine-induced syndrome, resembling anxiety neurosis, may follow ingestion of large quantities. Reports of a withdrawal syndrome of headache, anxiety, and muscle tension following abrupt cessation of caffeine after regular consumption of 500 to 600 mg/day indicate physiologic dependence; these symptoms usually occur between 12 to 18 hours after the last caffeine intake.

Methylphenidate. Methylphenidate, a mild cortical stimulant, has CNS actions similar to that of the amphetamines.

Mechanism of Action. Methylphenidate increases neuron activity in the ARAS. Theoretically, in attention deficit disorder (ADD), a neurologically immature situation exists. Increases in impulse activity from the ARAS to inhibitory centers in the cerebral cortex better control excessive restlessness and distractability.

Clinical Indications. Methylphenidate is effective in a total treatment program, including psychologic and sociologic therapy for ADD. Narcolepsy is another clinical application for this drug.

Adverse Effects/Precautions. Nervousness and insomnia are the most common adverse reactions. Anorexia and weight loss may occur during the first several weeks of methylphenidate therapy.

Pemoline. Pemoline is a CNS stimulant that has minimal sympathomimetic activity.

Mechanism of Action. Pemoline activates CNS dopaminergic pathways and does not possess appetite suppressant activity. Claims that pemoline increases RNA-polymerase activity and the rate of learning in humans are unsubstantiated.

Clinical Indications. Pemoline is employed as part of a total psychologic-sociologic treatment program for ADD. Because of its long half-life, pemoline can be administered once daily.

Adverse Effects/Precautions. Insomnia is a common side effect that occurs early in therapy. Dyskinesia involving the lips, tongue, face, and extremities has been reported after pemoline use. Anorexia and weight loss may occur during the first weeks of pemoline therapy.

MEDULLARY STIMULANTS

Medullary stimulants serve as an adjunct in treating respiratory depression. These drugs do not substitute for supportive artificial ventilation and symptomatic management which are the mainstays for treating drug-induced respiratory depression.

Doxapram. Doxapram is administered as a parenteral respiratory stimulant.

Mechanism of Action. Doxapram activates the peripheral carotid chemoreceptors to increase tidal volume; the respiratory rate also increases slightly. Higher doses of doxapram directly stimulate the medullary respiratory center.

Clinical Indications. Doxapram stimulates respiration in postanesthetic situations that are characterized by drug-induced respiratory depression. Although selected cases of CNS depressant overdose respond to doxapram, mechanical ventilation is the preferred treatment of the respiratory depression caused by CNS depressant overdosage.

Chronic obstructive pulmonary disease (COPD) with acute hypercapnia in hospitalized patients is amenable to short-term (approximately 2 hours) of doxapram therapy. The rate of doxapram infusion should not be increased to lower the pCO_2 in severely ill patients because of the increased work in breathing.

Adverse Effects/Precautions. Adverse reactions related to CNS and ANS effects include headache, dizziness, apprehension, disorientation, pupillary dilation, and hyperactivity. Decreases in hemoglobin, hematocrit, or RBC count have occurred in postoperative patients.

Nikethamide. Chemically related to the B vitamin nicotinamide, nikethamide is a CNS stimulant used primarily as a respiratory stimulant.

Mechanism of Action. Nikethamide acts directly to stimulate the medullary respiratory center. A peripheral activating effect on the carotid chemoreceptors also contributes to the respiratory stimulation that follows nikethamide administration. Nikethamide has limited clinical use.

Clinical Indications. Nikethamide is used primarily as a respiratory stimulant to counteract CNS depression, respiratory depression, and circulatory failure resultant from CNS depressants. Mechanical ventilation is the preferred method of treating respiratory depression due to CNS depressant overdosage. Nikethamide also restores respiration in patients undergoing electroshock therapy.

Adverse Effects/Precautions. Adverse effects attributed to nikethamide overdosage include burning or itching (especially at the back of the nose), flushing, nausea, vomiting, and changes in respiration depth and rate.

PSYCHOTHERAPEUTIC DRUGS

The first psychotherapeutic drugs (as distinguished from sedative-hypnotic agents) became clinically available in the early 1950s. Each year new agents are introduced in an attempt to identify more specific and effective drugs that have fewer and less severe adverse reactions. The types of psychotherapeutic drugs are divided into classes based upon the specific illness in which they find the greatest utility. Thus, the following contains the divisions of antidepressant, antimanic, antipsychotic, and antianxiety drugs (Tables 1.6, 1.7, 1.8).

ANTIDEPRESSANT DRUGS

During the 1950s, the antidepressant activity of the two major classes of drugs, the monoamine oxidase inhibitors (MAOIs) and the tricyclic antidepressants (TCADs)—both effective in the management of depression—was uncovered. The development of MAOIs as antidepressant drugs exemplifies the common pattern of a drug that was originally synthesized and screened for one disease yet was found useful for another condition.

To illustrate, effective use of isoniazid in tuberculosis patients prompted the clinical trial of a similar compound, iproniazid. Scientists discovered the first effective MAOI, i.e., iproniazid, unintentionally by noting the drug's euphoric and activating effects in tuberculosis patients. Upon biochemical investigation, iproniazid, a chemical relative of the antitubercular drug isoniazid, was found to inhibit monoamine oxidase, an enzyme (or related group of enzymes) that is widely distributed throughout the body and is responsible for inactivating aromatic amines, such as norepinephrine, dopamine, and 5-hydroxytryptamine.

The relationship of brain monoamines and monoamine oxidase activity to affective disorders is unclear, but a tenable monoamine hypothesis relates a depletion of CNS monoamines to depression and elevated central monoamine levels with excitation. Thus, one hypothesis states that MAOIs, such as ipronia-

Table 1.6 ANTIDEPRESSANT DRUGS

Available products	Trade names	Daily dosage range
Tricyclic antidepressants (TCADs):		
Amitriptyline HCl	Elavil; Amitril; others	75 mg
Amoxapine	Asendin	100–150 mg
Desipramine HCl	Norpramine; Pertofrane	75–200 mg
Doxepin HCl	Adapin; Sinequan	75 mg
Imipramine HCl	Tofranil; SK-Pramine; others	150 mg
Imipramine pamoate	Tofranil PM	75–150 mg
Nortriptyline HCl	Aventyl HCl; Pamelor	75–100 mg
Protriptyline HCl	Vivactil	60 mg
Trimipramine maleate	Surmontil	50–150 mg
Monoamine oxidase inhibitors (MAOIs):		
Isocarboxazid	Marplan	30 mg
Phenelzine	Nardil	30 mg
Tranylcypromine sulfate	Parnate	20 mg
Miscellaneous antidepressants:		
Maprotilene HCl	Ludiomil	150 mg
Trazodone	Desyrel	150 mg

Table 1.7 ANTIPSYCHOTIC DRUGS: MAJOR TRANQUILIZERS

Available products	Trade names	Daily dosage range
Phenothiazine Derivatives:		
Aliphatic Subgroup—		
Chlorpromazine HCl	Thorazine; others	10 mg–1 g
Promazine HCl	Sparine	40–800 mg
Triflupromazine HCl	Vesprin	30–150 mg
Piperazine Subgroup—		
Acetophenazine maleate	Tindal	40–80 mg
Carphenazine maleate	Proketazine	12.5–25 mg
Fluphenazine HCl	Permitil; Prolixin	0.5–10 mg in divided doses q. 6–8 hrs
Fluphenazine decanoate and enanthate	Prolixin decanoate; Prolixin enanthate	Initially, 12.5–25 mg IM or SC; 12.5–50 mg
Perphenazine	Trilafon	4–8 mg t.i.d.
Prochlorperazine	Compazine; Chlorazine	5 or 10 mg t.i.d. or q.i.d.
Trifluoperazine HCl	Stelazine; Suprazine	2–20 mg
Piperidyl Subgroup—		
Mesoridazine	Serentil	100–400 mg
Piperacetazine	Quide	20–160 mg
Thioridazine HCl	Mellaril; Millazine	50–800 mg
Butyrophenone:		
Haloperidol	Haldol	1–30 mg
Diphenylbutylpiperidine:		
Pimozide	Orap	0.2 mg/kg
Dibenzoxazepine:		
Loxapine succinate	Loxitane	20–100 mg
Dihydroindolone:		
Molindone	Moban	15–225 mg

Table 1.8 ANTIANXIETY AGENTS: MINOR TRANQUILIZERS

Available products	Trade names	Daily dosage range
Benzodiazepines:		
Alprazom	Xanax	0.25–0.5 mg t.i.d.
Chlordiazepoxide	Librium; A-poxide; others	15–40 mg
Clorazepate dipotassium	Tranxene	15–60 mg
Diazepam	Valium	2–10 mg
Halazepam	Paxipam	80–160 mg
Lorazepam	Ativan	2–6 mg
Oxazepam	Serax	30–60 mg
Prazepam	Centrax	20–60 mg
Other Misc. Chemical Classes:		
Chlormezanone	Trancopal	100–200 mg t.i.d. or q.i.d.
Hydroxyzine	Atarax; Atozine; others	50–100 mg q.i.d.
Meprobamate	Equabil; Miltown; SK-Bamate	1200–1600 mg

zid, prevent degradation of monoamines and elevate central monoamine levels, thereby counteracting the depressive state.

The accidental observation that imipramine (chemically related to the antipsychotic phenothiazine derivatives) effectively treated endogenous depression opened new areas for psychochemotherapy. Imipramine, an iminobenzyl derivative, has a triple ring structure (i.e., tricyclic) with the same side chain as chlorpromazine. Initial animal behavioral studies attributed a phenothiazine-like activity to imipramine.

Imipramine, the initial TCAD available, was first tested clinically after the discovery of chlorpromazine's antipsychotic activity. In 1957, Kuhn reported his study of 300 patients that indicated imipramine's effectiveness in the management of endogenous depression. Thus, imipramine's benefit in endogenous depression was only realized following its clinical screening.

The efficacy of antidepressant therapy is difficult to demonstrate. Studies indicate that one out of three depressed patients benefit from placebo, while two out of three show improvement with antidepressant therapy. Part of the difficulty in data interpretation lies in the high rate of spontaneous remission and the difficulty in assigning criteria for clinical improvement. The question concerning the remaining 1/3 of the patients who do not respond to antidepressant therapy remains unanswered.

TRICYCLIC ANTIDEPRESSANTS

The tricyclic antidepressants chemically resemble phenothiazines (Figure 1.22). Imipramine is identical to promazine except that the sulfur atom in the phenothiazine ring structure is replaced by a two carbon bridge (Figure 1.23). This molecular modification realigns the structure from a planar tricyclic ring complex to a skewed, three-dimensional, iminobenzyl ring system.

The planar type of psychoactive compound

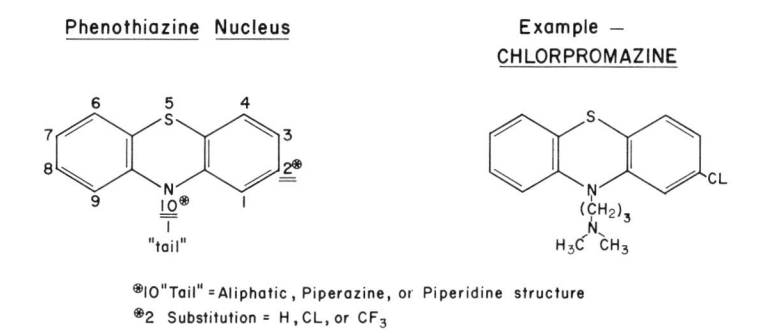

Fig. 1.22 Phenothiazine nucleus.

Fig. 1.23 Tricyclic antidepressant (TCAD) nucleus.

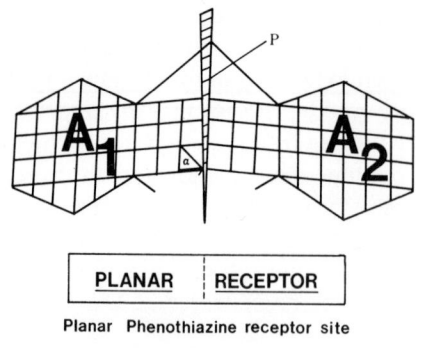

60 THERAPEUTIC PHARMACOLOGY

Fig. 1.24 Tricyclic psychotropic drug and planar phenothiazine receptor site. (Modified from Wilhelm, M., and Kuhn, R.: Pharmacopsychol. Neuropsychopharmacol., 3:317, 1970.)

Planar Phenothiazine receptor site
(α)-flexure angle α=30° 35° or less A₁ and A₂ are planar
Phenothiazine
Minimal "twisting" of three ring system - planar ("flat".)
P - Plane of symmetry

Nonplanar angled AD receptor site.
flexure angle α = 50-60° - nonplanar A₁ and A₂
Tricyclic AD
Pronounced "twisting" of three ring structure out of symmetry to fit - nonplanar.
P - Plane of symmetry

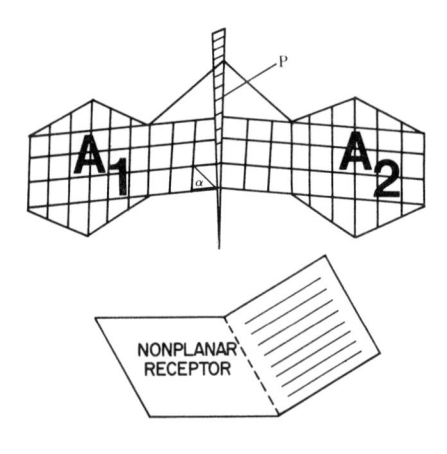

Fig. 1.25 Tricyclic psychotropic drug and nonplanar angled AD receptor site. (Modified from Wilhelm, M., and Kuhn, R.: Pharmacopsychol. Neuropsychopharmacol., 3:317, 1970.)

represented by a phenothiazine is characterized by a tricyclic 6-6-6 system in which all three rings contain 6 atoms. The structure activity relationship indicates that this planar ring system is consistent with antipsychotic effects. A more pronounced twisting of the ring system, producing a loss in coplanarity (as in imipramine), usually imparts an antidepressant action. This structure accounts for the hypothesis that the receptor site for antipsychotic activity is planar and accomodates a good fit with planar ring systems, e.g., those found in the phenothiazine derivatives (Figure 1.24). A nonplanar angled receptor more likely interfaces with antidepressant drugs if flexure (as a measure of the degree of nonplanarity) is more pronounced and the molecule is markedly twisted out of a plane (Figure 1.25).

The tricyclic antidepressants (TCADs) are found in relatively high concentrations in the brain after either oral or parenteral administration. Some of the tricyclic antidepressants are converted to active metabolites in vivo. The TCADs cause important changes in brain catecholamines and indoleamine activity and metabolism. Inhibition of synaptic reuptake mechanisms of brain monoamines is apparently an important component of the antidepressant effect. Inhibition of synaptic reuptake increases the monoamine neurotransmitter concentration in the synapse-receptor vicinity and enhances neuron circuit activity. Consistent with the prevention of monoamine reuptake is the observation that the TCADs increase the extraneuron and decrease the intraneuron metabolism of norepinephrine.

Amitriptyline, a tertiary amine TCAD, has a pronounced effect on serotonin reuptake and less effect on norepinephrine reuptake. Conversely, whereas the secondary amine TCAD desipramine has no effect on serotonin reuptake, it has a pronounced inhibitory activity on norepinephrine reuptake.

Evidence suggests that many depressions may have a biochemical basis in a relative deficiency in the central neurotransmitters norepinephrine and serotonin. Norepinephrine deficiency is asssociated with low urinary levels of MHPG (3-methoxy-4-hydroxyphenylglycol) while serotonin deficiency has been correlated with low spinal fluid levels of its metabolite, (5-OH IAA) 5-hydroxyindole acetic acid. Thus, depressed patients with norepinephrine deficiency, as determined by urinary excretion patterns, usually respond to the secondary amine TCADs and to imipramine (partially metabolized to the secondary amine, desipramine). On the other hand, depressed patients with normal norepinephrine, as indicated by metabolite excretion levels, are presumed to have serotonin deficiency and are preferentially treated with amitriptyline.

Clinical antidepressant effect activity is evidently associated not only with drugs that inhibit brain monoamine reuptake (e.g., the TCADs), but also with drugs such as iprindole and lithium that do not inhibit monoamine uptake. Also, no high correlation exists between monoamine reuptake inhibition by TCADs and clinical antidepressant efficacy.

In addition to their effects on monoamine reuptake, the TCADs also affect biogenic monoamine synthesis, storage, release, metabolism, and receptor functions. TCAD effect on amine reuptake occurs within the first days of therapy, whereas clinical antidepressant effects are often not observed for 2 to 3 weeks after initiation of drug administration. Also, both the plasma and brain drug levels plateau within the first several days of TCAD therapy. Thus, other delayed effects of the TCAD or a compensatory alteration of amine metabolism (such as synthesis) may reasonably explain the antidepressant action. Adaptive alterations in monoamine receptor function or topography possibly also contribute to the antidepressant activity.

Besides antidepressant activity, sedation, peripheral and central anticholinergic action, and potentiation of the biogenic monoamines characterize the pharmacologic profile for the TCADs. Peripheral anticholinergic activity accounts for common side effects reported with TCAD therapy. One hypothesis suggests involvement of a central anticholinergic effect in the TCAD antidepressant activity.

Amitriptyline. Amitriptyline is one of the most sedative of all the TCADs.

Mechanism of Action. Amitriptyline increases synaptic concentration of brain norepinephrine and serotonin by blocking their reuptake into the presynaptic neuron. The inhibitory effect on the membrane pump mechanism responsible for the reuptake of serotonin is more pronounced than that involved in norepinephrine reuptake.

Clinical Indications. Amitriptyline is particularly effective in cases of depression marked by anxiety and agitation. Endogenous depression is more amenable to amitriptyline therapy than are other depressive states. It generally improves anorexia, insomnia, physical complaints, and psychomotor retardation—which are all target symptoms of a depressive syndrome. Specific types of depression responsive to amitriptyline therapy are the depressed phase of manic-depressive syndrome, involutional melancholia, and selected reactive, neurotic, and schizoaffective depression.

Adverse Effects/Precautions. Anticholinergic side effects include dry mouth, blurred vision, constipation, and urinary retention. Amitriptyline is contraindicated in cases of glaucoma and prostate enlargement in males. Tachycardia, syncope, and orthostatic hypotension may occur. Patients on amitriptyline therapy should receive warnings about sustaining injuries from falls.

Drowsiness and impaired alertness are early CNS reactions; psychic and motor excitement are possible in prolonged therapy. Seizures, mania, and schizophrenic-like symptoms occasionally develop.

Patients using amitriptyline should avoid alcohol since amitriptyline potentiates alcohol's depressant effect. If amitriptyline replaces MAOI therapy in depression, a minimum of 14 days should elapse after discontinuation of the former. Initiation of amitriptyline therapy should begin cautiously with a gradual increase until optimal therapeutic response is achieved. This precaution is necessary since severe hyperpyrexia, convulsions, and deaths have occurred in patients concurrently receiving an MAOI and a TCAD.

Amoxapine. Amoxapine, a dibenzoxazepine-type TCAD, has antianxiety properties.

Mechanism of Action. Amoxapine probably reduces the reuptake of norepinephrine and serotonin into presynaptic neurons at central synapses. Additionally, by blocking dopamine receptors, amoxapine resembles the phenothiazines.

Clinical Indications. Amoxapine is indicated for patients with symptoms of neurotic or reactive depression. Although endogenous and psychotic depression are also amenable to amoxapine therapy, depressive states that are characterized by anxiety or agitation respond well to this drug.

Adverse Effects/Precautions. Some of the adverse effects that occur in more than 5% of the patients receiving amoxapine therapy are drowsiness, dry mouth, constipation, and blurred vision. Nausea, nervousness, insomnia, palpitations, tremors, and nightmares are less frequently reported reactions.

Desipramine. Desipramine, a metabolite of imipramine, is one of the least sedating of the TCADs.

Mechanism of Action. Desipramine preferentially increases the synaptic norepinephrine concentration of brain norepinephrine. By preferentially blocking norepinephrine reuptake, desipramine is theoretically effective in norepinephrine deficient depressive states (i.e., low urinary MHPG).

Clinical Indications. Desipramine relieves symptoms of various depressive states, especially those of endogenous depression. While earliest therapeutic effect occurs in 2 to 5 days, the full therapeutic benefit usually requires 2 to 3 weeks.

Adverse Effects/Precautions. Cardiovascular adverse reactions to desipramine include hypotension or hypertension, tachycardia, arrhythmias, heart block, myocardial infarction, and stroke. Among the neurologic and psychiatric reactions possible are confusion (especially in elderly patients), insomnia, nightmares, paresthesias of the extremities, tremors, extrapyramidal symptoms, and seizures.

Anticholinergic side effects, such as dry mouth, blurred vision, constipation, and urinary tension, are common with desipramine therapy.

Extreme caution is required when desipramine is administered to patients with cardiovascular disease, glaucoma, urinary retention, and hyperthyroid disease or those taking thyroid medication. The use of desipramine is discouraged in seizure-prone individuals since the drug lowers the seizure threshold.

Doxepin. Doxepin, a benzoxepin-type TCAD, has antianxiety properties.

Mechanism of Action. Doxepin inhibits the deactivation of norepinephrine and serotonin at central synapses by blocking their reuptake into presynaptic neurons. In contrast to the effect of the other TCADs, the blockade of guanethidine uptake in presynaptic neurons is not markedly reduced.

Clinical Indications. Doxepin is recommended in the management of psychoneurotic patients with depression and/or anxiety. Additional depressive or anxiety states amenable to doxepin include alcoholism recovery (when not taken concurrently with alcohol), depression that results from organic disease, involutional melancholia, and manic-depressive disease.

Adverse Effects/Precautions. Drowsiness, the most commonly noticed side effect, usually disappears with continued doxepin therapy. Anticholinergic side effects, such as blurred vision, dry mouth, constipation, and urinary retention, sometimes occur. Also, cardiovascular side reactions, such as hypotension and tachycardia, are encountered occasionally.

Doxepin is contraindicated in patients (especially the elderly) with glaucoma or a tendency toward urinary retention. Because of the lack of clinical experience with doxepin therapy in the pediatric population, use of the drug is discouraged in children under the age of 12.

Imipramine. Imipramine, one of the dibenzazepine group of TCADs, was the first TCAD available for clinical use.

Mechanism of Action. Imipramine potentiates central monoamine synapses by preventing the reuptake of norepinephrine and serotonin into presynaptic neurons. This activity apparently results from desipramine, a metabolite of imipramine. Although the mechanism of action in controlling childhood enuresis is unknown, it probably differs from the antidepressant effects.

Clinical Indications. Imipramine is especially valuable in controlling the symptoms of endogenous depression. As with other TCADs, 1 to 3 weeks of therapy usually elapse before any benefit is noted. Short-term imipramine therapy sometimes corrects childhood enuresis; exclusion of possible organic lesions is necessary before starting imipramine administration.

Adverse Effects/Precautions. Anticholinergic side effects are frequently noted with imipramine therapy. Cardiovascular adverse reactions include orthostatic hypotension, hypertension, tachycardia, palpitations, and arrhythmias. Elderly patients have reported confusion accompanied by hallucinations, disorientation, and delusions. Psychosis exacerbation by imipramine mandates detection of any signs of pre-existent psychotic disease.

In enuretic children treated with imipramine, the most common adverse effects include nervousness, sleep disorders, tiredness, and mild gastrointestinal disturbances.

Nortriptyline. Nortriptyline, the monomethyl metabolite of amitriptyline, has a minimal sedative effect compared to that of the parent compound amitriptyline.

Mechanism of Action. Nortriptyline interferes with the transport, release, and storage of catecholamines. The reuptake of norepinephrine and serotonin into presynaptic neurons is blocked at central monoamine synapses. Although nortriptyline increases the pressor effect of norepinephrine, it blocks the pressor effect of phenylethylamine, indicating a complex interaction with monoamine metabolism.

Clinical Indications. Because of its lack of sedating properties, nortriptyline is useful in treating the apathetic, depressed patient. The symptoms of endogenous depression are more amenable to this drug than are other depressive states.

Adverse Effects/Precautions. Anticholinergic side effects, including dry mouth, blurred vision, constipation, and urinary retention, are frequent patient complaints. Cardiovascular, psychiatric, and neurologic adverse reactions that are common to all TCADs may also occur with nortriptyline therapy.

Protriptyline. A nonsedating dibenzocycloheptene-type TCAD, protriptyline differs chemically from nortriptyline only by the presence of a double bond in the 2 carbon bridge of the center ring.

Mechanism of Action. Protriptyline has a marked blocking activity on norepinephrine and serotonin reuptake into presynaptic neurons at central monoamine synapses.

Clinical Indications. Protriptyline is indicated for the symptomatic treatment of patients with mental depression. Having significant activating properties, this drug is often useful in withdrawn depressed patients. Protriptyline's onset of action is more rapid than that of imipramine or amitriptyline.

Adverse Effects/Precautions. Protriptyline, more so than the other TCADs, aggravates agitation or anxiety and produces cardiovascular adverse reactions, such as tachycardia and hypotension. Anticholinergic side effects, e.g., dry mouth, blurred vision, constipation, and urinary retention, may also occur.

Trimipramine. Trimipramine, a dibenzazepine-type TCAD, has an anxiety-reducing sedative component.

Mechanism of Action. Trimipramine has only slight blocking activity on the reuptake of norepinephrine and serotonin by presynaptic neurons at central monoamine synapses.

Clinical Indications. Trimipramine, employed in the control of depression symptoms, is most useful if a component of the disease complex is either anxiety or agitation. Endogenous depression is the depressive state that responds best to trimipramine.

Adverse Effects/Precautions. The adverse effects and precautions for trimipramine include sedation and anticholinergic side effects, e.g., dry mouth, blurred vision, constipation, and urinary retention. Cardiovascular effects, as well as psychiatric and neurologic adverse reactions, are also possible.

MONOAMINE OXIDASE INHIBITORS (MAOIs)

The monoamine oxidase inhibitors (MAOIs) are a heterogenous group of drugs that inhibit the oxidative deamination (catabolism) of endogenous monoamines. One theory advocates that increased levels of brain norepinephrine and serotonin following MAOI administration explain the mechanism of antidepressant activity.

MAOIs, by decreasing the catabolism of monoamines (such as norepinephrine, serotonin, or dopamine), support accumulation of these monoamine neurotransmitters in presynaptic sites. Thus, more of the neurotransmitter is present for release from the presynaptic site into the synaptic cleft to activate receptors and consequently stimulate the neuron pathway.

Isocarboxazid. Isocarboxazid, a hydrazine-type MAOI, is used in the treatment of depression that is refractory to TCADs or electroconvulsive therapy.

Mechanism of Action. Isocarboxazid is a potent inhibitor of monoamine oxidase in the brain, heart, and liver. An increase in the presynaptic intraneuron concentration of endogenous amines, such as norepinephrine and serotonin, occurs. Thus, since relatively more of these monoamines are available for release at the synapse, pronounced activity in the monoaminergic pathway is expected. Also noted is an enhancement of the biologic and pharmacologic actions of these endogenous amines and exogenous monoamines, such as tyramine.

Clinical Indications. Depression that is refractory to TCADs or electroconvulsive therapy may respond well to isocarboxazid. Another possible use of this drug is in depressed patients where TCADs are contraindicated.

Adverse Effects/Precautions. Since MAO is an ubiquitous enzyme system, a wide variety of side effects occur with isocarboxazid therapy. The most frequently reported cardiovascular adverse reactions are orthostatic hypotension and disturbances in cardiac heart rate and/or rhythm. CNS reactions, often viewed as extensions of their pharmacologic activity, include insomnia, irritability, motor restlessness, and agitation.

The MAOIs, such as isocarboxazid, have the potential for serious adverse interactions with other drugs and certain foods.

Phenelzine. Usually employed in treatment-resistant depression, phenelzine is a hydrazine-type MAOI.

Mechanism of Action. By inhibiting MAOI, phenelzine increases the concentration of endogenous epinephrine, norepinephrine, and serotonin at presynaptic CNS storage sites.

Clinical Indications. Phenelzine may relieve symptoms in patients who exhibit "atypical," "nonendogenous," or "neurotic" depression. These conditions are often characterized by an anxiety component in the depressive complex and by phobic or hypochondriac features.

Adverse Effects/Precautions. Common adverse reactions to phenelzine include dizziness, constipation, dry mouth, postural hypotension, drowsiness, weakness and fatigue, edema, gastrointestinal disturbances, tremors, twitching, and hyperreflexia. Many of these side effects disappear or abate with continued treatment;

also, adjusting the phenelzine dosage minimizes these reactions. Phenelzine is not recommended for patients under age 16 because no controlled safety data are available for this age group.

Tranylcypromine. A nonhydrazine-type MAOI, tranylcypromine is usually employed for atypical depression.

Mechanism of Action. Tranylcypromine has a bimodal mechanism of antidepressant activity. In addition to the MAOI action that increases the amount of monoamines in the brain stem, a direct "stimulant" effect on central adrenergic receptors apparently occurs. The "stimulant" effect may result from tranylcypromine's structural similarity to amphetamine, which in turn may also explain the rapid initial antidepressant response. The MAOI activity accounts for sustained benefit in depressed patients.

Clinical Indications. Tranylcypromine has a more rapid onset of action than that noted with isocarboxazid or phenelzine. Tranylcypromine is recommended for drug treatment-resistant endogenous or severe reactive depression in closely supervised patients. Tranylcypromine has found new uses in phobias and as an adjunct to lithium therapy. This drug (once temporarily removed from the U.S. market because of toxicity) is a potent agent that is capable of producing serious side effects. Only patients who are either hospitalized or under close supervision and who have not benefited from other antidepressant therapy should receive tranylcypromine.

Adverse Effects/Precautions. Agitation, anxiety, and manic reactions indicate excessive tranylcypromine dosage. Other side effects include restlessness, dry mouth, nausea, diarrhea, tachycardia, and significant anorexia. Administration of this drug is contraindicated in patients over 60 years old and patients with cerebrovascular defects or cardiovascular disorders or with concurrent pheochromocytoma.

MISCELLANEOUS ANTIDEPRESSANT DRUGS

Maprotiline and trazodone are miscellaneous antidepressants that are often useful in the management of depression.

Maprotiline. A tetracyclic drug, maprotiline resembles the TCADs in activity.

Mechanism of Action. Maprotiline acts primarily by blocking norepinephrine reuptake into central adrenergic presynaptic sites. This drug apparently has no significant effect on serotonin reuptake at CNS sites.

Clinical Indications. Maprotiline is indicated in the treatment of depressive neurosis and manic-depressive illness. Depression, characterized by an anxiety component, also responds to maprotiline therapy.

Adverse Effects/Precautions. Frequently reported side effects are dry mouth (1 in 5 patients) and drowsiness (1 in 6 patients). Nausea or vomiting, seizures, and tremors may also occur. Hypotension, hypertension, tachycardia, palpitations, arrhythmia, heart block, and syncope are reported cardiovascular adverse reactions. CNS reactions include nervousness and anxiety. Extreme caution in maprotiline use is required for patients with myocardial infarction or patients with a history or presence of cardiovascular disease.

Trazodone. Trazodone, an effective antidepressant, is chemically unrelated to tricyclic, tetracyclic, or MAOI-type antidepressant agents.

Mechanism of Action. One hypothesis indicates that trazodone selectively inhibits serotonin reuptake into presynaptic neurons in the CNS, thereby increasing synaptic levels of this neurotransmitter. In animal studies, trazodone potentiates the activity of behavioral changes that are induced by the serotonin precursor, 5-hydroxytryptophan.

Clinical Indications. Trazodone is useful in the treatment of depression, especially in the absence of a prominent anxiety component. Patients benefited by this drug include those who exhibit several of the major depression criteria, e.g., changes in appetite or sleep, psychomotor agitation or retardation, loss of interest in usual activities or decrease in sexual drive, increased fatigue, guilt feelings, impaired concentration, and suicidal thoughts.

Adverse Effects/Precautions. Drowsiness, dizziness, fatigue, dry mouth, headache, and nausea or vomiting are the most frequently reported adverse effects. Trazodone is not recommended for use during the initial recovery phase of myocardial infarction; the drug is possibly arrhythmogenic in patients with pre-existing cardiac disease. It is not known whether interactions occur with MAOIs and trazodone.

ANTIMANIC DRUGS

Lithium salts are the only specific antimanic drugs. The first report of the efficacy of lithium in treating mania was recorded in Australia by Cade in 1949. Although his study on 10 manic patients went essentially unrecognized, the medical profession, in the mid-1960s, reconsidered the clinical application of lithium as an antimanic drug. Cade attributed the lag between discovery and application to the circumstances surrounding the primary investigation — specifically, a study that was conducted by an unknown scientist, working alone in a small chronic hospital with no research training and using primitive techniques and negligible equipment, was hardly credible, especially in the United States.

Lithium Carbonate. Lithium carbonate is the most frequently employed antimanic lithium salt.

Mechanism of Action. Lithium carbonate's mechanism of action is unknown. However, lithium acts as a substitute for the potassium and sodium cations that normally participate in ion flux to maintain an electrochemical gradient and osmotic balance. Additionally, lithium is critical in the cellular microenvironment that determines structure, energy supply, or timing of cellular processes.

Lithium alters sodium transport in neuron cells, resulting in a shift toward the intraneuron metabolism of catecholamines. This change accelerates the presynaptic destruction of norepinephrine and serotonin and increases the neuron uptake of norepinephrine.

Lithium-induced changes in cortisol levels relate to the drug's antimanic action. However, cortisol level changes may result from a basic mechanism, e.g., an alteration in catecholamine metabolism.

Lithium suppresses catecholamine-activated adenyl cyclase activity in the CNS. The benefit of lithium in manic patients may be associated with a drop in adenosine 3′, 5′-monophosphate (cyclic AMP) levels. Still another biochemical mechanism proposed for lithium's antimanic activity is interference with neuron carbohydrate metabolism, as represented by suppression of the uptake of myoinositol, glutamate, and gamma-aminobutyric acid in the CNS.

Clinical Indications. Lithium carbonate is indicated for use in the treatment of manic episodes of manic-depressive illness. Maintenance therapy prevents or diminishes the frequency and intensity of subsequent manic episodes in those manic-depressive patients who have a history of mania.

Adverse Effects/Precautions. Lithium use produces numerous side effects. Lithium toxicity relates closely to serum lithium levels and may occur at therapeutic doses; consequently, routine lithium serum determinations are necessary throughout lithium therapy.

Adverse reactions to lithium are rarely encountered at serum lithium levels less than 1.5 meq/L. Whereas mild to moderate toxic reactions may occur at levels from 1.5 to 2.0 meq/L, lithium levels greater than 2.5 to 3.0 meq/L are considered life-threatening. Since considerable variation in clinical response to lithium occurs, the serum level/adverse reaction correlation is not absolute.

Signs of lithium toxicity with a serum level of less than 1.5 meq/L include nausea, vomiting, thirst, polyuria, lethargy, slurred speech, muscle weakness, and fine motor tremor. At lithium levels between 1.5 to 2.0 meq/L, persistent gastrointestinal upset, coarse hand tremor, mental confusion, muscle hyperirritability, ECG changes, drowsiness, and incoordination characterize the clinical picture. Higher lithium levels (2.0 to 2.5 meq/L) often precipitate ataxia, giddiness, polyuria, serious ECG changes, muscle fasciculations, tinnitus aurium, blurred vision, clonic movements and seizures, stupor, severe hypotension, and coma. Fatalities usually result from pulmonary complications.

There is a narrow therapeutic window (i.e., toxic levels of lithium are close to therapeutic levels) with lithium carbonate. In addition, high risk patients (who are predisposed to lithium toxicity) include those with renal or cardiovascular disease, severe debilitation, and dehydration or sodium depletion. The ability to tolerate lithium is high during the acute manic phase and decreases when manic symptoms subside. Therefore, clinical expertise with this drug is required to determine if a patient's abnormal mood swings are significant enough to warrant continued long-term lithium treatment.

ANTIPSYCHOTIC DRUGS

The term antipsychotic drug is preferable to other designations, such as tranquilizer, antischizophrenic agent, and neuroleptic. "Antipsychotic drug" (Table 1.7) indicates the type of clinical action and connotes more than a tranquilizing action but less than a specific antischizophrenic action.

The primary chemical class of antipsychotic drugs is the phenothiazines. Other important chemical groups found in antipsychotic drugs include the thioxanthene and butyrophenone classes.

In the early 1950s in France, chlorpromazine was introduced into medicine as an adjunct to anesthesia because of the drug's sedative properties. One of a series of antihistamine-like drugs, the drug possessed a variety of autonomic blocking effects, principally on alpha-adrenergic receptors. Chlorpromazine was initially described as inducing "artificial hibernation" with retention of consciousness, marked indifference to surroundings, and hypothermia. The "lobotomie pharmacologique" produced by chlorpromazine led to its trial in conditions such as mania and schizophrenia. Clinical studies proved that chlorpromazine exhibited a varied profile of effects that were both novel and different from classical sedative drugs, such as the barbiturates.

Phenothiazine derivatives are the most numerous and widely prescribed antipsychotic drugs. Three chemical subclasses of phenothiazine derivatives (aliphatic, piperidine, and piperazine derivatives) exist, based upon differences in the sidechain "tail" from the basic phenothiazine nucleus (Figure 1.22).

All clinically effective antipsychotic phenothiazines have some substitution at the 2-position. The aliphatic and piperidine series are of low potency, whereas the piperazine sidechain results in high potency compounds.

Phenothiazines block dopamine receptors in the CNS. The nitrogen atom in the phenothiazine sidechain assumes the same spatial relationship to the center aromatic ring as the dopamine sidechain bears to the catecholamine ring structure, which could explain the dopamine receptor blocking action of the phenothiazines.

The phenothiazines exert some action on every organ system in the body and are among the most ubiquitously acting drugs in medicine. Of the spectrum of action on the CNS, the dopamine receptor blocking action is the only one that apparently correlates well with antipsychotic activity. A precise role for dopaminergic pathways in the etiology of schizophrenia remains undetermined.

Prior to the introduction of phenothiazines into medical practice, two of their pharmacologic actions were unknown: the capacity to ameliorate the symptoms of schizophrenia and to evoke extrapyramidal symptoms in susceptible patients. Extrapyramidal symptoms include a syndrome that resembles endogenous parkinsonism (paralysis agitans or "shaking palsy"). The biochemical mechanism operant in both of these situations is evidently impairment of dopaminergic influence in the brain.

Phenothiazines exert their activity on several subcortical areas of the brain. One region is the ascending reticular activating system (ARAS) of the midbrain where monitoring of sensory input occurs. The amygdala and the hippocampus, limbic system structures, influence emotional response and represent another prime site of phenothiazine activity. The hypothalamus, a center for autonomic control and pituitary endocrine function, is a third anatomic substrate for phenothiazine activity. Finally, the globus pallidus and corpus striatum are sites of phenothiazine activity, an action which relates to the extrapyramidal syndrome.

Phenothiazine Derivatives. Chlorpromazine is the phenothiazine prototype of contemporary antipsychotic drugs. Discovered in the search for anesthetic medications, chlorpromazine proved to have the unique property of calming patients without causing a pronounced degree of psychomotor depression which is characteristic of the classical sedative-hypnotics (such as the barbiturates). Further clinical trials demonstrated the drugs usefulness in treating psychotic patients.

Phenothiazine derivatives are divided into chemical subclasses based upon the "tail" from the phenothiazine nucleus. The aliphatic or dimethylamino subgroup, for example, contains promazine, chlorpromazine, and triflupromazine. The piperazine subgroup contains potent phenothiazine derivatives, including fluphenazine, prochlorperazine, and trifluoperazine. Representing the piperidine subgroup is thioridazine, a phenothiazine with pharmacologic properties dissimilar from drugs in the aliphatic and piperazine subgroups but possessing clinical effective antipsychotic properties.

As effective antipsychotic drugs, phenothiazines in all three subgroups resemble the prototype chlorpromazine; however, they differ mainly in their potency and in the types of side effects associated with their use.

Chlorpromazine. A dimethylamino-type phenothiazine, chlorpromazine has antipsychotic and antiemetic properties.

Mechanism of Action. Chlorpromazine blocks postsynaptic dopamine receptors in cortical and subcortical brain regions. This drug inhibits or alters dopamine release and increases dopamine turnover in the CNS. These processes are consistent with a theory chlorpromazine blocks postsynaptic dopamine receptors. Additionally, increased neuron firing rate in the midbrain appears to directly relate to antischizophrenic activity.

Chlorpromazine depresses the midbrain reticular formation, resulting in effects on body temperature, wakefulness, vasomotor tone, emesis, and hormone activity. Peripheral blockade of cholinergic and alpha-adrenergic receptors is common with chlorpromazine and contributes to the high incidence of patient complaints with chronic chlorpromazine therapy.

Clinical Indications. Chlorpromazine is a useful antipsychotic drug in the treatment and management of schizophrenia. The aliphatic phenothiazines, such as chlorpromazine, are more effective against the "positive" symptoms of schizophrenia (such as overactivity). Chlorpromazine is also indicated for the control of the manifestations of manic-depressive disease; other of this drug's clinical applications are in the treatment of tetanus, intractable hiccoughs, acute intermittent porphyria, and nausea and vomiting.

Adverse Effects/Precautions. Autonomic side effects related to adrenergic and cholinergic blockade are common with chlorpromazine therapy. Dry mouth, nasal congestion, salivation, perspiration, constipation, diarrhea, urinary retention, and urinary frequency are some adverse reactions.

Cardiovascular side effects, including hypotension, postural hypotension, tachycardia, and bradycardia, are also related to complex blocking effects on the autonomic nervous system (ANS).

Agranulocytosis, one of the most serious adverse effects of phenothiazine therapy, may occur between the fourth and tenth week of therapy. A reversible jaundice, sometimes appearing between the second and fourth weeks of phenothiazine therapy, occurs more frequently with chlorpromazine therapy than with other phenothiazines.

Eye changes, characterized by pigmentary

deposits in the anterior layers of the cornea, happen occasionally in patients exposed (for either short or long periods) to high dosage chlorpromazine. The chlorpromazine dosage evidently directly relates to ocular pigmentation.

Chlorpromazine has more autonomic side effects than the more potent phenothiazines in the piperazine group. Thus, hypotension and other side effects that result from autonomic blockade happen more frequently with chlorpromazine than with a piperazine-type, such as fluphenazine.

Drowsiness, lethargy, and malaise are induced by the more autonomic phenothiazines, such as chlorpromazine. Some patients subjectively describe chlorpromazine's action as a "chemical straight jacket."

Dose-related extrapyramidal symptoms occur in three different forms: pseudoparkinsonism, dystonia, and akathisia. Pseudoparkinsonism, the most common of the three, is characterized by stiffness, shuffling gait, mask-like faces, drooling, and cogwheel rigidity in the extremities. Regardless of the presence of pseudoparkinsonism, tremor (a common sign of endogenous parkinsonism) is often present in psychiatric patients. Thus, tremor is not clearly as indicative of pseudoparkinsonism as it is for endogenous parkinsonism. Women, especially the elderly, are more commonly affected by this condition which starts within a few weeks of therapy initiation and often lessens or disappears within 1 to 2 months. The incidence of pseudoparkinsonism is about 15 to 25% among patients who receive moderate doses of chlorpromazine.

Dystonia is an acute, rigid, or slowly fluctuating spasm, usually of the muscles of the neck, face, and tongue, that causes tightness and unusual placement of these muscles. This side effect appears during the first few days of treatment and occurs less frequently with chlorpromazine than with the piperazine derivatives, such as fluphenazine. Fortunately, antiparkinsonism drugs usually relieve this adverse reaction.

Akathisia ("restless leg syndrome") is indicated by a feeling of acute discomfort in the muscles of the extremities—sometimes in the entire body. Since only leg movement relieves this discomfort, afflicted patients get up and down frequently, move their legs and feet up and down, pace, and generally appear restless and agitated.

Tardive dyskinesia is a major side effect associated with prolonged use of the phenothiazines, including chlorpromazine. These "late appearing abnormal movements" occur commonly in chronic psychiatric patients. Frequently noted manifestations of tardive dyskinesia include abnormal movements of the tongue, mouth, jaw, and lips. Among these are vermicular tongue movements, chewing movements of the jaws, tongue protrusion, and smacking or puckering of the lips. Neck twisting, body rocking, or rhythmic pelvic movements are possible principal manifestations of this syndrome.

Neuroleptic malignant syndrome (NMS), first reported in the early 1960s, is associated with the use of phenothiazines, including chlorpromazine. Hyperpyrexia, rigidity, and tremors characterize NMS, a serious condition with an incidence rate of between 0.5 to 1% of all patients on antipsychotic drug therapy. Adult males under 40 years of age and patients who have organic brain disease are at great risk to develop NMS. Treatment consists of primarily supportive therapy; if untreated, NMS is fatal in 10 to 20% of such cases.

Because chlorpromazine lowers the seizure threshold, the drug is contraindicated in convulsion-prone patients. Epileptogenic effects are more common with sedative-type phenothiazines, such as chlorpromazine, than with other drugs.

Endocrine disorders with phenothiazine therapy occur frequently with the aliphatic group, such as chlorpromazine. Thus, females may experience lactation, breast engorgement, and menstrual disorders. Reports of gynecomastia in males have followed high doses of chlorpromazine. Dermatologic adverse effects include urticaria, maculopapular rash, and petechial skin reactions.

Chlorpromazine is unique among the phenothiazines for causing marked photosensitivity, and chronic patients sometimes show eye and skin pigmentation. The latter, a grayish, brownish, sometimes purplish hue, occurs on skin areas exposed to light and sun; this side effect, which relates to chlorpromazine therapy, fades with medication discontinuation.

Fluphenazine. Fluphenazine, a piperazine-type phenothiazine, produces less sedation than chlorpromazine and is referred to as a "stimulating" phenothiazine.

Mechanism of Action. Fluphenazine blocks postsynaptic dopamine receptors in the brain. Peripheral and central alpha-adrenergic blocking activity is prominent with fluphenazine, a drug which also inhibits the release of hypothalamic and pituitary hormones.

Clinical Indications. Fluphenazine is indicated in the management of the manifestations of psychotic disease. After several weeks of treatment with fluphenazine, patients with psychomotor retardation become less withdrawn, apathetic, and mute. Fluphenazine differs from other phenothiazines in that it is more potent on a milligram for milligram basis, has less potentiating effect on CNS depressants and anesthetics, is apparently less sedating, and is less likely than members of the aliphatic and piperdine phenothiazines to cause hypotension.

Adverse Effects/Precautions. Fluphenazine, more so than members of the aliphatic and piperidine phenothiazines, exerts extrapyramidal side effects. Adverse effects, related to anticholinergic and alpha-adrenergic blocking activity, occur less frequently with fluphenazine.

Thioridazine. A piperidine-type phenothiazine, thioridazine has strong sedative properties.

Mechanism of Action. Thioridazine blocks postsynaptic dopamine receptors in the CNS. In contrast to most other phenothiazines, thioridazine has minimal antiemetic activity and rarely produces extrapyramidal side effects, such as pseudoparkinsonism.

Clinical Indications. Thioridazine is used for the management of the manifestations of psychotic disorders and in the treatment of Alzheimer's disease. Patients who exhibit psychomotor excitement become tolerant to the sedative effects of thioridazine, yet their mental status improves, possibly indicating a direct effect on psychotic processes which are not related to general CNS depression.

Adverse Effects/Precautions. Many of thioridazine's adverse effects relate to its strong anticholinergic action. With the exception of rarely producing extrapyramidal side effects, adverse reactions resemble those of chlorpromazine.

THIOXANTHENE DERIVATIVES

Like the phenothiazines, the thioxanthenes consist of a tricyclic nucleus; however, the thioxanthenes differ from the phenothiazines in that a carbon atom replaces the nitrogen atom in the middle ring. CNS activity is noted in the thioxanthenes with a double bond between position-C_{10} and the side chain, as well as substitution in position-C_2.

Chlorprothixene and Thiothixene. Chlorprothixene and thiothixene are thioxanthene derivatives that have chemical and pharmacologic similarities to the piperazine-type phenothiazines. The first thioxanthenes were synthesized in the 1950s and, presently, two are clinically available in the United States.

Mechanism of Action. The thioxanthenes block postsynaptic dopamine receptors in the brain. The action of chlorprothixene on the brain stem following electrical stimulation of the reticular formation is characterized by a shortening of cortical activation. Other effects noted include a synchronization of the EEG tracings during rest and modifications of elicited potentials.

Clinical Indications. The thioxanthenes are indicated in the management of the manifestations of psychotic disorders. Whereas chlorprothixene is especially useful for schizophrenia treatment, thiothixene is recommended for a wide variety of psychotic states, including organic psychoses, schizophrenia, and psychotic depressions, and in the treatment of Alzheimer's disease.

Adverse Effects/Precautions. The thioxanthenes' adverse effects and precautions resemble those noted with the phenothiazines, especially the piperazine-type (such as fluphenazine).

BUTYROPHENONES

Two butyrophenones are available in the United States. One of these, haloperidol, was discovered in the middle 1950s and has found extensive use in the management of various psychotic conditions. The other available butyrophenone, droperidol, is employed only as an adjunct to general anesthesia because of the drug's rapid onset and relatively short duration of action.

Haloperidol. A butyrophenone derivative, haloperidol resembles the phenothiazines pharmacologically.

Mechanism of Action. Haloperidol blocks postsynaptic dopamine receptors in the brain.

Clinical Indications. Haloperidol is indicated for the management of the manifestations of psychotic disorders. The drug controls the tics and vocal utterances of Tourette's disorder in children and adults. Haloperidol also effectively treats severe behavioral problems in children who are combative and explosively excitable. Another of the drug's indications is in the short-term management of hyperactive children who exhibit excessive motor activity.

Adverse Effects/Precautions. Frequent side effects of haloperidol are pseudoparkinsonism, dystonia, and akasthesia. Oversedation, orthostatic hypotension, blood dyscrasias, and liver dysfunctions may also occur with haloperidol. Tardive dyskinesia appears in some patients (especially the elderly who receive high doses of haloperidol) on long-term therapy.

DIPHENYLBUTYLPIPERIDINES

Chemical alteration of the butyrophenone structure to produce diphenylbutylpiperidine results in a new group of antipsychotic drugs. Pimozide, an antipsychotic drug, is a member of the diphenylbutylpiperdine group that is available in the United States.

Pimozide. Pimozide, orally effective, is a long acting diphenylbutylpiperidine antipsychotic drug.

Mechanism of Action. Pimozide blocks dopaminergic receptors on postsynaptic neurons in the CNS. A series of secondary alterations in brain dopamine metabolism and function often accompany dopaminergic blockade. These ancillary effects on dopamine possibly cause some of the beneficial effects of pimozide as an antipsychotic drug.

Clinical Indications. Pimozide suppresses motor and phonic tics in patients with Tourette's disorder. Only those patients who have not responded favorably to standard therapy should receive pimozide, which is not a first choice drug treatment.

Adverse Effects/Precautions. Extrapyramidal reactions, often occurring within the first few days of pimozide therapy, are common. Persistent tardive dyskinesia may appear in some patients on long-term therapy or after drug therapy discontinuation. Other reported adverse reactions are sedation, dry mouth, and visual disturbances.

DIHYDROINDOLONE DERIVATIVES

Molindone is the only member of this group available for clinical use in the United States.

Molindone. Although structurally unrelated to the phenothiazines, thioxanthenes, or butyrophenones, molindone resembles the piperazine phenothiazines pharmacologically and in clinical application.

Mechanism of Action. Molindone's mechanism of action is unclear but probably involves blockade of postsynaptic dopamine receptors in the brain.

Clinical Indications. Molindone is indicated for the management of the manifestations of schizophrenia.

Adverse Effects/Precautions. The most frequently reported side effect is drowsiness; however, extrapyramidal symptoms and tardive dyskinesia may also occur.

DIBENZOXAPINES

Loxapine is the only member of this group available for clinical use in the United States.

Loxapine. Loxapine, chemically distinct from the thioxanthenes, butyrophenones, and phenothiazines, is employed as an antipsychotic drug.

Mechanism of Action. Loxapine's mechanism of action is unknown.

Clinical Indication. Loxapine is used in the management of psychotic disorders, including schizophrenia. It is also effective in the management of Alzheimer's disease.

Adverse Effects/Precautions. Frequent adverse reactions to loxapine are sedative and extrapyramidal effects, including drowsiness, rigidity, tremor, akathisia, and dystonic reactions. These adverse effects usually appear during the first few days of therapy or following a dosage increase.

ANTIANXIETY DRUGS

Anxiety is a common patient complaint made to clinicians. By referring to a heterogeneous collection of unpleasant feelings, the term frequently describes aspects of many different psychiatric syndromes. As a subjective mood, it is identical to the fearful feelings experienced under conditions of actual danger. Anxiety is further described as a state of uneasiness, which is characterized by apprehension and worry about possible events. This definition delineates subjective distress and anticipation focus, as opposed to the fear that ordinarily designates real danger.

Development of the benzodiazepines marked a major advance in psychochemotherapy. Although certain other classes of the antianxiety drugs were developed earlier (i.e., the propanediols, such as meprobamate), introduction of chlordiazepoxide into clinical medicine in 1960 heralded a new era in the control of anxiety and tension in neurotic patients. Of particular importance was the observation that beneficial results were sustainable with a minimum of side effects.

Benzodiazepines. Benzodiazepines depress subcortical areas of the CNS. The antianxiety effect may result from actions on the limbic system and reticular formation. In contrast to the barbiturates, the benzodiazepines do not significantly affect the cerebral cortex. Benzodiazepines apparently potentiate the CNS effects of gamma-aminobutyric acid (GABA). The wide therapeutic window (i.e., the significant difference between therapeutic and toxic doses) represents a definite advantage with these agents.

The diverse and complex pharmacologic properties of the benzodiazepines are attributed to their effects on the CNS. Although many of the compounds have a central muscle relaxant effect, diazepam is specifically indicated for certain spastic disorders, such as status epilepticus. Some benzodiazepines, like clorazepate and clonazepam, are clinically effective anticonvulsants. Flurazepam is recognized as an important nighttime sedative-hypnotic for insomniacs.

The major therapeutic utility of the benzodiazepines relates to their antianxiety effects. In this instance, loss of arousal is uncharacteristic. Early benzodiazepine studies determined that chlordiazepoxide, the first clinically available benzodiazepine derivative, has higher taming and antiaggressive properties than meprobamate, barbiturates, and even the phenothiazine derivatives.

Little clinical evidence suggests that one antianxiety benzodiazepine is more effective than another. The major differences are reflected in their onset and duration of action, as well as their biotransformation profile. Several of the benzodiazepines convert to active metabolites, thereby contributing to the overall pharmacologic response. Compounds such as oxazepam and lorazepam are metabolized to inactive compounds and consequently have relatively short half-lives.

Diazepam is metabolized to active compounds, including oxazepam and temazepam, that have a long half-life. Since hepatic biotransformation is the predominant route for benzodiazepine metabolism, the biotransformation of these drugs may be impaired in patients who have chronic liver disease. As oxazepam and lorazepam both undergo one-step hepatic inactivation, these drugs are often preferred in elderly patients and those with liver disease.

Proposed mechanisms of action for the antianxiety activity of the benzodiazepines vary. Emerging from these studies is a general acceptance that these drugs enhance or facilitate the inhibiting neurotransmitter action of gamma-aminobutyric acid (GABA). GABA mediates both pre- and postsynaptic inhibition in the CNS by interacting with specific membrane-bound receptors. The benzodiazepine receptor is considered part of a receptor-effector complex along with a GABA recognition/affinity site and a chloride ionophore. Activation of the benzodiazepine receptor, in concert with GABA influence, initiates biochemical results which culminate in an opening of neuron membrane chloride channels. These events manifest themselves as the neuron inhibitory action observed with the benzodiazepines. Thus, indirect influence on GABA receptors in the ARAS may block both cortical and limbic arousal following stimulation of the brain stem reticular formation. As noted earlier, a barbiturate recognition site probably exists as a component of this multimolecular GABA affinity site, benzodiazepine receptor, and chloride ionophore membrane-bound complex.

Alprazolam. Alprazolam is a benzodiazepine which is indicated only as an antianxiety drug.

Mechanism of Action. Alprazolam interacts with GABA-associated benzodiazepine receptors in the limbic system and brain stem reticular formation.

Clinical Indications. Alprazolam is indicated for the management of anxiety disorders or the short-term relief of anxiety symptoms. Anxiety associated with depressive states also responds to alprazolam.

Adverse Effects/Precautions. Drowsiness and dizziness or lightheadedness are frequently cited with alprazolam therapy.

Chlordiazepoxide. Chlordiazepoxide, the first clinically available benzodiazepine, is used as an antianxiety and antitremor drug.

Mechanism of Action. Chlordiazepoxide depresses the limbic system and ARAS by an interaction with benzodiazepine receptors. These receptors are part of a multimolecular membrane-bound complex that also contains a GABA recognition site and a chloride ionophore.

The drug's mechanism of antitremor activity is unknown.

Clinical Indications. Chlordiazepoxide is indicated for the management of anxiety disorders or for the short-term relief of anxiety symptoms, withdrawal symptoms of acute alcoholism, and preoperative apprehension and anxiety.

Adverse Effects/Precautions. Drowsiness, ataxia, and confusion may occur, especially in elderly patients. Agranulocytosis, a rare complication of chlordiazepoxide therapy, begins with a sore throat and fever. Hepatic dysfunction, recognizable by yellowing of the eyes or skin, is also possible with chlordiazepoxide.

Clorazepate. Clorazepate, a benzodiazepine, has anticonvulsant and antianxiety properties.

Mechanism of Action. Clorazepate depresses neuron activity in the limbic system and the reticular formation by interacting with

GABA-ergic pathways. This drug possesses clinically significant antiseizure activity and is converted to an active metabolite, demethyldiazepam, in vivo.

Adverse Effects/Precautions. The side effect most commonly reported is drowsiness. Less frequently reported reactions are dizziness, various gastrointestinal complaints, nervousness, blurred vision, dry mouth, headache, and mental confusion.

Diazepam. Diazepam is a benzodiazepine derivative that has antianxiety, anticonvulsant, antitremor, and central muscle relaxant properties.

Mechanism of Action. Diazepam interacts with specific benzodiazepine membrane-bound receptors that are coupled to GABA affinity sites in the limbic system, midbrain reticular formation, thalamus, and hypothalamus. This interaction affects GABA-ergic pathways in the CNS, which inhibit neuron action.

Diazepam has no significant peripheral autonomic blocking action. Transient analgesic activity occurs after intravenous administration of diazepam. A rapidly absorbed benzodiazepine, diazepam has a long half-life (20 to 70 hours). Accumulation of diazepam and its metabolites (such as oxazepam) may occur. Renal elimination is slow, which permits metabolites to remain in the blood for several days or even weeks.

Clinical Indications. Diazepam is indicated in the management of anxiety disorders or for the short-term management of anxiety. Other of its clinical uses include acute alcohol withdrawal, skeletal muscle spasm, status epilepticus, and preanesthetic anxiety. Parenteral diazepam is used as an adjunct before endoscopic procedures and prior to cardioversion. Spasms of facial muscles associated with problems of occlusion and temporomandibular joint disorders also respond to diazepam. Spasticity and athetosis in cerebral palsy patients are also treated wih diazepam.

Adverse Reactions/Precautions. Common reactions to diazepam therapy are drowsiness, fatigue, and ataxia. Redness, swelling, or pain at the injection site frequently accompany parenteral diazepam administration. Initiation or abrupt withdrawal of diazepam therapy may increase the incidence and/or severity of grand mal seizures. Use of diazepam for petit mal seizures may precipitate tonic status epilepticus. Acute narrow angle glaucoma is a contraindication for diazepam use.

Effectiveness for long-term clinical use (more than 4 months) of diazepam has not been assessed.

Halazepam. Halazepam is a benzodiazepine used in the treatment of anxiety.

Mechanism of Action. Halazepam depresses activity in the limbic system and reticular formation by interacting with specific benzodiazepine membrane-bound receptors. Activation of these receptors, which are coupled to GABA recognition sites, produces effects on GABA-ergic pathways, which open chloride ion channels and inhibit neuron action. Halazepam is biotransformed to an active metabolite, desmethyldiazepam.

Clinical Indications. Halazepam is indicated for the management of anxiety disorders or the short-term relief of anxiety symptoms.

Adverse Effects/Precautions. Although drowsiness is the most frequently reported side effect of halazepam therapy, gastrointestinal disturbances (nausea and vomiting) occur occasionally.

Lorazepam. Lorazepam is an intermediate acting hynoptic benzodiazepine with no conversion to active metabolites.

Mechanism of Action. Lorazepam interacts with specific benzodiazepine membrane-bound receptors in the limbic system and midbrain reticular formation to induce CNS depression (see halazepam). Metabolized to inactive compounds, lorazepam consequently has a relatively short half-life and duration of action. Lorazepam is sometimes preferred in patients with hepatic disease or the elderly because of its simple one-step degradation.

Clinical Indications. Although used primarily as an antianxiety drug, lorazepam possesses significant sedative-hypnotic activity. The drug is effective in the management of anxiety disorders or for short-term relief of anxiety symptoms or anxiety that is associated with depressive symptoms. Mutiple daily doses are necessary for sustained clinical effects. Significant accumulation does not occur with lorazepam.

Parenteral lorazepam is used as an amnesic and preanesthetic medication.

Adverse Effects/Precautions. If they occur, adverse reactions usually happen at the beginning of therapy; continued medication or dosage decreases cause the side effects to gradually disappear. Lorazepam's most frequent side effects are sedation, dizziness, weakness, and unsteadiness.

Parenteral benzodiazepine therapy (with diazepam or lorazepam) may produce coma or shock.

Oxazepam. Oxazepam, a metabolite of diazepam, is used primarily as an antianxiety agent.

Mechanism of Action. Oxazepam depresses the CNS by interacting with specific benzodiazepine membrane-bound receptors in the limbic system and midbrain reticular formation. Coupling the benzodiazepine receptor to GABA affinity sites and a chloride ionophore results in an effect on GABA-ergic pathways in the CNS. Slowly absorbed, oxazepam has a short to intermediate half-life. Minimal accumulation occurs with oxazepam and elimination rapidly follows therapy discontinuation. Oxazepam is often preferred in elderly patients because of the drug's simple one-step degradation and pharmacokinetic profile.

Clinical Indications. Oxazepam is indicated for the management of anxiety disorders, for the short-term relief of anxiety symptoms, and for relief of acute alcohol withdrawal. The drug is useful in treating elderly patients for anxiety, tension, agitation, and irritability.

Adverse Effects/Precautions. Occurring early in therapy, drowsiness is the most frequently reported adverse effect with oxazepam. Mild paradoxical reaction (i.e., excitement and stimulation of affect) is another side effect reported during the first few weeks of therapy. Leukopenia and hepatic dysfunction occasionally occur.

Prazepam. Prazepam is a benzodiazepine that is indicated only as an antianxiety agent.

Mechanism of Action. Prazepam interacts with specific benzodiazepine membrane-bound receptors in the limbic system and midbrain reticular formation. These receptors are coupled to GABA recognition sites and a chloride ionophore and, upon stimulation, produce effects on GABA-ergic pathways. Prazepam converts to an active metabolite, desmethyldiazepam, as a result of first pass hepatic biotransformation. This drug has a slow onset after a single dose.

Clinical Indications. Prazepam is used in the management of anxiety disorders or for the short-term relief of anxiety symptoms.

Adverse Effects/Precautions. Frequently reported side effects with prazepam therapy are fatigue, dizziness, weakness, drowsiness, lightheadedness, and ataxia. As with other benzodiazepines, transient and reversible aberrations of liver function tests may occur.

MISCELLANEOUS ANTIANXIETY DRUGS

Several alternate drugs to the benzodiazepines are available for the treatment of anxiety.

Hydroxyzine. Hydroxyzine is an H_1 histamine receptor blocker that has antianxiety properties.

Mechanism of Action. Hydroxyzine suppresses activity in the subcortical regions of the brain by an unknown mechanism. No cortical depressant action is observed with hydroxyzine. Additionally, this drug has significant antihistaminic, antispasmodic, skeletal muscle relaxant, and antiemetic action.

Clinical Indications. Hydroxyzine is useful in the symptomatic relief of anxiety and tension associated with psychoneurosis. The drug is also used as an adjunct in organic disease states in which anxiety is present.

Adverse Effects/Precautions. Dry mouth and drowsiness are frequently reported side effects. These adverse reactions are usually transient and disappear after several days of hydroxyzine therapy.

Meprobamate. A propanediol derivative, meprobamate has central muscle relaxant properties and is used as an antianxiety drug.

Mechanism of Action. Meprobamate depresses activity in the thalamus and the limbic system. These two cortical regions form a functional unit and are very rich in interneurons that interconnect them. The limbic system is considered the seat of emotion, whereas the thalamus is the area through which emotional stimuli enter consciousness.

Meprobamate reduces the incidence or shortens the duration of seizure discharges in the limbic system. In addition, meprobamate induces a synchronization of electrical activity of the thalamus. Meprobamate also has skeletal muscle relaxant and anticonvulsant properties.

Clinical Indications. Meprobamate is used in the treatment of psychoneurotic disease, insomnia, certain depressive states, and psychosomatic conditions.

Adverse Effects/Precautions. Adverse effects on the CNS include drowsiness, ataxia, and dizziness. Nausea, vomiting, and diarrhea are frequently noted gastrointestinal complaints. Reported cardiovascular adverse reactions include palpitations, tachycardia, and arrhythmias. Allergic or idiosyncratic responses may also occur with meprobamate therapy. Physical dependence may result from chronic meprobamate use.

Propranolol. Propranolol, a beta-adrenergic receptor blocking drug, readily enters the CNS. See Chapters 2 and 3 for complete discussions on propranolol.

Mechanism of Action. Propranolol apparently reduces anxiety by blocking central beta-adrenergic receptors.

Clinical Indications. Propranolol is used as an antianxiety drug when the anxiety is associated with overt sympathetic action (e.g., palpitations in stage fright, etc.). Propranolol also effectively controls akathisia, a form of motor restlessness which sometimes follows antipsychotic drug therapy, as with phenothiazine.

Adverse Effects/Precautions. See Chapters 2 and 3 for descriptions of the adverse reactions to propranolol therapy.

Buspirone (BuSpar^R). Buspirone, an anxiolytic agent that is chemically unrelated to the benzodiazepines, produces minimal sedation and euphoria and apparently does not affect motor skills. Dizziness, nausea, headache, and occasional nervousness and excitement have occurred with buspirone.

ANTIPARKINSONISM DRUGS (TABLE 1.9)

The goal of therapy for parkinsonism patients is relief of debilitating symptoms since there is no known cure for the disorder. Two main classes of drugs used in parkinsonism treatment are the anticholinergic drugs and the dopaminergic drugs.

ANTICHOLINERGIC DRUGS

Naturally occurring cholinergic blocking drugs (obtained from belladonna and botanically related plants), such as atropine, scopolamine, and hyoscyamine, were the earliest drugs used to treat parkinsonism. Certain synthetic anticholinergic drugs, including benztropine, biperiden, procyclidine, and trihexyphenidyl, have a more selective CNS effect and have largely replaced the naturally occurring anti-

Table 1.9 ANTIPARKINSONISM DRUGS

Available products	Trade names	Daily dosage range
Anticholinergic Drugs:		
Benztropine mesylate	Cogentin	0.5–6 mg
Biperiden	Akineton	2–8 mg
Diphenhydramine HCl	Benadryl; others	75–150 mg
Ethopropazine HCl	Parsidol	50–100 mg
Orphenadrine HCl	Disipal	50 mg t.i.d.
Procyclidine	Kemadrin	10–20 mg
Trihexyphenidyl HCl	Artane; Aphen; Tremin; others	6–10 mg
Dopaminergic Drugs:		
Amantadine HCl	Symmetrel	100–200 mg
Bromocriptine mesylate	Parlodel	2.5–100 mg
Carbidopa	Lodosyn; in Sinemet	70–100 mg
Levodopa	Dopar; Larodopa; Levodopa	Initial: 0.5–1 g
		Maintenance: 4–6 g

cholinergic alkaloids. Anticholinergic drugs mainly reduce the tremor component of parkinsonism.

Benztropine. Benztropine, a synthetic cholinergic blocking drug, has selective antiparkinsonism activity.

Mechanism of Action. Benztropine blocks cholinergic receptors in the basal ganglia and neutralizes the relative excess in cholinergic activity at this site.

Clinical Indications. Effective as an adjunct in the treatment of parkinsonism, benztropine is also useful in alleviating drug-induced extrapyramidal symptoms, except tardive dyskinesia.

Adverse Effects/Precautions. CNS side effects include disorientation, confusion, nervousness, and dizziness. More severe reactions, such as psychoses, hallucinations, and delirium, have occurred. Peripheral anticholinergic adverse reactions to benztropine are dry mouth, blurred vision, urinary retention, and tachycardia.

Biperidin. A synthetic cholinergic blocking drug, biperidin has selective antiparkinsonism activity.

Mechanism of Action. Biperidin blocks cholinergic receptors in the basal ganglia, thereby neutralizing excessive cholinergic influence.

Clinical Indications. Biperidin, used in the symptomatic treatment of parkinsonism, is also effective in treating drug-induced extrapyramidal disorders.

Adverse Reactions/Precautions. Biperidin may produce adverse CNS reactions, including confusion, delirium, and hallucinations. Anticholinergic side effects, such as dry mouth, blurred vision, urinary retention, and tachycardia, may occur.

Procyclidine. Procyclidine, a synthetic cholinergic blocking drug, has selective antiparkinsonism activity.

Mechanism of Action. Procyclidine blocks cholinergic receptors in the basal ganglia to counteract excess acetylcholine influence.

Clinical Indications. Useful in the treatment of parkinsonism, procyclidine also relieves the symptoms of drug-induced extrapyramidal dysfunction.

Adverse Effects/Precautions. Adverse effects include signs of CNS stimulation, including nervousness, confusion, hallucinations, and delirium. Anticholinergic side effects are blurred vision, dry mouth, urinary retention, and tachycardia.

DOPAMINERGIC DRUGS

A basic premise in parkinsonism therapy is that benefit occurs with increased dopaminergic activity. This theory is based upon the assumption that parkinsonism symptoms result from depletion of striatal dopamine. The immediate precursor of endogenous dopamine is l-dihydroxyphenylalanine (levodopa). Dopamine does not readily cross the blood brain barrier and is susceptible to plasma enzyme degradation. Levodopa passes in the CNS and is decarboxylated in the brain to dopamine, thus elevating levels of this neurotransmitter in the basal ganglia. Theoretically, this action balances a central cholinergic predominance (seen in parkinsonism) by activating dopaminergic pathways.

Levodopa. Levodopa is the immediate precursor of dopamine.

Mechanism of Action. Levodopa penetrates the blood brain barrier and enters the CNS where it is converted to dopamine. About 95% of the orally administered levodopa is rapidly decarboxylated to dopamine so that only a small percentage of levodopa is spared to enter the CNS.

Dopamine causes cyclic AMP accumulation in the corpus striatum by activating a dopamine sensitive adenyl cyclase. Thus, cyclic AMP is the intracellular mediator of levodopa action. Levodopa may cause cardiac stimulation by the action of dopamine on beta-adrenergic receptors. Levodopa and dopamine inhibit prolactin secretion, probably due to a direct action on the secretory cells of the anterior pituitary gland.

Clinical Indications. Levodopa is indicated in the treatment of idiopathic, postencephalitic, arteriosclerotic parkinsonism, and symptomatic parkinsonism following carbon monoxide and manganese intoxication. Bradykinesia and rigidity usually respond more quickly than tremors to levodopa, improving patient overall function ability. Posture, gait, and facial expression improve and a sense of well-being replaces the lethargy and apathy associated with parkinsonism. Incidences of levodopa side effects require a highly individualized dosage regimen; also, gradual increases in dosage achieve the desired therapeutic level.

Adverse Effects/Precautions. The majority of patients treated with levodopa experience adverse effects. Early in therapy, patients frequently experience anorexia, nausea, and vomiting. Although about 4 out of 5 patients experience these gastrointestinal side effects (which usually disappear with continued therapy), phenothiazine antiemetics are not recommended to avoid interference with the mechanism of dopamine action. Orthostatic hypotension occurs in about one in three patients.

Abnormal involuntary movements and reversible psychiatric disturbances may occur in long-term therapy. About 50% of these cases develop within 2 to 4 months of levodopa therapy; 4 out of 5 patients eventually show some abnormal movements (faciolingual tics, grimacing, head bobbing, rocking movements) which may necessitate limiting the levodopa dose. Behavioral disturbances (hallucinations, paranoia, mania, and depression) may also restrict levodopa therapy. The drug's effect on the hypothalamus probably accounts for the renewal of sexual interest sometimes noted by patients receiving levodopa.

Carbidopa. Used clinically only in combination with levodopa, carbidopa inhibits peripheral decarboxylation of levodopa.

Mechanism of Action. Carbidopa, a decarboxylase inhibitor, prevents the peripheral decarboxylation of levodopa. By not crossing the blood brain barrier, carbidopa does not affect levodopa metabolism in the brain. Administration of carbidopa makes more peripheral levodopa available for transport into the CNS. Carbidopa does not increase the intrinsic efficacy of levodopa and has no significant pharmacologic effect in recommended doses.

Clinical Indications. Carbidopa is used in conjunction with levodopa to treat idiopathic parkinsonism, postencephalitic parkinsonism, and symptomatic parkinsonism associated with carbon monoxide and manganese intoxication.

The dosage of levodopa may be reduced by about 70 to 80% with concomitant carbidopa administration. In such cases, the two drugs should be started at the same time, using no more than 20 to 25% of the previous daily dosage of levodopa. At least 8 hours should elapse between the last dose of levodopa and starting combined carbidopa/levodopa therapy, a regimen sometimes used in the management of neuroleptic malignant syndrome (NMS).

Adverse Effects/Precautions. Although problems occur with combination carbidopa/levodopa therapy, adverse reactions are not apparent with carbidopa alone. Carbidopa does not decrease the adverse effects due to the CNS effects of levodopa. Some evidence indicates that carbidopa may protect against the development of dopamine-induced cardiac arrhythmias.

Additional Dopaminergic Drugs. Amantidine and bromocryptine mesylate are alternative antiparkinsonism drugs that act by increasing dopaminergic influence in the nigrostriatal region of the brain.

ANTI-INFECTIVES

The choice of drugs used in the treatment of meningitis and encephalitis (caused by various organisms), mechanisms of antibiotic action, and related information are discussed in Chapter 7.

DRUG INTERACTIONS

Many of the drug interactions that occur with CNS drugs result in additive or superadditive CNS depression; other clinically significant drug interactions result in excessive CNS stimulation or hypertension. Some interactions with oral anticoagulants may be life-threatening, due to effects on blood coagulation.

SEDATIVES AND HYPNOTICS

CHLORAL HYDRATE

Oral Anticoagulants. Due to displacement from protein binding sites, increased hypoprothrombinemic effects may occur in patients taking both drugs, necessitating adjustment of the coumarin dosage.

Furosemide. Some patients who receive chloral hydrate followed by IV furosemide may experience sweating, hot flashes, hypotension or hypertension, and tachycardia.

Alcohol and CNS Depressants. Since additive effects occur with alcohol and CNS depressants, delayed administration of chloral hydate or reduced dosage are recommended for patients who have ingested alcohol in the preceding 12 to 24 hours.

GLUTETHIMIDE

Alcohol and CNS Depressants. As with chloral hydrate, additive effects occur with CNS depressants and glutethimide.

Coumarin Anticoagulants. Since glutethimide induces hepatic microsomal enzymes, the metabolism of coumarin anticoagulants may increase, resulting in decreased anticoagulant response.

Other Anticholinergic Drugs. Additive effects result from concomitant administration of glutethimide and other anticholinergic agents.

METHYPRYLON

Alcohol and CNS Depressants. Concomitant use of methyprylon and alcohol or other CNS depressants produces additive depressant effects.

ETHCHLORVYNOL

Alcohol, Barbiturates, and Other CNS Depressants. Exaggerated depressant effects result from concomitant use of ethchlorvynol and CNS depressants.

Coumarin Anticoagulants. Since ethchlorvynol may cause decreased prothrombin time, coumarin anticoagulants dosage usually requires adjustment at either the initiation or discontinuation of therapy.

Tricyclic Antidepressants. Due to reports of transient delirium following concomitant use of ethchlorvynol and amitriptyline, ethchlorvynol should be administered with caution to patients also receiving tricyclic antidepressants.

ETHINAMATE

Alcohol and CNS Depressants. Additive depressant effects occur after concomitant use of ethinamate and drugs having CNS depressant or hypnotic effects.

FLURAZEPAM

Alcohol and CNS Depressants. Concomitant use of flurazepam and CNS depressants results in additive depressant effects. If the patient consumes alcohol during the day following administration of flurazepam for nighttime sedation, this additive reaction also occurs.

TEMAZEPAM

Alcohol and CNS Depressants. Concomitant use of temazepam with alcohol and other CNS depressants may produce additive effects.

TRIAZOLAM

Psychotropic Drugs, Anticonvulsants, Antihistamines, Alcohol, Ethanol, and Other CNS Depressant Drugs. Coadministration with these drugs may produce possible additive CNS depressant effects.

SEDATIVES AND HYPNOTICS (BARBITURATES)

DRUGS INCREASING THE EFFECTS OF BARBITURATES

Valproic Acid. Since valproic acid decreases barbiturate metabolism, dosage adjustments may be required.

Volatile Anesthetics or Curare-like Drugs. Concomitant use with barbiturates produces additive respiratory depressant effects.

CNS Depressants. Additive depressant effects follow concomitant use with other CNS depressants (sedatives and hypnotics, antihistamines, tranquilizers, phenothiazines, or alcohol).

MAO Inhibitors. By inhibiting metabolism of the barbiturate, MAOIs prolong the effects of barbiturates.

Chloramphenicol. This drug inhibits the metabolism of phenobarbital.

DRUGS INHIBITED BY THE EFFECTS OF BARBITURATES

Coumarin Anticoagulants. By inducing hepatic microsomal enzymes, barbiturates increase metabolism and decrease anticoagulant responses of these drugs, necessitating dosage adjustment if barbiturates are either initiated or withdrawn from the patient's therapy.

Digitoxin and Tricyclic Antidepressants. Increases occur in the metabolism of these drugs since barbiturates induce hepatic microsomal enzymes.

Corticosteroids. By hepatic microsomal enzyme induction, barbiturates may enhance the metabolism of exogenous corticosteroids.

Doxycycline. Phenobarbital shortens the half-life of doxycycline for periods as long as 2 weeks following discontinuation of barbiturate therapy. Thus, concomitant use of these drugs requires close monitoring of clinical responses to the antibiotic.

Estradiol. Since estradiol's effects apparently decrease with either pretreatment with or concurrent administration of phenobarbital, patients should use an alternate contraceptive method.

Quinidine. Hepatic enzyme induction and reduction of quinidine's serum half-life result from concurrent administration of phenobarbital.

Furosemide. Concomitant administration of barbiturates and furosemide may either produce or aggravate orthostatic hypotension.

ANTICONVULSANTS

DRUGS INCREASING THE EFFECTS OF PHENYTOIN

Coumarin Anticoagulants, Disulfiram, Phenylbutazone, Isoniazid, Chloramphenicol, Cimetidine, and Sulfonamides. Since these agents inhibit phenytoin metabolism, nystagmus, ataxia, or other toxic signs of phenytoin may occur.

Isoniazid. Concomitant use may produce phenytoin intoxication in patients who are slow acetylators.

Chloramphenicol. Significant increases in phenytoin serum levels result from chloramphenicol use.

Dexamethasone. Reports following concomitant use of these drugs indicate increases in phenytoin serum levels since both agents compete for hydroxylation by hepatic microsomal enzymes.

Salicylates. High doses of salicylates displace phenytoin from protein binding sites and increase the concentration of free phenytoin in the plasma.

DRUGS DECREASING THE EFFECTS OF PHENYTOIN

Barbiturates. Barbiturates evidently enhance phenytoin's metabolism rate. Excessive response to phenytoin may follow discontinuation of barbiturate therapy.

Carbamazepine. Increased phenytoin metabolism rate may result from concomitant administration of carbamazepine.

Folic Acid. Reports of increased seizure frequency have followed the addition of folic acid in patients also receiving phenytoin.

Alcohol and CNS Depressants. Additive effects may occur with alcohol and any CNS depressant, including phenytoin. Acute alcohol intoxication may increase the anticonvulsant effect because of decreased metabolic breakdown of phenytoin. Enzyme induction often decreases anticonvulsant effect in cases of chronic alcohol abuse.

Antacids. Reports suggest that decreased GI absorption and decreased phenytoin bioavailability follow antacid administration.

DRUGS INHIBITED BY THE EFFECTS OF PHENYTOIN

Dicumarol. Phenytoin decreases dicumarol's anticoagulant effect.

Disopyramide and Quinidine. Maintenance of these antiarrhythmics' therapeutic effects may necessitate larger doses since phenytoin apparently induces their metabolism.

Corticosteroids. Larger doses are evidently needed during phenytoin therapy since reports indicate that phenytoin inhibits the effect of prednisolone and dexamethasone.

Oral Contraceptives. Concomitant administration with phenytoin reduces the efficacy of oral contraceptives. Also, another reported adverse reaction involves breakthrough bleeding.

Furosemide. Phenytoin evidently impairs the absorption of furosemide.

ANTIDEPRESSANTS

MONOAMINE OXIDASE INHIBITORS (MAOIs)

Amphetamines. MAOIs tend to increase the amount of norepinephrine in storage sites of the adrenergic neuron and amphetamines cause catecholamine release, freeing larger amounts of norepinephrine to react with the receptor. Thus, concomitant use of these drugs is highly dangerous and may produce fatalities.

Tricyclic Antidepressants (TCADs). Although concomitant use with an MAOI may produce adverse reactions which vary from excitation to death, other evidence indicates safe use of the two drugs together when the following precautions are followed: avoidance of large doses, oral administration, avoidance of clomipramine and imipramine, and close patient monitoring.

Ephedrine. Concomitant admnistration with a MAOI may produce hypertensive reactions.

Alcohol. MAOIs impair the metabolism of tyramine (contained in some alcoholic beverages) in the intestine and liver, producing an enhanced pressor response to tyramine. Patients should avoid alcoholic beverages because the tyramine content of alcoholic drinks varies.

Levodopa. Concomitant administration may result in hypertension, facial flushing, palpitations, and lightheadedness. Also, worsening of akinesia and tremor may also occur with use of both levodopa and a MAOI.

Meperidine. Severe immediate reactions (excitation, sweating, rigidity, and hypertension) may occur following concomitant administration of meperidine and MAOIs.

Phenothiazines. Although some combinations of a MAOI and phenothiazines are beneficial, concomitant use produces increased side effects in some patients.

Phenylpropanolamine. Since phenylpropanolamine resembles ephedrine pharmacologically, the same cautions apply as with ephedrine because of potential hypertensive reactions.

TRICYCLIC ANTIDEPRESSANTS (TCADs)

Amphetamines. Since amphetamine abuse in patients receiving TCADs has reportedly resulted in death, caution should be exercised in administering both drugs.

Anticholinergics. Excessive anticholinergic activity may result from concomitant use. An antidepressant drug with low anticholinergic activity is less likely to show this interaction.

Barbiturates. When used with therapeutic doses of TCADs, barbiturates apparently stimulate the TCAD metabolism and decrease their blood levels.

Cimetidine. Cimetidine may impair the hepatic metabolism of TCADs, resulting in adverse effects that include urinary retention, tachycardia, and constipation.

Methylphenidate. An enhanced antidepressant effect may result from concomitant use.

ANTIPSYCHOTICS

PHENOTHIAZINES

Amphetamines. Concurrent use is not advised because of a mutually inhibitory effect.

Anticholinergics. Patients should probably not routinely receive both drugs since anticholinergics may reduce the therapeutic response to phenothiazines. Other potential problems include additive anticholinergic effects and inhibition of gastrointestinal absorption of phenothiazine by anticholinergics.

Tricyclic Antidepressants. Increased toxicity and reduced phenothiazine therapeutic response may result from concomitant use.

Lithium Carbonate. Concomitant use is discouraged in patients with acute manic symptoms due to the potential problem of neurotoxicity or extrapyramidal symptoms.

HALOPERIDOL

Lithium Carbonate. Since a combined inhibitory effect on striatal adenylate cyclase may result, concomitant use is discouraged to avoid possible neurotoxicity.

ANTIANXIETY DRUGS

BENZODIAZEPINES

Alcohol. Alcohol and the benzodiazepines have additive CNS depressant effects.

Cimetidine. With either initiation or discontinuation of cimetidine therapy, altered benzodiazepine response may occur due to cimetidine's inhibition of the hepatic metabolism of some benzodiazepines.

Disulfiram. As with cimetidine, disulfiram inhibits the hepatic metabolism of some benzodiazepines, enhancing benzodiazepine response.

Levodopa. Reduction of the antiparkinsonism effect of levodopa necessitates discontinuation of benzodiazepine therapy.

ANTIMANIA DRUGS

LITHIUM CARBONATE

Neuromuscular Blocking Agents. Prolongation of the action of neuromuscular blocking agents is possible in patients receiving chronic lithium carbonate therapy.

Piroxicam. Initiation or discontinuation of piroxicam therapy may alter the effect of lithium, which necessitates monitoring serum lithium levels.

NARCOTIC ANALGESICS

Neuromuscular Blocking Agents. Concomitant use of narcotic analgesics and skeletal muscle relaxants may result in an increased degree of respiratory depression and lung collapse.

CNS STIMULANTS

AMPHETAMINES

Haloperidol. Haloperidol may antagonize the stimulant effect of amphetamines.

ANTIPARKINSONISM DRUGS

LEVODOPA

Methionine. Large doses of methionine are discouraged in patients also receiving levodopa due to possible worsening of the parkinsonism.

Pyridoxine. By apparently enhancing levodopa metabolism, pyridoxine decreases the amount of levodopa available to the site of action in the brain.

SUMMARY

Significant advances in understanding brain function and dysfunction have occurred in the last four decades. Especially noted are developments in fundamental and clinical principles of mental processes and the use of drugs to correct aberrant CNS processes. For instance, although a cure for a complex psychiatric illness such as schizophrenia is not available, the control of symptoms with maintenance pharmacotherapy allows the patient to function effectively. The discovery of endogenous peptides that activate opiate receptors in the CNS has improved our understanding of biofeedback and placebo response, as well as permitting molecular design for specific agonist and antagonist opiate-like compounds.

CNS disorders that usually occur in later life (such as parkinsonism and Alzheimer's disease) challenge biochemists and pharmacologists to determine causative factors and treatment approaches. This research thrust is especially important because of the increasing geriatric population and the need to offer optimal health care for this segment of the population.

Effective symptom control in epilepsy, psychiatric illness, resistant severe chronic pain, and other debilitating CNS disorders represents modern therapeutic achievements. Although our present understanding of mental processes is incomplete and rudimentary, clinical successes encourage additional work. Undoubtedly, many forthcoming major advances in medical treatment will occur in CNS neuropharmacology.

SUGGESTED READINGS

Akil, H., et al.: Endogenous opioids: Biology and function. Annu Rev Neurosci, 7:223, 1984.

Berger, J.G., (ed.): Antianxiety Agents. New York, John Wiley and Sons, 1986.

Cherry, L.: The good news about depression. New York, 19:32, June 2, 1986.

Clark, W.G., and del Guidice, J. (eds.): Principles of Psychopharmacology. 2nd Ed. New York, Academic Press, Inc., 1978.

Covino, B.G., and Vasallo, H.G.: Local Anesthetics: Mechanisms of Action and Clinical Use. New York, Grune and Stratton, Inc., 1976.

Curatolo, P.W., and Robertson, D.: Health consequences of caffeine. Ann Intern Med, 98:641, 1983.

Eichelman, B.S.: Analyzing the elusive schizophrenias. Am Pharm, NS18:18, 1978.

Ellenor, G.L.: Reducing irrational antipsychotic polypharmacy prescribing. Hosp Pharm, 12:369, 1977.

Frey, H.H., and Janz, D. (eds.): Antiepileptic Drugs. In Handbook of Experimental Pharmacology. Vol. 74. Berlin, Springer-Verlag, 1985.

Hoffman, R.P., Moore, W.E., and O'Dea, L.: Medication problems confronted by the schizophrenic patient. J APhA, NS14:252, 1974.

Kessler, K.A., and Walstzky, J.P.: Clinical use of antipsychotic drugs. Am J Psychiatry, 138: 202, 1981.

Manschreck, T.C.: Drug treatment of schizophrenia. Drug Ther, 13:185, 1983.

Melzack, R., and Wall, P.D.: Pain mechanisms: A new theory. Science, 150:971, 1965.

Minuck, M.: Reaction to drugs during surgery and anesthesia. Can Med Assoc J, 82:1008, 1960.

Neuropsychopharmacology: A series from Roche Laboratories. Nutley, NJ, Hoffmann-La Roche, Inc., 1976.

Quinn, N.P.: Anti-parkinsonism today. Drugs, 28:236, 1984.

Rall, T.W.: Evolution of the mechanism of action of methylxanthines: From calcium mobilizers to antagonists of adenosine receptors. Pharmacologist, 24:277, 1982.

Rhodes, P.J., Rhodes, R.S., Jahnigen, D.W., and Piepho, R.W.: Pain management in the elderly. Colorado J Pharm, 28:47, 1985.

Snyder, S.H.: Drugs and neurotransmitter receptors in the brain. Science, 224:22, 1984.

Solomon, G.E., Kutt, H., and Plum, F.: Clinical Management of Seizures: A Guide for the Physician. 2nd Ed. Philadelphia, W.B. Saunders Co., 1983.

Study, R.E., and Barker, J.L.: Cellular mechanisms of benzodiazepine action. JAMA, 247:2147, 1982.

Usdin, E., et al.: Pharmacology of Benzodiazepines. Deerfield Beach, FL, Verlag chemie, 1983.

Weissman, M.M.: Why do more women than men suffer from depression? Pharm Times, 48:63, March 1982.

White, J.P.: Meeting pain head on. Drug Topics, 127:54, 1983.

Wincor, M.Z.: Insomnia and the new benzodiazepines. Clin Pharm, 1:425, 1982.

Wizwer, P.I., and Carvalho, M.G.: Anxiety management: Medication as a component of therapy. NARD J, 106:61, Oct. 1984.

CHAPTER EXAMINATION

An elderly patient with idiopathic parkinsonism has taken levodopa for approximately 1 year with successful control of symptoms. Lately, behavioral changes in the patient have prompted the clinician to consider antipsychotic drug therapy.

1. Levodopa
   a. cures idiopathic parkinsonism in over 70% of patients receiving the drug
   b. gives symptomatic relief in a high percentage of patients with idiopathic parkinsonism
   c. is more effective in controlling a drug-induced parkinsonism-like syndrome than in idiopathic parkinsonism
   d. is noted for a lower incidence of adverse reactions

2. The antiparkinsonism activity of levodopa is best explained by
   a. restoration of striatal dopaminergic influence
   b. blockade of striatal cholinergic receptors
   c. the ability of levodopa to release endogenous catecholamines
   d. blockade of serotonin receptors in the spinal cord

3. Introduction of a phenothiazine antipsychotic drug into the patient's therapeutic regimen
   a. would probably antagonize the action of levodopa
   b. is the best initial clinical choice to counteract the behavioral changes observed in the patient
   c. should be followed by a reduction of the levodopa dosage since a synergistic response is likely
   d. is preferred to use of a butyrophenone, such as haloperidol

4. Frequent adverse effects seen with levodopa therapy include
   a. gingival hyperplasia, xerostomia, and a SLE-like syndrome

    b. blurred vision, constipation, and urinary retention
    c. dystonic movements, anorexia, and nausea/vomiting
    d. salivation, hypotension, and bradycardia
5. A drug that increases levodopa activity by preventing its degradation is
    a. pyridoxine
    b. chlorpromazine
    c. chlorprothixene
    d. carbidopa

A severely depressed patient has received desipramine for 1 week with no positive clinical response. The physician decides to change the patient's medication to tranylcypromine.

---

6. Onset of antidepressant action with initial desipramine therapy usually occurs in
    a. 4 hours
    b. 2 months
    c. 2 weeks
    d. 1 day
7. Changing the medication from desipramine to tranylcypromine
    a. necessitates a desipramine "wash-out" period of about 2 weeks before starting the tranylcypromine
    b. is long overdue
    c. is unacceptable under any clinical situation
    d. represents a change to a drug that is less likely to cause adverse reactions or to interact with food or other drugs
8. Desipramine
    a. is a monoamine oxidase inhibitor
    b. blocks presynaptic neuron reuptake of endogenous norepinephrine
    c. produces cholinergic side effects in a high percentage of patients
    d. is biotransformed to an active monomethyl derivative
9. Tranylcypromine is a monoamine oxidase inhibitor that
    a. is commonly used in combination with tricyclic antidepressants
    b. preferentially inhibits extraneuron monoamine oxidase in the reticular activating system
    c. is commonly used as an OTC weight control product
    d. interacts adversely with tyramine-containing food and tricyclic antidepressants

---

A 21-year-old university student has taken diazepam for several weeks for anxiety associated with academic and personal problems. After learning that alcohol also relieves her anxiety, she decides to have a few drinks each evening to help her sleep. Additionally, after talking to her parents, her hometown family doctor, who is also a family friend, sends her a prescription for flurazepam to ease her over her stress.

---

10. Diazepam is a benzodiazepine derivative that has preferential depressant activity on the
    a. medullary vital centers
    b. limbic system
    c. motor cortex
    d. cerebellum
11. Benzodiazepine receptors are located in the CNS in close proximity to
    a. GABA receptors and chloride ionophores
    b. serotonin ligands
    c. nicotinic receptors
    d. muscarinic receptors
12. Flurazepam
    a. antagonizes the action of diazepam on the CNS
    b. is a barbituric acid derivative
    c. adds to the combined depressant effects of diazepam and alcohol on the CNS
    d. is contraindicated for the control of insomnia
13. Concomitant use of alcohol and diazepam
    a. is potentially life-threatening
    b. is always better for anxiety than nondrug therapy, such as biofeedback
    c. antagonizes the benefit of flurazepam in insomnia
    d. illustrates pharmacologic antagonism

A teenage boy with a history of grand mal convulsions takes phenytoin and phenobarbital with excellent clinical control of the epileptic seizures. Recently, he has become extremely agitated and has shown symptoms of paranoid schizophrenia. Chlorpromazine is considered as an addition to his treatment regimen.

14. Chlorpromazine is an antipsychotic drug that
    a. activates dopamine receptors in the reticular activating system
    b. is most effective in retarded psychoses
    c. is always safe in patients with a history of seizures
    d. lowers the seizure threshold
15. Phenytoin suppresses
    a. the spread of aberrant cortical excitation
    b. is more effective in controlling petit mal seizures than grand mal seizures
    c. is a specific adrenergic agonist in reticular formation pathways
    d. preferentially blocks the chemoreceptor trigger zone of the medullary vomiting center
16. Symptoms of paranoid schizophrenia resemble those that occur with
    a. a chlorpromazine overdose
    b. a phenytoin-phenobarbital drug interaction
    c. an amphetamine abuser
    d. excessive phenytoin dosage
17. A good clinical decision before initiating any treatment for psychotic behavior is
    a. dropping the phenobarbital from the therapeutic regimen
    b. increasing the phenytoin and phenobarbital dosage
    c. trying high doses of chlorpromazine for one week
    d. taking a careful history of the patient and the possibility of "social drug" use

A middle-aged male patient has taken high doses of phenelzine for several months to treat reactive depression. This patient, who has a history of gouty arthritis, also takes probenecid. His only complaint is difficulty in talking due to "dry mouth" and this problem has lessened in recent weeks. After developing excruciating pain in his side and back, the patient is taken to the emergency room of the local hospital where meperidine IM 100 mg is prescribed for suspected kidney stones.

18. Meperidine given concomitantly with a monoamine oxidase inhibitor
    a. produces increased analgesic potency of meperidine with an elevation of the pain threshold
    b. may result in coma and death
    c. lowers blood uric acid levels
    d. blocks the uricosuric action of probenecid
19. Meperidine
    a. interacts with the same receptors as enkephalins and endorphins
    b. is found in Papaver somniferum
    c. is used extensively for detoxification and temporary maintenance treatment of narcotic addiction
    d. none of the above
20. During the time the depressed patient received phenelzine, his reported side effects were minimal. The patient was probably warned to
    a. not exercise or do aerobics
    b. take aspirin
    c. reduce sexual activity
    d. not eat foods with a high concentration of tyramine, such as Camembert or Stilton cheese
21. Conditions in which meperidine is contraindicated or used only with extreme caution include
    a. nursing mothers
    b. head injury and increased intracranial pressure
    c. preoperative procedures
    d. a and b

A housewife habitually drinks a pot or two of coffee a day and claims the caffeine helps her finish her housework. She decides to take an OTC weight control product containing phenylpropanolamine because summer swimsuit season is approaching. On top of this, she develops a terrible cold and purchases a cough-cold preparation that contains the nasal decongestant, pseudoephedrine. She calls her pharmacy one afternoon and complains of dizziness and anxiety.

22. The amount of caffeine in a cup of coffee is approximately
    a. 1 mg
    b. 100 mg
    c. 500 mg
    d. 10 mg
23. Caffeine
    a. blocks adenosine receptors in the CNS
    b. is routinely found in OTC weight control products in combination with phenylpropanolamine
    c. inhibits CNS adenyl cyclase
    d. is a chemical isomer of amphetamine
24. Phenylpropanolamine and pseudoephedrine are
    a. sympathomimetics
    b. effective antitussive drugs
    c. considered safe and effective, at recommended doses, as oral nasal decongestants
    d. a and c
25. Symptoms of phenylpropanolamine or pseudoephedrine overdosage include
    a. hepatic necrosis
    b. restlessness and confusion
    c. a SLE-like syndrome
    d. excessive sedation
26. Caffeine, in excessive amounts (approximately 700 mg daily)
    a. can produce a type of physiologic dependence
    b. is a CNS depressant
    c. potentiates the action of insulin
    d. none of the above

A middle-aged patient has taken pentazocine for the short-term management of severe pain. Although presently physically healthy, this patient has a history of narcotic and alcohol dependence.

27. Patients with this type of medication history are
    a. resistant to pentazocine analgesia
    b. likely to develop psychological and physical dependence to pentazocine
    c. likely to react adversely to pentazocine
    d. a and c
28. Pentazocine
    a. could precipitate withdrawal symptoms in patients who take narcotic analgesics regularly
    b. is a pure narcotic agonist analgesic
    c. has extensive clinical utility as an antitussive
    d. has a greater abuse potential than morphine
29. Pentazocine
    a. owes its activity to the d-isomer
    b. lacks sedative activity
    c. is a potent mu receptor agonist
    d. exerts its narcotic agonist effect on kappa and sigma opiate receptors
30. The analgesic that most closely resembles pentazocine pharmacologically is
    a. morphine
    b. codeine
    c. butorphanol
    d. methadone

ANSWER KEY

1. b	16. c
2. a	17. d
3. a	18. b
4. c	19. a
5. d	20. d
6. c	21. d
7. a	22. b
8. b	23. a
9. d	24. d
10. b	25. b
11. a	26. a
12. c	27. b
13. a	28. a
14. d	29. d
15. a	30. c

chapter 2

AUTONOMIC NERVOUS SYSTEM

CHAPTER OBJECTIVES

After studying this chapter, you should be able to:
1. Diagram the anatomic characteristics of the autonomic nervous system (ANS).
2. List the criteria that distinguish a chemical as a neurotransmitter.
3. Briefly describe classic experiments that support the theory of chemical transmission in neuron activity.
4. Describe the sites along neuron pathways that drugs affect most often.
5. Differentiate between presynaptic and postsynaptic sites as prime targets for drug activity.
6. Outline the biosynthetic and catabolic pathways for acetylcholine and norepinephrine metabolism.
7. Define and give an example of end product negative feedback involving a neurotransmitter.
8. Outline the autonomic innervation to the following: iris musculature; gastrointestinal tract; myocardium; bronchiolar smooth muscle; ciliary muscle; peripheral blood vessels; genitalia; and sweat glands. Describe the effects that cholinergic or adrenergic activation produce on receptors at these sites.
9. Using examples of muscarinic and nicotinic activity, define and illustrate cholinergic activation.
10. List several therapeutic uses of the cholinergic stimulants.
11. Discuss the theoretical clinical applications of cholinergic blocking agents and describe their actual therapeutic uses.
12. Differentiate between the mechanism of action of choline esters (e.g., bethanechol Cl) and cholinesterase inhibitors (e.g., physostigmine salicylate).
13. Describe the mechanisms whereby metoclopramide alleviates gastroparesis.
14. Discuss the mechanism of action and therapeutic indications of cholinesterase reactivators.
15. Define or briefly describe the following: Electrophorus electricus; mydriasis; cycloplegia; EPSP; IPSP; miotic agent; iridocyclitis; choroiditis; paralytic ileus; and "Vagusstoff."
16. Describe the limitations of the ganglionic blocking drugs in the treatment of hypertension.
17. Name two ganglionic blocking drugs employed in hypertensive crisis.
18. Contrast the sites and mechanisms of action of d-tubocurarine and succinylcholine.
19. Describe the therapeutic uses of the neuromuscular blocking drugs and list several adverse effects that may occur with these drugs.
20. Discuss, in detail, the concept of alpha- and beta-adrenergic receptors.
21. Compare and contrast the selective activity of epinephrine, norepinephrine, and isoproterenol on alpha- and beta-adrenergic receptors.
22. Describe the "fight or flight" reaction in terms of physiologic responses.

23. State whether alpha-, beta$_1$- or beta$_2$-, or mixed alpha-beta-adrenergic receptors are involved in adrenergic stimulation of the following: heart; radial muscle of the iris; bronchial muscle; stomach; intestine; liver; pancreas; urinary bladder sphincter; arterioles; and adipose tissue.
24. Name several beta$_2$-adrenergic stimulants and give their therapeutic uses.
25. Discuss the clinical uses and adverse effects of alpha-adrenergic blocking drugs.
26. State whether the following adrenergic blockers are nonselective (blocks both beta$_1$- and beta$_2$-receptors) or are cardioselective (preferentially blocks beta$_1$-receptors in low doses): nadolol; metoprolol; atenolol; propranolol; timolol; labetalol; and acebutolol.
27. Discuss the therapeutic applications of beta-adrenergic blockers.
28. Name several disease states or clinical situations in which sympathomimetics are contraindicated.
29. Name several OTC adrenergic drugs and describe precautions that should be exercised in their use.
30. Name several drug interactions that may result from concurrent use of OTC drugs and prescription autonomic drugs.

INTRODUCTION

The autonomic nervous system (ANS) supplies innervation to smooth muscles, glands, and visceral organs. Termed the "involuntary nervous system" because of its control of physiologic reactions not under conscious regulation, this communications network maintains homeostasis and facilitates appropriate bodily responses to environmental influences. An example of nonvolitional control is pupillary size regulation for appropriate light introduction to the retina. To illustrate, the pupil dilates in dim light and constricts in bright light for optimal visual acuity and for the prevention of retinal damage from excessive light exposure, respectively.

The need for sunglasses or "dark glasses" after dilation of the pupils by atropine or a similar drug in an ophthalmic examination best illustrates the pupillary light reaction. In this instance, drug-induced blockade of the pupillary light reflex prevents constriction in bright light and produces an uncomfortable reaction (photophobia). Excessive exposure to light may cause serious retinal damage. This reflex functions normally unless a unique situation (such as drug-induced blockade) occurs.

A more dramatic example is the activation of the ANS in a crisis situation. To illustrate, if an individual is trapped in a burning building, an "alarm reaction" involving a massive epinephrine (adrenalin) discharge occurs. A myriad of biochemical and physiologic responses result from this adrenalin surge, which allows the individual to cope better with the emergency.

Examination of the "burning building" example reveals an analogy between the building's regulatory mechanisms and those of the human body. Specifically, before the building's emergency (i.e., fire), other regulatory mechanisms (i.e., thermostatic temperature regulation and automatic control mechanisms for air circulation and electrical lighting) probably maintained the building's homeostatic environment in noncrisis situations, just as the ANS ordinarily functions in humans. However, when a fire triggered the building's smoke detector, an alarm amd automatic sprinklers were activated to counteract the emergency. Thus, an "alarm system" is an essential component of a well-regulated building environment, just as the human's biologically-activated "alarm" system (i.e., adrenalin reaction) is vitally important to set off critical compensatory reactions to threatening emergencies.

ANATOMY AND PHYSIOLOGY OF THE AUTONOMIC NERVOUS SYSTEM (ANS)

The autonomic (or involuntary) nervous system is separated into two divisions based upon anatomic and physiologic criteria: the parasympathetic and sympathetic (Figure 2.1). Both ANS divisions innervate many organs (Table 2.1). The dual autonomic innervation of the heart and intestines is important because of the opposing action of these two divisions. Effector

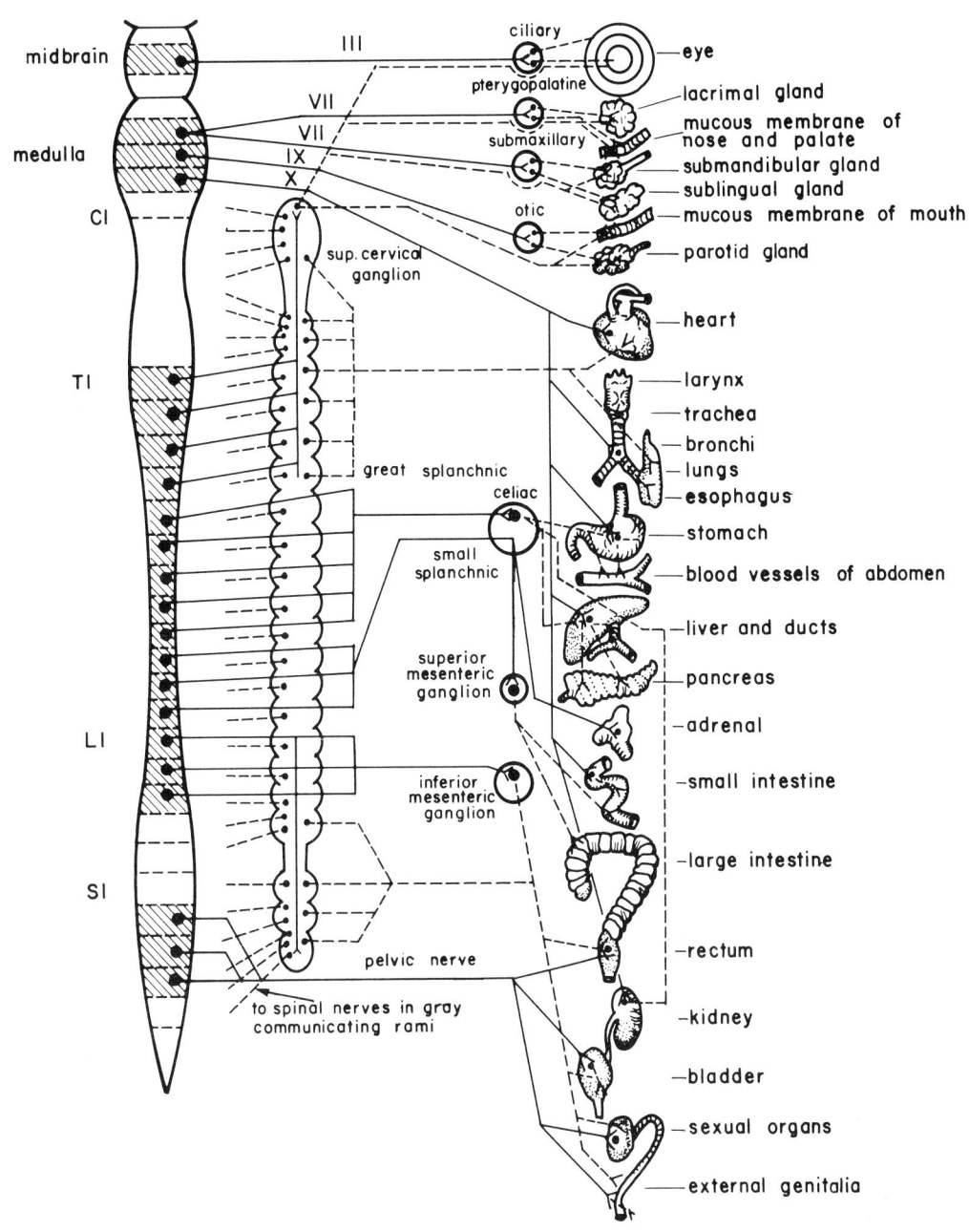

Fig. 2.1 Autonomic nervous system. (From Crouch, J.E.: Essential Human Anatomy. Philadelphia, Lea & Febiger, 1982.)

Table 2.1 COMPARISON OF SYMPATHETIC AND PARASYMPATHETIC IMPULSES ON SOME ORGANS.*

Organ	Sympathetic	Parasympathetic
Eye		
iris	increase in pupil size	decrease in pupil size
ciliary muscle	relaxation, to accomodate for distant vision	contraction, to accomodate for near vision
lacrimal gland	excessive secretion	normal secretion
Salivary Glands	secretion of mucus-rich saliva	large quantities of watery saliva
Respiratory System	relaxation of smooth muscle, increasing volume	contraction of smooth muscle, decreasing volume
blood vessels	dilation	constriction
Heart (cardiac muscle)	increased rate, output, and blood pressure	decreased rate, output, and blood pressure
coronary vessels	dilation	constriction
Peripheral Blood Vessels	dilation in skeletal muscles	constriction in skeletal muscles
	constriction in skin	dilation in skin
	constriction in viscera, except in heart and lungs	dilation in viscera, except in heart and lungs
Stomach and Intestines		
glands	inhibited secretion	increased secretion
sphincter valves	stimulation	inhibition
wall	decreased action	increased action
Pancreas	inhibition of both exocrine and endocrine cells	stimulation of both exocrine and endocrine cells
Liver	promotion of glycogen breakdown; inhibition of bile secretion	promotion of both glycogen formation and bile secretion
Spleen	contraction and release of stored blood	minimal effect
Adrenal Medulla	stimulation of secretion of epinephrine and norepinephrine	no effect
Uterus	stimulation of pregnant uterus; inhibition of nonpregnant uterus	little effect
Urinary Bladder	inhibition of wall; stimulation of sphincter	stimulation of wall; inhibition of sphincter
Sweat Glands	stimulation of secretion	normal secretion

* Reprinted from Crouch, J.E.: Essential Human Anatomy. Lea & Febiger, Philadelphia, 1982.

cells in these organ systems may be activated to either elevate or suppress the characteristic inherent activity of the heart and intestines. Thus, an increased force of contraction and higher heart rate indicate the sympathetic influence on the heart; bradycardia, on the other hand, results from parasympathetic predominance. In the iris musculature, pupillary size reflects opposite activity of the sympathetic and parasympathetic divisions.

Changes in the organ system activity result from the interplay between the sympathetic and parasympathetic divisions. Drugs that affect the ANS may mimic the activity of one of the systems, thereby eliciting a pharmacologic effect by an "active" mechanism. Conversely, a "passive" mimetic effect on one of the divisions may result from blocking the influence of the opposing division.

The parasympathetic division of the ANS usually predominates under basic daily undemanding life situations, including sleep. The sympathetic division, however, shocks the mammalian physiologic processes into action in situations of environmental or internal stress. Thus, if confronted with danger, the individual experiences the following: the heart beat increases and becomes more forceful; the pupils dilate, allowing more light to the retina; the blood flow to skeletal muscle increases; the blood sugar elevates; the intestines quiet down; the sphincters of the alimentary tract close; and general perception of the environment heightens.

PARASYMPATHETIC DIVISION

Preganglionic cell bodies of the parasympathetic division lie in the brain (midbrain and medulla oblongata) and the sacral portion of the spinal cord. The oculomotor (III), facial (VII), glossopharyngeal (IX), vagal (X), and bulbar accessory (XI) nerves constitute the cranial outflow of the parasympathetic division. The cranial nerves synapse with terminal ganglia that lie near and within the structures of the head, neck, thoracic cavity, and selected areas in the abdominal viscera. Discrete ganglia separated from the innervated structure are found only in the head. The sacral outflow (S2 to S4) of the parasympathetic division supplies the pelvic nerve that synapses in terminal ganglia in or near the descending colon and the pelvic viscera.

Efferent preganglionic fibers that emanate from the cranial-sacral origin supply fibers to smooth muscle, glands, and visceral organs. The parasympathetic preganglionic fibers make synaptic union with postganglionic neurons in ganglia located near the innervated smooth muscle, organ, or gland. Thus, the parasympathetic preganglionic fibers are relatively long, as compared to the postganglionic fibers. The usual ratio of preganglionic fibers to postganglionic fibers is 1:2 or 1:1, resulting in more discrete responses upon parasympathetic activation.

SYMPATHETIC DIVISION

The sympathetic division of the ANS is anatomically characterized by a thoracic-lumbar outflow of efferent fibers that innervate smooth muscle, glands, and visceral organs. Preganglionic fibers emerge from the spinal cord, and many synapse with postganglionic fibers in sympathetic ganglia that lie in a vertical chain along the vertebral column (Figure 2.2). The sympathetic preganglionic fibers leave the spinal cord by the ventral root as tiny medullated

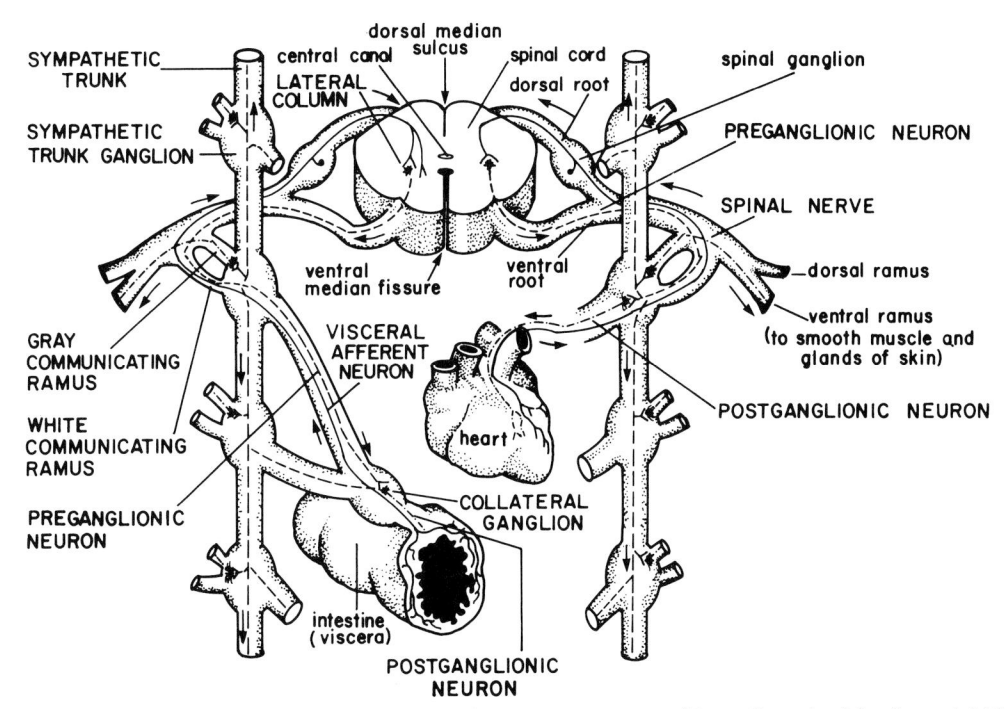

Fig. 2.2 Sympathetic division of the autonomic nervous system. (From Crouch, J.E.: Essential Human Anatomy. Philadelphia, Lea & Febiger, 1982.)

nerves and enter the ganglia chain through the white rami communicantes. Of the two chains of the sympathetic ganglia, one chain of 22 ganglia lies on each side of the spinal cord. These chain ganglia (or paravertebral ganglia) are the origin of many postganglionic sympathetic fibers, although important sympathetic ganglia may also occur as collateral (or prevertebral) ganglia and terminal ganglia. The mesenteric ganglia and the celiac ganglia, located near the innervated organ, represent prevertebral ganglia. Terminal sympathetic ganglia lie near or in the innervated organ and are represented by ganglia that supply fibers to the urinary bladder and rectum. The ratio of sympathetic preganglionic fibers to postganglionic fibers approaches 1:20; this factor, along with the widespread distribution of sympathetic ganglia, accounts for the diffuse, generalized response following activation of the sympathetic division.

CHARACTERISTICS OF THE AUTONOMIC NERVOUS SYSTEM

Ganglia and plexuses are distinguishing factors in the ANS. Their presence contrasts with the somatic motor (voluntary) nervous system in which fibers pass unintercepted from the spinal cord to the motor end plate of striated muscle.

Afferent autonomic nerves represent the sensory portion of the reflex arcs in the ANS. Certain autonomic nerves (such as the vagus) contain a large proportion of afferent fibers that carry sensory information to the medulla. These fibers are important in reflex blood pressure regulation, as well as in other physiologic responses like heart rate and respiration. The central nervous system (CNS) functions in concert with the ANS in both the maintenance of homeostasis and the body's reaction to environmental or internal stresses. Thus, centers in the medulla oblongata influence the integration of blood pressure control and respiration.

The hypothalamus, generally considered the central site of autonomic integration, contains regulating loci that monitor and react to maintain the balance of body temperature, water balance, carbohydrate and fat metabolism, and blood pressure. Emotional reactivity is influenced by the cerebral cortex that has neuronal communication with the hypothalamus and limbic system via the Papez circuit (see Chapter 1). The ascending reticular activating system (ARAS), important in the transition from wakefulness to sleep, also has interconnecting neuron contact with the hypothalamus, limbic system, and cerebral cortex, as seen in the Papez circuit relationship.

Chemical mediators transmit information (nerve action potential) across gaps or spaces in the autonomic neuron pathways. These interruptions in physical communication are represented by autonomic ganglia (in which a synaptic cleft separates the preganglionic fibers from postganglionic fibers) and by the neuroeffector junction (in which the autonomic postganglionic fibers do not physically attach to effector cells or receptor sites on smooth muscles, glands, and visceral organs). After release into the autonomic synapse or neuroeffector junction upon passage of a nerve action potential, these chemicals (transmitters or neurohormones) attach to receptor sites on postganglionic membranes or effector cells on smooth muscles, glands, and visceral organs. Combining a chemical transmitter with a receptor site initiates biochemical events that culminate in a physiologic effect or response.

Acetylcholine is the chemical neurotransmitter at the following: all autonomic ganglia; the neuroeffector junction of postganglionic parasympathetic fibers and effector cells on smooth muscle, glands, and visceral organs; the junction of autonomic fibers and the adrenal medulla; and the autonomic nerve-effector cell union on sweat glands and vasodilator vessels. Thus, these fibers are designated as cholinergic —as a consequence of the specific chemical (acetylcholine) released from their endings upon passage of a nerve action potential.

Norepinephrine (noradrenalin) is the neurotransmitter released from postganglionic sympathetic nerves that innervate smooth muscles, glands, and visceral organs. Thus, these fibers are termed "adrenergic fibers," indicating the chemical transmitter released from these sympathetic nerve endings.

Certain criteria must be met before a chemical is defined as a neurotransmitter. Specifically, the neurotransmitter must be present in the neuron and receptor pathway together with enzymes responsible for its production and destruction. The postulated neurotransmitter must induce the same physiologic effect as that which occurs in nerve stimulation to that site. The neurotransmitter must actually be released into the synaptic space upon nerve stimulation. Additionally, the blockade of nerve stimulation by selected drugs that also block the neurotransmitter's action lends further credence to other evidence supporting a chemical's designation as a neurotransmitter.

The neurotransmitter is synthesized in the nerve endings or at proximal sites for transportation to the nerve terminal. Enzymes and the precursor molecules, required for neurotransmitter synthesis, must therefore be present in sufficient quantities. Once synthesized, the neurotransmitter is protected from enzymatic degradation by vesicle storage. The neurotransmitter, taken up in vesicular storage sacs, is thus protected from enzymatic destruction by cytoplasmic or mitochondrial enzymes.

A nerve action potential causes the release of neurotransmitter into the synaptic space or the neuroeffector junction. The liberated neurotransmitter then attaches to the postsynaptic membrane or effector cell membrane, resulting in depolarization and a "postgap" activation, which generates a nerve action potential. A prolonged attachment of the neurotransmitter to the postsynaptic or effector cell membrane results in a loss of reactivity. Consequently, rapid neurotransmitter destruction or its removal from the receptor vicinity is imperative. Otherwise, an immediate paralysis of function in the innervated structures would follow all receptor activation.

Following transient "postgap" depolarization and the action potential translation into biologic response, a period of membrane repolarization must take place. Unless repolarization occurs, the membrane receptor sites are refractory to additional stimulation. Thus, persistent depolarization prevents a biologic response since subsequent nerve action potentials are ineffective until effective repolarization of the "postgap" membrane has transpired.

DRUG ACTION ON ANS NEUROTRANSMISSION

Upon the passage of a nerve impulse, neurotransmitters, such as acetylcholine and norepinephrine, are released from presynaptic sites and nerve terminals. Pharmacologic agents alter neurotransmitter events at one or more sites in the neurotransmission sequence. Most drugs owe their activity to an effect on the synaptic or neuroeffector milieu and act either directly or indirectly in the "breaks" or "gaps" in the neuron pathway by altering neurotransmitter influence at receptor sites on effector cells.

A direct agonist or antagonist attaches to a receptor site to either elicit or block a neurotransmitter response, respectively. For example, isoproterenol is a direct acting beta-adrenergic receptor agonist that mimics the action of the neurotransmitter norepinephrine. A direct cholinergic receptor antagonist, e.g., atropine, blocks cholinergic receptors to prevent the attachment of the neurotransmitter acetylcholine. On the other hand, indirect agents do not themselves attach to receptors; instead they alter the amount of neurotransmitter available. To illustrate, tyramine displaces norepinephrine from presynaptic storage sites, thereby increasing the amount of neurotransmitter in the synaptic cleft that is available for adrenergic receptor attachment. Conversely, a depletion of norepinephrine stores in adrenergic nerve terminals, e.g., that which occurs with guanethidine, elicits an adrenergic neuron blocking effect. Thus, an indirect effect relates to an increased or decreased amount of neurotransmitter available for attachment to receptors.

A hybrid, combined direct/indirect interaction may also occur. For instance, clonidine attaches to presynaptic central alpha$_2$-adrenergic receptors in a "direct" manner, but the reduction in sympathetic tone results from an inhibition of presynaptic norepinephrine release following the alpha$_2$-adrenergic receptor activation. Thus, the final "indirect" consequence

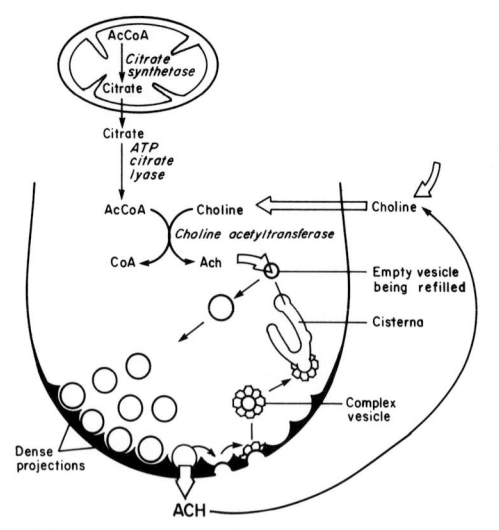

Fig. 2.3 Postulated mechanisms of synthesis, storage, and release of acetylcholine and the recycling of vesicles in cholinergic nerve endings. (Modified from Bowman, W.C., and Rand, M.J.: Textbook of Pharmacology, 2nd Ed. Oxford, Blackwell Scientific Publications, 1980.)

is the presence of less norepinephrine in the synaptic cleft or adrenergic nerve terminal-effector cell junction. This "bottom-line" feature of the drug's activity illustrates a combination "direct and indirect" receptor-neurotransmitter mechanism.

CHOLINERGIC TRANSMISSION

Acetylcholine is synthesized from acetyl Coenzyme A (CoA) and choline by the action of choline acetyltransferase (Figure 2.3). The source of acetyl CoA is citrate, an intermediate in oxidative carbohydrate metabolism. Choline is either obtained from exogenous sources or "recycled" following synaptic hydrolysis of acetylcholine by active transport into the cholinergic nerve terminals. Choline acetyltransferase is found in the cytoplasm of nerve ending particles. The enzyme actually originates in the perikaryon and travels to the nerve terminal where it catalyzes acetylcholine synthesis. Choline is the limiting factor in the synthesis of acetylcholine and about 50% of the choline produced by cholinesterase activity is reutilized to synthesize new acetylcholine.

After acetylcholine synthesis, the neurotransmitter is stored in vesicles. This "depot" acetylcholine in vesicles is the storage form primarily released by nerve impulses and accounts for about 85% of the original store. "Stationary" acetylcholine constitutes the remaining 15% that is not released by a nerve impulse.

A third storage form of acetylcholine is termed "surplus" acetylcholine. This intracellular form accumulates only in physostigmine (eserine) treated autonomic ganglia and is not released by nerve stimulation but rather by K^+.

The vesicles that house the newly synthesized acetylcholine are one of the most consistent ultrastructural features of junctional tissues. In cholinergic nerve endings, the synaptic vesicles range in diameter from 200 to 400 A units. These neurohumoral containers migrate toward the nerve terminal synaptic membrane during nerve stimulation and disgorge their acetylcholine contents by exocytosis. Thus, the vesicle and synaptic membrane essentially fuse prior to the exocytotic emptying of acetylcholine into the synaptic cleft.

Acetylcholine reversibly attaches to the postsynaptic membrane receptor and induces changes in the membrane character (Figure 2.4). The rate of dissociation of the neurotransmitter-receptor union occurs rapidly to actuate neuron activity with succeeding impulses.

Upon release from cholinergic nerve endings, acetylcholine is inactivated by several means. Enzymatic degradation of acetylcholine is accomplished by cholinesterase, including true or specific cholinesterase. This enzyme, associated with neural structures, is preferential in its catabolism of acetylcholine. Other sites containing true or specific cholinesterase (acetylcholinesterase) include the red blood cells and the placenta. Nonspecific cholinesterase catalyzes the hydrolysis of other choline esters, especially butyrylcholine. Plasma, liver, and glial cells contain the nonspecific cholinesterase. Nonenzymatic means of acetylcholine inactivation involve binding to nonreceptor sites, diffusion away from the neuron receptor site, and dilution in extracellular fluids.

Otto Loewi's classic experiments in 1921 es-

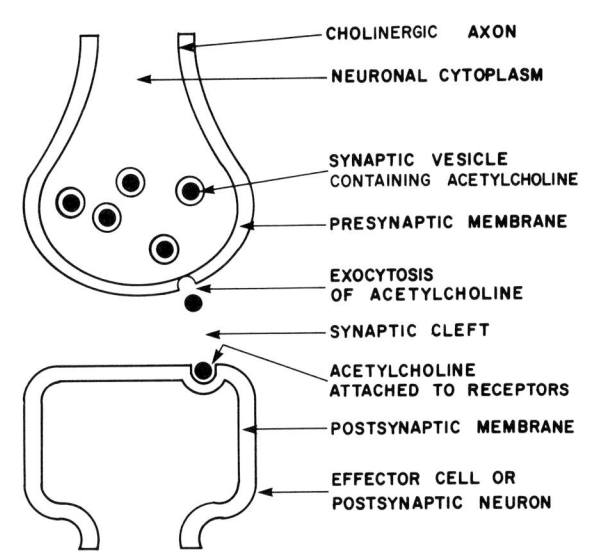

Fig. 2.4 Cholinergic transmission.

tablished the role of acetylcholine as a neurotransmitter. The following outlines Loewi's fundamental studies that were conducted on the perfused frog heart:
1. Vagal stimulation resulted in the release of a substance (Vagusstoff) into the perfusion fluid of the frog heart that slowed the rate of a second or recipient heart.
2. Atropine prevented the inhibiting effect of vagal stimulation on the frog heart.
3. Although atropine blocked the inhibitory effect of vagal stimulation, it did not block the release of Vagusstoff as perfusate collected from the donor heart after vagal stimulation slowed the rate of the second or recipient heart.
4. If the perfusate-containing Vagusstoff was incubated with ground-up frog heart tissue, the activity was lost. This indication of the inactivation of Vagusstoff was attributed to enzymatic destruction by cholinesterase.
5. Physostigmine (eserine), a cholinesterase inhibitor, reversed the inhibiting effect noted when the perfusate containing Vagusstoff was incubated with frog heart tissue.

Accordingly, the hypothesis that parasympathetic nerve endings (vagus) release acetylcholine (which then attaches to receptor cells on the heart muscle) emerged as a tenable explanation. Additionally, these data indicated that atropine blocks the effects of acetylcholine on the muscle cells but does not prevent its release after vagal stimulation. Physostigmine was noted to prevent destruction of acetylcholine but has no effect on the release of acetylcholine from vagal nerve endings.

ACETYLCHOLINE RECEPTOR

The acetylcholine receptor translates acetylcholine binding into changes in ionic permeability of the postsynaptic membrane. Membrane-bound, the acetylcholine receptor is concentrated mainly at synaptic sites. The isolation and characterization of the acetylcholine receptor was accomplished by using materials with a high acetylcholine receptor concentration, such as the intact electroplax of the electric eel (Electrophorus electricus) and frog skeletal muscle.

Isolation by subcellular fractionation techniques purifies the receptor material five to ten fold. Certain snake neurotoxins, such as bungarotoxin, bind specifically to postsynaptic acetylcholine receptors. Acetylcholine receptor affinity labels (such as "bungarotoxin") are introduced in situ to irreversibly bind to the membrane-bound acetylcholine receptors.

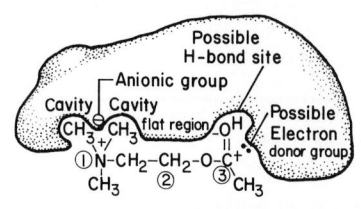

Fig. 2.5 Acetylcholine (ACh) and its postulated interaction with a receptor. (From Goldstein, A., Aronow, L., and Kalman, S.M.: Principles of Drug Action. The Basis of Pharmacology, 2nd Ed. Copyright © 1974, John Wiley & Sons, Inc. Reprinted with permission.)

NICOTINIC ACETYLCHOLINE RECEPTOR

Three points of attraction exist between acetylcholine and the nicotinic acetylcholine receptor. The affinity triad on the acetylcholine molecule consists of the quaternary nitrogen (1), the atom bridge separating the quaternary nitrogen from the carbonyl oxygen (2), and the carbonyl function (3), as indicated in Figure 2.5.

An anionic function on the receptor surface attracts the quaternary nitrogen of the acetylcholine molecule. The anionic receptor function is probably the carboxylate anions of aspartic or glutamic acids. These dicarboxylic amino acids are negatively charged at physiologic pH and are strong candidates as the anionic affinity source on the acetylcholine receptor. Two of the methyl groups on the quaternary nitrogen apparently add stability by enhancing the receptor cavity fit and binding through van der Waals forces.

The acetylcholine receptor topography contains a "flat" region adjacent to the anionic cavity. This area accomodates the atom bridge connecting the quaternary nitrogen and the carbonyl function. The atom span between the nitrogen and carbonyl function is relatively linear, and attraction by van der Waals forces occurs on the flat region of the receptor.

The carbonyl function of the acetylcholine receptor represents the last of the affinity triad that characterizes the acetylcholine molecule. The carbonyl oxygen forms hydrogen bonds with NH groups of peptide bonds on the receptor membrane surface. The carbonyl carbon interacts with an electron-rich area of the receptor. One hypothesis indicates that the epsilon-NH_2 group of a lysine residue is the interacting functional moiety.

Thus, electrostatic attraction, van der Waals forces, and hydrogen bonding collectively bind acetylcholine and its receptor together for the formation of a stable complex to initiate a biologic response. The bond tenacity of the acetylcholine-receptor combination is not strong enough to be irreversible.

Utilizing test compounds with two quaternary functions in the same molecule allows for certain postulations concerning the nicotine receptor topography. Specifically, one quaternary function reacts with the anionic site on the receptor active center, and the second one evidently causes a reaction at an additional anionic site outside the active center area on the receptor. The blockade of the second anionic site apparently causes nicotinic blockade at acetylcholine receptors on autonomic ganglia and at the neuromuscular junction.

The distance between the quaternary nitrogens on the methonium compounds (R_3-N^+-$(CH_2)_n$-N^+-R_3), as determined by the number of the methylene groups (CH_2), differentiates between nicotinic receptors at autonomic ganglia and neuromuscular junctions (Figure 2.6). A four to eight group carbon separation in the quaternary nitrogen functions produces compounds that are primarily autonomic ganglia blockers. The optimum distance for autonomic ganglionic blockade is either a five or six carbon separation.

Data suggest that the two nicotinic receptor anionic sites at the neuromuscular junctions are located farther apart. Thus, a separation of $(CH_2)_{10}$ is the preferred distance for blocking nicotinic receptors at the neuromuscular junctions. A linear separation of the quaternary functions is not necessarily required for neuromuscular blockade, but a distance of 14.5 to 15.0 Å units is critical. For example, neuromuscular nicotinic blocking drugs include d-tubocurarine, characterized by a complex interstial chemical structure between the cationic nitrogen functions, and pancuronium, in which a steroid nucleus separates the quaternary nitrogens.

The biologic translation of the acetylcholine-receptor combination is initially evidenced by a rapid influx of sodium ions and efflux of potas-

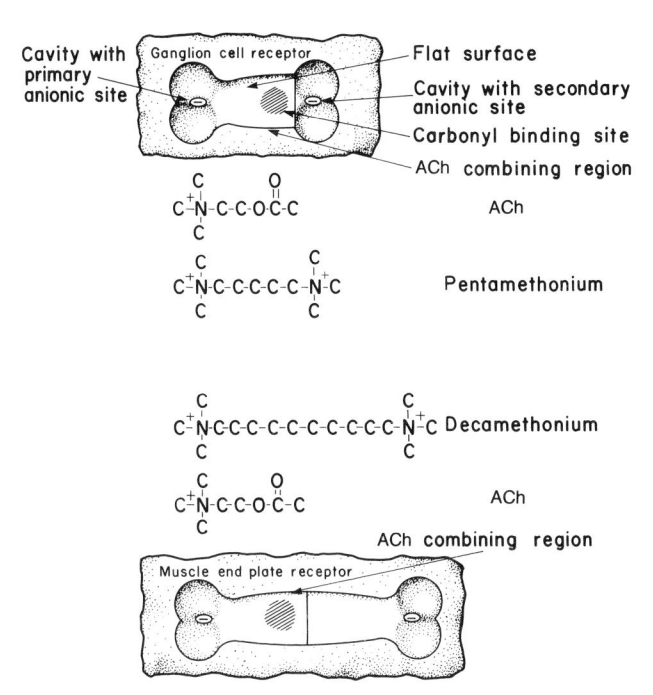

Fig. 2.6 Hypothetical acetylcholine (ACh) receptors. (Modified from Goldstein, A., Aronow, L., and Kalman, S.M.: Principles of Drug Action. The Basis of Pharmacology, 2nd Ed. Original figure copyright © 1974, John Wiley & Sons, Inc. Used with permission.)

sium ions through channels in the synaptic membrane. Depolarization of the synaptic membrane results from the ion flux and a specific physiologic event occurs.

Characterization of the properties of the nicotinic receptor at neuromuscular junctions on a molecular level indicates that the holoreceptor is a pentamer surrounding an ion channel (Figure 2.7). The receptor is composed of four subunits defined in the stoichometric ratio of alpha (2), beta, gamma, and delta subunits. Only the two alpha subunits contain the primary recognition sites for acetylcholine, acetylcholine antagonists, and snake toxins (such as bungarotoxin). Since acetylcholine binding of the alpha subunits is mutually exclusive of one another, the binding of two acetylcholine molecules results in a rapid transformational change that opens the ion channel for Na^+ influx and K^+ efflux.

MUSCARINIC ACETYLCHOLINE RECEPTOR

Physiologic responses to muscarinic receptor activation usually occur more slowly and less

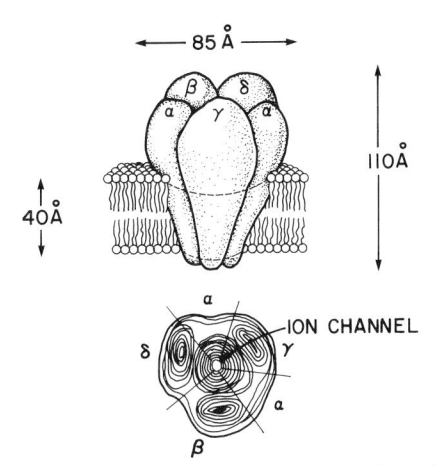

Fig. 2.7 Molecular structure of the cholinergic receptor at the neuromuscular junction. (Modified from Kistler, J., et al.: Structure and function of an acetylcholine receptor. Biophys. J., 37:371, 1982.)

dramatically than with nicotinic stimulation. Studies on the structural-activity relation of muscarinic receptor blocking drugs, such as atropine sulfate, have demonstrated certain features of the muscarinic receptor. The distance between the nitrogen atom and the carbonyl oxygen of the ester portion of atropine approaches the separation distance of these functional groups in the acetylcholine molecule (Figure 2.8). Consequently, the positively-charged nitrogen on acetylcholine agonists or antagonists forms an ionic bond with an anionic subsite on the muscarinic receptor (Figure 2.5). Hydrogen bonding occurs between the carbonyl function of acetylcholine agonists and antagonists and a cavity located at the esteratic subsite on the receptor substance.

The relative "fit" at this cavity subsite determines whether a compound is a muscarinic agonist or an antagonist. Smaller groups substituted on the carbonyl function elicit an agonist reaction (for example, acetylcholine), whereas if the substituted groups are bulky (such as

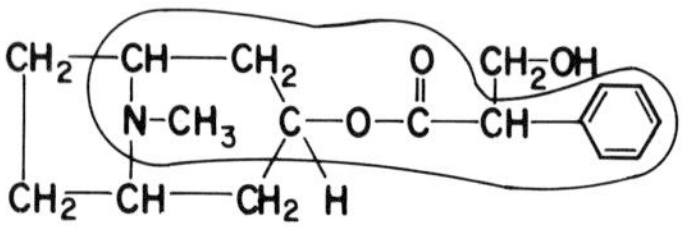

Fig. 2.8 Atropine structure

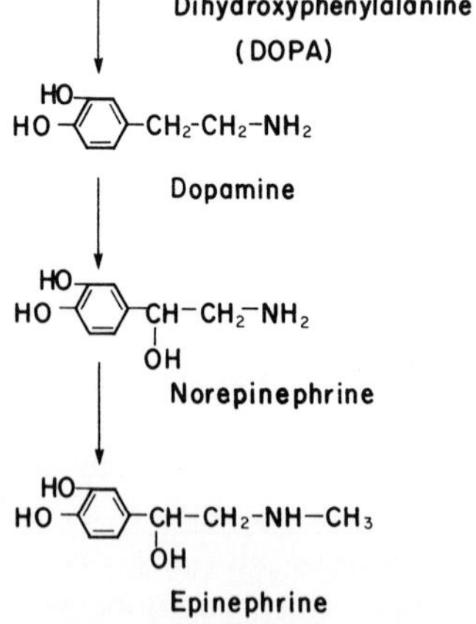

Fig. 2.9 Epinephrine biosynthesis

atropine), muscarinic receptor antagonism occurs. Stated another way, atropine and related compounds compete with muscarinic agonists (acetylcholine) for identical binding sites on muscarinic receptors.

Muscarinic receptors are subdivided into M_1 and M_2 designations. M_1 receptors are present on interneurons in autonomic ganglia and in certain regions of the central nervous system, whereas M_2 receptors are primarily present in cardiac tissue and gastrointestinal smooth muscle.

Biochemical changes at postsynaptic sites are noted upon muscarinic agonist attachment to the receptor substance. M_2 receptors may be linked to adenyl cyclase, in which inhibition of this enzyme occurs when these receptors are activated. M_2 receptor interaction with a guanine nucleotide-binding regulatory protein that binds guanosine triphosphate (GTP) may explain the adenyl cyclase inhibition. Another related theory hypothesizes that the combination of acetylcholine (or other cholinergic agonists) with the M_2 receptor activates guanylate cyclase, which forms guanosine 3', 5'-monophosphate (cyclic GMP).

Muscarinic receptor activation is also characterized by calcium ion influx across synaptic membranes. M_1 receptors probably regulate Ca^{++} fluxes and the synthesis of phosphorylated derivatives of inositol.

ADRENERGIC TRANSMISSION

The amino acid tyrosine is the immediate precursor in the formation of the endogenous catecholamines (Figure 2.9). Tyrosine hydroxylation is the rate limiting step in the synthesis of the adrenergic neurotransmitter, norepinephrine. Tyrosine hydroxylase, a unique constituent of adrenergic neurons and chromaffin cells, catalyzes the formation of dihydroxyphenylalanine (DOPA) from tyrosine.

DOPA, through the action of DOPA decarboxylase and pyridoxal phosphate, is converted to dopamine, the first non-amino acid intermediate in the biosynthesis scheme. DOPA decarboxylase, a fairly general decarboxylase, is also termed "L-aromatic amino acid decarboxylase." DOPA decarboxylase and dopamine-beta-hydroxylase are present in 100 to 1000 greater amounts than is tyrosine hydroxylase. These initial reactions, which convert tyrosine to dopamine, occur in the cytoplasm of the neuron terminal (Figure 2.10). Dopamine then enters the vesicles and undergoes hydroxylation (dopamine-beta-hydroxylase) to form norepinephrine. Virtually all norepinephrine is found in postganglionic sympathetic nerve terminals.

Further metabolic transmethylation of norepinephrine occurs in the chromaffin cells of the adrenal medulla to form epinephrine. Phenylethanolamine-N-methyltransferase catalyzes the formation of epinephrine from norepinephrine. The methyl group donor that functions as a cofactor in this conversion is S-adenosyl-L-methionine (SAM). Having a unique distribution, phenylethanolamine-N-methyltransferase is largely confined to the adrenal medulla.

Norepinephrine is the neurotransmitter released from adrenergic nerve terminals in the ANS. Norepinephrine is stored in highly specialized subcellular vesicles found in adrenergic nerve endings and chromaffin cells. These catecholamine storage vessels range in diameter from 400 to 1300 A units and are generally larger than their cholinergic counterparts, which store acetylcholine.

Monoamine oxidase (MAO) and catechol-o-methyltransferase (COMT) are the main enzymes involved in the catabolism of norepinephrine and epinephrine. The speed of degradation is considerably slower than that of acetylcholine hydrolysis by acetylcholinesterase. Intraneuronal MAO is important in catecholamine metabolism although the enzyme is also found extraneuronally. Whereas MAO is localized in the mitochondria, COMT is a relatively nonspecific enzyme that is found in the cytoplasm of most tissues.

The norepinephrine storage vesicles have an outer-limiting membrane that is selectively permeable to dopamine. Dopamine enters the vesicles and converts to norepinephrine by the action of dopamine-beta hydroxylase. A high concentration of catecholamine and ATP in a 4:1 ratio characterizes the granular storage of

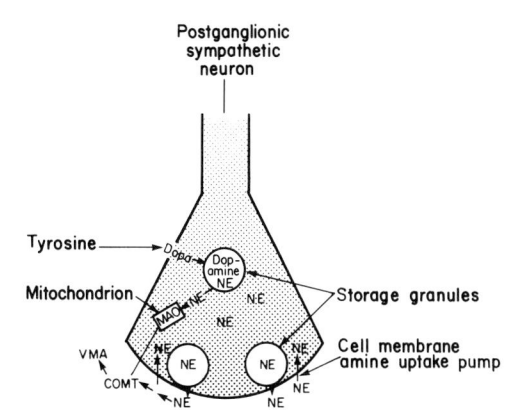

Fig. 2.10 Norepinephrine metabolism in the postganglionic sympathetic neuron. (Modified from Abrams, W.B.: The mechanisms of action of antihypertensive drugs. Dis. Chest, **55**:148, 1969.)

norepinephrine. Also contained in the vesicles is a soluble protein, chromogranin, which is somehow involved in the storage process.

The vesicles undergo an influx of Ca^{++} prior to norepinephrine release. The Ca^{++} influx into the norepinephrine vesicles is possibly the main stimulus responsible for both the mobilization of the norepinephrine vesicles toward the nerve terminal membrane during nerve stimulation and for their release of norepinephrine into the synaptic cleft. The entire contents of the norepinephrine vesicles empty into the adrenergic synapse by the process of exocytosis (Figure 2.11).

Inhibition of norepinephrine synthesis by norepinephrine end product feedback occurs in the presynaptic neuron. Mechanisms involved in the stimulation of norepinephrine synthesis include activation of tyrosine hydroxylase by cyclic AMP-dependent protein kinase and perhaps by Ca^{++}-dependent protein kinase. In addition, norepinephrine that has undergone active re-uptake from the junctional cleft into the adrenergic terminal (Uptake-1) is taken up into the synaptic storage vesicles.

The functions of catecholamine storage vesicles include the taking up of dopamine from the cytoplasm to protect it from enzymatic degradation by MAO and the subsequent oxidation of dopamine to the neurotransmitter substance norepinephrine. The vesicles bind and store norepinephrine to retard its diffusion out of the

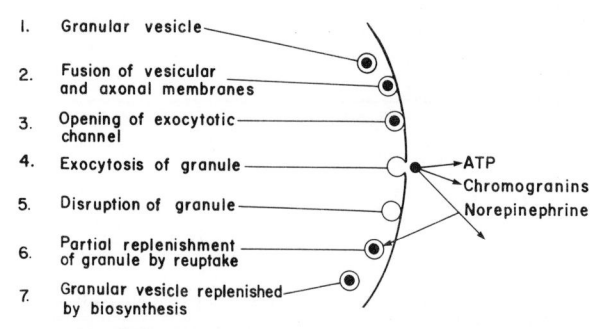

1. Granular vesicle
2. Fusion of vesicular and axonal membranes
3. Opening of exocytotic channel
4. Exocytosis of granule → ATP, Chromogranins, Norepinephrine
5. Disruption of granule
6. Partial replenishment of granule by reuptake
7. Granular vesicle replenished by biosynthesis

Fig. 2.11 Sequence of events in transmitter release at the sympathetic postganglionic neuron. (Modified from Bowman, W.C., and Rand, M.J.: Textbook of Pharmacology, 2nd Ed. Oxford, Blackwell Scientific Publications, 1980.)

neuron and protect it from the action of intra-neuron MAO. Finally, the vesicles serve as a depot of neurotransmitter, which is released upon the appropriate stimulus.

The following describes other important aspects of norepinephrine distribution and metabolism prior to its release from the presynaptic adrenergic neuron. Displacement of norepinephrine from storage vesicles by sympathomimetic amines (such as tyramine) is an important phenomenon. This represents an indirect mechanism whereby foodstuffs and beverages with a high tyramine content can have a pronounced adrenergic effect. Clinically significant food-drug interactions may involve this mechanism.

The displaced norepinephrine may be taken up into the storage vesicle (to contribute to a larger storage pool) or may diffuse out of the presynaptic neuron to interact with adrenergic receptors. Norepinephrine that is displaced by indirect acting amines and that which diffuses out of the vesicles is metabolized by mitochondrial monoamine oxidase.

The release of the vesicle-bound norepinephrine into the junctional space depends upon the Ca^{++} since in Ca^{++} deprivation, norepinephrine release fails. Pronounced Ca^{++} influx into neuronal sites occurs during norepinephrine release and Ca^{++} apparently precipitates the breakdown of the vesicle catecholamine-ATP (4:1) complex.

Fusion of the vesicle with the synaptic membrane results in subsequent discharge of the vesicle contents into the neuroeffector junction. Several different interactions of the released norepinephrine molecule with junctional structures are possible. First, the combination of norepinephrine with postsynaptic receptors on effector cells may occur, producing the appropriate physiologic response. A second course of norepinephrine distribution is its penetration into the effector cell (Uptake-2) in which its inactivation by catechol-o-methyltransferase (COMT) forms normetanephrine. Thirdly, norepinephrine may produce an activation of presynaptic adrenergic receptors (alpha$_2$) that inhibits norepinephrine release into the neuroeffector junction. A fourth mechanism operant in norepinephrine disposition is re-uptake into the presynaptic neuron (Uptake-1) and storage vesicles. This most important process terminates norepinephrine activity in the junctional space.

Thus, MAO and/or COMT activity is not a primary mechanism for terminating norepinephrine activity at adrenergic nerve terminals; rather, norepinephrine re-uptake mechanisms into the neuron and storage vesicles remove the neurotransmitter from receptor site proximity to reduce the likelihood of effector cell activation. The re-uptake mechanism for norepinephrine is an energy-requiring membrane transport process and can be blocked by inhibiting Na^+, K^+-activated ATPase.

ADRENERGIC RECEPTORS

In 1948, Ahlquist classified adrenergic receptors as alpha and beta, based upon the nature and degree of pharmacologic responses to agonists at various receptor sites and by studies that employed specific blocking agents. Responses associated with alpha-adrenergic receptors are vasoconstriction, mydriasis, and intestinal relaxation. Beta-adrenergic receptor functions include vasodilation, cardioacceleration, positive inotropic response, intestinal relaxation, and bronchiolar relaxation.

Sympathomimetics vary in the degree of activation of specific receptors and are designated as pure alpha-adrenergic agonists, mixed alpha-beta-adrenergic agonists, and pure beta-adrenergic agonists. For example, phenylephrine is mainly an alpha-adrenergic agonist, epinephrine has mixed alpha- and beta-adrenergic activity, and isoproterenol is an almost pure beta-adrenergic agonist.

Adrenergic receptors are located in the CNS and at the junction of postganglionic sympathetic nerve fibers and effector cells on smooth muscles, glands, amd visceral organs. Alpha-adrenergic receptors are subdivided into alpha$_1$ and alpha$_2$, depending upon their location and the function associated with their activation. For example, presynaptic alpha$_2$-adrenergic receptors in the (CNS) exert a negative feedback on sympathetic outflow from the CNS. Thus, clonidine, an alpha$_2$-adrenergic receptor agonist, reduces sympathetic outflow from the CNS by activating central alpha$_2$-adrenergic receptors. Central reduction of sympathetic influence inhibits peripheral adrenergic activity on arteriolar smooth muscle, thereby reducing vasoconstrictive predominance.

Alpha$_1$-adrenergic receptors, found at peripheral postsynaptic sites, have a major role in the regulation of adrenergic activity, including vasoconstrictive influence. Alpha$_1$-adrenergic receptors are also found in the CNS.

Postsynaptic alpha$_2$-adrenergic receptors are found in extrasynaptic sites in blood vessels and the CNS. As previously noted, alpha$_2$-adrenergic receptors are also found at presynaptic sites, as well as on postjunctional membranes. Activation of presynaptic alpha$_2$-adrenergic receptors causes a reduction of both neurotransmitter release and sympathetic influence.

Beta-adrenergic receptors are of two types: beta$_1$ and beta$_2$. Beta$_1$-adrenergic responses include cardiac stimulation and lipolysis, whereas beta$_2$-adrenergic receptor activation results include bronchodilation. The latter response accounts for the specific usefulness of beta$_2$-adrenergic agonists in bronchial asthma since bronchodilation is achieved with minimal cardiac stimulation.

ALPHA-ADRENERGIC RECEPTORS

The alpha-adrenergic receptor has four areas of affinity for the attachment of norepinephrine (Figure 2.12). The quartet of affinity sites on the receptor includes an anionic portion, an atom that donates a pair of electrons, an organometallic group, and a van der Waals binding site. The cationic protonated amino group of norepinephrine forms an ionic bond with the anionic portion of the receptor. Hydrogen bonding occurs with the receptor atom, which donates the electron pair. The catechol nucleus represents a third norepinephrine-receptor attachment that is bound by chelate formation between the catechol hydroxyl groups and an organometallic group on the receptor. Finally, binding of the aryl group of the catechol nucleus by van der Waals forces strengthens the adjacent chelate formation.

The anionic site on the alpha-adrenergic receptor is shielded in some manner, perhaps by steric hindrance, to prevent the formation of an ion pair with catecholamines that have large substituent groups on the amino nitrogen (such as isoproterenol).

The activation of alpha-adrenergic receptors elicits a contraction of most smooth muscles. The agonist-alpha-adrenergic receptor interaction is characterized by an increase in perme-

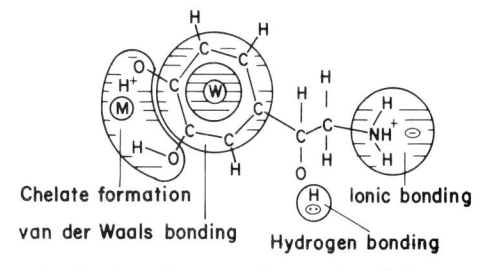

Fig. 2.12 Attachment of norepinephrine to an adrenoreceptor. (From Bowman, W.C., and Rand, M.J.: Textbook of Pharmacology, 2nd Ed. Oxford, Blackwell Scientific Publications, 1980.)

ability of the neuroeffector membrane to Na^+, K^+, Ca^{++}, and Cl^-, resulting in depolarization. In arterioles, for example, the smooth muscle contractile mechanisms are activated by the Ca^{++} influx that occurs during the passage of the action potential and depolarization.

Activation of the alpha-adrenergic receptors in intestinal smooth muscles causes relaxation. At these sites, the agonist-alpha-adrenergic receptor interaction causes a selective K^+ influx, resulting in hyperpolarization of the neuroeffector membrane.

BETA-ADRENERGIC RECEPTORS

The beta-adrenergic receptor does not exhibit the "shielding" phenomenon of the anionic binding site that characterizes the alpha-adrenergic receptor (Figure 2.13). Consequently, isoproterenol and other catecholamines with bulky substituent groups on the amino nitrogen unobtrusively attach to the receptor. Also, these agonists are even stronger beta-adrenergic receptor activating agents than is norepinephrine. One theory indicates that the substituent groups (such as the methyl groups) engage in additional van der Waals binding with the receptor substance.

A characteristic feature of beta-adrenergic

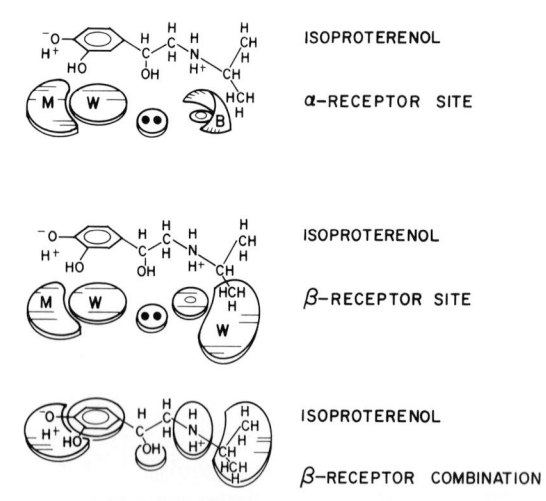

Fig. 2.13 Isoproterenol and adrenoreceptors. (Modified from Bowman, W.C., and Rand, M.J.: Textbook of Pharmacology, 2nd. Ed. Oxford, Blackwell Scientific Publications, 1980.)

receptor agonists is their ability to form quinone methides. Thus, when a beta-adrenergic agonist aligns to the receptor, the formation of this intermediate occurs with the subsequent methide reaction with the receptor. This combination constitutes the active agonist-receptor complex.

Beta-adrenergic receptors are either of the beta$_1$ (chiefly cardiac) or beta$_2$ (smooth muscle and metabolic effects) type. Adenosine 3', 5'-monophosphate (cyclic AMP) is the key compound involved in smooth muscle relaxation and metabolic effects. Smooth muscle inhibition, cardiac excitatory effects, and glandular secretory responses all relate to increases in the intracellular concentration of cyclic AMP.

Activation of beta$_1$-adrenergic receptors increases the rate and force of the heart beat. The agonist-receptor interaction increases the depolarization rate that precedes the cardiac action potential. Thus, an increased heart rate results from the increase in frequency of action potential firing. Additionally, an elevation of Ca^{++} in the cardiac cell promotes a positive inotropic action.

Stimulation of beta$_2$-adrenergic receptors relaxes the smooth muscles that possess tone and exhibit spontaneous activity. The rate of depolarization that precedes the action potential decreases, inhibiting spike generation. Activation of beta-adrenergic receptors also impairs smooth muscle excitation-contraction coupling by increasing Ca^{++} binding to the sarcoplasmic reticulum. Thus, less free Ca^{++} is available to activate the contractile mechanism. If a source of ATP is not available for conversion to cyclic AMP, beta-adrenergic receptor attachment will not result in smooth muscle relaxation.

The catecholamine recognition site of beta-adrenergic receptors (described earlier) relates functionally to the stimulation of adenyl cyclase (AC). The AC activation occurs through an adjacent bridging, which utilizes a guanine nucleotide-binding regulatory protein (Gs). All of these moeities are membrane-bound and function in unison upon beta-adrenergic receptor activation. Cyclic AMP is synthesized from adenosine triphosphate (ATP) in the cytoplasmic milieu that interfaces with the neuroeffector membrane.

The intracellular cytoplasmic receptor for cyclic AMP is a protein kinase (Figure 2.14). The subsequent activation of the protein kinase, following its interaction with cyclic AMP, results in several metabolic effects. Practically all of the actions of catecholamines appear linked to the activation of adenyl cyclase and the resultant increase in the intracellular concentration of cyclic AMP. However, studies have defined the pathway between the accumulation of cyclic AMP and response in only the case of the metabolic changes induced by catecholamines.

The intracellular protein kinase that acts as a receptor for cyclic AMP is a tetramer, consisting of two regulatory and two catalytic subunits. The activation reaction with cyclic AMP results in a dissociation of the enzyme that isolates the catalytic subunit. The cleaved catalytic subunit phosphorylates a number of enzymes, including those involved in the regulation of glycogenolysis and lipolysis.

The activation of the enzyme phosphorylase kinase by the catalytic subunit affects glucogenolysis. Phosphorylase kinase catalyzes the conversion of "inactive" phosphorylase to "active" phosphorylase, thus promoting glycogenolysis by the "active" phosphorylase and favoring glucose formation. The hyperglycemia so induced relates to the activation of hepatic glycogen phosphorylase.

The catalytic subunit formed by the cyclic AMP-protein kinase also phosphorylates glycogen synthase. In this case, inhibition of the enzyme reduces glycogen synthesis. The phosphorylation of glycogen synthase functions in concert with phosphorylase kinase activation to produce increased glycogenolysis, causing hyperglycemia.

Phosphorylation of triglyceride lipase by the catalytic subunit results in an increased lipolysis in adipose tissue, increasing circulation levels of lipids (hyperlipidemia). Thus, catacholamines increase amounts of circulating substrates, namely glucose and fatty acids, for energy utilization by a complex biochemical cascade set in motion by the initial agonist-beta-adrenergic receptor interaction.

DISORDERS TREATED WITH AUTONOMIC DRUGS

A variety of disorders respond to autonomic drug therapy. The ability of autonomic drugs to correct disorder symptoms largely depends upon their agonist or antagonist action at autonomic receptors on the affected structure.

DISEASES TREATED WITH CHOLINERGIC DRUGS

Cholinergic drugs correct certain disorders by activating muscarinic receptors on target struc-

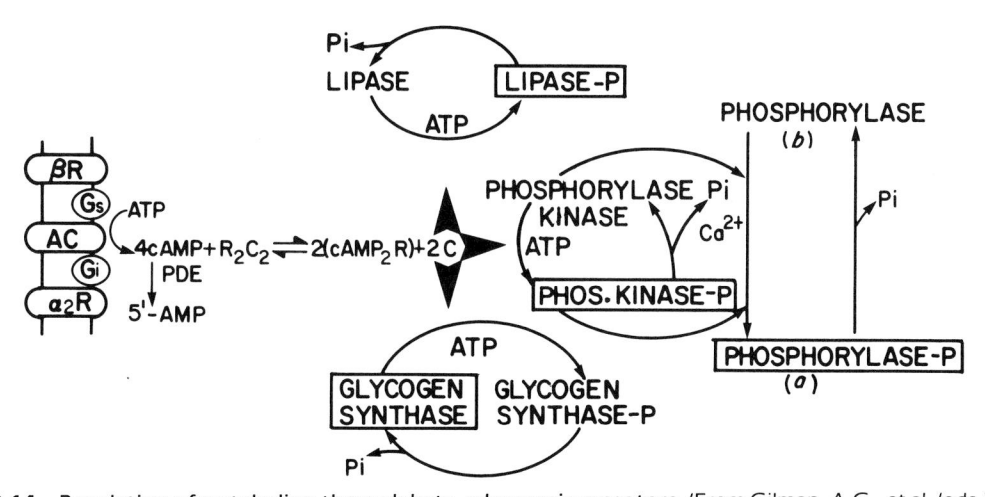

Fig. 2.14 Regulation of metabolism through beta-adrenergic receptors. (From Gilman, A.G., et al. (eds.): The Pharmacological Basis of Therapeutics, 7th Ed. New York, Macmillan Publishing Co., Inc., 1985.)

tures, such as the iris musculature (sphincter iridis) and the urinary bladder (detrusor urinae). Certain diseases involving the skeletal muscles (voluntary) also respond to cholinergic drugs. Their use is based upon the drug's direct or indirect stimulation of nicotinic receptors at the motor end plate on skeletal muscle. Additionally, some cholinergic drugs act on nicotinic receptors to induce skeletal muscle relaxation.

GLAUCOMA

Glaucoma, a group of eye diseases characterized by increased intraocular pressure, affects 2% of all Americans over the age of 40. Pathologic changes induced in the optic disk probably relate to ischemia of the ocular blood vessels and damage to the optic nerve, which sometimes leads to blindness. Glaucoma is the primary cause of blindness in the United States.

Aqueous humor forms at the ciliary processes by filtration and active secretion (Figure 2.15). The aqueous humor flows through the pupil and into the anterior chamber of the eye and is then reabsorbed through the trabecular meshwork, a specialized area of the corneal-iris angle. Increased intraocular pressure results from either increased formation or decreased absorption of aqueous humor.

The canal of Schlemm, an aqueous humor drainage channel, and the trabecular meshwork are located in the proximity of the cornea-iris angle. Fluid normally filters through perforations in the meshwork (spaces of Fontana) and then channels out of the angle region to venous outlets on ocular surfaces.

Glaucoma is designated as primary or secondary. Structural defects or degenerative changes take place in the anterior chamber of the eye; these interfere with the normal circulation of the ocular aqueous humor and result in primary glaucoma. If the elevation of intraocular pressure occurs subsequent to infection or inflammation, the condition is termed "secondary" glaucoma. Primary glaucoma, the most common form, exists as two variations: (1) chronic open-angle glaucoma and (2) acute narrow-angle or closed glaucoma. The angle refers to the space between the base of the corneal contact site with the sclera and is also called the cornea-iris angle and "critical angle."

Chronic Open-angle Glaucoma. In this form of glaucoma, the angle is normal, but a defect in the trabecular meshwork decreases drainage into the canal of Schlemm. This condition often has an insidious onset as the intraocular pressure gradually increases without symptoms.

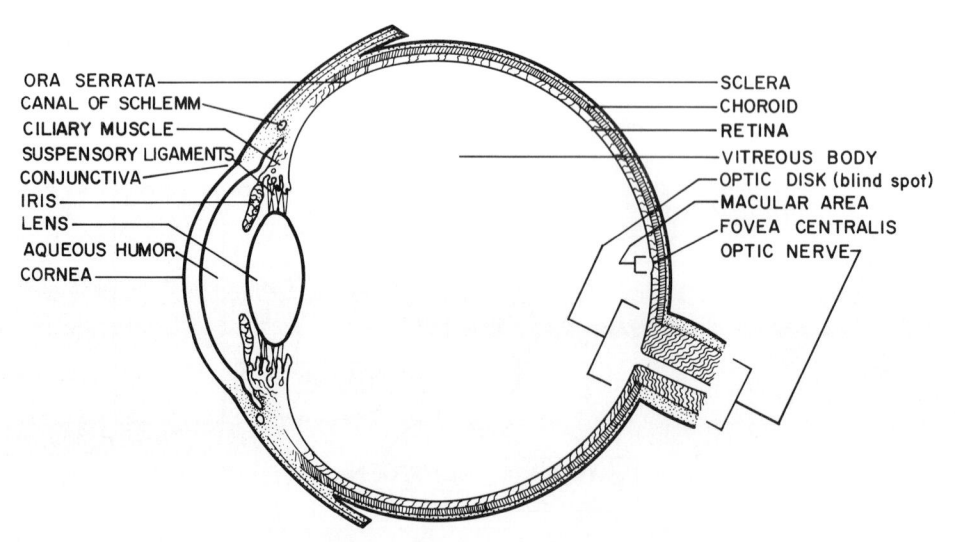

Fig. 2.15 Schematic section of the human eye. (Illustration courtesy of the American Optometric Association, St. Louis, Mo.)

Diagnosis is sometimes made only after some damage to the optic nerve has occurred. "Tunnel vision" (loss of peripheral vision) characterizes progression of this condition. Miotics, such as pilocarpine and physostigmine, cause ciliary muscle contraction, resulting in a pulling on the scleral spur. The miotic effect opens drainage paths in the trabecular meshwork and facilitates aqueous humor outflow.

Acute Narrow-angle Glaucoma. In acute narrow-angle glaucoma, the anterior chamber of the eye is shallow and the trabecular area at the cornea-iris critical angle occludes because of the sharp angle present. Initial pressure change causes an iris bulge that blocks the flow of aqueous humor through the pupil, a condition that makes immediate treatment imperative. Pressure elevation following angle closure can occur suddenly; also, permanent ocular damage results within a few hours after the onset of an attack.

Dilation of the pupils always aggravates narrow-angle glaucoma because the folds of the iris (i.e., the circular pigmented membrane surrounding the pupil) further block the narrow angle as the pupil enlarges. Constriction of the pupil pulls the iris musculature away from the critical cornea-iris angle, thereby relieving blockage of the trabecular meshwork where fluid (aqueous humor) drains into the canal of Schlemm. Thus, miotics are indicated in the treatment of acute narrow-angle glaucoma.

Emotional reactions that cause pupillary dilation sometimes precipitate acute attacks of this disease. Also, accidental ingestion of drugs that cause the pupil to dilate (such as mydriatics) sets off acute attacks.

Secondary Glaucoma. If infection and subsequent inflammatory processes cause secondary glaucoma, reduction in the intraocular pressure usually follows treatment with an antibiotic (or anti-infective) and an anti-inflammatory agent (such as a corticosteroid).

Other forms of secondary glaucoma, similar to that which results from dislocation of the lens, usually require surgical intervention.

MYASTHENIA GRAVIS

A chronic disease, myasthenia gravis is characterized by variable degrees of skeletal muscle weakness. Abnormalities of the thymus gland are often present. This disease frequently begins in the muscles of the eye, and ptosis of the eyelids is a common finding in the early stages. Marked skeletal muscle fatigue is another characteristic of this disease. Myasthenia gravis may result from an autoimmune reaction, which damages acetylcholine receptors at the neuromuscular end plate.

Antibodies that are present in the plasma of patients with myasthenia gravis reduce the number of acetylcholine receptors present at the postjunctional end plate. Abnormalities are also noted in the ultrastructural framework of the postsynaptic membrane.

Myasthenia gravis diagnosis is usually accomplished by a thorough examination of the history, signs, and symptoms in the patient. The disease is differentiated from other neuromuscular disorders by a pharmacologic test that utilizes the acetylcholinesterase inhibitor, edrophonium. A positive confirmation of myasthenia gravis consists of the immediate improvement of the extraocular muscle strength after an intravenous test dose of edrophonium. Neostigmine is sometimes substituted for edrophonium.

POSTOPERATIVE GASTROINTESTINAL ATONY AND PARALYTIC ILEUS (ADYNAMIC ILEUS)

Paralysis or atony of the intestinal walls with abdominal distention is a consequence of a variety of physiologic disorders and surgical causes. Paralytic ileus is produced by peritoneal irritation that results from mechanical disruption of the abdominal viscera during surgical procedures, peritonitis, peptic ulcer perforation, and other such traumatic stimuli. Inhibition of ilium movement occurs because of a spinal reflex termed the "intestino-intestinal reflex". Adrenergic sympathetic neurons comprise the efferent leg of the reflex loop. The efferent adrenergic fibers relay information to cell bodies of excitatory cholinergic neurons, subsequently reducing cholinergic influence and inhibiting intestinal activity.

Stasis of the gastrointestinal contents may lead to gas formation and distention, a situation further aggravating the ileus by accentuating the intestino-intestinal reflex. The clinical consequence of paralytic ileus includes malabsorption of foodstuffs and fluid loss into the ileum lumen.

URINARY BLADDER ATONY

Postoperative dysuria results from atony of the detrusor muscle of the urinary bladder. The time period between the surgery and spontaneous urination shortens by the use of cholinergic agents (direct or indirect). Determining that the urinary retention is nonobstructive before cholinergic drugs are administered is important because inducing urinary bladder contraction when excretion of urine is blocked presents a clinical emergency.

DISEASES TREATED WITH CHOLINERGIC BLOCKING DRUGS

Hypermotility and/or increased muscle tone are associated with gastrointestinal disorders, such as peptic ulcer, pylorospasm, and spastic colitis. Antispasmodic cholinergic blocking drugs are often used as adjunctive therapy in these diseases. Cholinergic blocking drugs are also used in ophthalmic procedures to dilate the pupil and to dry secretions prior to surgical procedures.

PEPTIC ULCER

The term "peptic ulcer" designates a gastrointestinal ulceration that is bathed with gastric secretions (including pepsin and hydrochloric acid). Affected areas include the stomach, duodenum, and esophagus. The latter two regions are not routinely in contact with gastric contents and the presence of gastric secretions (such as esophageal reflux) causes inflammation and possibly ulceration.

Most ulcers in the duodenum and esophagus occur in the area adjacent to the stomach. These proximal areas receive a high concentration of the leaked or regurgitated gastric juice. Self-digestive processes become operant and are evidenced by the erosion of the mucosa of the affected area, as well as by digestive damage to the muscle layer below the mucosa. The stomach lining, normally bathed in gastric juice, is protected from its digestive action by a mucosal barrier. Nevertheless, gastric ulcers may result if a breakdown in this mucosal protection occurs.

DUODENAL ULCER

Occurring five times as often as gastric ulcers, duodenal ulcers affect males four times more frequently than females. Practically all (95%) duodenal ulcers occur in close proximity (within 5 cm) of the pyloric opening into the stomach. The incidence of malignancy in duodenal ulcers is low.

Factors involved in the development of duodenal ulcers include stress, diet, excessive alcohol use, and the chronic use of irritating medicinal drugs (for example, aspirin). Common symptoms of duodenal ulcer are a burning sensation in the center of the abdomen, heartburn, and nausea. Food, milk, or antacids sometimes temporarily relieve these symptoms, which are most noticeable about an hour after eating.

GASTRIC ULCER

Gastric ulcers are not as common as duodenal ulcers. Most gastric ulcers appear within a few centimeters of the pyloric sphincter along the lesser curvature of the antrum. Pyloric sphincter dysfunction, which allows reflux of bile acids from the duodenum into the stomach, has been implicated in the pathogenesis of gastric ulcer. Chronic gastritis and genetic factors may be predisposing influences. The symptoms and treatment of gastric ulcer are similar to those of duodenal ulcer.

ESOPHAGEAL ULCER

Regurgitation of gastric contents can inflame and irritate the immediate esophageal lining to the point of causing ulceration. The symptoms and treatment of esophageal ulcer resemble those for both duodenal and gastric ulcer.

DISEASES TREATED WITH ADRENERGIC DRUGS

The role of cyclic nucleotides (e.g., cyclic AMP and cyclic GMP) in the causation of bronchial asthma is an active research area. Beta$_2$-adrenergic receptor agonists elevate cyclic AMP, a biochemical response which relates to bronchodilation and benefits bronchial asthma. The beta$_1$-adrenergic receptor agonists produce cardiac stimulation and are used in the treatment of various heart disorders. Additional clinical uses of adrenergic drugs relate to alpha-adrenergic receptor activation and include maintenance of blood pressure in hypotensive states and relief of nasal congestion.

BRONCHIAL ASTHMA

A chronic condition, bronchial asthma is marked by recurrent attacks of paroxysmal dyspnea. Spasmodic contraction of the bronchi causes wheezing; other clinical manifestations are production of mucoid sputum and coughing. The characteristic labored or difficult breathing can progressively worsen, leading to an acidosis due to an accumulation of carbon dioxide in the blood. Also, electrolyte imbalance may occur.

Patients with bronchial asthma are a special risk if concurrent cardiac disease exists. The frequent respiratory infections common in asthma patients can spark acute emergency situations such as congestive heart failure and cardiac arrest. Airway obstructions that block the free flow of air out of the lungs can precipitate acute pulmonary failure.

Asthma is classified into two types: extrinsic asthma and intrinsic asthma. Extrinsic asthma relates to immunologic and biochemical abnormalities; the causes of intrinsic asthma are not well understood.

Extrinsic asthma occurs in genetically susceptible individuals ranging in age from 5 to 35. These patients apparently become sensitized to one or more antigens that are absorbed transmucosally. Exposure to the antigen (or antigens) forms a skin-sensitizing (reaginic) antibody, designated as "IgE" (immunoglobulin E), which characterizes allergic disease.

The interaction of an IgE with the antigen produces a series of cellular changes, particularly in mast cells. The release of substances, including histamine, from mast cells increases capillary permeability as evidenced by edema formation. Hypersecretion of mucous glands and contraction of bronchiolar smooth muscle also characterize the IgE-antigen interaction.

In addition to histamine, other substances that are released from mast cells have been identified in the asthmatic attack. Slow-reacting substance of anaphylaxis (SRS-A) is a possible chemical mediator in asthma pathology. Regardless of the precipitating mediator, the subsequent narrowing of the airway passages and obstruction of air flow characterize the clinical asthma attack.

Intrinsic asthma affects a different age group, as compared to extrinsic asthma; i.e., intrinsic asthma patients are younger than 5 and older than 35 and characteristically have no previous history of allergy or positive reaction to skin test antigens. In contrast to extrinsic asthma, an immunologic mechanism for intrinsic asthma has not been proven.

Both types of bronchial asthma patients respond favorably to bronchodilators, such as epinephrine. This positive response to bronchodilator drugs distinguishes asthma from other disease states that are characterized by a fixed obstruction of pulmonary passages. The latter condition does not respond favorably to bronchodilator chemotherapy.

SHOCK

Shock is a general term that designates inadequate blood perfusion of tissues. Acute peripheral circulatory failure results from derangement of circulatory control or loss of circulatory fluid (i.e., hypovolemia). This condition is marked by hypotension, as well as by an increase in heart rate. Coldness of the skin and anxiety are other clinical signs of shock.

Shock is not always accompanied by low arterial blood pressure or reduced cardiac output; thus, other signs of inadequate perfusion to vital organs must be monitored. These additional indications include reduced urine output, mental confusion, cardiac abnormalities, and increased blood levels of the products of anaerobic metabolism, including lactic acid. Once shock is diagnosed on the basis of decreased tissue perfusion, assessment of the primary hemodynamic abnormalities is necessary. Plasma expanders that increase intravascular volume are required if hypovolemia is a major determinant of the shock.

Adrenergic agents and other drugs that affect the autonomic nervous system are often useful in shock because of their effects on the cardiac output and peripheral resistance.

DISEASES TREATED WITH ADRENERGIC BLOCKING DRUGS

Disorders of the blood vessels and cardiovascular disease often respond to adrenergic blocking drugs.

BUERGER'S DISEASE (THROMOANGITIS OBLITERANS)

Buerger's disease, an inflammatory disease of the peripheral arteries, usually affects the arteries of the legs (particularly the tibial artery). Pain is felt in the instep and often phlebitis is present. Circulatory problems that characterize Buerger's disease are not due to a buildup of fatty material in the blood vessels (atherosclerotic processes). The disease, frequently associated with heavy smoking, occurs predominantly in young to middle-aged men (24 to 45 years). Severe pain and ischemic disorders of the legs may result in gangrene, necessitating amputation.

Nicotine or some other component in tobacco smoke apparently sensitizes the peripheral arteries and produces inflammation. Thrombosis, accompanied by abscess formation and tissue necrosis, results from the inflammation and arterial blockage.

Vasodilators are somewhat beneficial although the response to these agents is often poor since arterial spasm is not a characteristic of this disease.

RAYNAUD'S DISEASE (RAYNAUD'S PHENOMENON)

Raynaud's disease is characterized by spasm in the superficial peripheral arteries, resulting in numbness and pain in the hands or fingers and occasionally in the feet or tip of the nose. In contrast to Buerger's disease, smoking is not directly involved in the etiology of Raynaud's disease; however, the smoking habit contributes to arterial constriction, necessitating avoidance. Vasodilators, often useful in treating Raynaud's disease, directly counteract the arterial spasm.

The exact cause of Raynaud's disease is not yet known although exaggerated sympathetic nervous system activity in the periphery is a likely etiologic factor. Exposure to cold or emotional stress aggravate this disease.

MIGRAINE

Migraine is a symptom complex of periodic vascular headaches, which are usually temporal and unilateral. These "throbbing" headaches are often associated with irritability, nausea, vomiting, constipation or diarrhea, and photophobia. Migraine headache, usually attributed to the recurrent dilation of cranial arteries, is the most common of all neurologic disorders with an estimated prevalence rate ranging from 4 to 30%.

The pathophysiology of migraine is associated with an initial intracranial vasoconstriction that is evidenced by resultant prodromal (usually ocular) symptoms. Vasodilation and local edema then follow to produce the characteristic headache.

Precipitating factors, such as anxiety and physical or emotional stress, probably release catecholamines (epinephrine and norepinephrine), indoleamines (tryptamine and 5-hydroxy tryptamine), and prostaglandins ($PGF_{2\ alpha}$). Depletion of vascular serotonin and norepinephrine, along with histamine and neurokinin release, apparently produce the cerebral vasodilation and edema that occur in migraine headaches.

The severe pain, which results from distended, dilated cranial and extracranial arteries, occurs when pain receptors in the stretched arterial smooth muscle are stimulated. Histamine and neurokinin release also contribute to activation of pain receptors and vasodilation in migraine headaches.

MIGRAINE NEURALGIA (CLUSTER HEADACHE)

Cluster headaches are characterized by severe pain, mainly retro-orbital, associated with lacrimation and blockage of the nostril on the same side of the face. These headaches last for days or weeks and each attack persists from less than an hour to several hours.

CARDIOVASCULAR DISEASES

Cardiovascular diseases and other vascular disorders amenable to beta-adrenergic blocking drugs are discussed in Chapters 3 and 4.

AUTONOMIC DRUGS

Autonomic drugs are classified as cholinergic drugs, cholinergic blocking drugs, adrenergic drugs, and adrenergic blocking drugs. Agonist activity on autonomic receptors is achieved by either direct or indirect means. Antagonist action is usually a competitive and reversible process in which the receptor blocking drug prevents the neurotransmitter from attaching to the postsynaptic receptor substance. Thus, physiologic activities including membrane permeability to ions (e.g., Na^+, Ca^{++}, and Cl^-), biochemical reactions (e.g., glycogenolysis, lipolysis), and mechanical events (e.g., myocardial contraction, vascular smooth muscle relaxation) are accomplished (agonist) or prevented (antagonist), depending upon the nature of the autonomic drug.

CHOLINERGIC DRUGS

Cholinergic drugs (Table 2.2) elicit their pharmacologic responses by activating cholinergic receptors. These acetylcholine receptors are classified as either muscarinic or nicotinic. The muscarinic or nicotinic receptor agonist activity is classically defined in terms of pharmacologic response. Thus, a muscarinic action (i.e., neuroeffectors on glands, smooth muscles, and visceral organs) is characterized by salivation, lacrimation, increased gastrointestinal motility, and a slow heart rate. Nicotinic responses, in contrast, include rapid heart beat and hypertension (autonomic ganglia) and skeletal muscle contractions (motor end plate).

Muscarinic and nicotinic receptors have been extensively described in the periphery, but their

Table 2.2 CHOLINERGIC STIMULANTS

Available products	Trade names	Daily dosage range
Direct acting:		
Bethanechol Cl	Urecholine; Duvoid	10–50 mg b.i.d.–q.i.d ; 2–5 mg SC
Carbachol	Carbacel; Isopto Carbachol	0.75–3% topically
Pilocarpine HCl	various	0.5–3% solution ophthalmic
Pilocarpine nitrate	P.V. Carpine Liquifilm	0.5–3% solution ophthalmic
Indirect acting:		
Ambenonium Cl	Mytelase	5–25 mg t.i.d. or q.i.d.
Demecarium Br	Humorsol	Ophthalmic 1–2 drops: 0.25% b.i.d.
Edrophonium Cl	Tensilon	5–20 mg
Echothiophate iodide	Phospholine iodide	Ophthalmic instillation not to exceed 0.25% and b.i.d.
Isoflurophate	Floropryl	Ophthalmic ointment
Neostigmine Br	Prostigmin Br	10–30 mg orally
Neostigmine	Prostigmin methylsulfate	0.25–1 mg IM or SC methylsulfate
Physostigmine	Eserine sulfate; Isopto Eserine	Ointment: 0.25%; Ophthalmic solution: 0.25%
Physostigmine salicylate	Antilirium	1 or 2 mg t.i.d.

role in the CNS is less clear. Research in central acetylcholine neuron pathways is important for the study of novel pharmacologic activity. For example, an acetylcholine precursor, dimethylethanolamine, has been promoted for its effects on mood and learning.

Cholinergic drugs act on the ANS by either a direct action on acetylcholine receptors or by an indirect effect that increases endogenous acetylcholine concentration at synaptic and neuroeffector junctions.

DIRECT ACTING CHOLINERGIC DRUGS

Direct acting cholinergic drugs are agonists at muscarinic and nicotinic receptor sites.

Acetylcholine. Acetylcholine, the endogenous neurotransmitter at cholinergic synapses, is rarely employed as a therapeutic agent. Rapid hydrolysis by plasma cholinesterase causes the transient and fleeting action of acetylcholine.

Mechanism of Action. Acetylcholine directly stimulates both muscarinic and nicotinic receptors, depending upon accessibility to the receptor site and dosage. This drug produces rapid and complete miosis by intraocular administration.

Clinical Indications. Acetylcholine, administered by intraocular instillation (not topical) into the anterior chamber, induces pupillary constriction in cataract surgery, penetrating keratoplasty, iridectomy, and other anterior segment procedures. A miotic effect facilitates iridectomy and is also valuable after removal of the lens (e.g., cataract surgery) in which case a necessary and rapid pupillary closure prevents forward displacement of the vitreous humor and subsequent retinal detachment.

Adverse Effects/Precautions. No significant reactions are expected because of acetylcholine's localized activity.

Methacholine. Methacholine, a choline ester, has a methyl group on the beta carbon of choline.

Mechanism of Action. A direct acting cholinergic drug, methacholine preferentially activates muscarinic receptors. Smooth muscles, glands, and the heart respond to methacholine, a drug that is essentially devoid of activity on autonomic ganglia and skeletal muscle (nicotinic sites). The duration of response of methacholine is longer and more persistent than that of acetylcholine because of the slower rate of hydrolysis by acetylcholinesterase. Methacholine resists hydrolysis by nonspecific cholinesterase.

Clinical Indications. Methacholine is used in selected cases of atrial tachycardia that are unresponsive to other forms of therapy. Because of its dilator effect, methacholine has been used to treat peripheral vascular disease. The drug's ionic nature allows effective administration by electrophoresis to produce vasodilation. The degree of response to methacholine is difficult to predict, thus limiting its therapeutic acceptability.

Adverse Effects/Precautions. Muscarinic side effects, such as salivation, nasal stuffiness, and diarrhea, may occur with this drug.

Carbachol. Carbachol is an ester of carbamic acid (rather then acetic acid, as in acetylcholine) and choline.

Mechanism of Action. Carbachol is a potent muscarinic agonist that is not readily hydrolyzed by acetylcholinesterase or nonspecific choline esterase (because of the resistance of the carbamoyl group to degradation). Carbachol's nicotinic agonist action limits its therapeutic utility. The release of endogenous acetylcholine from cholinergic nerve terminals contributes to the cholinergic response.

Vasodilation, bradycardia, increased motility and tone of smooth muscles, and stimulation of salivary, lacrimal, and sweat glands are muscarinic responses noted with carbachol. Additionally, nicotinic receptors at autonomic ganglia are stimulated, producing unpredictable autonomic responses. Nicotinic receptor activation also occurs at the motor end plate on skeletal muscle. Carbachol, because of the ancillary nicotinic action, resists the cholinergic blocking activity of atropine. Carbachol selectively activates muscarinic receptors in the gastrointestinal and urinary tracts.

Clinical Indications. The principal therapeutic use of carbachol is as a miotic agent in ophthalmology procedures; the drug is used either topically for the treatment of glaucoma or intraocularly in ocular surgery. Use of a wetting agent, such as benzalkonium chloride, facilitates corneal penetration of carbachol.

Adverse Effects/Precautions. Side effects are minimal and unlikely due to the localized application of carbachol.

Bethanechol. Bethanechol, structurally similar to both methacholine and carbachol, has selective muscarinic agonist properties and is not readily hydrolyzed by either acetylcholinesterase or nonspecific cholinesterase.

Mechanism of Action. Bethanechol selectively activates muscarinic receptors in the gastrointestinal and urinary tracts, increasing the tone and amplitude of contraction of the stomach and intestines. Peristalsis is stimulated and the secretions of the gastrointestinal tract increase. The detrusor urinae muscle of the urinary bladder contracts and the vesical trigone and external sphincter relax. These actions, as well as an increase in ureteral peristalsis, result in urinary evacuation.

Clinical Indications. Bethanechol, used as a stimulant to the urinary bladder, aids postoperative and postpartum urinary retention. Selected cases of chronic hypotonic myogenic or neurogenic bladder are also amenable to bethanechol therapy. Another of this drug's clinical applications is in postoperative abdominal distention and gastric atony.

Adverse Effects/Precautions. Adverse reactions are uncommon with bethanechol. Possible muscarinic side effects include a fall in blood pressure, involuntary defecation, urinary urgency, and salivation.

Contraindications for bethanechol use are bronchial asthma, severe cardiac disease, and mechanical obstruction of the urinary or gastrointestinal tracts. Hyperthyroid patients have developed atrial fibrillation following bethanechol administration.

Pilocarpine. Pilocarpine is an alkaloid found in the leaves of various species of South American shrubs, genus Pilocarpus. Because of its tertiary amine structure, the alkaloid has better penetration across membranes, but its muscarinic activity is weaker than that exhibited by acetylcholine.

Mechanism of Action. The cholinergic agonist actions of pilocarpine are mainly on muscarinic receptors. Additional nicotinic actions of pilocarpine include facilitating impulses across autonomic ganglia and stimulating epinephrine release from the adrenal medulla.

Optimal requirements of a muscarinic agonist include an ether oxygen situated about 0.3 nm from a methonium group and a methyl group at a distance of 0.54 nm from the methonium group. Consequently, compounds other than choline esters (but having these structural characteristics) exhibit significant muscarinic activity. The absence of an ether oxygen in the pilocarpine molecule probably accounts for the considerably weaker muscarinic action of pilocarpine when compared to acetylcholine.

Pilocarpine, upon local application to the eye, is well absorbed through the cornea. The subsequent miosis pulls away the iris musculature from the critical cornea-iris angle and decreases resistance to the outflow of aqueous humor. Contraction of the ciliary muscle opens the intertrabecular spaces and facilitates aqueous humor outflow. A fall in intraocular pressure occurs in chronic open-angle glaucoma, as well as in acute angle-closure or chronic glaucoma.

Clinical Indications. Pilocarpine is generally the initial cholinergic agonist employed in the treatment of glaucoma. The drug acts synergistically with anticholinesterase drugs in the reduction of intraocular pressure. The combination of pilocarpine with anticholinesterase therapy enables a reduction in the concentration of the anticholinesterase agent. Clinical benefit accrues since the adverse effects of anticholinesterase agents are dose-related.

Additional uses of pilocarpine, based upon its miotic effect, include the reversal of atropine-induced pupillary dilation and the breaking of adhesions between the iris and the lens (alternate use of mydriatics and pilocarpine). Sustained release of pilocarpine is achieved with a copolymer ellipically-shaped unit containing pilocarpine that is placed in the cul de sac of the eye. The relatively constant release of drug in the pilocarpine ocular unit approximates a 1 to 2% solution of a pilocarpine salt. Each pilocarpine ocular unit is effective for 7 days and should be placed in the eye at bedtime so that stable myopia can occur by morning.

Adverse Effects/Precautions. Ocular side effects include pain from excessive smooth muscle spasm and conjunctival and uval hyperemia. Systemic side effects, evidenced by muscarinic activity, are rare. The patient should press a finger to the lacrimal sac for 1 to 2 minutes following the pilocarpine instillation to minimize systemic absorption. The use of pilocarpine is contraindicated in bronchial asthma.

Aceclidine. A synthetic muscarinic drug resembling arecoline, aceclidine is employed as an alternative to pilocarpine.

Mechanism of Action. Aceclidine is a cholinergic agonist that acts directly on muscarinic receptors.

Clinical Indications. This drug is used in the treatment of glaucoma in cases that are refractory to pilocarpine therapy.

Adverse Effects/Precautions. The adverse effects and precautions are the same as those for pilocarpine.

Metoclopramide. A cholinergic agent, metoclopramide acts on peripheral muscarinic sites. The drug also acts centrally to block dopamine receptors.

Mechanism of Action. Metoclopramide counteracts the gastrointestinal stasis that occurs prior to the emetic response. Cholinergic stimulation by metoclopramide increases esophageal sphincter tone and gastric emptying. The increase in gastric motility, combined with a central antiemetic effect, makes the drug useful as an antiemetic.

Clinical Indications. Metoclopramide is used as an antiemetic agent in cancer chemotherapy, in the control of gastroparesis in diabetics, and esophageal reflux.

Adverse Effects/Precautions. Dystonias or extrapyramidal effects may occur with metoclopramide therapy.

ANTICHOLINESTERASE DRUGS (INDIRECT ACTING CHOLINERGIC DRUGS)

Anticholinesterase drugs block the enzymatic degradation of acetylcholine and cause its accumulation at cholinergic receptor sites. Several of the anticholinesterase drugs are toxic agents employed as insecticides or promoted as potential "nerve-gases" in chemical warfare. However, some of these agents (including physostigmine, neostigmine, and pyridostigmine) are useful in therapeutics because of their indirect cholinergic action.

The active center of acetylcholinesterase consists of anionic and esteratic subsites (Figure 2.16). The anionic subsite on acetylcholinerase combines with the positive nitrogen charge of choline by means of electrostatic or ionic bonding, comprising one of the attachment sites of acetylcholine to the enzyme.

At the esteratic subsite, a covalent bond forms with the carbonyl group of the acetate portion of acetylcholine. The attachment of acetylcholine to acetylcholinesterase in this manner orients the acetylcholine molecule so that nucleophillic attack on the acyl carbon occurs. Thus, acetylation of the enzyme is followed by rupture of the ester linkage of acetylcholine and the elimination of choline. The acetylated enzyme then reacts with water to form regenerated active enzyme and acetic acid.

Acetylcholinesterase is an extremely efficient enzyme that has the capacity to hydrolyze 3×10^5 acetylcholine molecules per enzyme molecule per minute.

ACETYLCHOLINESTERASE INHIBITION

Reversible inhibitors of acetylcholinesterase combine with the active anionic subsite or with a peripheral anionic subsite that is spatially removed from the active center of the enzyme. Quaternary reversible acetylcholinesterase inhibitors interact by means of the quaternary nitrogen with the anionic subsite on the active site and by hydrogen bonding to the nitrogen at the esteratic subsite (for example, edrophonium).

Reversible acetylcholinesterase inhibitors that contain a carbamyl ester grouping, such as physostigmine and neostigmine, attach to the anionic subsite because of their quaternary (neostigmine) or tertiary (physostigmine) nitrogen (Figure 2.17). A carbamylated enzyme forms by the bonding at the esteratic subsite of acetylcholinesterase. The carbamylated intermediate is stable and its formation precludes the rapid enzymatic hydrolysis of acetylcholine for a period of time (in vivo, 3 to 4 hours). The interaction of a reversible inhibitor (substrate) with acetylcholinesterase (enzyme) depends upon the anionic site attraction and the nature of the esteratic site interaction. Subsequent rapid reversibility of binding (edrophonium) or the formation of a stable carbamylated intermediate (physostigmine and neostigmine) characterize the reversible inhibitor-acetylcholinesterase interaction.

Irreversible inhibitors of acetylcholinesterase (organophosphates) do not routinely interact with the anionic subsite at the active center of acetylcholinesterase (Figure 2.18). Rather, the organophosphates form a stable complex by phosphorylating the enzyme. Irreversible inhibitors of cholinesterase have limited use in clinical practice.

REVERSIBLE ANTICHOLINESTERASE DRUGS

Reversible anticholinesterase drugs inhibit the degradation of acetylcholine and permit its accumulation at muscarinic and nicotinic receptor sites.

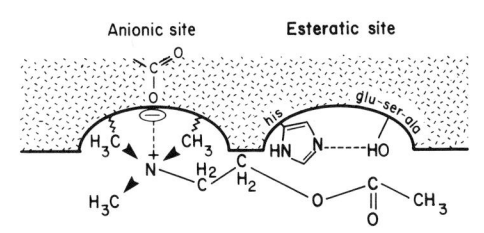

Fig. 2.16 Binding sites of acetylcholinesterase. (From Bowman, W.C., and Rand, M.J.: Texbook of Pharmacology, 2nd Ed. Oxford, Blackwell Scientific Publications, 1980.)

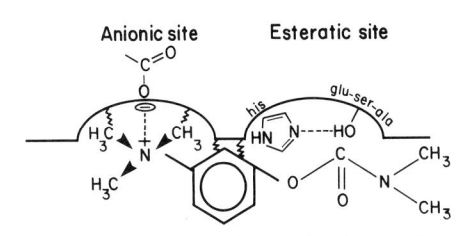

Fig. 2.17 Interaction of neostigmine and acetylcholinesterase. (From Bowman, W.C., and Rand, M.J.: Textbook of Pharmacology, 2nd Ed. Oxford, Blackwell Scientific Publications, 1980.)

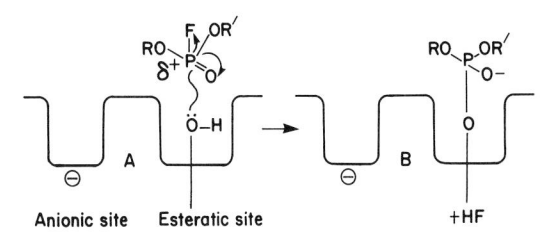

Fig. 2.18 Irreversible acetylcholinesterase phosphorylation. (Modified from Gringuaz, A.: Drugs. How They Act and Why. St. Louis, C.V. Mosby, 1978.)

Physostigmine (Eserine). Physostigmine is a naturally occurring alkaloid obtained from the Calabar bean, the dried ripe seed of Physostigmine venenosum. This perennial plant, once used by natives in witchcraft trials by ordeal, grows in Western Africa. The alkaloid was introduced as eserine in 1877 for use in glaucoma, one of its few clinical uses in modern therapeutics.

Mechanism of Action. Physostigmine is a reversible inhibitor of acetylcholinesterase that forms a carbamylated intermediate with the enzyme. Physostigmine reacts primarily with the true cholinesterase (acetylcholinesterase). The carbamylated intermediate of the enzyme so formed prevents the acetylcholine-acetylcholinesterase interaction and spares endogenous acetylcholine from enzymatic hydrolysis. The accumulation of acetylcholine at autonomic ganglia and cholinergic neuroeffector junctions causes the pharmacologic responses to physostigmine. The predominant effects that occur in therapeutic doses of physostigmine are muscarinic in nature.

Physostigmine contains a tertiary amine and readily passes the blood brain barrier. Consequently, it possesses both peripheral and central cholinergic activity.

Clinical Indications. The major therapeutic application of physostigmine relates to its effects on the eye. This drug induces intense miosis and contraction of the ciliary muscle, increasing facility for aqueous humor outflow and reducing intraocular pressure. In addition to physostigmine's value in reducing intraocular pressure in glaucoma, it is also used parenterally to reverse the effects of toxic doses of anticholinergic drugs, including tricyclic antidepressants.

Adverse Effects/Precautions. Ocular side effects, such as stinging, burning, and lacrimation, may occur with physostigmine therapy. Chronic physostigmine administration may cause follicular conjunctivitis. Systemic effects (possibly due to excessive dosage) result from peripheral cholinesterase inhibition; these adverse reactions include salivation, diarrhea, and bradycardia.

Neostigmine. A reversible cholinesterase inhibitor, neostigmine contains a quaternary nitrogen. This structural feature limits its passage into the CNS and imparts a direct action on peripheral cholinergic receptor sites.

Mechanism of Action. Neostigmine inhibits the hydrolysis of acetylcholine by competing with acetylcholine for attachment sites on acetylcholinesterase. By forming a carbamylated intermediate with acetylcholinesterase, neostigmine elicits anticholinesterase activity. Additionally, neostigmine has a direct action at the motor end plate on skeletal muscle. This direct cholinomimetic activity sets the drug apart from physostigmine and makes the neuromuscular actions of neostigmine more pronounced than those of physostigmine. As well as augmenting gastric secretions, neostigmine also increases the motor activity of the gastrointestinal tract.

Clinical Indications. Neostigmine is indicated in the treatment of myasthenia gravis. By both prejunctional and postjunctional effects, neostigmine counteracts the low vesicular acetylcholine concentration and reduced acetylcholine receptor population noted in this disease.

Difficulty in dosage titration is a problem observed with neostigmine therapy for myasthenia gravis. The irregular absorption of oral neostigmine, due to its quaternary amine structure, complicates achievement of the clinical goal of maintaining a stable level of muscular strength with minimal side effects.

Neostigmine reverses the action of curare-type muscle relaxants that act to block acetylcholine receptors at the motor end plate on skeletal or striated muscle. Thus, neostigmine may be useful in the postsurgical reversal of neuromuscular blocking agent activity.

Neostigmine's additional therapeutic uses include the prevention and treatment of postoperative distention and urinary retention (after mechanical obstruction has been ruled out).

Adverse Effects/Precautions. Common side effects generally relate to excessive peripheral cholinesterase inhibition and include salivation, muscle fasciculations, intestinal cramps, and diarrhea. Neostigmine sometimes causes a skin rash that disappears upon discontinuation of therapy.

Neostigmine should be used with caution in patients with bronchial asthma. Patients with concurrent epilepsy and cardiovascular disease also require careful scrutiny before neostigmine therapy is initiated.

Edrophonium. Edrophonium, an anticholinesterase drug, has a rapid onset and short duration of action.

Mechanism of Action. Edrophonium, a reversible inhibitor of cholinesterase, interacts with the anionic subsite on the enzyme. The cholinergic action of edrophonium primarily results from the accumulation of acetylcholine at sites of cholinergic transmission. Compared to neostigmine, edrophonium has a wider margin between the dose required to affect neuromuscular transmission and the dose required to stimulate the heart, smooth muscle cells, and glands.

Clinical Indications. Edrophonium is indicated as a diagnostic aid in the differential diagnosis of myasthenia gravis; however, the drug's brevity of action renders it unacceptable for maintenance therapy in this disease. Postsurgical use of edrophonium antagonizes the neuromuscular blocking action of curare-type muscle relaxants.

Adverse Effects/Precautions. Cholinergic reactions may occur in patients who are hyperreactive to cholinergic drugs. Ordinarily, the short duration of action precludes excessive side effects.

Ambenonium. Ambenonium, a bis-quaternary anticholinesterase drug, has a pharmacologic profile similar to that of neostigmine.

Mechanism of Action. Ambenonium is a reversible inhibitor of acetylcholinesterase. This drug does not form a covalent linkage at the esteratic subsite, as occurs with physostigmine and neostigmine; nonetheless, ambenonium demonstrates a marked affinity for the enzyme.

Ambenonium is similar in action to neostigmine in that it acts on prejunctional and postjunctional sites at the neuromuscular junction in skeletal muscle. Ambenonium has a selective and prolonged action against acetylcholinesterase.

Clinical Indications. Ambenonium is used clinically for the treatment of myasthenia gravis.

Adverse Effects/Precautions. Hyperreactive patients may exhibit cholinergic reactions, including bradycardia and other evidence of muscarinic activation.

Pyridostigmine. Pyridostigmine, a close congener of neostigmine, contains a quaternary nitrogen moiety that is incorporated into a pyridyl nucleus.

Mechanism of Action. Pyridostigmine is a reversible anticholinesterase that interacts with the anionic and esteratic subsites of the active center of acetylcholinesterase.

Clinical Indications. Pyridostigmine, which is indicated in the treatment of myasthenia gravis, also effectively reverses the effects of curare-like muscle relaxants.

Adverse Effects/Precautions. Cholinergic reactions are possible in hyperreactive individuals. The skin rash which sometimes occurs usually disappears upon cessation of therapy.

Demecarium. Demecarium consists of two neostigmine molecules connected by a bridge of ten methylene groups. This effective linking of two quaternary ammonium nuclei results in an anticholinesterase drug of increased potency and duration of action.

Mechanism of Action. Demecarium interacts with the anionic subsite at the active center of acetylcholinesterase. In addition, the second quaternary functional group of the demecarium molecule is attracted to negative subsites that are removed from the active center. Demecarium, a potent and long acting inhibitor of acetylcholinesterase, produces a long acting miosis. The outflow of aqueous humor improves in open angle glaucoma. Demecarium induces "spasm" of accommodation by its muscarinic action on the ciliary muscle, thereby reducing the amount of convergence associated with a given amount of accommodation.

Clinical Indications. Demecarium is administered topically in the conjunctival sac for the treatment of chronic open-angle glaucoma. This drug is also indicated in the diagnosis and treatment of accommodative esotropia ("cross eye").

Adverse Effects/Precautions. Side effects include periorbital pain, ocular burning sensation, and blurred vision. Systemic adverse effects related to hyperparasympathetic action may occur, but these reactions are uncommon with therapeutic doses.

Demecarium is contraindicated in narrow-angle glaucoma because of the local congestion that occurs with this drug.

IRREVERSIBLE ANTICHOLINESTERASE DRUGS

Most irreversible anticholinesterase drugs are too toxic for medical use. Echothiophate and isofluorophate, used in ophthamology, are characterized by their prolonged cholinergic activity.

Echothiophate. An extremely potent organophosphorus choline derivative, echothiophate irreversibly inhibits acetylcholinesterase.

Mechanism of Action. Echothiophate phosphorylates the esteratic subsite of the active center of acetylcholinesterase (Figure 2.18). The phosphorylated derivative is extremely stable and not readily subject to hydrolysis; therefore, acetylcholinesterase activity does not generally return until new acetylcholinesterase is synthesized.

Clinical Indications. Echothiophate is a long acting miotic commonly used in the treatment of chronic open-angle glaucoma. Less frequent administration is a definite advantage of this drug. Echothiophate is used in subacute or chronic angle-closure glaucoma after iridectomy or in glaucoma following cataract surgery and in the treatment of accommodative esotropia.

Adverse Effects/Precautions. Ocular stinging, lacrimation, and burning may occur. Systemic side effects, which relate to muscarinic activation, are possible.

Isofluorophate. Isofluorophate, an irreversible cholinesterase inhibitor, is commercially available only in ointment form.

Mechanism of Action. Isofluorophate forms a stable phosphorylated complex with acetylcholinesterase by reacting with the esteratic subsite on the active center of the enzyme.

Clinical Indications. Used primarily in the treatment of chronic open-angle glaucoma, isofluorophate has a prolonged duration of action. It is also used in angle-closure glaucoma after iridectomy and in the diagnosis and treatment of accommodative esotropia.

Adverse Effects/Precautions. Ocular and systemic side effects related to cholinergic activation, such as salivation, bradycardia, and diarrhea, may occur. Caution should be exercised to prevent overdosage. Isofluorophate opthalmic ointment may retard corneal healing. When exposed to water (i.e., moisture), isofluorophate forms hydrofluoric acid.

MUSCARINIC RECEPTOR BLOCKING DRUGS

Antimuscarinic drugs (Tables 2.3, 2.4) exert their pharmacologic effects by competitive blockade of acetylcholine receptors at the neuroeffector junction of postganglionic parasympathetic fibers and effector cells on smooth muscles, glands, and visceral organs. The classical prototype antimuscarinic drug is atropine, an alkaloid obtained by extraction from Atropa belladonna.

NATURALLY OCCURRING ALKALOIDS AND THEIR DERIVATIVES

Alkaloids with muscarinic blocking action (Table 2.3) are found in Atropa belladonna (deadly nightshade), Hyoscyamus niger (henbane), and Datura stramonium (jimsonweed).

The botanical name, "Atropa belladonna," reflects two of the main uses of this plant in earlier times. In Greek mythology, Atropa, the oldest of the three Fates, cut the thread of life;

Table 2.3 MUSCARINIC BLOCKING DRUGS (NATURALLY OCCURRING)

Available products	Trade names	Daily dosage range
Atropine sulfate	Atropine sulfate; Dey-Dose Atropine sulfate;	0.4–0.6 mg; 0.025 mg/kg diluted with 3 to 5 ml saline, inhalant;
	Atropine-Care Ophthalamic	Instill 1 or 2 drops up to 3 times daily
Belladonna extract	Belladonna Extract	15 mg t.i.d. to q.i.d.
Belladonna tincture	Belladonna tincture	0.6–1.0 ml t.i.d. or q.i.d.
Homatropine HBr	Homatropine HBr; Homatrocel; Isopto Homatropine	Ophthalmic for refraction, instill 1 or 2 drops; for uveitis, instill 1 or 2 drops up to every 3–4 hr
l-Hyoscyamine sulfate	Anaspaz; Levsin; Cystospaz	0.125–0.25 mg every 3 to 4 hr, orally or sublingually
Methscopolamine Br	Pamine	2.5–5 mg
Scopolamine HBr	Scopolamine HBr; Isopto Hyoscine	Injection, 0.32–0.65 mg; Antiemetic tablets, 0.25–0.8 mg 1 hr before travel

Table 2.4 MUSCARINIC BLOCKING DRUGS (SYNTHETIC).

Available products	Trade names	Daily dosage range
Anticholinergics:		
Anisotropine MBr	Valpin 50; Anisotropin MBr	50 mg t.i.d.
Clidinium Br	Quarzan	2.5–5 mg t.i.d. or q.i.d.
Glycopyrrolate	Robinul; Glycopyrrolate	1 mg t.i.d.
Hexocyclium methylsulfate	Tral Filmtabs	25 mg q.i.d.
Isopropamide iodide	Darbid	5 mg every 12 hrs
Mepenzolate Br	Cantil	25–50 mg q.i.d.
Methantheline Br	Banthine	50–100 mg every 6 hrs
Oxyphenonium Br	Antrenyl Br	10 mg q.i.d.
Propantheline Br	Pro-Banthine; Norpanth; SK-Propantheline Br	15 mg 30 min. before meals and 30 mg at bedtime
Tridihexethyl Cl	Pathilon	25–50 mg t.i.d. or q.i.d.
Antispasmodics:		
Dicyclomine HCl	Bentyl; Di-spaz; Dicyclomine HCl	10–20 mg t.i.d. or q.i.d.
Flavoxate HCl	Urispas	100 or 200 mg t.i.d. or q.i.d.
Methixene HCl	Trest	1 or 2 mg t.i.d.
Oxybutynin Cl	Ditropan	5 mg b.i.d. or t.i.d.
Oxyphencyclimine HCl	Daricon	10 mg b.i.d.
Thiphenamil HCl	Trocinate	400 mg initially

Atropa's namesake, the deadly nightshade, was a popular plant used in the Middle Ages to poison adversaries. Belladonna translates to "beautiful lady," apparently signifying the early cosmetic use of the plant leaves as a beauty aid, i.e., pupil dilation resulted when leaf preparations were introduced into the eye. As corroborated by recent scientific research, dilated pupils are still equated with beauty, just as they were in the Roman and Egyptian eras.

Atropine. Atropine, found in Atropa belladonna and Datura stramonium, is a racemic mixture of equal parts of d- and l-hyoscyamine that is formed during extraction procedures. The antimuscarinic activity results almost entirely from the naturally occurring l-hyoscyamine.

Mechanism of Action. Atropine inhibits the action of acetylcholine on smooth muscles, glands, and visceral organs by blocking muscarinic receptors. Due to its structural similarity to acetylcholine, atropine binds to muscarinic receptors, but does not elicit the response noted when acetylcholine-receptor interaction occurs. The atropine-receptor combination prevents access of acetylcholine to receptor sites, which produces an effective muscarinic block. The degree of muscarinic block depends upon the relative concentrations of atropine and acetylcholine present in the receptor vicinity and represents a classic example of competitive inhibition in drug mechanisms.

The atropine molecule does not produce the identical conformational changes in the muscarinic receptor substance that acetylcholine elicits. Rather, atropine produces molecular perturbations in the receptor substance that are sufficiently different from acetylcholine so that the typical pharmacologic response is absent. In summary, atropine is structurally similar enough to acetylcholine to bind to muscarinic receptors, but the receptor fit is not as "tight" and does not produce the response noted with the acetylcholine-receptor interaction. The bulky substituent group connected to the carbonyl function in the atropine molecule apparently prevents a "proper" fit in the receptor substance cavity that accepts this molecular portion of muscarinic agonists and antagonists.

Atropine produces a passive dilation of the pupil by blocking muscarinic receptors on the circular or sphincter muscle of the iris. By removing the parasympathetic influence (that tends to constrict the pupil), the sympathetic predominance of dilation occurs as the radial musculature contracts without counterbalancing parasympathetic resistance. Thus, the term "passive dilation" is appropriate since one of two opposing systems in a reciprocating function (pupillary size) is blocked (parasympathetic), allowing the other (sympathetic) to predominate.

The ciliary muscle also contains muscarinic receptors. The tone of this muscle determines the curvature of the crystalline lens. The loss of parasympathetic influence on the ciliary muscle relaxes the muscle, increases the tension of suspensory ligaments, and "flattens" the crystalline lens. This condition is termed "loss of accommodation" or "cycloplegia"; thus, atropine is termed a "cycloplegic drug."

Atropine produces an extended reduction in tone and motility of the gastrointestinal tract by virtue of its muscarinic blocking action. This activity occurs along the entire gastrointestinal tract.

Atropine's prevention of exocrine gland secretions is a consequence of the drug's ability to block muscarinic receptors on the secretory cells of these glands. The salivary glands and the mucus glands lining the respiratory tract are markedly affected by atropine, resulting in a pronounced drying effect in the mouth and respiratory tract.

Atropine, in moderate doses, produces tachycardia due to the drug's blockade of muscarinic receptors in the heart. Thus, the inhibitory effect of the vagus (parasympathetic) is blocked and a more rapid heart beat occurs. Low doses of atropine produce bradycardia by an unknown mechanism.

In usual therapeutic doses, atropine has little effect on the CNS. In large doses, the drug produces signs of central nervous stimulation, including restlessness, irritability, disorientation, hallucinations, and delirium.

Atropine does not have selective affinity for M_1 or M_2 receptors, but it has especially marked muscarinic antagonist activity at the muscarinic receptors on smooth and cardiac muscle, as well as those of exocrine gland cells.

Clinical Indications. Atropine is valuable in the treatment of gastric hypermotility, spasticity of the small intestine amd colon, amd pylorospasm. Although atropine reduces gastric acid secretion in peptic ulcer, the dose required to diminish gastric acid often results in significant side effects, thus limiting its clinical use in hypersecretory gastric disorders.

Ophthalmic preparations of atropine produce mydriasis and cycloplegia for refraction of the eyes for corrective lens. Used in iritis, atropine is also employed alternately with physostigmine to prevent the formation of adhesions between the iris and cornea.

Bradycardia amd atrioventricular block associated with increased vagal (parasympathetic) tone are treated with atropine. When used as preanesthetic medication, this drug decreases salivary and bronchial secretions.

Adverse Effects/Precautions. Tachycardia and xerostomia are common side effects that occur with atropine. Other adverse reactions related to muscarinic receptor blockade include constipation, urinary retention, and blurred vision. Glaucoma patients should not take atropine because of the aggravation of increased intraocular pressure that is characteristic of this condition.

Scopolamine (l-hyoscine). The alkaloid scopolamine is found primarily in Hyoscyamus niger (henbane).

Mechanism of Action. The peripheral antimuscarinic actions of scopolamine resemble those of atropine, but the effects of scopolamine on the eye and on secretions are more marked. In contrast to the CNS stimulation that often occurs with atropine, scopolamine depresses the CNS.

Scopolamine is frequently used instead of atropine when some CNS depressant is desired (such as in preanesthetic medication). When given together, scopolamine and morphine produce an amnesic condition termed "twilight sleep."

Clinical Indications. Scopolamine reduces gastrointestinal hypermotility and hypertonicity in the irritable colon syndrome; related therapeutic indications are diverticulitis, pylorospasm, and cardiospasm. Scopolamine, available in a transdermal drug release system for use in motion sickness, is applied to the postauricular skin at least 4 hours before the antiemetic effect is needed.

Parenteral scopolamine is also employed for preanesthetic sedation and in obstetrics together with analgesics to induce amnesia ("twilight sleep"). Other clinical applications are in ophthalmic preparations to produce mydriasis and cycloplegia and in the treatment of iridocyclitis.

Adverse Effects/Precautions. The most common side effects, including xerostomia, drowsiness, and blurred vision, relate to muscarinic blockade. Patients taking scopolamine should avoid potentially hazardous tasks due to drug-induced decreased alertness and mental acuity. Decreased sweating may cause heat prostration in individuals in high environmental temperatures. Also, patients with narrow-angle glaucoma should avoid scopolamine.

l-Hyoscyamine. A naturally occurring alkaloid in Atropa belladonna, l-hyoscyamine exhibits a preferential blocking effect on peripheral muscarinic receptors.

Mechanism of Action. l-Hyoscyamine blocks peripheral muscarinic receptors on smooth muscles, glands, and visceral organs.

Clinical Indications. l-Hyoscyamine is used in the treatment of gastric hypersecretion, visceral spasm, gastrointestinal hypermotility, spastic colitis, and pylorospasm. The drug also reduces respiratory secretion in rhinitis and related conditions. Renal colic and cystitis are other therapeutic indications for l-hyoscyamine.

Adverse Effects/Precautions. Practically all of the adverse effects of l-hyoscyamine (such as dry mouth, blurred vision, constipation, and urinary retention) relate to the drug's peripheral antimuscarinic action.

Levorotatory Alkaloids of Belladonna. This preparation is a mixture of the l-alkaloids of Atropa belladonna, including l-hyoscyamine.

Mechanism of Action. This drug preparation effectively blocks peripheral muscarinic receptors with minimal effects on the CNS.

Clinical Indications. Therapeutic uses for this drug preparation include gastrointestinal spasm, peptic ulcer, spastic colitis, and biliary colic. Other clinical applications include the treatment of enuresis, dysmenorrhea, and hypersecretory conditions of the respiratory tract, such as bronchial asthma.

Adverse Effects/Precautions. Noted side effects relate to the peripheral muscarinic blocking action and include dry mouth, blurred vision, constipation, and urinary retention.

Belladonna Extract and Tincture. These products, which are galenical preparations of Atropa belladonna, contain antimuscarinic alkaloids.

Mechanism of Action. Belladonna extract and belladonna tincture contain alkaloids that block muscarinic receptors on smooth muscles, glands, and visceral organs.

Clinical Indications. Therapeutic uses include gastrointestinal spastic conditions, peptic ulcer, dysmenorrhea, and nocturnal enuresis.

Adverse Effects/Precautions. Antimuscarinic side effects include xerostomia, blurred vision, urinary retention, and constipation.

ANTICHOLINERGICS CLOSELY RELATED TO NATURALLY OCCURRING ALKALOIDS

These drugs include synthetic molecular variants of the naturally occurring alkaloids.

Homatropine. Two salts of homatropine are available commercially for clinical use. Homatropine methylbromide is used for gastrointestinal disorders, whereas homatropine hydrobromide is employed as a rapidly acting mydriatic with a shorter duration of action than that of atropine.

Mechanism of Action. Homatropine blocks the effects of acetylcholine on peripheral muscarinic receptors. In ophthalmology, the drug blocks the muscarinic receptors on the circular (sphincter) muscle of the iris and the ciliary muscle, resulting in mydriasis and loss of accommodation (cycloplegia).

Clinical Indications. Homatropine methylbromide is used to treat peptic ulcer, pylorospasm, hyperchlorhydria, and spastic colitis. Homatropine hydrobromide produces mydriasis and cycloplegia for cycloplegic refraction. Inflammatory conditions of the uveal tract also respond to homatropine hydrobromide.

Adverse Effects/Precautions. The side effects of homatropine are the same as those of atropine.

Methscopolamine. Methscopolamine is a quaternary ammonium derivative of scopolamine.

Mechanism of Action. Methscopolamine has peripheral muscarinic blocking activity, but it lacks the central nervous action of scopolamine because of the drug's inability to cross the blood brain barrier. Although less potent than atropine, methscopolamine has a more prolonged duration of action.

Clinical Indications. The main therapeutic use of methscopolamine is in the treatment of gastrointestinal disorders (such as hypermotility and hypertonicity).

Adverse Effects/Precautions. Antimuscarinic side effects may occur with methscopolamine therapy.

Tropicamide. Tropicamide is a synthetic tropic acid derivative with a tertiary amine structure.

Mechanism of Action. Tropicamide has peripheral antimuscarinic activity, particularly on receptors in the iris circular muscle and the ciliary muscle. The drug is mainly utilized in ophthalmic preparations in the refraction of eyes for corrective lens.

Clinical Indications. Tropicamide is used clinically as a mydriatic and cycloplegic.

Adverse Effects/Precautions. Antimuscarinic side effects are uncommon with tropicamide.

Cyclopentolate. Cyclopentolate is a synthetic tertiary-amine antimuscarinic drug.

Mechanism of Action. Cyclopentolate blocks muscarinic receptors, chiefly in the iris circular musculature and the ciliary muscle.

Clinical Indications. Cyclopentolate produces rapid cycloplegia and mydriasis in the refraction of eyes for corrective lens.

Adverse Effects/Precautions. Antimuscarinic side effects occur infrequently with cyclopentolate.

SYNTHETIC MUSCARINIC BLOCKING DRUGS

Many synthetic muscarinic blocking drugs (Table 2.4) have a direct musculotropic action on smooth muscles and some demonstrate significant nicotinic receptor blocking activity.

Atropine-like Tertiary Amines with Direct Spasmolytic Activity. Dicyclomine, oxyphencyclimine, thiphenamil, and adiphenine are examples of antimuscarinic compounds with a lesser degree of specificity in blocking acetylcholine receptors.

Mechanism of Action. As well as blocking muscarinic receptors, these drugs possess an extra component of antispasmodic activity in that they have a direct musculotropic action on smooth muscle. Their nonspecific nature renders these compounds less likely to produce atropine-like side reactions. Also, these drugs are less potent in their antispasmodic action when compared to atropine.

Clinical Indications. Dicyclomine and related compounds are used chiefly in the treatment of mild disturbances of the gastrointestinal tract.

Adverse Effects/Precautions. Antimuscarinic side effects are infrequent with this class of compounds.

Atropine-like Quaternary Ammonium Compounds with Antinicotinic Activity. Propantheline, methantheline, anisotropine, clidinium, and glycopyrrolate are examples of antispasmodic drugs in this category. These agents have ancillary autonomic ganglionic blocking action, as well as the predominant antimuscarinic activity.

Mechanism of Action. Propantheline and the related drugs in this class have a high degree of autonomic ganglionic blocking action. Neuromuscular block at the motor end plate in skeletal muscles may also occur at higher doses of these agents, indicating another nicotinic blocking site. These drugs block a wide spectrum of autonomic acetylcholine receptor sites and show both marked antispasmodic activity and an antisecretory action.

Clinical Indications. Propantheline and other atropine-like quaternary ammonium drugs are used primarily in the treatment of gastrointestinal disorders, such as peptic ulcer and gastrointestinal hypermotility.

Adverse Effects/Precautions. Antimuscarinic and antinicotinic side effects may occur with this class of antispasmodics. Nicotinic blocking adverse effects (usually encountered from high doses of these drugs) include impotence and respiratory muscle paralysis.

DRUGS BLOCKING NICOTINIC RECEPTORS

Drugs that block nicotinic receptors (Tables 2.5, 2.6), including nicotine, lobeline, and succinylcholine, usually produce a transient stimulation at these sites. Their therapeutic application depends upon a rather diffuse blockade at either autonomic ganglia or neuromuscular nicotinic receptor sites.

Table 2.5 SYNTHETIC GANGLIONIC BLOCKING DRUGS.

Available products	Trade names	Daily dosage range
Mecamylamine HCl	Inversine	2.5–25 mg orally
Trimethaphan camsylate	Arfonad	3–4 mg/min IV drip at first in a solution containing 1 mg/ml

Table 2.6 NICOTINIC NEUROMUSCULAR RECEPTOR BLOCKING DRUGS.

Available products	Trade names	Daily dosage range
Nondepolarizing muscle relaxants:		
Atracurium besylate	Tracrium	0.4–0.5 mg/kg initially as an IV bolus injection
Gallamine triethiodide	Flaxedil	1.0 mg/kg; total dose of 40–80 mg
Hexafluorenium Br	Mylaxen	0.4 mg/kg; total dose < 36 mg
Metocurine iodide	Metubine Iodide	0.2–0.4 mg/kg for endotracheal intubation; 1.75–5.5 mg for electroshock therapy
Pancuronium Br	Pavulon	0.04–0.1 mg/kg initially
Tubocurarine Cl	Tubocuratine Cl	0.1–0.3 mg/kg initially
Vecuronium Br	Norcuron	0.08–0.1 mg/kg initially as an IV bolus injection
Depolarizing muscle relaxant:		
Succinylcholine chloride	Anectine; Quelicin; Sucostrin	20–80 mg after initial test dose of 10 mg

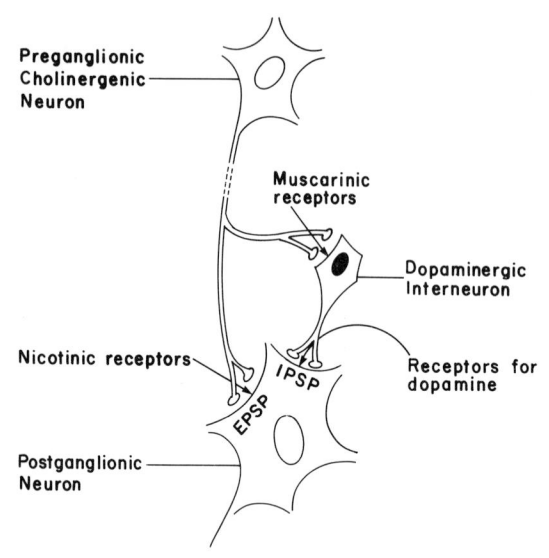

Fig. 2.19 Possible mechanisms of inhibitory modulation by dopaminergic interneurons. EPSP, excitatory postsynaptic potential; IPSP, inhibitory postsynaptic potential. (Modified from Bowman, W.C., and Rand, M.J.: Textbook of Pharmacology, 2nd Ed. Oxford, Blackwell Scientific Publications, 1980.)

DRUGS THAT BLOCK NICOTINIC RECEPTORS IN AUTONOMIC GANGLIA

These compounds (Tables 2.5, 2.6) have limited clinical utility because of their generalized blocking action on autonomic ganglia. Newer agents that are more selective and less toxic have replaced many antihypertensive drugs in this category.

Ganglionic Stimulants and Blocking Agents. Autonomic ganglia contain mainly nicotinic receptors, although muscarinic and alpha-adrenergic receptors (dopamine receptors) are also present (Figure 2.19). Nicotinic blocking drugs either prevent the depolarizing action of acetylcholine or produce a persistent depolarization of the postsynaptic membrane receptor substance. Some drugs (such as the nicotine and lobeline alkaloids) produce an initial stimulation of ganglionic nicotinic receptors before effecting a final blockade of these same receptors. Ganglionic blocking drugs find limited use as hypotensive drugs to lower blood pressure by decreasing the sympathetic tone to various vascular regions of the body. Thus, an apparent affinity for sympathetic ganglia results, which reduces the vasoconstricting influence of adrenergic nerves on arterioles.

Naturally Occurring Alkaloids with Biphasic Action. Nicotine. Found in tobacco (Nicotiana tabacum), nicotine produces dependence in habitual users. Nicotine, one of the most toxic substances known to man, is a colorless liquid alkaloid which turns brown upon exposure to air and develops a tobacco odor. The acute lethal dose for an adult is about 60 mg.

Mechanism of Action. Nicotine has a biphasic action on autonomic ganglia. An initial stimulation of ganglionic nicotinic receptors occurs, which is followed by a more prolonged depression. The immediate effect is depolarization of the postsynaptic membrane in a manner similar to the neurotransmitter, acetylcholine. The initial transient activation of nicotinic receptors is followed by a persistence of nicotine attachment to the receptor and an impedence of ganglionic transmission. The reactivity of autonomic ganglia decreases with increased nicotine ingestion.

Nicotine produces an increase in heart rate and blood pressure in nonsmoking individuals. CNS stimulation is also usually evident. In smokers, tolerance to nicotine develops and these effects may not be noticed.

Nicotine promotes the release of catecholamines from the adrenal medulla and isolated organs. Tolerance to this effect of nicotine does not occur.

Clinical Indications. Nicotine gum is available for use as a temporary aid in withdrawal from cigarette smoking.

Adverse Effects/Precautions. Nicotine gum has a slightly peppery taste, and some patients complain about burning or soreness in the mouth following use of this product. Nausea and vomiting have also been reported, and dependence upon this gum may occur in some patients.

Lobeline (Indian tobacco). Lobeline, an alkaloid found in the herb, Lobelia inflata, has many of the same actions of nicotine but is less potent.

Mechanism of Action. Lobeline produces an initial stimulation of autonomic ganglia and the CNS followed by depression.

Clinical Indications. Lobeline is used as an over-the-counter (OTC) smoking cessation aid. These products were available for decades before the introduction of nicotine gum as a smoking deterrent.

Adverse Effects/Precautions. Few adverse effects are associated with lobeline-containing products.

SYNTHETIC GANGLIONIC BLOCKING DRUGS

These compounds (Table 2.5) have very limited clinical application in modern therapeutics.

Hexamethonium. Hexamethonium is the prototype C_6 compound that led to the development of newer ganglionic blocking drugs. The drug acts as a competitive inhibitor of acetylcholine at nicotinic receptor sites in autonomic ganglia. Currently, the drug is not used clinically.

Pentolinium. Pentolinium is more potent than hexamethonium and the duration of action of pentolinium is also longer. Presently, pentolinium is not used clinically in the U.S.A.

Mecamylamine. Mecamylamine is an orally effective ganglionic blocking drug.

Mechanism of Action. Mecamylamine blocks nicotinic receptors in autonomic ganglia. Tolerance develops to the blood pressure lowering effects of mecamylamine.

Clinical Indications. The routine use of mecamylamine in severe hypertension is no longer necessary because of newer antihypertensive drugs. However, mecamylamine is a valuable drug for a few selected, hypertensive patients and for a small group of patients with spinal cord injury who suffer from autonomic hyperreflexia.

Adverse Effects/Precautions. Mild side effects include visual disturbances, xerostomia, gastrointestinal disorders, and postural hypotension with syncope. Marked hypotension, constipation, paralytic ileus, urinary retention, and cycloplegia are more severe reactions to this drug. Since mecamylamine can pass the blood brain barrier, large doses produce central nervous stimulation or depression.

Trimethaphan. A parenteral ganglionic blocking drug, trimethaphan is a useful hypotensive agent.

Mechanism of Action. Trimethaphan blocks nicotinic receptors in autonomic ganglia.

Clinical Indications. Trimethaphan is used for controlled hypotension to reduce bleeding in surgical procedures of the head and neck. The drug is also employed for the short-term control of blood pressure in hypertension and in the emergency treatment of pulmonary edema in hypertensive patients.

Adverse Effects/Precautions. Caution should be exercised in using this drug in the elderly or debilitated, as well as in children. Cautious use is also advocated in patients prone to allergic reactions since the drug promotes histamine release.

DRUGS BLOCKING NICOTINIC RECEPTORS AT THE NEUROMUSCULAR JUNCTION

These agents (Table 2.6) insure adequate skeletal muscle relaxation for surgical procedure, endotracheal intubation, and electroconvulsive therapy. Neuromuscular blocking agents are either nondepolarizing drugs (e.g., d-tubocurarine) which act by competitive inhibition of acetylcholine or depolarizing drugs (e.g., succinylcholine) which produce persistent depolarization of the receptor membrane of the motor end plate.

NONDEPOLARIZING OR COMPETITIVELY BLOCKING DRUGS (CURARE ALKALOIDS AND RELATED DRUGS)

The curare-like alkaloids competitively block the attachment of acetylcholine to nicotinic receptors. "Curare" is the term applied to crude extracts of plants in the genuses Strychnos and Chondrodendron, which are used by some South American Indian tribes as arrowhead poisons. Curare was originally marketed as a dark brown plant extract of variable composition. After a century of use of this crude product as a pharmacologic tool to elicit skeletal muscle paralysis, the alkaloid d-tubocurarine was determined to be the active principle. Following this discovery in 1935, only a few years passed before the clinical possibilities of d-tubocararine as a muscle relaxant to supplement general anesthesia were examined.

The curare alkaloid, d-tubocurarine, competitively inhibits acetylcholine at nicotinic receptors at the motor end plate on skeletal muscle. Competitive inhibitors of the curare-type produce a nondepolarizing block to cause the skeletal muscle relaxation. Competitive neuromuscular blockers (e.g., d-tubocurarine and related drugs) are generally used in situations which require an intermediate or prolonged duration of action. Anticholinesterase drugs usually antagonize the action of nondepolarizing neuromuscular blocking agents.

Tubocurarine. A pure alkaloid from curare, tubocurarine is administered by intravenous or intramuscular injection, usually as an adjunct to general anesthesia.

Mechanism of Action. The receptor blockade by tubocurarine prevents the critical end plate depolarization by acetylcholine. The tubocurarine molecules compete with acetylcholine for receptors according to the law of mass action; also, tubocurarine elicits a parallel shift in the log-dose response curves of acetylcholine, a characteristic of competitive antagonism.

Clinical Indications. Tubocurarine is used as an adjunct to general anesthesia to produce skeletal muscle relaxation. The drug also diminishes the risk of injury in electroconvulsive therapy by reducing the intensity of muscle contractions. Used in patients requiring mechanical ventilation for easing intubation with an endotrachial tube, tubocurarine is also employed in such procedures as bronchoscopy and laryngoscopy. Tubocurarine is usually administered intravenously over a period of 1 to 1.5 minutes; its onset of action occurs within a minute and lasts for 25 to 90 minutes.

Adverse Effects/Precautions. The most common adverse effect is an exaggerated and prolonged skeletal muscle relaxation that increases the danger of respiratory depression.

Rapid intravenous injection of tubocurarine increases histamine release, which causes bronchospasm. A decreased respiratory capacity results from the histamine-induced bronchospasm, possibly aggravated by paralysis of the respiratory muscles.

Metocurine. Metocurine iodide is a curare-like nondepolarizing skeletal muscle relaxant which is given by intravenous injection.

Mechanism of Action. Metocurine blocks nerve impulses to skeletal muscles by competing for acetylcholine receptors on the motor end plate. Compared to tubocurarine, metocurine possesses less autonomic ganglia blocking action. Metocurine is approximately twice as potent as tubocurarine in inducing skeletal muscle paralysis.

Clinical Indications. Metocurine is used as an adjunct in surgical procedures that require profound skeletal muscle relaxation and in electroshock therapy to reduce skeletal muscle contractions. Metocurine passes the placental barrier, an important consideration in pregnant patients.

Adverse Effects/Precautions. Prolonged skeletal muscle relaxant action is the most frequently reported adverse effect. Hypersensitivity reactions to iodine may occur with metocurine iodide injection.

Gallamine. Gallamine triethiodide is an intravenous nondepolarizing skeletal muscle relaxant.

Mechanism of Action. Gallamine competes with acetylcholine for nicotinic receptors at the neuromuscular junction but has no effect on autonomic ganglia. In contrast to tubocurarine, this drug does not cause histamine release and resultant problems (such as bronchospasm).

Clinical Indications. Gallamine is used as an adjunct to anesthesia to induce skeletal muscle relaxation in surgical procedures. The drug also facilitates the management of patients undergoing mechanical ventilation.

Adverse Effects/Precautions. Patients sensitive to iodine should not receive gallamine triethiodide. An absolute contraindication of gallamine usage is in myasthenia gravis patients. Exaggerated muscle relaxant activity is the most common adverse effect noted.

Pancuronium. Pancuronium bromide, a nondepolarizing skeletal muscle relaxant, is approximately five times as potent (milligram for milligram) as tubocurarine.

Mechanism of Action. By blocking the nicotinic receptor-acetylcholine interaction, pancuronium induces skeletal muscle relaxation. This drug has little effect on histamine release.

Clinical Indications. Pancuronium is an adjunct to general anesthesia to assure sufficient skeletal muscle relaxation for surgical procedures. Judicious use of this drug also aids in the management of mechanical ventilation.

Adverse Effects/Precautions. The extension of skeletal muscle relaxation after anesthesia and surgery is the most frequent adverse reaction.

Atracurium. Atracurium besylate, a nondepolarizing skeletal muscle relaxant, is available as an unequal mixture of isomers with a consistent ratio that insures pharmacologic uniformity in the manufactured product.

Mechanism of Action. Atracurium is a competitive blocker of the acetylcholine-nicotinic receptors at the neuromuscular junction. The drug is a less potent histamine releaser when compared to tubocurarine or metocurine. Nonetheless, histamine release occurs, accompanied by moderate effects on the circulation, as evidenced by a fall in blood pressure. The duration of action is about $1/3$ to $1/2$ that of tubocurarine.

Clinical Indications. Atracurium is employed as an adjunct to general anesthesia because of its skeletal muscle relaxant properties. Atracurium also facilitates endotracheal intubation.

Adverse Effects/Precautions. Cardiovascular side effects, e.g., flushing and hypotension, are minimal. Adverse reactions which relate to histamine release have been reported with this drug, although the necessity for discontinuation of atracurium therapy is rare.

Vecuronium. Vecuronium, a nondepolarizing skeletal muscle relaxant, has the same pharmacologic characteristics as d-tubocurarine.

Mechanism of Action. Vecuronium competes with acetylcholine for nicotinic receptors at the neuromuscular junctions.

Clinical Indications. Used as an adjunct to general anesthesia, vecuronium facilitates endotracheal intubation and more extensive skeletal muscle relaxation in selected surgery. Vercuronium should only be administered by intravenous injection.

Adverse Effects/Precautions. An extension of the skeletal muscle relaxant effect of vecuronium beyond the surgical and anesthetic period is the most frequent adverse reaction noted.

DEPOLARIZING BLOCKING DRUGS (SUCCINYLCHOLINE AND RELATED COMPOUNDS)

Depolarizing neuromuscular blockers, such as succinylcholine and decamethonium, interact with acetylcholine receptors to induce a persistent depolarization of the motor end plate. This action results in an inactivation of the sodium transport process necessary for generation of a propagated impulse along the skeletal muscle fiber. An additional component of the depolarization blockade involves a desensitization phenomenon or refractoriness of end plate acetylcholine receptors that follows the initial end plate depolarization by the drug. Depolarizing neuromuscular blockers are used for endotracheal intubation or short surgical procedures. The action of these drugs is not reversed by anticholinesterase and in fact, succinylcholine paralysis may be enhanced.

Succinylcholine. Chemically characterized as the combination of two molecules of acetylcholine, succinylcholine is an ultra-short acting skeletal muscle relaxant that produces a persistent depolarization of the motor end plate.

Mechanism of Action. Succinylcholine combines with the nicotinic receptors at the motor end plate on skeletal muscle. Initially, an acetylcholine-like action is evidenced by muscle fasciculations, but this action is replaced by a blockade of neuromuscular transmission for as long as succinylcholine occupies the nicotinic receptors. This initial stimulation does not occur with the nondepolarizing competitive blockers (such as curare-like drugs).

Succinylcholine is rapidly metabolized by plasma pseudocholinesterase, thus accounting for the drug's ultra-short duration of action of 4 to 10 minutes. About 1 in 3,000 persons has an atypical pseudocholinesterase that is relatively ineffective in destroying succinylcholine. In these individuals, prolonged apnea may occur after succinylcholine administration (requiring artificial ventilation), and the duration of drug action extends from 2 to 4 hours. This situation illustrates the importance of pharmacogenetics in medical practice.

Clinical Indications. Succinylcholine is used as an adjunct to general anesthesia to facilitate endotracheal intubation or to insure sufficient skeletal muscle relaxation in surgery. Additionally, succinylcholine, when employed in electroconvulsive shock therapy, diminishes the possibility of injury due to excessive contractions of the skeletal muscles. Although usually given intravenously, succinylcholine may be administered intramuscularly if required.

Adverse Effects/Precautions. Succinylcholine has been associated with an acute onset of malignant hyperthermia characterized by hypermetabolism of skeletal muscle. Clinical signs of this emergency include spasm of the jaw muscles, tachycardia, rapid breathing, and high fever. Consequently, succinylcholine should be used only when measures to counteract this reaction are available.

Decamethonium. A C_{10} compound, decamethonium specifically blocks nicotinic receptors at the neuromuscular junction. Primarily used as a pharmacologic tool to study nicotinic receptor blockade, this drug is mainly of theoretical interest.

CHOLINESTERASE REGENERATORS

A "cholinesterase regenerator," such as pralidoxime, can reduce the toxicity of the anticholinesterases. Consequently, the destruction of accumulated acetylcholine can proceed normally, which returns function to neuromuscular and muscarinic sites. Reversing respiratory muscle paralysis is a critical effect of cholinesterase regeneration.

Pralidoxime. Pralidoxime is a cholinesterase reactivator that is used in the treatment of anticholinesterase drug overdosage.

Mechanism of Action. Pralidoxime regenerates cholinesterase that has been inactivated by "irreversible" cholinesterase inhibitors such as the organophosphates (Figure 2.20). This drug also slows the process of "aging" of phosphorylated cholinesterase to a nonreactive form and detoxifies certain organophosphates by direct chemical reaction.

Clinical Indications. Indicated as an adjunctive antidote with atropine in the treatment of organophosphate poisoning, pralidoxime is also effective in cases of overdosage of anticholinesterase drugs that are used in myasthenia gravis.

Adverse Effects/Precautions. Dizziness, blurred vision, diplopia, headache, drowsiness, nausea, tachycardia, hyperventilation, and muscular weakness have all been reported after pralidoxime use. It is very difficult, however, to ascertain whether these adverse reactions are the result of pralidoxime therapy or of organophosphate/anticholinesterase activity.

ADRENERGIC DRUGS

As direct agonists, adrenergic drugs (Tables 2.7, 2.8, 2.9) interact with adrenergic receptors; as indirect agonists, they increase the amount of

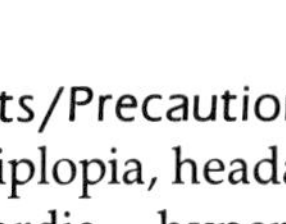

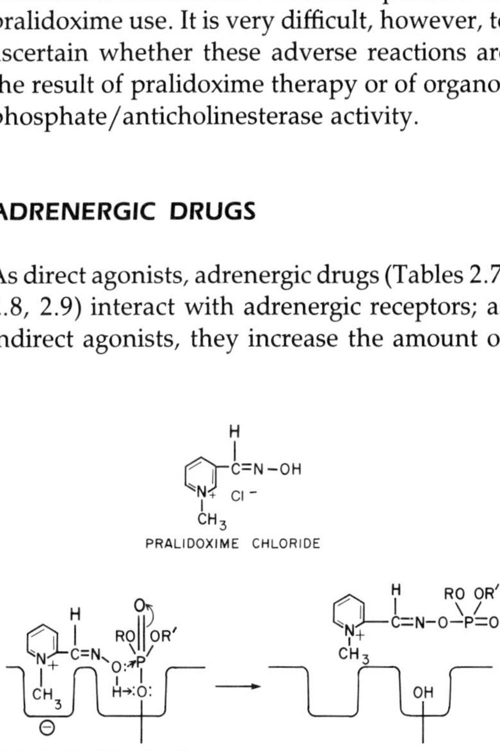

Fig. 2.20 Possible mechanism of phosphorylated acetylcholinesterase reactivation. (From Gringuaz, A.: Drugs. How They Act and Why. St. Louis, C.V. Mosby, 1978.)

Table 2.7 ADRENERGIC DRUGS: BRONCHODILATORS.

Available products	Trade Names	Daily dosage range
Epinephrine (as bitartrate)	Epitrate	Instill 1 drop once or b.i.d.
Epinephrine	Adrenalin HCl; Asthma Nefrin; Dey-Dose Epinephrine; Adrendin Cl; Epinephrine HCl	0.3–0.5 mg IM, SC, or by inhalation for broncho-dilation Instill 1 or 2 drops, as in ophthalmics; 0.5–1 mg in cardiac arrest
Ephedrine sulfate	Ephedrine Sulfate	25–50 mg orally
Isoproterenol	Isuprel	10–15 mg sublingually
Metaproterenol sulfate	Alupent; Metaprel	0.65 mg per inhalation (2–3 inhalations) or 20 mg orally
Pseudoephedrine HCl	Sudafed; others	60 mg every 6 hrs
Terbutaline sulfate	Brethine; Bricanyl	5 mg orally t.i.d. or 0.25 mg SC

Table 2.8 ADRENERGIC DRUGS: DRUGS THAT ELEVATE BLOOD PRESSURE.

Available products	Trade names	Daily dosage range
Catecholamines:		
Dobutamine HCl	Dobutrex	Infuse from 2.5–10 mcg/kg/min
Dopamine HCl	Intropin; Dopamine HCl; Dopastat	Initial IV infusion at 2–5 mcg/kg/min.; increase to rates 20–50 mcg/kg/min.
Isoproterenol	Isuprel; Isoproterenol	Dilute a 1:5000 solution to 1:500,000 and infuse at rates adjusted to the patient's response
Norepinephrine	Levophed	IV infusion of a 4 mcg per ml dilution at a rate of 2–3 ml/min.
Sympathomimetic amines:		
Ephedrine sulfate	Ephedrine sulfate	25–50 mg orally; 25–50 mg SC, IM, or slow IV
Metaraminol	Aramine; Metaraminol Bitartrate	2–10 mg IM or SC; 0.5–5 mg IV bolus, followed by an infusion of 15–100 mg in the form of a dilute solution
Methoxamine HCl	Vasoxyl	3–5 mg slow IV
Phenylephrine	Neo-Synephrine	2–5 mg IM or SC; 0.2 mg IV

Table 2.9 ADRENERGIC DRUGS: NASAL DECONGESTANTS.

Available products	Trade names	Daily dosage range
Ephedrine	Vatronol Nose Drops; Ephedrine Sulfate; Efedron Nasal	Instill 2 or 3 drops or apply a small amount of jelly in each nostril b.i.d. or t.i.d.
Epinephrine HCl	Adrenalin Cl	Instill 1–2 drops in each nostril every 4–6 hrs
Naphazoline HCl	Privine	2 drops or sprays of the 0.05% solution in each nostril
Oxymetazoline HCl	Afrin; others	2 or 3 drops of sprays of the 0.05% solution in each nostril
Phenylephrine HCl	Neo-Synephrine; others	0.25% in each nostril every 3–4 hrs
Phenylpropanolamine HCl	Propadrine; others	25 mg t.i.d. or q.i.d.
Propylhexedrine HCl	Benzedrex	Topically by inhaler
Pseudoephedrine HCl	Sudafed, others	60 mg every 6 hrs
Tetrahydrozoline HCl	Tyzine	2–4 drops of 0.1% solution in each nostril
Xylometazoline HCl	Otrivin; others	2 or 3 drops or sprays in each nostril every 8–10 hrs

neurotransmitter available for attachment to adrenergic receptors.

ENDOGENOUS ADRENERGIC DRUGS

Three adrenergic agents (epinephrine, norepinephrine, and dopamine) are endogenous entities that are present either as neurotransmitters or as their precursors in the sympathetic nervous system.

Epinephrine. Epinephrine is the endogenous catecholamine that the adrenal medulla synthesizes and releases. The adrenal glands of domestic animals are the chief source of commercial epinephrine.

Mechanism of Action. Epinephrine is a direct acting adrenergic drug that activates both alpha- and beta-adrenergic receptors. Epinephrine, the most potent alpha-adrenergic agonist, mimics all actions of the sympathetic nervous system except those on the sweat glands and facial blood vessels.

Local effects of epinephrine include vasoconstriction of blood vessels in mucosal membranes, resulting in nasal congestion relief. Aerosol administration of epinephrine relaxes constricted bronchiolar smooth muscle like that found in the paroxyms of bronchial asthma. The systemic effects of epinephrine are reflected by the drug's role as an "emergency substance" and activation of effector cells connected with adrenergic nerve fibers.

The systemic effects of epinephrine are largely determined by the dose and its routes of administration. The most striking effect of intravenous injection of epinephrine is a rise in blood pressure due to peripheral vasoconstriction and myocardial stimulation.

Metabolic effects of epinephrine result from the formation of cyclic AMP. These include mobilization of fats and an increase in free fatty acids in the blood as a result of an increase in adipose cell lipase activity. Hyperglycemia occurs due to stimulation of glycogenolysis and inhibition of glycogen synthase. These metabolic effects result from beta-adrenergic receptor activation.

Clinical Indications. The main therapeutic uses of epinephrine are in the relief of bronchospasm and in hypersensitivity reactions. Epinephrine also prevents capillary bleeding, diminishes conjunctival hyperemia, and inhibits the synthesis of aqueous humor for benefit in open-angle glaucoma. Epinephrine enhances the action of local anesthetics by its vasoconstrictor action; thus, the local anesthetic remains at the site of action for a prolonged period. Heart block or cardiac arrest is yet another clinical indication for epinephrine.

Adverse Effects/Precautions. Increased nervousness, muscular tremor, palpitations, and headache often occur with epinephrine administration. This drug increases the work of the heart by its positive inotropic and chronotropic effects. Therefore, the heart's oxygen consumption increases, a situation that further aggravates the disorder in congestive heart failure (CHF) or in hyperthyroidism. Epinephrine should not be used (or be used with caution) in patients with nervous instability, diabetes mellitus, cardiovascular disease, and/or hyperthyroidism.

Norepinephrine. Norepinephrine is the endogenous catecholamine neurotransmitter released from postganglionic adrenergic nerve terminals. It differs from epinephrine by the absence of a methyl group on the nitrogen atom.

Mechanism of Action. Norepinephrine has a powerful effect on alpha-adrenergic receptors to produce peripheral vasoconstriction. Norepinephrine is equipotent to epinephrine in stimulating the beta-adrenergic receptors, but compensatory mechanisms slow the heart. Norepinephrine minimally affects beta$_2$-adrenergic receptors.

Clinical Indications. Norepinephrine elevates blood pressure in acute hypotensive states in which blood volume is not compromised. Correction of the blood volume deficit is indicated preceding norepinephrine administration.

Adverse Effects/Precautions. Hypertension and reflex bradycardia are adverse reactions that may occur with norepinephrine. Patients with a blood volume deficit should not receive this drug except in certain emergency instances to maintain coronary and cerebral artery perfusion.

Dopamine. An endogenous catecholamine, dopamine is formed by the decarboxylation of the amino acid, dihydroxyphenylalanine (DOPA). Dopamine is the immediate precursor in norepinephrine biosynthesis.

Mechanism of Action. Dopamine is a direct acting beta-adrenergic receptor agonist. It also has an indirect action which promotes norepinephrine release from adrenergic nerve terminals (Figure 2.21). Dopamine's direct inotropic effect on the heart minimally affects systemic blood pressure or heart rate.

Clinical Indications. Dopamine is given by intravenous infusion to treat shock, as in cases of trauma, myocardial infarction, and endotoxic septicemia. Before administering dopamine to patients in shock, the hypovolemia

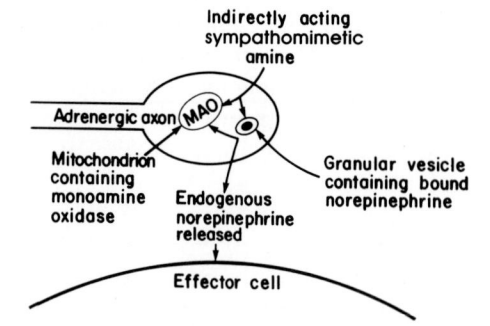

Fig. 2.21 Indirect acting sympathomimetic amine. (Modified from Bowman, W.C., and Rand, M.J.: Textbook of Pharmacology, 2nd Ed. Oxford, Blackwell Scientific Publications, 1980.)

must be corrected by the transfusion of whole blood, plasma, or appropriate fluids. Dopamine is also used in the treatment of chronic refractory CHF.

Adverse Effects/Precautions. Nausea, vomiting, and headache are common untoward effects. Cardiac side effects include tachycardia, ectopic beats, and precordial pain.

MISCELLANEOUS NATURAL AND SYNTHETIC ADRENERGIC DRUGS

Numerous clinically employed adrenergic drugs are chemical modifications of catecholamine compounds; these synthetic derivatives are either catecholamines or noncatecholamines. Naturally occurring alkaloids or their derivatives, such as ephedrine and pseudoephedrine, are additional important adrenergic drugs.

Dobutamine. A chemical relative of dopamine, dobutamine is characterized by the presence of an aromatic group on the amino group of the catecholamine nucleus.

Mechanism of Action. Dobutamine primarily activates beta$_1$-adrenergic receptors in the heart. The drug has minimal peripheral alpha$_1$-adrenergic receptor activity (e.g., vasoconstriction). Likewise, beta$_2$-adrenergic receptors are only slightly affected. No pronounced peripheral vascular effects are elicited.

Clinical Indications. Dobutamine is used for the short-term treatment of cardiac decompensation or reduced contractility, such as that which occurs in CHF or results from cardiac surgery.

Adverse Effects/Precautions. Cardiovascular responses, such as tachycardia, hypertension, and ventricular arrhythmias, are the most frequent adverse reactions.

Ephedrine. Ephedrine is a naturally occurring alkaloid contained in certain Ephedra species. The plant was used in China for at least 5000 years before its introduction into Western medicine by K.K. Chen in 1924. The Chinese called preparations from E. sinica "ma-huang," meaning "yellow horse" and referring to the color and shape of the Ephedra flower.

Mechanism of Action. Ephedrine releases norepinephrine from adrenergic nerve terminals. Alpha- and beta-adrenergic receptors are also directly stimulated by ephedrine. Several characteristics differentiate ephedrine's activity from that of epinephrine. First, ephedrine is effective orally, a definite advantage in ambulatory patients. Second, ephedrine has a longer duration of action. Third, ephedrine is less potent (about 1/100 on a weight basis) as a sympathomimetic agent. And lastly, ephedrine has a more pronounced stimulant effect on the CNS. Tachyphylaxis is characteristic of frequent ephedrine administration.

Clinical Indications. Therapeutic indications for ephedrine include bronchial asthma, nasal congestion, and as a mydriatic in ocular procedures. The pressor effects of ephedrine make it a valuable agent to maintain blood pressure and combat acute hypotensive states in spinal anesthesia. Narcolepsy and Stokes-Adams syndrome are also sometimes treated with ephedrine.

Adverse Effects/Precautions. Nausea, vomiting, and anorexia may occur with ephedrine. Palpitations, tachycardia, precordial pain, and cardiac arrhythmias are frequent adverse effects on the cardiovascular system. CNS adverse effects include headache, insomnia, nervousness, anxiety, and delirium and hallucinations. Convulsions are the principal manifestation of ephedrine overdose. Ephedrine should be used cautiously in patients with cardiovascular disease, hypertension, diabetes mellitus, and hyperthyroidism.

Pseudoephedrine. Pseudoephedrine is a stereoisomer of ephedrine.

Mechanism of Action. Although pharmacologically similar to ephedrine, pseudoephedrine has weaker pressor effects. Clinically, pseudoephedrine exhibits relative freedom from pressor effects in normotensive patients. The stimulation of alpha-adrenergic receptors is the principal mechanism for decongestant action, whereas its beta-adrenergic receptor agonist action manifests itself in bronchodilation.

Clinical Indications. Pseudoephedrine is used as a nasal decongestant and bronchodilator.

Adverse Effects/Precautions. Ephedrine-like reactions on the cardiovascular system (e.g., palpitations, tachycardia, and hypertension) and on the CNS (e.g., anxiety and nervousness) may occur. Patients who are particularly sensitive to sympathomimetic drugs may experience mild stimulation.

Phenylephrine. Phenylephrine, a synthetic sympathomimetic, has minimal effects on the CNS.

Mechanism of Action. Phenylephrine acts principally by stimulating alpha-adrenergic receptors on vascular smooth muscle. The resultant vasoconstriction increases the peripheral resistance which characterizes the drug's pressor response. Blood vessels in mucous membranes are markedly constricted with subsequent shrinkage by direct application of phenylephrine, which promotes drainage in nasal passages, the eustachian tubes, and paranasal sinuses.

Clinical Indications. Phenylephrine is used as a nasal decongestant in treating the symptoms of sinusitis, acute coryza, hay fever (i.e., allergic rhinitis), and the common cold.

Adverse Effects/Precautions. Fear, anxiety, tremors, and other manifestations of central nervous stimulation may occur with phenylephrine. Cardiac effects, such as irregular heart beat, are infrequent.

Rebound congestion is a common phenomenon that occurs with topical decongestants, such as phenylephrine. To avoid this effect, patients should not administer phenylephrine chronically, but rather they should limit its use to 3 to 5 days.

Phenylpropanolamine. Phenylpropanolamine (PPA) is a synthetic sympathomimetic that is a mixture of the D and L forms of norephedrine. It possesses anorectic properties.

Mechanism of Action. Phenylpropanolamine is a direct alpha-adrenergic receptor agonist that has an additional indirect action on both alpha- and beta-adrenergic receptors. The vasoconstrictor activity on alpha-adrenergic receptors causes the drug's beneficial nasal decongestant action.

The anorectic effect of PPA (central in nature) is probably mediated through hypothalamic norepinephrine pathways, activating a "satiety center" that decreases hunger. PPA's effects on glucostatic satiety mechanisms in the hypothalamus may account for some of its anorectic effects.

Clinical Indications. PPA is valuable as a nasal decongestant in treating symptoms of allergic rhinitis, sinusitis, and the common cold. Reports of small but consistent weight loss account for the drug's acceptance as an OTC weight control product for short-term (12 weeks) programs.

Adverse Effects/Precautions. Nervousness, restlessness, insomnia, headache, and nausea are some of the drug's side effects. Adverse effects on the cardiovascular system (e.g., hypertension and strokes) and the CNS (e.g., hallucinations and psychotic episodes) have been reported. At recommended oral therapeutic doses, however, the incidence of adverse side effects is low. Since PPA is a sympathomimetic, it should be used cautiously, if at all, in patients with cardiovascular disease, hypertension, hyperthyroidism, or diabetes mellitus.

ANOREXIANT ADRENERGIC DRUGS

Amphetamines (see Chapter 1) comprise the group of drugs that has the longest history of use in the treatment of obesity; however, the adverse effects of amphetamines (i.e., psychologic and physical dependency) occur with alarming frequency and have practically halted amphetamine use as anorectics. Their use in weight reduction programs is limited to patients for whom alternative therapy has proven ineffective. Nonamphetamine adrenergic drugs that are used in short-term (up to 12 weeks) weight loss programs include benzphetamine, diethylpropion, phenmetrazine, phentermine, fenfluramine, and mazindol. Although these drugs are available, drug treatment of obesity is of limited value since the only satisfactory means of weight control is caloric reduction and physical activity.

Mechanism of Action. Appetite suppression by the anorexiant adrenergic drugs probably relates to an effect on the satiety center in the hypothalamus and limbic system. Fenfluramine, unlike the other drugs in this group, produces CNS depression rather than stimulation, possibly resulting from a reduction in brain serotonin (5-HT). By acting primarily on the limbic system, mazindol differs from the other agents which mainly affect hypothalamic sites.

Clinical Indications. Anorexiant adrenergic drugs, as an adjunct to reduced caloric intake, are used in short-term (up to 12 weeks) weight reduction programs.

Adverse Effects/Precautions. Secondary actions of these drugs include CNS stimulation and blood pressure elevation. Cardiovascular adverse effects include palpitations, tachycardia, arrhythmias, and hypertension or hypotension. The use of anorexiant adrenergic agents with CNS stimulants is contraindicated. Fenfluramine may induce CNS depression; withdrawal symptoms after drug discontinuation may also occur. Mazindol may potentiate the pressor effects of exogenous catecholamines.

ADDITIONAL VASOCONSTRICTOR ADRENERGIC DRUGS

The sympathomimetics (i.e., naphazoline, oxymetazoline, propylhexedrine, tetrahydrozoline, and xylometazoline) are used primarily for their alpha-adrenergic agonist properties that result in vasoconstriction of the vessels in nasal mucosa. Tetrahydrozoline and naphazoline produce this same effect in the ocular vessels.

ADDITIONAL PRESSOR ADRENERGIC DRUGS

Metaraminol. Metaraminol is a synthetic sympathomimetic amine that has potent pressor properties.

Mechanism of Action. Metaraminol stimulates alpha- and beta-adrenergic receptors, resulting in a positive inotropic effect on the heart and vasoconstriction in peripheral blood vessels. Release of norepinephrine from adrenergic nerve terminals is also a component of metaraminol action. This drug minimally affects the CNS.

Clinical Indications. Metaraminol is used as a pressor agent during spinal anesthesia to prevent and treat acute hypotension.

Adverse Effects/Precautions. The possibility of excessive hypotensive action must be recognized with metaraminol. Cardiac arrhythmias, especially in myocardial infarction patients, may occur with this drug.

Mephenteramine. A synthetic sympathomimetic, mephenteramine possesses a significant prolonged pressor activity.

Mechanism of Action. Mephenteramine acts directly on both alpha- and beta-adrenergic receptors. Mephenteramine also indirectly releases endogenous norepinephrine, an important component of mephenteramine's activity. Its positive inotropic effect on the heart increases cardiac output. Vasoconstriction, resulting from peripheral alpha-adrenergic receptor stimulation, and cardiac stimulation produce a prolonged pressor response of up to 4 hours if the drug is given intramuscularly. Mephenteramine has only a mild stimulant effect on the CNS.

Clinical Indications. Mephenteramine maintains blood pressure in controlled hypotensive states. Another clinical application is as a nasal decongestant.

Adverse Effects/Precautions. Mephenteramine produces minimal side effects that include anxiety and other signs of minor CNS stimulation.

Hydroxyamphetamine. Although pharmacologically similar to ephedrine, hydroxyamphetamine elicits no significant effects on the CNS.

Mechanism of Action. Hydroxyamphetamine activates alpha- and beta-adrenergic receptors; the alpha-adrenergic responses primarily account for this drug's therapeutic application.

Clinical Indications. Hydroxyamphetamine, a pressor adrenergic drug, is chiefly used clinically in the United States as a mydriatic. The drug has also been used in the treatment of Stokes-Adams syndrome for its cardiac stimulant property and as a nasal decongestant.

Adverse Effects/Precautions. Photophobia and blurred vision may result from the marked pupillary dilation this drug produces. Hydroxyamphetamine is contraindicated in narrow-angle glaucoma.

Methoxamine. A noncatecholamine adrenergic agonist, methoxamine has pharmacologic properties similar to phenylephrine.

Mechanism of Action. Methoxamine directly activates alpha-adrenergic receptors, resulting in vasoconstriction and increased blood pressure. This drug minimally affects beta-adrenergic receptors and produces little activity on the CNS.

Clinical Indications. Methoxamine is used primarily as a pressor agent in hypotensive states and to treat paroxymal atrial tachycardia.

Adverse Effects/Precautions. Excessive blood pressure elevation accompanied by headache may occur with methoxamine, especially in high doses.

ADDITIONAL BRONCHODILATOR ADRENERGIC DRUGS

Isoproterenol. A structural relative of epinephrine, isoproterenol is a synthetic sympathomimetic amine that possesses a selectivity for beta-adrenergic receptor stimulation.

Mechanism of Action. Isoproterenol preferentially activates both beta$_1$- and beta$_2$-adrenergic receptors. The beta$_1$-adrenergic response of the myocardium is responsible for the drug's effectiveness in hypoperfusion shock syndrome and cardiac arrest or standstill. The beta$_2$-adrenergic activity results in marked bronchial dilation and therefore is beneficial in bronchospastic diseases, such as bronchial asthma.

Clinical Indications. Isoproterenol is valuable in the treatment of bronchospasm associated with acute and chronic bronchial asthma, pulmonary emphysema, bronchitis, and bronchiectasis. Parenteral administration of isoproterenol is indicated as an adjunct in the management of shock (hypofusion syndrome). Isoproterenol is also indicated in cardiac arrest, Stokes-Adams syndrome, and certain ventricular arrhythmias that respond to increased cardiac activity.

Adverse Effects/Precautions. Serious reactions with isoproterenol therapy are uncommon. Tachycardia, precordial pain, nausea, vomiting, and minimal CNS stimulation have been reported.

Ethylnorepinephrine. Ethylnorepinephrine is a synthetic sympathomimetic amine that is available for parenteral administration.

Mechanism of Action. Ethylnorepinephrine has selective beta-adrenergic receptor agonist activity. Although less potent, its action is similar to that of isoproterenol.

Clinical Indications. Ethylnorepinephrine is indicated in the treatment of bronchial asthma and in reversible bronchospastic diseases, such as bronchitis and emphysema.

Adverse Effects/Precautions. Side effects attributed to sympathomimetic activity include elevation or depression of blood pressure, palpitations, dizziness, and/or nausea.

Metaproterenol. Metaproterenol resembles isoproterenol structurally except that the catecholamine moiety is not present and thus, metaproterenol is not metabolized by COMT.

Mechanism of Action. Metaproterenol is primarily a beta$_2$-adrenergic receptor stimulant that has little activity on beta$_1$-adrenergic receptors.

Clinical Indications. Metaproterenol is used for its bronchodilator activity in bronchial asthma and other bronchospastic diseases, including bronchitis and emphysema.

Adverse Effects/Precautions. Nausea, vomiting, and signs of sympathetic stimulation (e.g., tremors, palpitations, nervousness, and hypertension) are side effects reported with metaproterenol administration.

Albuterol. Albuterol (international generic name—salbutamol) resembles isoproterenol in action but is longer acting.

Mechanism of Action. Albuterol selectively activates beta$_2$-adrenergic receptors.

Clinical Indications. Albuterol is used as a bronchodilator in chronic or acute bronchial asthma, bronchitis, or other chronic obstructive pulmonary disease (COPD).

Adverse Effects/Precautions. Nervousness and muscle tremors are common side effects of albuterol therapy.

Terbutaline. A noncatecholamine sympathomimetic, terbutaline is a selective beta$_2$-adrenergic agonist.

Mechanism of Action. Terbutaline selectively activates beta$_2$-adrenergic receptors. The specificity of terbutaline for beta$_2$-adrenergic receptors is not as absolute when the drug is given by subcutaneous injection.

Clinical Indications. Terbutaline is used as a bronchodilator in the management of asthma and other bronchospastic diseases.

Adverse Effects/Precautions. Sympathomimetic reactions, such as nervousness and muscle tremors, are the most frequently reported adverse effects of terbutaline administration.

Isoetharine. Isoetharine is a sympathomimetic amine that has preferential affinity for beta$_2$-adrenergic receptors.

Mechanism of Action. Isoetharine is a selective beta-adrenergic receptor agonist. It has less preferential affinity for beta$_2$-adrenergic receptors when compared to other beta$_2$-adrenergic receptor agonists, such as metaproterenol and albuterol.

Clinical Indications. Isoetharine is employed as a nebulized solution in the treatment of bronchospastic disease.

Adverse Effects/Precautions. Isoetharine is relatively free of toxic side effects. Adverse effects related to adrenergic activity include palpitations, tachycardia, muscle tremors, and mild CNS stimulation. Excessive use of this drug has caused parodoxical airway resistance.

Ritodrine. Ritodrine activates beta$_2$-adrenergic receptors and has clinical application as a uterine muscle relaxant.

Mechanism of Action. Ritodrine is a selective beta$_2$-adrenergic receptor agonist with consequent relaxation of the bronchiolar and uterine smooth muscle.

Clinical Indications. The main therapeutic application of ritodrine is as a uterine relaxant to stop premature labor. Administered intravenously initially, the drug is subsequently given orally if the initial IV administration achieves positive response.

Adverse Effects/Precautions. Side effects (usually controlled by dosage adjustments) include palpitations, tremor, nausea, vomiting, headache, and erythema.

ADRENERGIC BLOCKING DRUGS

Alpha-adrenergic receptor blockers (Table 2.10), once used in the treatment of hypertension, find limited use in modern therapy (with the exception of prazosin). The advent of beta-adrenergic receptor blockers marked an important advance in the treatment of cardiovascular disease and hypertension.

DRUGS BLOCKING ALPHA-ADRENERGIC RECEPTORS

By interfering with the ability of sympathomimetic amines to initiate a physiologic response, these drugs produce significant effects on smooth muscles, glands, and organ systems that contain alpha-adrenergic receptors. Two subtypes of alpha-adrenergic receptors (alpha$_1$ and alpha$_2$) may be blocked, and blocking agents often show a preference for one subtype. For instance, prazosin has selective blocking activity on alpha$_1$-adrenergic receptors, whereas the alkaloid yohimbine preferentially blocks alpha$_2$-adrenergic receptors.

Alpha-adrenergic receptor blockers have limited therapeutic value because they block sympathetic cardiovascular responses and prevent the necessary physiologic adjustments when patients change from a prone or resting posture to an upright or standing position. Additionally, alpha-adrenergic blocking drugs inhibit ejaculation in many male patients.

Phenoxybenzamine. Phenoxybenzamine, a haloalkylamine, has a specific alpha-adrenergic receptor blocking action. No alpha-adrenergic agonist activity is noted with phenoxybenzamine.

Mechanism of Action. Phenoxybenzamine interacts with alpha-adrenergic receptors by forming a covalent bond with the receptor substance (Figure 2.22). Agonists capable of interacting with the alpha-adrenergic receptor are ineffective in the presence of phenoxybenzamine blockade.

Clinical Indications. Phenoxybenzamine controls episodes of hypertension and sweating in pheochromocytoma.

Adverse Effects/Precautions. Side effects that result from blockade of alpha-adrenergic responses include nasal congestion, miosis, postural hypotension, tachycardia, and ejaculation inhibition. With continued therapy, these reactions to alpha-adrenergic blockade decrease.

The selective blocking of alpha-adrenergic

Table 2.10 ALPHA-ADRENERGIC RECEPTOR BLOCKING DRUGS.

Available products	Trade name	Daily dosage range
Phenoxybenzamine HCl	Dibenzyline	Initially, 10 mg/day; increase gradually to 20–60 mg/day
Phentolamine	Regitine	50 mg orally 4–6 times daily
Tolazoline HCl	Priscoline	10–50 mg q.i.d. SC, IV, IM

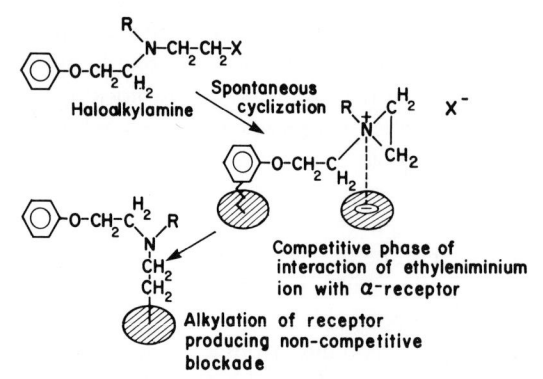

Fig. 2.22 Mechanism of alpha-adrenergic receptor blocking action of haloalkylamines. (Modified from Bowman, W.C., and Rand, M.J.: Textbook of Pharmacology, 2nd Ed. Oxford, Blackwell Scientific Publications, 1980.)

receptors by phenoxybenzamine leaves the beta-adrenergic receptors unoccupied. Consequently, a compound that has both alpha- and beta-agonist action produces an exaggerated effect on the beta-adrenergic response system since alpha-adrenergic receptors are blocked. Epinephrine (a mixed alpha- and beta-agonist), administered after phenoxybenzamine, thus induces unopposed beta-adrenergic responses, including hypotension and tachycardia.

Phentolamine. Phentolamine is a competitive inhibitor of the effects of endogenous and exogenous alpha-adrenergic agonists.

Mechanism of Action. Phentolamine, a competitive inhibitor of adrenergic agonists, blocks both alpha$_1$- and alpha$_2$-adrenergic receptors. The drug's action at both the arterial tree and venous bed reduces total peripheral resistance.

Clinical Indications. Phentolamine prevents and controls hypertensive episodes prior to surgical procedures in patients who have pheochromocytoma. Parenteral phentolamine also prevents and treats skin necrosis and sloughing after extravasation of norepinephrine or dopamine intravenous solutions.

Adverse Effects/Precautions. Hypotensive reactions, tachycardia, and cardiac arrhythmias have been reported after phentolamine administration. Phentolamine is contraindicated in patients with myocardial infarction, coronary insufficiency, or other signs of coronary artery disease.

Tolazoline. Tolazoline, an alpha-adrenergic blocker that has ancillary histamine-like effects, is marketed as a parenteral preparation for intravenous, intramuscular, or subcutaneous administration.

Mechanism of Action. Tolazoline produces peripheral vasodilation by transient alpha-adrenergic blockade and by a direct action on vascular smooth muscle. The drug also produces an oversecretion of gastric acid and pepsin and pulmonary vasodilation by stimulating histamine H$_2$-receptors.

Clinical Indications. Tolazoline is indicated for spastic peripheral vascular disorders, such as thromboangitis obliterans (Buerger's disease), diabetic arteriosclerosis, and Raynaud's disease.

Adverse Effects/Precautions. The most common clinical side effects of tolazoline relate to cardiac and gastrointestinal stimulation. Tolazoline may precipitate myocardial infarction, as well as induce tachycardia, angina, and cardiac arrhythmias. Other reported adverse reactions to tolazoline therapy include nausea, vomiting, and worsening of peptic ulcer.

Concurrent use of epinephrine or norepinephrine with tolazoline may result in severe hypotension ("epinephrine reversal"), followed by an exaggerated rebound.

Prazosin. Prazosin, a selective alpha$_1$-adrenergic (postsynaptic) blocking drug, is used to treat hypertension.

Mechanism of Action. Prazosin blocks postsynaptic alpha$_1$-adrenergic receptors and induces a direct relaxant effect on vascular smooth muscle. In contrast to classical alpha-adrenergic blockers, prazosin does not routinely produce reflex tachycardia and tolerance does not develop after continued therapy.

Clinical Indications. Prazosin is indicated in the treatment of hypertension.

Adverse Effects/Precautions. The most common adverse reactions observed with prazosin therapy are dizziness, headache, drowsiness, and weakness. Prazosin is also associated with a phenomenon known as "first dose syncope." In approximately 1% of the patients receiving an initial dose of 2 mg or greater, syncope usually occurs within 30 to 90 minutes of the initial drug dose.

MISCELLANEOUS NATURAL AND SYNTHETIC DRUGS BLOCKING ALPHA-ADRENERGIC RECEPTORS

Various other drugs block alpha-adrenergic receptors in addition to having other pharmacologic effects.

Ergot Alkaloids. A myriad of complex and diverse pharmacologic effects characterize ergot alkaloids, the first adrenergic blocking drugs that were discovered. The ergot alkaloid ergonomine, an oxytocic drug, is essentially devoid of alpha-adrenergic blocking activity. Chapter 9 contains additional information on these alkaloids and their derivatives.

Ergotamine and Dihydroergotamine. Ergotamine and dihydroergotamine block alpha-adrenergic receptors and are used to treat certain vascular diseases, such as vascular headache.

Mechanism of Action. Ergotamine causes direct vasoconstriction of cranial and extracranial arteries with a concurrent reduction in arterial pulsations. This direct action on arterial smooth muscle is unrelated to the alpha-adrenergic blocking activity of ergotamine. Additionally, by probably inhibiting norepinephrine re-uptake at adrenergic nerve endings, ergotamine increases the vasoconstrictor effect.

Clinical Indications. Ergotamine (oral, sublingual, or inhalation) and dihydroergotamine (parenteral) effectively treat acute migraine attacks and cluster headaches. Dihydroergotamine is used for its rapid onset of action or when other administration routes are unacceptable.

Adverse Effects/Precautions. Numbness and tingling of the extremities are common reactions. Also, gastrointestinal effects, such as nausea, vomiting, and diarrhea, may occur. Prolonged use should be avoided because of the danger of ergotism or gangrene. Vascular complications, usually involving the legs, signal chronic toxicity. Ergotamine derivatives are contraindicated in peripheral vascular disease and in pregnancy.

Methysergide. A semisynthetic ergot derivative, methysergide has significant antiserotonin activity.

Mechanism of Action. Methysergide blocks the peripheral action of serotonin on vascular smooth muscle but promotes the enhanced sensitivity of cephalic arteries to norepinephrine. Methysergide may also be a central serotonin agonist.

Clinical Indications. Methysergide is used in the prophylactic therapy of migraine and cluster headaches. This drug's effectiveness depends upon regular therapy; thus, it should not be used intermittently. Because of methysergide's poor margin of safety, it should be used only in severe cases.

Adverse Effects/Precautions. Adverse effects occur in 2 out of 5 patients. Nausea, vomiting, diarrhea, and cold, numb, and painful extremities are frequently cited side effects. CNS adverse effects, such as drowsiness and "dissociation," have also been reported. Additional reactions include papuloerythematous skin rashes, hair loss, and weight gain. Prolonged therapy may result in retroperitoneal fibrosis, pleuropulmonary fibrosis, and fibrotic thickening of cardiac valves. Methysergide is contraindicated in peripheral vascular disease and in pregnancy.

PHENOTHIAZINES AND OTHER NEUROLEPTIC AGENTS

Chlorpromazine and other phenothiazine tranquilizers have significant adrenergic blocking activity. Also, the butyrophenone derivative, haloperidol, possesses adrenergic blocking activity.

DRUGS BLOCKING BETA-ADRENERGIC RECEPTORS

The beta-adrenergic blocking drugs (Table 2.11) are valuable in the treatment of cardiovascular disorders, including hypertension, angina pectoris, and cardiac arrhythmias (see Chapter 3). Additional uses for specific beta-adrenergic blockers include anxiety (propranolol), glaucoma (timolol), and migraine (propranolol).

NONSELECTIVE BETA-ADRENERGIC BLOCKING DRUGS

Propranolol, nadolol, pindolol, and timolol are nonselective beta blockers since they inhibit both beta$_1$- and beta$_2$-adrenergic receptors. Selective beta$_1$-adrenergic receptor blockers include metoprolol, atenolol, and acebutolol. The following presents propranolol as the prototype beta-adrenergic receptor blocker.

Propranolol. Propranolol, the first beta-adrenergic receptor blocking drug that achieved widespread clinical use, is a nonselective beta-adrenergic blocking drug that is characterized by a variety of clinical indications, including hypertension, angina pectoris, hyperthyroidism, and migraine.

Mechanism of Action. By attaching to beta-adrenergic receptors, propranolol prevents the interaction of the adrenergic neurotransmitters, norepinephrine and epinephrine.

Clinical Indications. Propranolol, often used in combination with a diuretic, effectively treats hypertension. The drug is also valuable in the management of certain supraventricular and ventricular arrhythmias. Reports indicate that propranolol has reduced the incidence of reinfarction and mortality after myocardial infarction. Additional clinical applications of propranolol include migraine, hyperthyroidism, pheochromocytoma, and anxiety.

Adverse Effects/Precautions. Most of the adverse reactions to propranolol extend from its pharmacologic effects. Myocardial depression, resulting from beta-adrenergic receptor blockade, can result in heart failure, a special problem in patients who have inadequate cardiac function.

Specifically, hypersensitivity to catecholamines has been observed in some patients withdrawn from beta-adrenergic blocker therapy. The abrupt withdrawal of propranolol has precipitated angina pectoris and, in some cases, myocardial infarction.

Propranolol reduces the compensatory sympathetic-adrenal (hyperglycemic) reaction to insulin, thereby augmenting insulin's hypoglycemic action. Propranolol masks the tachycardia and anxiety often interpreted by the diabetic as an early sign of an insulin reaction, sometimes resulting in severe hypotension before the diabetic recognizes the problem.

Bronchial asthma or related pulmonary

Table 2.11 BETA-ADRENERGIC RECEPTOR BLOCKING DRUGS.

Available products	Trade names	Daily dosage range
Acebutolol	Sectral	400–800 mg/day
Atenolol	Tenormin	50 mg once daily
Labetalol	Normodyne Trandate	400–800 mg/day
Metoprolol tartrate	Lopressor	Initially, 100 mg/day; Maintenance dose, 100–450 mg/day
Nadolol	Corgard	80–240 mg once daily
Pindolol	Visken	15 mg/day
Propranolol HCl	Inderal	Varies according to clinical condition
Timolol maleate	Blocadren	20–40 mg/day

diseases are contraindications to propranolol therapy.

Nadolol. Nadolol, a nonselective beta-adrenergic receptor blocker, has a long duration of action.

Mechanism of Action. Nadolol is a competitive blocking drug at both $beta_1$- and $beta_2$-adrenergic receptors. Nadolol does not possess significant membrane-stabilizing activity and, because of its low lipid solubility, does not readily enter the CNS. This drug has no clinically significant partial agonist activity and, unlike most of the beta-adrenergic blockers, is not metabolized. Nadolol is excreted unchanged in the urine.

Clinical Indications. Used in the management of angina pectoris and hypertension, nadolol is effective in once a day dosage.

Adverse Effects/Precautions. Most of the adverse effects seen with nadolol are mild and transient; however, bradycardia, bronchospasm, dizziness, fatigue, nausea, and gastrointestinal disturbances are possible. Since a worsening of angina pectoris or myocardial infarction occurs in some patients abruptly withdrawn from beta-adrenergic blocker therapy, gradual reduction of nadolol dosage is indicated in those who have received the drug for an extended period.

Pindolol. A nonselective beta-adrenergic blocking drug, pindolol has significant intrinsic sympathomimetic activity.

Mechanism of Action. Pindolol blocks both $beta_1$- and $beta_2$-adrenergic receptors. Additionally, pindolol has partial agonist activity, evidenced by a smaller reduction in cardiac output and heart rate as compared to other beta-adrenergic blockers.

Clinical Indications. Pindolol is useful in the treatment of hypertension.

Adverse Effects/Precautions. Side effects include bradycardia, sedation, abnormal response to hypoglycemia, hyperglycemia, blood lipid changes, and gastrointestinal symptoms. The clinical problems associated with beta-adrenergic blocking agents (such as exacerbation of ischemic heart disease following abrupt withdrawal of therapy, masking of hypoglycemic symptoms in diabetics, and precipitation of congestive heart failure) also apply to pindolol.

Timolol. A nonselective beta-adrenergic blocking drug, timolol is used to treat hypertension, glaucoma, and postmyocardial infarction.

Mechanism of Action. Timolol blocks both $beta_1$- and $beta_2$-adrenergic receptors, thus preventing the effects of adrenergic agonists. This drug is several times more potent (milligram for milligram) than propranolol as a beta-adrenergic blocking agent. Like propranolol, timolol undergoes considerable first-pass hepatic metabolism. Timolol has neither significant adrenergic agonist activity nor membrane-stabilizing action. The mechanism of action responsible for the drug's benefit in glaucoma treatment apparently involves a decrease in the secretion and outflow of aqueous humor.

Clinical Indications. Timolol is effective in the management of hypertension and in the reduction of the incidence of recurring myocardial infarction after an initial attack. This drug is also available as an ophthalmic preparation for use in the treatment of chronic open-angle glaucoma, secondary glaucoma, and glaucoma that accompanies aphakia. Pupillary constriction and spasm of accommodation, routinely encountered with cholinergic agents used in glaucoma, do not occur with timolol.

Adverse Effects/Precautions. The common side effects that occur with timolol use in hypertension treatment (such as bradycardia, fatigue, tiredness, dizziness, dyspnea, and eye irritation) are usually mild and transient. As with all systemically administered beta-adrenergic blockers that have been chronically employed, the possibility of exacerbation of ishemic heart disease following abrupt timolol withdrawal exists.

The ocular side effects noted with the ophthalmic preparation include keratitis, discomfort, and rarely, corneal anesthesia. About 50% of the side effects that occur with the use of the ophthalmic solution are systemic in nature; these include bradycardia, hypotension, cardiac abnormalities, bronchospasm, and CNS depression.

SELECTIVE BETA$_1$-ADRENERGIC RECEPTOR BLOCKING DRUGS

These drugs block beta$_1$-adrenergic receptors in doses that are ineffective in blocking beta$_2$-adrenergic receptors.

Acebutolol. Acebutolol is a cardioselective (beta$_1$) adrenergic receptor blocker.

Mechanism of Action. Acebutolol selectively blocks beta-adrenergic receptors and has both membrane-stabilizing effects and partial adrenergic agonist activity.

Clinical Indications. Acebutolol is used in the treatment of hypertension.

Adverse Effects/Precautions. Bradycardia, sedation, abnormal response to hypoglycemia, hyperglycemia, blood lipid changes, and gastrointestinal disturbances may occur with acebutolol therapy. The precautions in acebutolol use are the same as those of propranolol treatment.

Atenolol. Atenolol, a selective beta$_1$-adrenergic blocking drug, is used as an antihypertensive agent.

Mechanism of Action. Atenolol specifically blocks beta$_1$-adrenergic receptors. The drug possesses no clinically significant membrane-stabilizing action, nor does it exhibit intrinsic sympathomimetic activity.

Clinical Indications. Usually administered in once a day doses, atenolol is indicated in the treatment of hypertension. Although the plasma half-life of atenolol is from six to eight hours, its antihypertensive action persists longer.

Adverse Effects/Precautions. Fatigue and depression may occur although atenolol does not enter the CNS readily because of the drug's low lipid solubility. Atenolol, since it does not significantly block beta$_2$-adrenergic receptors, rarely potentiates insulin-induced hypoglycemia. However, a masking of the hypoglycemia-induced reflex tachycardia in the hypoglycemic diabetic patient may occur.

Atenolol should be used cautiously in patients who have bronchial asthma or other bronchoconstrictor disease. Also, atenolol may precipitate congestive heart failure and should not be employed in these instances without close patient monitoring. The presence of cardiac conduction disturbances also necessitates special precautions if atenolol is used.

Metoprolol. A selective beta$_1$-adrenergic receptor blocker, metoprolol is available in oral and parenteral dosage forms.

Mechanism of Action. Metoprolol preferentially blocks beta$_1$-adrenergic receptors, thus representing a cardioselective activity. The dose of metoprolol required for beta$_2$-adrenergic response blockade, such as vasodilation, induced by isoproterenol (a beta-adrenergic receptor agonist) is 50 to 100 times that of propranolol. This contrasts with the essentially equivalent potency of metoprolol or propranolol to block cardiovascular beta$_1$-adrenergic responses to isoproterenol.

Clinical Indications. Indicated in the treatment of hypertension, metoprolol is frequently administered with other drugs for this condition. A reduction in the incidence of recurrent myocardial infarction and mortality has been reported for patients undergoing metoprolol therapy following their initial myocardial infarction.

Adverse Effects/Precautions. The most frequent side effects of metoprolol use are fatigue, headache, dizziness, and insomnia. Metoprolol should be used cautiously (if at all) in asthmatic patients or patients who have a risk for congestive heart failure. Cardiac conduction disease also represents a relative contraindication for this drug.

An impairment of glucose tolerance in diabetic patients results from the partial inhibition of the beta-adrenergic receptor mediated release of insulin by metoprolol. This drug can also mask early warning signs of hypoglycemia (such as tachycardia) in the hypoglycemic diabetic patient.

BETA-ADRENERGIC BLOCKING DRUGS WITH ALPHA-ADRENERGIC BLOCKING ACTIVITY

Certain beta-adrenergic blockers possess an additional alpha-adrenergic blocking component.

Labetalol. Labetalol, a beta-adrenergic and alpha-adrenergic blocking drug, is effective in the management of essential hypertension. It is also available in a parenteral form for the intravenous treatment of hypertensive crisis.

Mechanism of Action. Labetalol exhibits nonselective beta-adrenergic receptor blocking action, as well as selectively blocking alpha$_1$-adrenergic receptors. The drug is not a particularly potent blocker of either type of receptor when compared to prototype alpha and beta blocking drugs. For instance, labetalol is 1/3 as potent as propranolol in blocking beta-adrenergic receptors, and it has only 1/10 the alpha-adrenergic receptor blocking potency of phentolamine. Resulting from the alpha-adrenergic receptor blockade, the vasodilation reduces peripheral resistance and lowers blood pressure, whereas the blocking of beta-adrenergic receptors protects the heart against stress and exercise-induced increases in blood pressure and heart rate.

Clinical Indications. Labetalol, indicated in the treatment of essential hypertension, is also effective in the treatment of hypertension that is associated with pheochromocytoma and that encountered after the abrupt withdrawal of clonidine.

Adverse Effects/Precautions. Adverse effects include nausea, vomiting, paresthesias, sweating, dizziness, flushing, and headache. Orthostatic hypotension, related to alpha-adrenergic receptor blockade, is another reported side effect. Labetalol should not be used in patients with bronchial asthma, congestive heart failure, cardiac conduction block, cardiogenic shock, or severe bradycardia.

MISCELLANEOUS DRUGS THAT INTERFERE WITH ADRENERGIC NEURON FUNCTION

According to their clinical indications, the drugs included in this category are discussed in detail in Chapter 3.

DRUGS THAT BLOCK ADRENERGIC NEURONS

Certain drugs, such as guanethidine and bretylium, interfere with the presynaptic release of norepinephrine into the synaptic cleft. This reduces sympathetic tone due to a lesser amount of the neurotransmitter available for attachment to adrenergic receptors. Additionally, reserpine depletes the stores of presynaptic norepinephrine, resulting in less neurotransmitter for release after sympathetic nerve stimulation. The net result resembles the effects of guanethidine and bretylium in that less neurotransmitter is released into the adrenergic synaptic cleft. Either case achieves blockade of the adrenergic neuron.

DRUGS THAT REDUCE CENTRAL ADRENERGIC OUTFLOW

Clonidine and methyldopa are two drugs that interfere with central control of peripheral adrenergic influences. The mechanisms involved are complex, but one probably involves central presynaptic alpha$_2$-adrenergic agonist activity. These interactions of clonidine and methyldopa with the central adrenergic receptors reduce the sympathetic impulse traffic to peripheral adrenergic neurons. An outcome is inhibition of the sympathetic innervation to vascular smooth muscle with subsequent vessel relaxation and reduction of peripheral resistance.

DRUGS THAT INHIBIT MONOAMINE OXIDASE

The accumulation of catecholamines at critical neuron sites (by inhibiting their metabolic breakdown) forms the basis for the pharmacologic efficacy of monoamine oxidase inhibitors, a class of drugs introduced into psychochemotherapy as antidepressant drugs in the 1950s. Paradoxically with these drugs, reduction in blood pressure occurs possibly due to a central presynaptic alpha$_2$-adrenergic agonist action or peripheral accumulation of a "false transmitter" at adrenergic neuron synapses.

DRUGS THAT INHIBIT CATECHOLAMINE SYNTHESIS

By blocking the synthesis of epinephrine and norepinephrine, metyrosine directly reduces adrenergic influence since less neurotransmitter is synthesized at presynaptic sites. Metyrosine is effective in the management of patients with pheochromocytoma.

DRUG INTERACTIONS

Clinically significant drug interactions may occur with the autonomic drugs. Individuals taking anticholinesterase drugs, in either an ophthalmic or oral dosage form, may experience toxic reactions after exposure to carbamate or organophosphate-type pesticides and insecticides. Taking antispasmodic muscarinic receptor blocking drugs with other drugs (including OTC products) which have cholinergic blocking activity may intensify the side effects of the antispasmodics. Also, skeletal muscle relaxant nicotinic blocking drugs interact with other agents.

The activity of adrenergic drugs (sympathomimetics) on the cardiovascular system may be either enhanced or inhibited by the concurrent use of other drugs. Beta-adrenergic receptor blocking drugs have clinically significant interactions with other drugs.

CHOLINERGIC DRUGS

MIOTICS, CHOLINESTERASE INHIBITORS

Carbamate or Organophosphate-type Insecticides and Pesticides. Added systemic effects are possible from absorption through the respiratory tract or skin; thus, persons receiving cholinesterase inhibitors should take precautionary measures (respiratory masks, frequent washing and clothing changes) in case of exposure to carbamate or organophosphate-type products.

Succinylcholine. Before or during general anesthesia, this drug should be administered cautiously in patients who also receive cholinesterase inhibitors due to the possibility of respiratory and cardiovascular collapse.

Systemic Anticholinesterase Drugs. Concurrent administration in myasthenia gravis may produce adverse additive effects.

CHOLINERGIC BLOCKING DRUGS

MUSCARINIC BLOCKING DRUGS
GASTROINTESTINAL ANTICHOLINERGICS

Antacids. Since these drugs interfere with absorption, simultaneous administration with muscarinic blocking drugs is discouraged.

Antihistamines, Benzodiazepines, and Tricyclic Antidepressants (TCADs). Due to their anticholinergic effects, these drugs may enhance the side effects of atropine and its derivatives.

Cholinesterase Inhibitors. Anticholinergics antagonize the miotic actions of cholinesterase inhibitors.

Corticosteroids. Increased ocular pressure can result from concurrent long-term therapy with corticosteroids and anticholinergics.

Guanethidine, Histamine, and Reserpine. These drugs antagonize the inhibition of gastric acid secretion by anticholinergics.

MAO Inhibitors. These drugs block detoxification of anticholinergics and may potentiate their actions.

Sympathomimetics. Anticholinergics enhance the bronchial relaxation that results from sympathomimetics.

NICOTINIC BLOCKING DRUGS

NONDEPOLARIZING SKELETAL MUSCLE RELAXANTS

Antibiotics. Parenteral use of antibiotics may either intensify or mask the action of curare. Unexpected prolongation of respiratory depression may occur in patients who receive both drugs simultaneously.

Inhalation Anesthetics. Both the intensity of blockade and duration of action of curare preparations increase in patients who also receive these drugs.

Thiazide Diuretics. Increased sensitivity to curare preparations may result from the potassium depletion that thiazide diuretics produce.

DEPOLARIZING SKELETAL MUSCLE RELAXANTS

Diazepam. Administration of this drug may reduce the duration of neuromuscular blockade that succinylcholine produces.

Digitalis. Since succinylcholine may cause a sudden loss of potassium from muscle cells, it may also cause arrhythmias in patients who also receive digitalis.

Furosemide. This drug may potentiate the action of succinylcholine.

GANGLIONIC BLOCKERS

Mecamylamine. Anesthesia, diuretics, other antihypertensive drugs, and alcohol may potentiate the action of mecamylamine.

ADRENERGIC DRUG INTERACTIONS

BRONCHODILATORS

Digitalis. Concomitant use with heavy doses of digitalis is not recommended because of the possible induction of anginal pain that results from coronary insufficiency.

Halothane. Halogenated hydrocarbon anesthetics that sensitize the myocardium can potentiate the arrhythmic effects of sympathomimetics.

Insulin. Diabetic patients who receive epinephrine should possibly have their dose of insulin or oral hypoglycemic agents increased.

MAO inhibitors. Patients who receive MAO inhibitors should use vasopressors cautiously.

Propranolol. Beta-adrenergic blocking agents antagonize the cardiostimulating and bronchodilating effects of sympathomimetics.

Phentolamine. Alpha-adrenergic blocking agents antagonize the vasoconstricting and hypertensive effects of epinephrine and ephedrine.

Phenothiazines. These drugs (and ergot alkaloids) may reverse the pressor effects of ephedrine.

Tricyclic Antidepressants and some Antihypertensives. These drugs may potentiate the effects of sympathomimetics. However, sympathomimetics may lessen the effects of antihypertensive agents, e.g., guanethidine. Drugs that reduce the amount of norepinephrine in sympathetic nerve endings (such as reserpine and methyldopa) may reduce the pressor response to ephedrine.

NASAL DECONGESTANTS

Beta-adrenergic Blocking Agents and MAO Inhibitors. Since these drugs increase the effects of sympathomimetics, patients who receive both MAO inhibitors and sympathomimetics may experience severe hypertensive reactions.

Methyldopa, Mecamylamine, and Reserpine. Sympathomimetics reduce the antihypertensive effects of these drugs.

Isoproterenol. Because of possible induction of serious arrhythmias, simultaneous administration of isoproterenol and epinephrine (both cardiac stimulants) is discouraged.

ALPHA-ADRENERGIC BLOCKING DRUGS

Prazosin. Since prazosin is highly protein-bound, it may interact with other highly bound drugs.

Tolazoline. Concomitant use with alcohol may produce a disulfiram-like reaction. Also, "epinephrine reversal," evidenced by a fall in blood pressure, may result from concurrent use of large doses of tolazoline with epinephrine or norepinephrine.

BETA-ADRENERGIC BLOCKING DRUGS

Drug interactions with beta-adrenergic blocking drugs are listed in Chapter 3.

SUMMARY

The autonomic nervous system (ANS) governs the activity of smooth muscle, cardiac muscle, visceral organs, and glands. Although initially perceived as an efferent system, newer research recognizes that the ANS contains afferent pathways that are essential in the regulation of physiologic processes. The autonomic afferent-efferent reflexes are important in such functions as heart rate and blood pressure. These reflex pathways combine with the usual reciprocating double autonomic nerve supply (i.e., parasympathetic and sympathetic) to maintain homeostatic balance and to permit appropriate response in emergency and/or stress situations.

There are many possibilities for drug intervention in the functional activity of the ANS. Specifically, drugs may mimic the activation of either one of the two ANS divisions or agents may block the effects of parasympathetic or sympathetic nervous system stimulation. Additionally, drugs that affect autonomic function may act at sites common to both ANS divisions, for example, the autonomic ganglia, in which less specificity in action occurs. Finally, selected drugs, which are ordinarily designated as autonomic drugs, activate receptors in both the peripheral voluntary nervous system and the CNS.

The diverse pharmacologic effects of autonomic drugs are reflective of the extensive neuron supply to smooth muscles, cardiac muscle, visceral organs, and glands. Autonomic drugs, therefore, often cross over into another organ system (e.g., cardiovascular system) creating a complex network of interactions.

SUGGESTED READINGS

Appelt, G.D.: Weight Control Products. *In* Handbook of Nonprescription Drugs. Vol. 8. Washington, American Pharmaceutical Association, 1986.

Appelt, G.D.: Anorectic drugs. Wellcome Trends in Hospital Pharmacy, 6:8, 1984.

Atracurium. Med Lett Drugs Ther, 26:53, 1984.

Glass, D.B., and Krebs, E.G.: Protein phosphorylation catalyzed by cyclic AMP-dependent and cyclic GMP-dependent protein kinases. Annu Rev Pharmacol Toxicol, 20:263, 1980.

Ingelfinger, F.J.: Anticholinergic therapy of gastrointestinal disorders. N Engl J Med, 268:1454, 1963.

Koelle, G.B.: Acetylcholine. Current status in physiology, pharmacology and medicine. N Engl J Med, 286:1086, 1972.

Lindstrom, J., and Dau, P.: Biology of myasthenia gravis. Annu Rev Pharmacol Toxicol, 20:337, 1980.

Loh, H.H., and Law, P.Y.: The role of membrane lipids in receptor mechanisms. Annu Rev Pharmacol Toxicol, 20:201, 1980.

Nicotine Gum. Med Lett Drug Ther, 26:27, 1984.

Potter, D.E.: Adrenergic pharmacology of aqueous humor dynamics. Pharmacol Rev, 33:133, 1981.

Rahwan, R.G.: Cyclic nucleotides: Their roles in disease processes, drug action and drug design. US Pharmacist, 11:49, 1986.

Shore, P.A.: Transport and storage of biogenic amines. Annu Rev Pharmacol, 12:209, 1972.

Starke, K: Presynaptic receptors. Annu Rev Pharmacol Toxicol, 21:7, 1981.

Steer, M.L., Atlas, D., and Levitzki, A.: Interrelations between beta-adrenergic receptors, adenyl cyclase, and calcium. N Engl J Med, 292:409, 1975.

Weiner, N.: Regulation of norepinephrine synthesis. Annu Rev Pharmacol, 10:273, 1970.

CHAPTER EXAMINATION

A patient who has chronic glaucoma is being treated with pilocarpine HCl ophthalmic solution 8%. A friend recommends that she ask her pharmacist for a phenobarbital/belladonna alkaloids preparation to relieve the gastrointestinal distress that she (the patient) has experienced lately.

1. Pilocarpine
   a. directly stimulates nicotinic receptors
   b. inhibits cholinesterase
   c. activates cholinesterase
   d. directly stimulates muscarinic receptors

2. In narrow angle glaucoma, pilocarpine
   a. pulls the iris musculature away from the trabeculum
   b. causes constriction of the iris radial musculature
   c. relaxes the iris sphincter (circular) muscle
   d. produces cycloplegia

3. In chronic open angle glaucoma, pilocarpine
   a. facilitates synthesis of aqueous humor
   b. opens the intertrabecular spaces to facilitate aqueous humor outflow (apparently by causing contraction of the ciliary muscle)
   c. is of no value
   d. relaxes the iris sphincter (circular) muscle

4. The patient's recent gastrointestinal symptoms
   a. are obviously not related to the pilocarpine medication
   b. represent the nicotinic activity that sometimes occurs with pilocarpine
   c. may be accompanied by muscle tremors, troubled breathing, and excessive salivation
   d. indicate muscarinic blockade induced by pilocarpine

5. The belladonna alkaloids/phenobarbital preparation
   a. is a good choice to counteract the gastrointestinal distress and will not compromise the therapeutic benefit in glaucoma
   b. is contraindicated in the patient's case
   c. is often used with pilocarpine to control chronic open-angle glaucoma
   d. none of the above

A 40-year-old male patient wants to purchase an OTC weight control product that contains phenylpropanolamine. Recently, because of overtime employment, he has routinely bought an OTC stimulant preparation that contains caffeine.

6. Phenylpropanolamine
   a. is an indirect acting sympathomimetic
   b. is an effective nasal decongestant
   c. activates alpha-adrenergic receptors
   d. all of the above

7. Conditions in which phenylpropanolamine should be used either with caution or not at all are
   a. otitis media and vertigo
   b. hypertension and hyperthyroidism
   c. diabetes mellitus and hypothyroidism
   d. diabetes insipidus and renal disease

8. Mixtures of phenylpropanolamine and caffeine as OTC weight control products
   a. have been associated with hypertension and CNS stimulation
   b. are no longer marketed in the United States due to a FDA ruling
   c. are contraindicated in severe cardiovascular disease
   d. all of the above

9. As a pharmacist, your recommendation to the patient should
   a. include a warning relative to the possible phenylpropanolamine-caffeine interaction
   b. be an explanation that caffeine blocks the appetite suppressant action of phenylpropanolamine
   c. offer encouragement to buy more OTC stimulants
   d. advise him of the benefit of drinking several cups of coffee daily

10. Phenylpropanolamine is
    a. a beta-adrenergic blocking drug
    b. especially active on presynaptic alpha$_2$-adrenergic receptors in the CNS

c. pharmacologically and chemically related to ephedrine
d. a potent cycloplegic drug

A patient has just entered the hospital ER for the treatment of tricyclic antidepresssant overdosage.

---

11. A recommended antidote to counteract the anticholinergic and cardiovacular toxicity is
    a. pralidoxime
    b. atropine sulfate
    c. physostigmine salicylate
    d. edrophonium
12. The antidote of choice
    a. activates cholinesterase
    b. inhibits cholinesterase
    c. blocks muscarinic receptors
    d. blocks nicotinic receptors
13. A drug that chemically and pharmacologically resembles the antidote is
    a. pilocarpine
    b. scopolamine
    c. pyridostigmine
    d. propantheline
14. The mechanism of action of the antidote involves the interaction of the drug at
    a. a nicotinic receptor
    b. a muscarinic receptor
    c. the anionic and esteratic sites on acetylcholinesterase
    d. the beta$_1$-adrenergic receptor
15. Anticholinergic side effects are evidenced by
    a. excessive salivation and tremor
    b. xerostomia and tachycardia
    c. diarrhea and pupillary constriction
    d. constipation and rhinorrhea

Dicyclomine is prescribed as an antispasmodic for a female patient. She complains that the drug "just isn't doing the job" and asks that you call her physician and request a change to a more "potent" drug.

---

16. The pharmacologic classification of dicyclomine is a
    a. muscarinic drug
    b. alpha-adrenergic blocker
    c. beta-adrenergic blocker
    d. muscarinic blocker
17. The biochemical mechanism of dicyclomine action apparently involves an inhibition of the formation of
    a. cyclic AMP
    b. cyclic GMP
    c. an organometallic chelate
    d. a covalent bond at the esteratic site on cholinesterase
18. An alternative drug to dicyclomine you might recommend to the physician is
    a. bethanechol
    b. propantheline
    c. pralidoxime
    d. propranolol
19. Dicyclomine
    a. completely abolishes the secretion of gastric HCl
    b. markedly inhibits spasticity in both skeletal and smooth muscle
    c. may produce dry mouth and blurred vision
    d. commonly produces diarrhea
20. The physician decides to prescribe a product containing bellafolline (the levo-alkaloids of belladonna). This preparation
    a. acts preferentially on peripheral sites
    b. acts preferentially on the CNS
    c. is too potent to be used therapeutically
    d. will selectively block beta-adrenergic receptors

ANSWER KEY

1. d	11. c
2. a	12. b
3. b	13. c
4. c	14. c
5. b	15. b
6. d	16. d
7. b	17. b
8. d	18. b
9. a	19. c
10. c	20. a

chapter 3

CARDIOVASCULAR SYSTEM

CHAPTER OBJECTIVES

After studying this chapter, you should be able to:
1. Describe the action potential in a cardiac cell, especially the ion fluxes that occur during the phases.
2. Relate the waves and complexes of the electrocardiogram (ECG) with the electrophysiologic events of the heart.
3. Discuss the major pharmacologic actions of quinidine sulfate on the heart.
4. Compare the actions of bretylium, propranolol, and lidocaine on excitability and conduction in the atria, A-V node, and ventricles.
5. Compare the use of digitalis to verapamil for particular cardiac arrhythmias.
6. Describe toxic reactions that sometimes occur with quinidine.
7. Give the major routes of administration, range of onset and duration of action, specific cardiac conditions treated, and possible side effects for lidocaine, propranolol, phenytoin, disopyramide, and procainamide.
8. Discuss three clinically significant drug interactions that occur with the antiarrhythmic drugs.
9. Name several untoward responses that may occur in organic nitrate therapy.
10. Describe the clinical applications of Ca^{++} channel blocking drugs.
11. Evaluate the therapeutic effectiveness of glyceryl trinitrate, diltiazem, erythrityl tetranitrate, dipyridamole, and isosorbide dinitrate.
12. Describe three major pharmacologic effects of the digitalis glycosides on the heart.
13. Name the major pathologic condition for which digitalis is employed and describe the clinical characteristics of this disease.
14. Compare digitoxin to digoxin with respect to degree of gastrointestinal absorption, protein binding, onset and duration of action, biotransformation, and toxicity.
15. Name two drugs sometimes used for intravenous digitalization and state the dosage range usually employed.
16. Compare the potency of digitalis leaf with that of digitoxin.
17. Name two clinically significant drug interactions that occur with digoxin and describe the mechanisms involved.
18. Describe the ECG changes, clinical signs, and implications of digitalis intoxication.
19. Elaborate on the relationship of digitalis activity on the heart to calcium (Ca^{++}) and potassium (K^+) blood levels.
20. Discuss the proposed mechanism of action of digitalis on myocardial Na^+-K^+ ATPase.
21. Describe the mechanisms whereby the organic nitrates appear beneficial in the treatment of "typical" angina pectoris.
22. Discuss the biochemical mechanisms which may explain the vasodilator activity of verapamil.
23. Outline the various sites whereby a drug may act to lower an elevated blood pressure.
24. Compare the effective antihypertensive activity of hydralazine with that of reserpine.
25. Discuss the rationale of thiazide combinations with other hypertensive drugs.

26. Name several clinical signs of potassium deficiency.
27. Discuss the major pharmacologic properties of minoxidil, nadolol, methyldopa, clonidine, atenolol, diazoxide, sodium nitroprusside, metoprolol, and prazosin.
28. Describe the drug regimens employed in hypertensive crisis, moderate to severe hypertension, and mild hypertension.
29. Discuss the proposed mechanisms of antihypertensive activity for methyldopa, guanethidine, prazosin, guanadrel, clonidine, hydrochlorthiazide, sodium nitroprusside, acebutomol, labetalol, captopril, propranolol, pindolol, and diazoxide.
30. Discuss the major signs of toxicity that occur with the antihypertensive drugs.

INTRODUCTION

The heart has always been associated with emotions and romance; melodies such as "My Heart Cries for You," "Your Cheating Heart," and "Heart of My Heart" are a few of the hundreds of song titles attesting to the importance of the heart in the human psyche. Phrases like "let's get to the heart of the matter" and "you've got to have heart" encourage one to cope with and confront life's everchanging events. Indeed, as legend supports, the heart is the basis for human life, symbolically and physically.

The heart, a muscular blood pump, lies within the chest cavity. Bearing little resemblance to the traditional shape of the St. Valentine's Day heart, this hollow organ, weighing about 300 g, is pear-shaped and about the size of a clenched adult fist.

The heart pumps more than 10 L of blood per minute with its 70 or so beats. In one day, this amounts to approximately 14,000 L of blood. This pumping function, which totals 2 to 3 billion beats in an average lifetime, provides the body tissues with a fresh supply of oxygenated blood from the lungs and carries carbon dioxide back to the lungs for excretion (Figure 3.1).

The heart's pumping action also provides the body's tissues and cells with nutrients absorbed into the blood from foodstuffs in the small intestine. The blood carries the waste products of cellular metabolism to the kidneys, where they are excreted in the urine. Hormones that regulate bodily processes are also transported by the blood to target tissues. Additionally, disease-fighting cells (such as leukocytes) must be supplied to infected tissue by the constant circulation of pumped blood.

Thus, the frail, fetal heart beat first detected a month after conception initiates an essential, multifaceted process that lasts the lifetime of the individual.

ANATOMY AND PHYSIOLOGY OF THE HEART AND BLOOD VESSELS

The cardiovascular system consists of the cardiac component (the heart) and the vascular element (the blood vessels). Contained within this closed system is the blood that the cardiovascular system distributes.

HEART

The human heart has four chambers; the upper two are the atria (from the Latin "atrium," an entrance hall) and the lower are the ventricles (from the Latin "ventriculus," belly). A septum, or partition, extends from the top to the bottom, and this structure, together with the valves that lie between the atria and ventricles, produces the four chambers and accounts for the "right heart" and "left heart" designations (Figure 3.2). Not held in place by ligaments or tendons, the heart hangs from the vessels that lead away

CARDIOVASCULAR SYSTEM   **151**

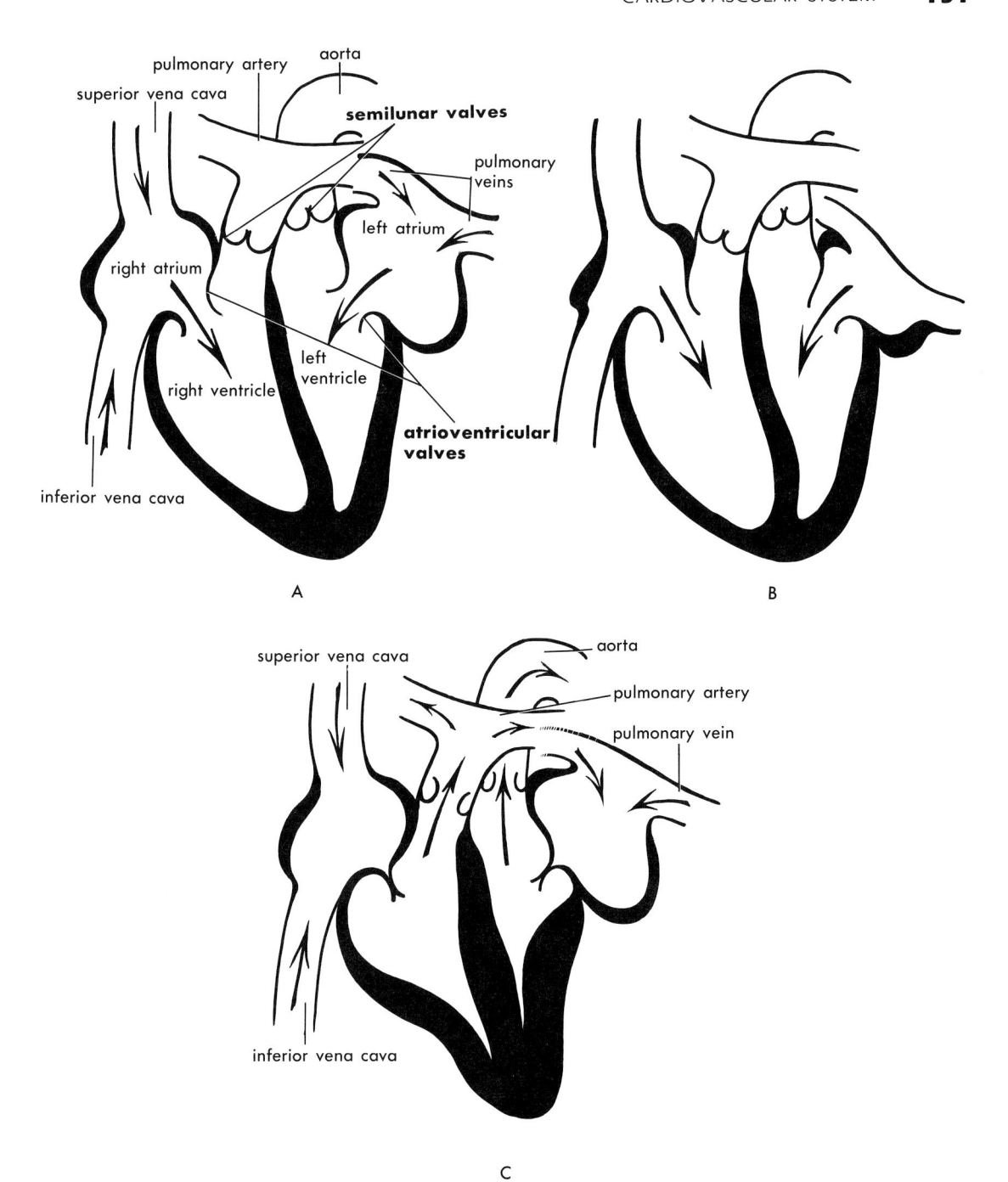

Fig. 3.1 Stages in the cardiac cycle. **A,** Heart is relaxed; semilunar valves are closed; atrioventricular valves are open. Atria and ventricles are filling with blood. **B,** Atria are contracting; ventricles are relaxed and filling. Semilunar valves remain closed; atrioventricular valves are open. **C,** The atria are relaxed as the ventricles contract. The atrioventricular valves are closed, the semilunar valves are open, and blood is pumped into the pulmonary artery and the aorta. (From Crouch, J.E.: Essential Human Anatomy. Philadelphia, Lea & Febiger, 1985.)

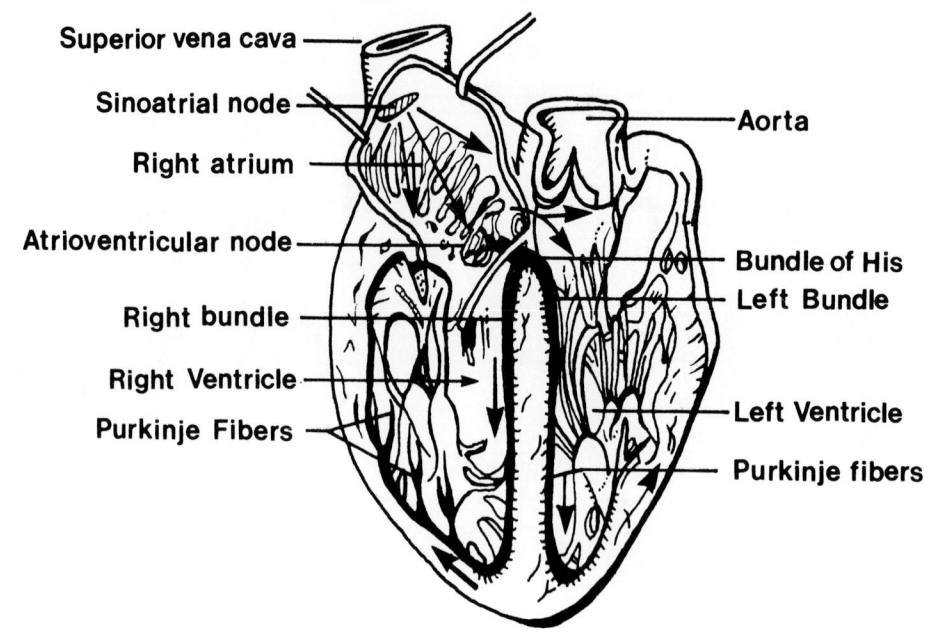

Fig. 3.2 Anatomy of the heart and its conducting system. (From Simon, H., and Bloomfield, D.A.: Cardioactive Drugs. Baltimore, Urban and Schwarzenberg, 1983.)

from and into it. The heart is enclosed in the pericardium, a thin but tough membranous pouch.

The heart muscle (myocardium) is a structurally and functionally unique organ. Myocardial fibers form an intertwining system which permits, upon the passage of a nerve action potential, atrial contractions which are immediately followed by ventricle contractions. The atria, whose walls are quite thin, perform no significant work. The wall of the left ventricle is thicker than that of the right ventricle; thus, the left ventricle accomplishes most of the heart's work.

Valves separate the atria from the ventricles; the bicuspid (mitral) valve is between the left atrium and the left ventricle, and the tricuspid valve (named for its three points or cusps) separates the right atrium from the right ventricle. As the atria fill with blood, the valves open, allowing the blood to flow into the working portion of the heart, the ventricles. When the ventricles have filled, the cuspid valves snap closed simultaneously with initiation of the heart beat. As the ventricles contract to expel the blood from the heart, the tightly closed valves prevent the blood from backing up into the atria. Semilunar (half-moon) valves are in the large vessels that emerge from the heart; these close at the end of ventricular contraction to prevent the expelled blood from returning to the ventricle.

In the normal heart, two sounds (lub-dub) are usually detected with a stethoscope: the first (lub), which is the loudest and most prolonged, is caused by the rapid closing of the cuspid valves; the second (dub) results from closure of the semilunar valves in the vessels at the point where they emerge from the heart (Figure 3.1).

The efficiency of the heart as a pump is important. In a healthy individual, it is the chief factor limiting the capacity for muscle exertion that lasts for more than a few seconds. Another outstanding feature of the healthy heart is its power of reserve. Its performance during bodily rest represents only a fraction of its full capacity; when necessary, the heart can rapidly increase its output manyfold.

The heart beat is characterized by contraction (systole) and relaxation (diastole) of the cardiac muscle. The heart's pumping efficiency is described in terms of force of contraction and heart rate. Cardiac output, for instance, directly relates to the force of systole. Thus, a "positive inotropic activity" designates an increase in the contractile force of the heart. An increase in the heart rate is termed a "positive chronotropic effect." Negative inotropism and chronotropism are characterized by a weakly contracting heart with a slow heart rate.

Certain drugs, like digitalis, affect both the inotropic and chronotropic properties of the myocardium. Digitalis increases the force of systole in a decompensated heart (positive inotropism) and slows the heart rate (negative chronotropism). Epinephrine also produces a positive inotropic effect on the heart, but in contrast to digitalis, it also speeds the heart rate, which represents a positive chronotropic action.

CARDIAC NERVES

Some muscles (such as skeletal muscles) are absolutely dependent upon intact innervation for physiologic function. The heart muscle, in contrast, possesses the unique property of automaticity and continues to beat for a limited time in the complete absence of extrinsic nerve supply. In the normal life situation, however, adjustments in heart rate in response to various stimuli are accomplished mainly by the cardiac nerves.

Changes in heart rate occur as a result of the interaction between two reciprocating efferent nerve pathways (Figure 3.3). The double innervation consists of an accelerator pathway and an inhibiting influence exerted by the vagus nerves (vagi). Cardio-accelerator nerves are part of the sympathetic nervous system and arise from the thoracic (chest) portion of the spinal cord. They originate from cell bodies in the medulla and spinal cord. Increased impulse activity due to stimulation of the cell bodies speeds the heart rate (tachycardia). Cardio-inhibitory fibers emanate from the vagal center in the medulla and travel to the heart via the vagi.

Activation of the efferent vagus fibers slows (bradycardia) and even stops the heart if sufficient stimulation of the vagal centers occurs. Because of the reciprocating nature of the cardiac innervation, tachycardia occurs if the ac-

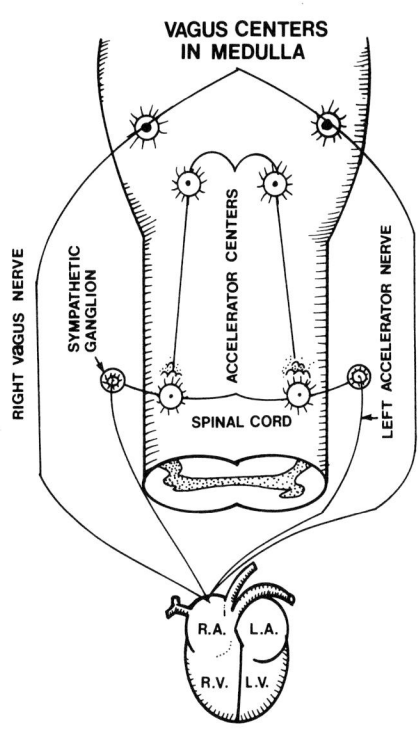

Fig. 3.3 Efferent nerves of the heart. (Modified from Carlson, A.J., and Johnson, V.: The Machinery of the Body. Chicago, University of Chicago Press, 1953.)

celerator mechanism is activated or if the continuous vagal activity is diminished. Thus, removal of the "braking" influence of the vagi results in an unopposed accelerator mechanism.

The sympathetic accelerator nerves apparently exercise no constant action on the heart; instead, they cause rapid acceleration of the heart in excitement. The vagi, however, exercise continual control of the heart so that the pulse rate is not the frequency of the uncontrolled pacemaker, but is the frequency of the pacemaker under a considerable amount of vagal control.

CARDIAC REFLEXES

Cardiac reflexes are important in determining heart rate in response to physiologic activity (such as exercise) or changes in blood pressure or blood volume.

Bainbridge Reflex. A cardiac reflex, originating in the right atrium and the veins that empty into the atrium, figures prominently in the cardiac acceleration seen during exercise (Figure 3.4). Contracting muscles force blood faster through the veins and the blood flows back to the heart more rapidly. The right atrium becomes distended with the increase in blood volume, and the stretch of the atrial wall stimulates afferent vagal fibers that travel to the medulla. A reflex stimulation of the cardiac accelerator nerve then occurs, resulting in tachycardia and a greater quantity of blood being pumped. Thus, the active muscles are supplied with the extra blood without which the muscular work could not continue.

Aortic Depressor Reflex. The control of the heart rate by nerve activation in states other than exercise also involves cardiac reflexes. The vagi function as an afferent information limb to the brain, as illustrated by the Bainbridge reflex. In other reflexes (such as the depressor reflex and carotid sinus reflex), the vagi transmit impulses away from the brain after activation of vagal centers in the medulla. An increased impulse activity along the efferent pathway results in cardiac slowing.

An automatic reflex governor exists involving the afferent depressor nerves that terminate in the aortic arch and ventricular muscle at the base of the aorta and the efferent vagal limb. If the heart accelerates, more blood is pumped into the aorta, thereby stretching the aortic walls. This blood-volume induced distention of the aortic walls stimulates the depressor nerves and a slowing of the heart occurs due to reflex activation of the vagal centers in the medulla (Figure 3.5). The depressor reflex mechanism is critical when sudden changes in heart rate occur; it is also an important factor in maintaining the normal heart rate of about 70. Thus, any tendency to exceed this rate is counteracted by this reflex correction.

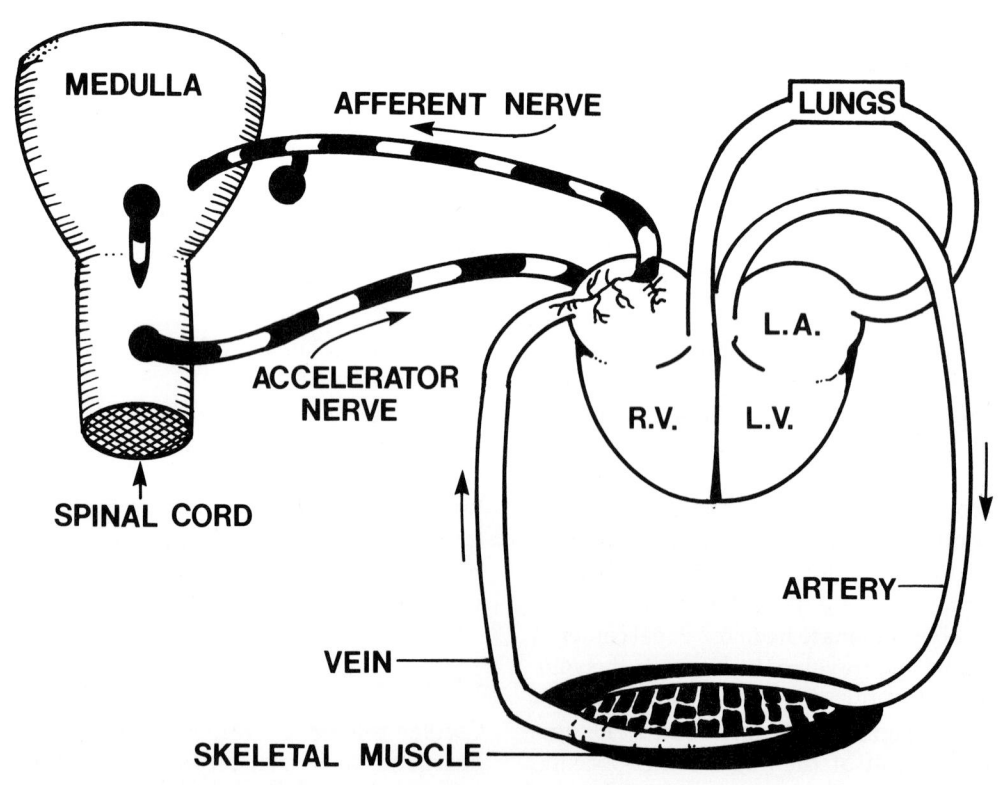

Fig. 3.4 Reflex mechanisms operant during exercise. (Modified from Carlson, A.J., and Johnson, V.: The Machinery of the Body. Chicago, University of Chicago Press, 1953.)

Carotid Sinus Reflex. The carotid sinus reflex has essentially the same function as the aortic depressor reflex. The carotid sinus is a special structure located at the bifurcation of the common carotid artery into internal and external branches (Figure 3.6). The carotid sinus exists as a small thin-walled swelling of the internal carotid artery. The walls of the carotid sinus are supplied with afferent nerve fibers which represent the sensory component of the reflex.

Increased blood pressure at the carotid sinus activates the afferent carotid sinus nerves that send increased impulse activity to the medulla. The vagal center is thus stimulated resulting in an increased vagal activity as demonstrated by a slowing of the heart. The efferent limb of the carotid sinus reflex is thereby represented by the vagi.

A fall in blood pressure at the carotid sinuses inhibits the cardio-inhibitory center (vagal center) and stimulates the cardio-accelerator and the vasomotor centers; it also stimulates increased epinephrine secretion, augmenting the latter's effects. This interrelationship of blood pressure and heart rate is important because a fall in blood pressure without a compensatory increase in heart rate (and vasoconstriction) could result in syncope.

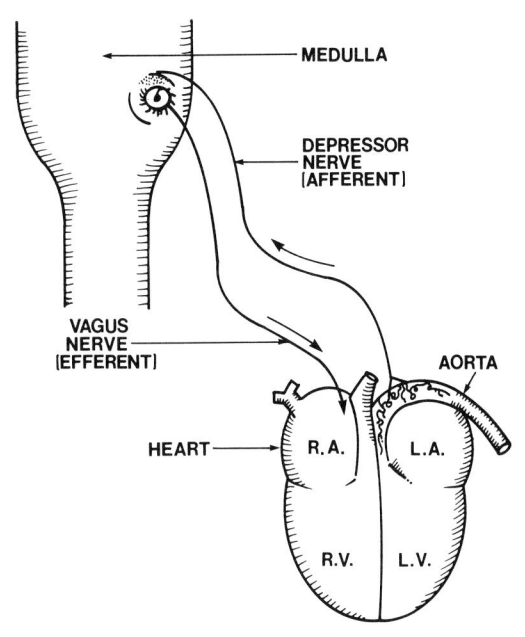

Fig. 3.5 *Aortic depressor reflex.* (Modified from Carlson, A.J., and Johnson, V.: The Machinery of the Body. Chicago, University of Chicago Press, 1953.)

ELECTROPHYSIOLOGY

Normal contraction of the heart depends upon a wave of electrical excitation. Spontaneous "pacemaker" tissue in the sinoatrial node (S-A node) of the right atrium initiates this activity that spreads over the atria and ventricles.

The wave of excitation spreads from the S-A node throughout the atria at a rate of about one meter per second. A short time delay occurs when the wave reaches the atrioventricular node (A-V node) before it proceeds through the bundle of His and Purkinje system of the ventricles (Figure 3.2). The Purkinje system, formed by division of the bundle of His into left and right "bundle branches," forms a specialized conduction pathway between the atria and ventricles. The time interval between the beginning of the atrial contraction and ventricle contraction is about 0.15 seconds. Thus, the wave of excitation is delayed at the A-V node

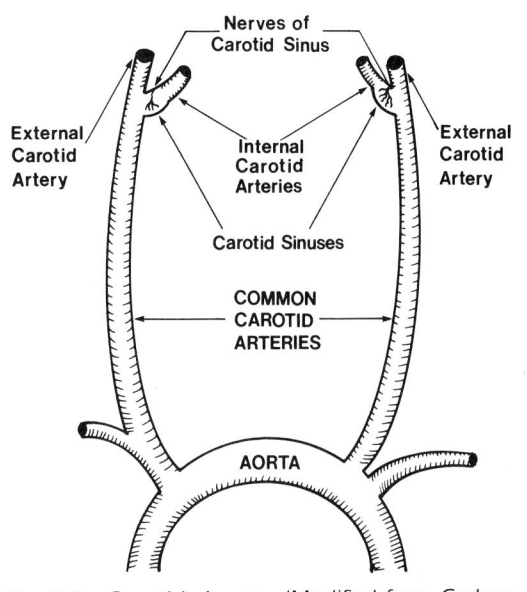

Fig. 3.6 *Carotid sinuses.* (Modified from Carlson, A.J., and Johnson, V.: The Machinery of the Body. Chicago, University of Chicago Press, 1953.)

156 THERAPEUTIC PHARMACOLOGY

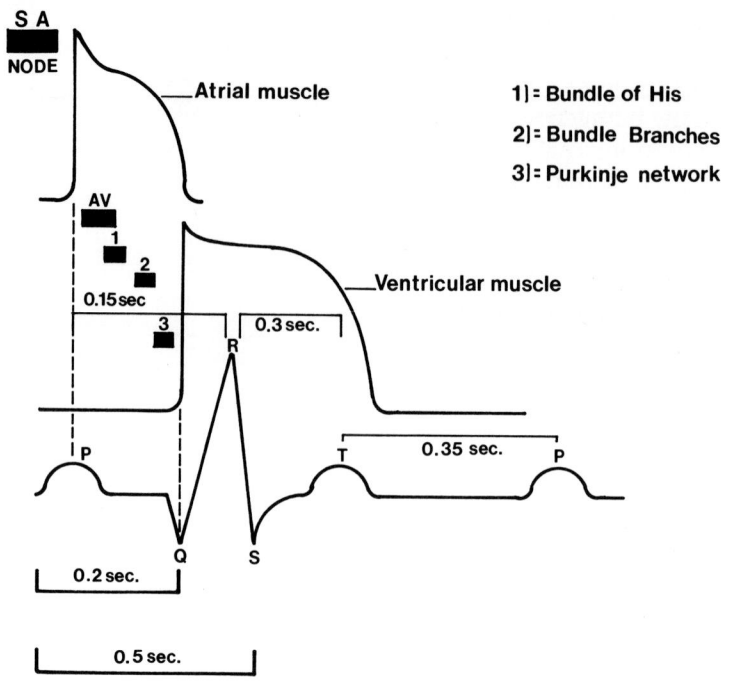

Fig. 3.7 Action potential correlation with ECG.

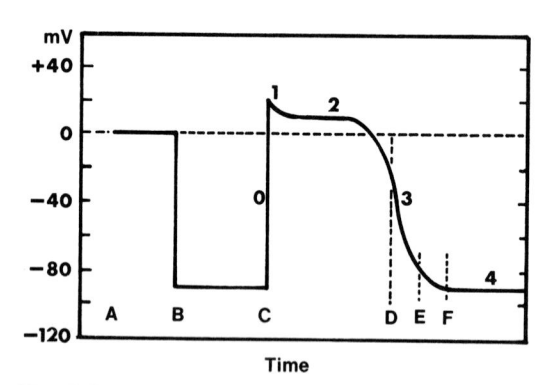

Fig. 3.8 Excitation process in cardiac cell. (Modified from Berne, R.M., and Levy, M.N.: Cardiovascular Physiology. 5th Ed. St. Louis, C.V. Mosby, 1986.)

and subsequently is transmitted through the bundle of His and bundle branches of the ventricular muscle. The delay between the atrial and ventricular contraction allows time for the atrial blood to fill the ventricles before it is pumped into the pulmonary and systemic circulation.

The muscle contraction is characterized by a change in electrical potential that can be recorded by electrophysiologic monitoring (ECG,EKG). By means of the ECG, it is possible to observe the electrical potential changes and follow their time relation to the passage of an excitation wave (Figure 3.7). The passage of the action potential through the atrial muscle is represented by the P wave on the ECG. The QRS complex designates the continuation of the excitation wave through the ventricles. Ventricular repolarization results in the T wave. Atrial repolarization is not evident in the ECG record since it is masked by the QRS complex.

Action Potential and Ion Fluxes. Figure 3.8 illustrates the cardiac action potential and Figure 3.9 shows its relation to contraction (systole) and relaxation (diastole) of the heart. The action potential is divided into five phases with the graphic representation indicating differences in potential between the intracellular and extracellular space. The changes in potential (mV) are due to transmembrane ion fluxes (Figure 3.10). These changes are detected by a microelectrode inserted intracellularly in a single cardiac cell. The action potential tracing also applies to the changes in potential that occur in the atria and ventricles as a wave of electrical excitation passes through those tissues, as represented by an ECG (Figure 3.7).

The basis of excitability in cardiac "pacemaker" tissue (S-A node) and excitation-conduction tissue is the spontaneous increase in cell membrane permeability to sodium ions (Na^+) and potassium ions (K^+). Changes in potential occur between the intracellular and extracellular spaces when the Na^+ and K^+ are transferred across the membrane. The spontaneous changes in Na^+ and K^+ permeability are accompanied by corresponding mechanical changes, resulting in the systole and diastole of the heart beat (Figure 3.9).

Permeability and conductivity in the resting cardiac cell are much higher for K^+ than for Na^+, so the resting potential is determined by the K^+ gradient. The intracellular concentration of K^+ of a resting cardiac cell is 160 meq/L compared to an extracellular concentration of 4 meq/L. The interior of the resting cardiac cell is negative with respect to the exterior, and the -90 mV resting intracellular potential represents the relatively high K^+ concentration.

Phase 0 of the action potential represents depolarization and is characterized by an increased Na^+ permeability, resulting in an intense Na^+ influx into the cell interior. This causes a reversal in transmembrane potential as illustrated in Figure 3.8. The "fast" Na^+ channels that are activated or "opened" during depolarization are quickly "closed" and cannot be reactivated until Phase 3 repolarization occurs.

The Phase 1 membrane potential is determined by the Na^+ potential of $+20$ mV, but quick repolarization occurs due mainly to inactivation of the Na^+ influx and activation of an active chloride (Cl^-) current. The increased Na^+ permeability is short and transient and the transmembrane potential begins to recover. Phase 1 is thus characterized by a short and rapid decrease in potential that passes into a Phase 2 plateau.

In Phase 2, only a small or zero transmembrane potential can be determined. Phase 2 represents activation of the "slow" calcium ion (Ca^{++}) channel resulting in an inward Ca^{++} current. The "slow" Ca^{++} channels are "closed" much more slowly than the "fast" Na^+ channels in Phase 0, and, therefore, the plateau

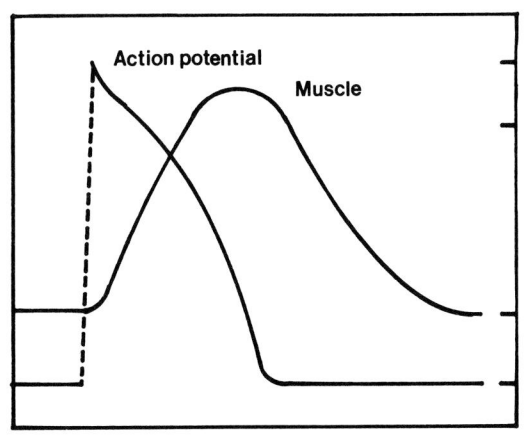

Fig. 3.9 Time relationship of action potential to muscle contraction and relaxation. (Modified from Berne, R.M., and Levy, M.N.: Cardiovascular Physiology. 5th Ed. St. Louis, C.V. Mosby, 1986.)

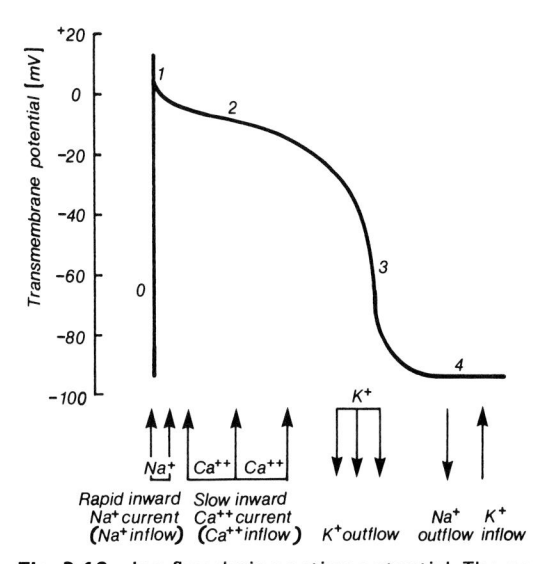

Fig. 3.10 Ion flux during action potential. The action potential phases are indicated 0–4. (From Nayler, W.G., and Merrilles, N.C.R.: Cellular exchange of calcium. In Calcium and the Heart. Edited by P. Harris and L.H. Opie. New York and London, Academic Press, 1971.)

nature of Phase 2 results. Also during the Phase 2 plateau, membrane conductance is reduced due to an inwardly directed reversal of the outward background current of K^+.

The plateau in Phase 2 is terminated by activation of a K^+ current that repolarizes the cell to normal values of diastolic membrane potential.

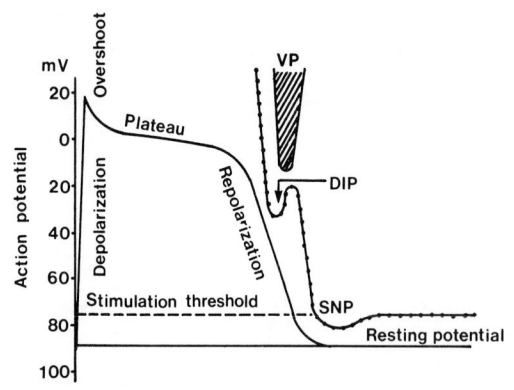

Fig. 3.11 Vulnerable and supernormal periods in the action potential. (Modified from Friedemann, M.: Die Kardioversion. Berne and Stuttgart, H. Huber, 1968.)

Thus, Phase 3 represents a repolarization process and ends with the inactivation or closing of the K^+ channel.

In Phase 4, or diastole, the resting cardiac cells await a stimulus to reinitiate Phase 0. However, some cardiac cells exhibit spontaneous Phase 4 depolarization and self-excitatory properties. The automaticity of certain cardiac tissue, including the pacemaker and His-Purkinje excitation-conduction system, is reflected in spontaneous Phase 4 diastolic depolarization. During Phase 4, a Na^+-K^+ pump mechanism that maintains the intracellular concentration of Na^+ and K^+ becomes operant. This pump mechanism actively extrudes Na^+ from the cell in exchange for the influx of the K^+. The energy required to operate these Na^+-K^+ pumps is provided by the splitting of energy-rich phosphates through the action of Na^+-K^+ membrane ATPase.

Characteristics of the Excitation Process. During Phases 1 and 2, a period of absolute refractoriness occurs when stimulation of the cell or fiber cannot be restimulated to produce a further depolarization. Hence, this is known as the absolute refractory period. A relative refractory period exists during Phase 3 of the action potential. During this period, only a strong stimulus will elicit excitation of the myocardial cell or fiber. The total refractory period includes both the absolute and relative refractory periods. For ventricular tissue, it occurs from the beginning of depolarization, represented by the R peak on the ECG and Phase 0 of the action potential, until the end of repolarization, represented by the T peak on the ECG and Phase 3 of the action potential.

A vulnerable period for ventricular and atrial fibrillation lies between Phases 2 and 3 of the action potential (Figure 3.11). This corresponds to the ascending limb of the T wave in the ECG for ventricular tissue and in the RS interval for the atria (atrial repolarization is hidden in the QRS complex). Depolarization may be triggered during this period by a stimulus such as an extrasystole. Following repolarization, a short-lived increased excitability in cardiac cells occurs. During this supernormal period, relatively weak stimuli can initiate depolarization.

BLOOD VESSELS

Blood is pumped out of the heart into the arteries and returns to the heart through the veins. In 1628, William Harvey discovered the circulation of the blood by observing the direction in which flow occurred in the arteries and veins. The missing link in Harvey's discovery was that he could not offer an explanation as to how the arteries and veins were connected. The Italian physiologist, Marcello Malpighi, 1628–94, illustrated that the capillaries (visible only through the microscope) connected the arteries and the veins.

ARTERIES

Arteries are tubes having thick walls which contain muscle fibers. The largest, the aorta, emerges from the left ventricle and serves as the pathway for blood delivery from the brain to the toes. The pulmonary arteries, which emerge from the right ventricle, transport blood from the heart to the lungs. Branching from the aorta, the coronary arteries supply the heart with the blood it requires.

In cross section, an artery resembles Figure 3.12. The outer coat, or layer, is connective tissue which holds the artery in place, and the thick middle layer (the working part of the artery) contains a large number of muscle fibers which normally contract and relax. The inner layer, the endothelium, is a very thin tissue which provides a smooth surface offering minimal resistance to the flow of blood. The only valves in the arterial system are located at the point where the arteries leave the heart. After emerging from the heart, the arteries branch extensively to supply blood to all parts of the body. Due to this branching, the arteries become smaller as the distance from their point of emergence from the heart increases. They finally become so small that they are called arterioles; these further branch to become capillaries.

The fact that arteries have a muscular structure enables them to perform work. As the heart beats, the expelled blood causes the muscle fibers in the arteries to stretch. When the fibers contract in response to the stretch, they exert a force on the blood within the artery; this force tends to push the blood away from the heart. Blood is prohibited from re-entering the heart due to the valves, located at the point where the arteries emerge from the heart, which snap closed with completion of the heart beat. Therefore, the driving force of the heart causes blood to be discharged into the arterial system, but the work performed by the arteries (contraction of arterial muscle) helps to keep it flowing.

The assistance provided by the arterial muscle lessens the workload placed upon the heart. Since the artery alternately bulges and contracts (dilates and relaxes with each heart beat), it seems only logical that the flow of blood in the arteries pulsates with the pulses yielding a measurement of heart rate. However, a pulse can be detected only in the larger arteries because as the blood in the arterial system gets farther from the heart, the flow becomes practically continuous.

The driving power of the heart, which forces blood into the arteries, results in considerable pressure in the arterial system. Referring to the fact that the heart beat, coupled with arterial muscle contraction, keeps blood flowing efficiently, it follows that the pressure has two components: one results from the heart's driving force and the other results from tension exerted by arterial muscle. Blood pressure measurements present two values; the higher one

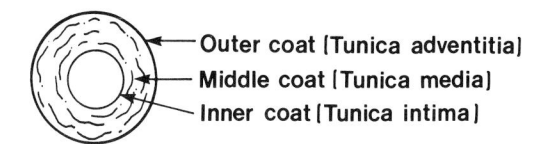

Fig. 3.12 Cross section of an artery.

(systolic) is a measure of the force exerted by the heart beat and the lower value (diastolic) represents the pressure to which the arterial system is constantly subjected.

Several factors influence blood pressure. Among these are the elasticity of the arteries, the pumping efficiency of the heart, the viscosity or "thickness" of the blood, the volume of the blood, and the various nerve controls which involve the brain sending impulses to the heart as well as to the arterial system. As the demands of the body increase during exercise, the blood pressure rises somewhat as the heart rate increases, but after a short period of rest, the heart rate slows and the pressure does not continue to rise (a phenomenon known as Marey's Law).

CAPILLARIES

By the time blood reaches the capillaries (tiny, hairlike vessels), flow is constant and slow since the capillaries are so small. While the arteries have muscular walls, the capillaries' walls are one cell thick. Many miles of capillaries are in the body and within these microscopic vessels the blood performs its functions: furnishing nutrients and oxygen to the cells in exchange for waste products from the cells. The slow rate at which blood flows in the capillaries favors the exchange of nutrients for waste products.

VEINS

After the blood passes through the capillaries, it enters the veins to begin its return to the heart. Capillaries merge to form venules (very small veins) and these, in turn, further merge to become larger veins. Most of the arterial pressure disappears as blood flows through the arterioles and capillaries and, therefore, the pressure in the veins is quite low. Furthermore, the driving force of the heart, as well as that of arterial muscle, has been almost completely expended in forcing blood through the capillaries. Hence, some other mechanism must be involved in returning blood to the heart by way of the veins. To illustrate, consider a rubber tube, plugged at one end, filled with water, and suspended vertically. If the tube is compressed at any point, water flows from the open end. The squeezing or "milking" action of skeletal muscles as they move against the veins filled with blood causes a flow to occur, but the veins in the outer parts of the body have numerous valves which allow the flow to occur only toward the heart. Flow in the veins is much slower than in the arteries, but since more blood is in the veins than in the arteries, the blood return to the heart is very efficient.

In contrast to the arteries, the veins contain little muscular tissue. They are considered as nonworking tubes that provide a means of returning blood to the heart from the capillaries.

DISEASES OF THE HEART AND BLOOD VESSELS

Normally, the heart beat is rhythmic with a ventricular contraction occurring each time the S-A node sends out a wave of excitation (Figure 3.13). When the contraction of the ventricles is not synchronized with that of the atria at a normal rate, the condition broadly known as an arrhythmia results.

ARRHYTHMIAS

A cardiac arrhythmia occurs when there is a disturbance in the normal regular rhythm of impulse generation or conduction. Even if the heart rate is normal, an irregular rhythm can disrupt cardiac output because of uncoordinated contraction of the atria and ventricles.

Cardiac arrhythmias may exist with or without disturbances in heart rate. Conversely, heart rate abnormalities (excessively fast or slow) can occur without a disorder in rhythm. Cardiac arrhythmias are classified according to the cardiac rate and rhythm characteristics of the particular disorder. Therefore, the mechanisms responsible for cardiac arrhythmias involve disorders in impulse generation, faulty or aberrant impulse conduction, or simultaneous abnormalities of both impulse generation and conduction.

SINOATRIAL (S-A) NODE DISORDERS

Sinoatrial (S-A) node disorders are represented by changes in sinus discharge rate or by complete sinus arrest.

Sinus Tachycardia. Physiologic situations, such as stress, can activate the sympathetic system resulting in sinus tachycardia (over 100 beats/minute). Disease conditions, including hyperthyroidism, fever, shock, congestive heart failure, and anemia, can also activate the sympathetic cardio-accelerator system, which increases the heart rate (Figure 3.13a).

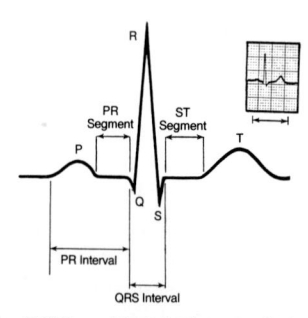

Fig. 3.13 ECG with designated intervals. A through M. Cardiac arrhythmias. (From Stein, E.: Interpretation of Arrhythmias. Philadelphia, Lea & Febiger, 1988.)

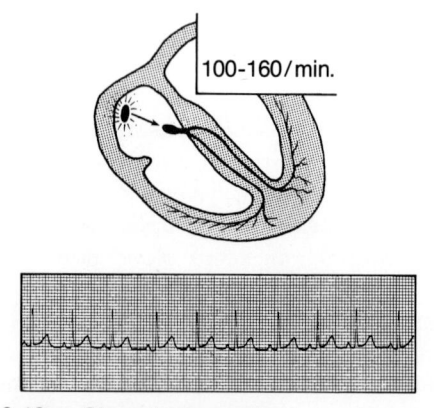

Fig. 3.13a Sinus tachycardia.

Sinus Bradycardia. A sinus rate below 60 beats/minute without a change in rhythm is called sinus bradycardia (Figure 3.13b). Disease conditions such as hypothyroidism and myocarditis can precipitate this condition. Additionally, extensive physical conditioning (like that of marathon runners) may result in sinus bradycardia.

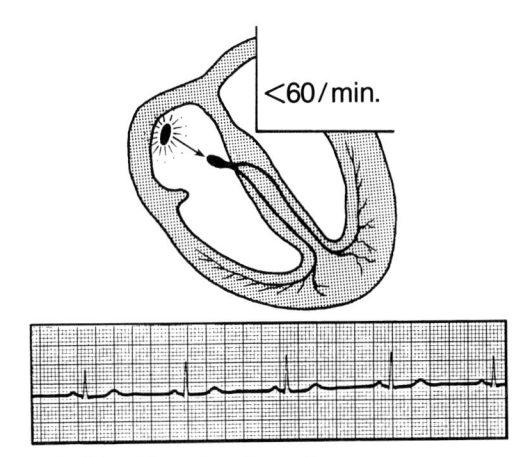

Fig. 3.13b Sinus bradycardia.

Sinus Arrhythmia. A disturbance of the normal cardiac rhythm that originates in the sinus node and does not have adverse consequences is called sinus arrhythmia. This condition is characterized by a normal conduction sequence with an irregular rhythm (Figure 3.13c). The heart rate varies with respiration (increases with inspiration and decreases with expiration). This irregularity is common in children and may also occur in adults with respiratory disease.

Sick Sinus Syndrome (Tachy-Brady Arrhythmia). Usually occurring in cardiac hypoxia, this serious condition results in a disturbance in normal cardiac rhythm. It is characterized by erratic function of the sinus node with either marked slowing, cessation, or blockade of impulse generation. Alternating sinus tachycardia and sinus bradycardia may occur; thus, tachy-brady arrhythmia is a synonym for sick sinus syndrome.

Sinus Tachyarrhythmia. Tachyarrhythmia, originating in the sinoatrial node, is characterized by an excessively rapid heart rate of over 100 beats/minute combined with a rhythm disorder. An inability to maintain the cardiac output is a common consequence of this arrhythmia.

Sinoatrial (S-A) Arrest. Conduction impairment in the S-A node with S-A function failure results in sinus arrest. "Escape beats" from secondary pacemaker tissue serve as an auxillary system to maintain cardiac output.

ATRIAL ARRHYTHMIAS

Atrial arrhythmias occur frequently in concert with rheumatic heart disease, cardiomyopathy, and coronary artery disease. Additionally, atrial flutter or fibrillation can be precipitated by toxic, metabolic, or inflammatory conditions.

Extrasystoles. Hypoxia and disturbances in electrolyte balance are among the conditions that spark cells other than normal pacemaker cells to spontaneously depolarize. If an impulse originates in a site other than the S-A node, this site is called an ectopic focus. The impulses spreading from the ectopic focus or foci can cause an early, additional contraction of the atria. Hence, the term extrasystole is applicable.

Premature Atrial Contraction (PAC). An early contraction of the heart due to stimulation from an ectopic focus is called a premature atrial con-

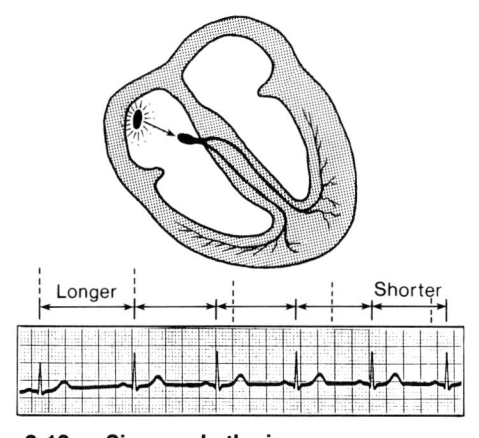

Fig. 3.13c Sinus arrhythmia.

traction (PAC). The ECG shows this pattern (Figure 3.13d).

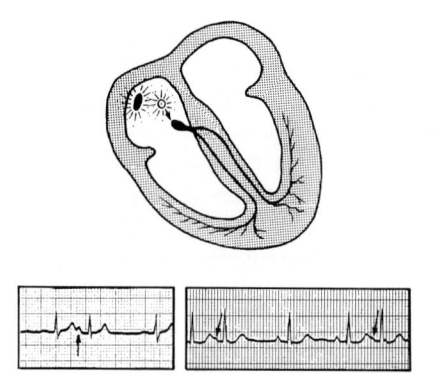

Fig. 3.13d Premature atrial contraction [PAC].

Paroxysmal Atrial Tachycardia (PAT). Repetitive firing of an atrial ectopic focus or multiple foci that produces a heart rate of more than 100 beats/minute results in atrial ectopic tachycardia. These episodes of tachycardia often start suddenly and end abruptly; thus, the term "paroxysmal atrial tachycardia (PAT)" is applied, even though technically the cardiac condition is a tachyarrhythmia (Figure 3.13e).

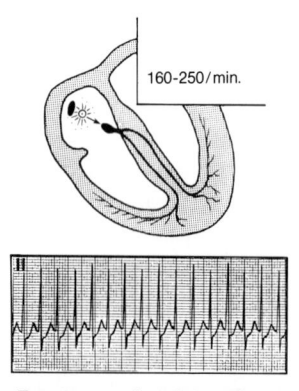

Fig. 3.13e Paroxysmal atrial tachycardia [PAT].

Atrial Flutter. An atrial tachyarrhythmia, atrial flutter occurs when impulses (200 to 350 beat/minute) generate from an ectopic focus or multiple foci, inducing uncoordinated atrioventricular activity.

Blood passes from the atria to the ventricles less efficiently than during the coordinated contraction of the atria in normal sinus rhythm. The ECG shows a characteristic regular "sawtooth" flutter wave pattern (Figure 3.13f).

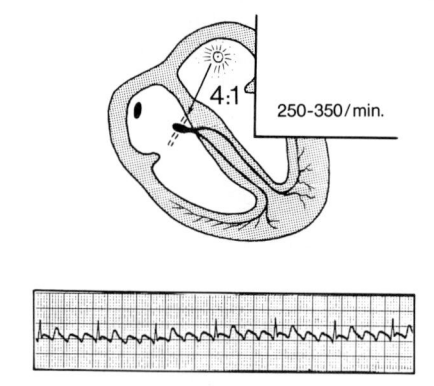

Fig. 3.13f Atrial flutter.

Atrial Fibrillation. Atrial fibrillation, an atrial tachyarrhythmia, is characterized by a heart rate of 300 to 600 beats/minute. Because of multiple foci firing independently throughout the atria, no coordinated contraction of atrial tissue occurs; also, blood passively moves from the atria to the ventricles. The irregular ventricular rate significantly reduces cardiac output.

In atrial fibrillation, the ECG shows an irregular wave in contrast to the "saw tooth" pattern seen in atrial flutter (Figure 3.13g). With chronic atrial fibrillation, clot formation may occur due to the blood stasis. These clots may dislodge to circulate in the blood stream resulting in possible vessel obstruction in highly critical areas of the body.

Because of the filtering effect of the A-V

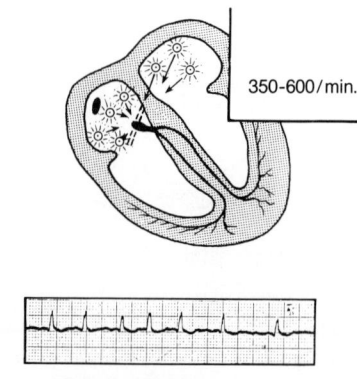

Fig. 3.13g Atrial fibrillation.

node, only every second to fourth atrial impulse is conducted into the ventricles. Rapid ventricular response (a ventricular rate above 120 beats/minute) requires therapy and may necessitate emergency treatment. Indeed, if all the ectopic impulses generated in the atria in flutter or fibrillation were conducted to the ventricles, ventricular fibrillation would occur. This could result in a significant reduction in cardiac output, circulatory arrest, and death.

Paroxysmal Supraventricular Tachycardia (PSVT). By definition, a supraventricular tachyarrhythmia is any tachyarrhythmia originating above the ventricles, i.e., paroxysmal atrial tachycardia (PAT). Since it is often difficult to determine if the origin of the arrhythmia is the S-A node, atrial tissue, the A-V node, or at the junction of the atria and ventricles, the term "supraventricular" is appropriate (Fig. 3.13h).

Tachyarrhythmias (such as PSVT) may result from a disorder in impulse conduction. A re-entry mechanism is apparently involved in the etiology of conduction defect tachyarrhythmias. Anterograde impulse conduction from the atria to the ventricles is the normal pathway through the A-V node. Under certain conditions retrograde conduction of the impulse from the ventricles to the atria occurs. The same impulse may then recirculate via the A-V node anterograde pathway to the ventricles resulting in ventricular tachycardia. Thus, the cycle of anterograde and retrograde conduction of the same impulse results in a tachyarrhythmia, such as PSVT.

An impulse from the atria may be conducted anterogradely to the ventricles through the "normal" A-V nodal pathway but return (re-entry) through an extranodal accessory pathway. The same impulse then stimulates the atria resulting in an activated A-V nodal pathway and ventricular contraction. A circular conduction of a single impulse thus results in re-entrant tachycardia.

Wolff-Parkinson-White Syndrome (WPW). This disease state occurs when an accessory pathway becomes active and conducts impulses from ventricles to atria (or less commonly, from atria to ventricles) bypassing the

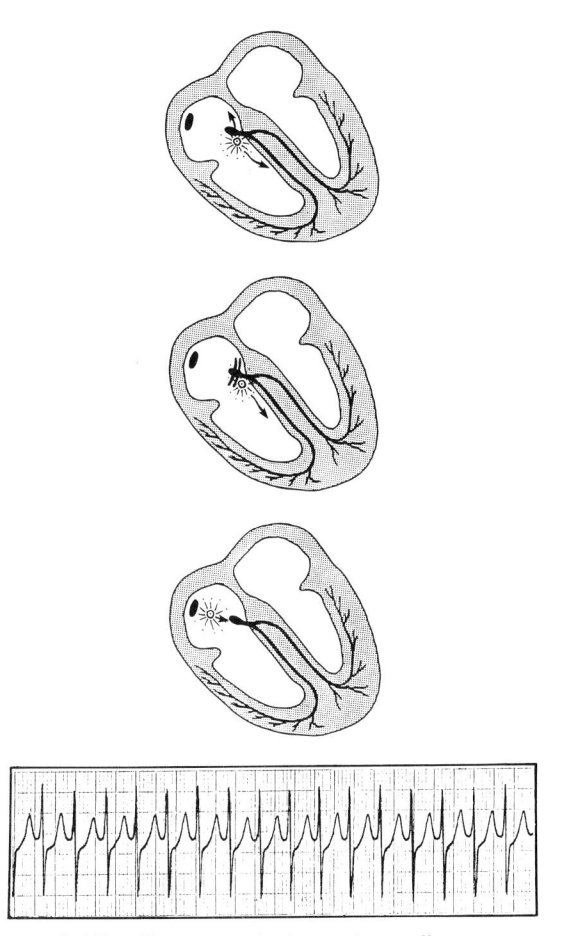

Fig. 3.13h Supraventricular tachycardia.

A-V node. This accessory pathway results in circular conduction and re-entrant supraventricular tachycardia.

Premature activation of the ventricles sometimes results from the WPW syndrome, indicated by the appearance of a delta wave just preceding the QRS complex (Figure 3.13i).

Lown-Ganong-Levine Syndrome (LGL). Another type of extranodal accessory pathway is Lown-Ganong-Levine syndrome. In this condition, an impulse travels from the atria to the ventricles through an accessory pathway around the A-V node but enters the normal conduction pathway below the A-V node. LGL syndrome predisposes the heart to the development of supraventricular tachyarrhythmias.

164 THERAPEUTIC PHARMACOLOGY

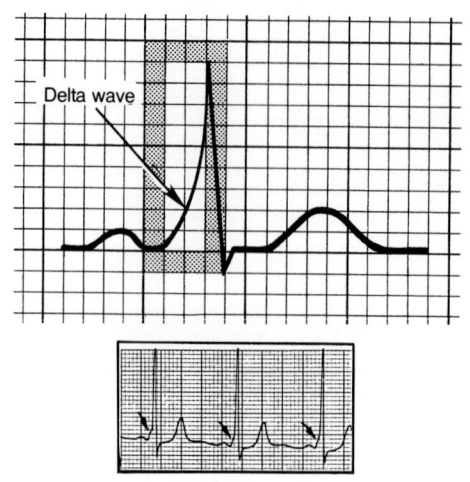

Fig. 3.13i Wolff-Parkinson-White syndrome [WPW].

ATRIOVENTRICULAR (A-V) NODE DISORDERS

Atrioventricular (A-V) node disorders are characterized by either an ectopic focus or an impaired conduction in the A-V junctional tissue.

Premature Junctional Contraction (PJC). An extrasystole or premature beat is due to an impulse from an ectopic focus in the A-V junctional tissues (Figure 3.13j).

A-V Conduction Block. The impaired conduction of an impulse slowed at a site in the A-V node is called a first degree A-V block, whereas blockade of conduction of some impulses is referred to as a second degree A-V block. Thus, if only one of every two atrial impulses enters the A-V node and results in ventricular contraction, a second degree A-V block with a 2:1 ratio occurs.

Third degree A-V block describes a blocking of all impulses and no atrial stimuli are transmitted to the ventricles. Immediate activation of a subsidiary pacemaker and initiation of a junctional rhythm are necessary for life to continue.

VENTRICULAR ARRHYTHMIAS

Ventricular arrhythmias occur more frequently as a person ages; their incidence also increases with a patient history of prior myocardial infarction and cardiac hypertrophy. Ventricular tachycardia and ventricular fibrillation are the most common causes of sudden cardiac death.

Premature Ventricular Contraction (PVC). An early contraction resulting from an ectopic site in the ventricular conduction system is called a premature ventricular contraction (PVC). This is represented in the ECG by Figure 3.13k.

Ventricular Tachycardia. Ventricular tachycardia results from ectopic impulse formation in the ventricles and is indicated by an accelerated heart rate with a significant reduction of cardiac output and stroke volume. This is due to the

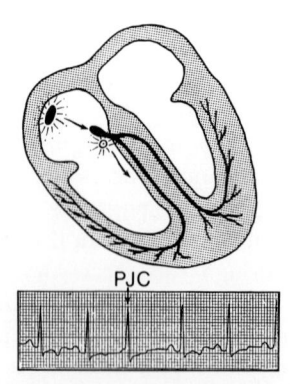

Fig. 3.13j Premature junctional contraction [PJC].

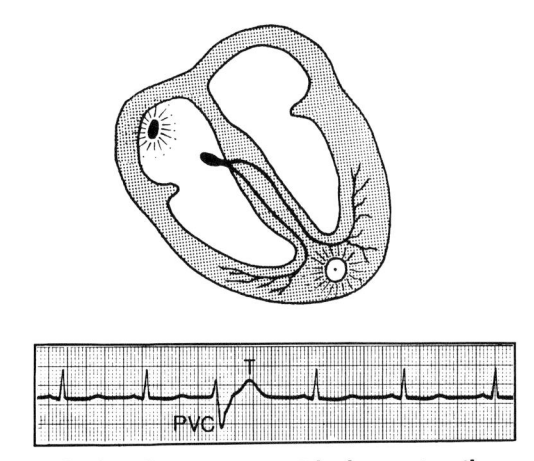

Fig. 3.13k Premature ventricular contraction [PVC].

decreased ventricular filling time that results from the increased ventricular rate.

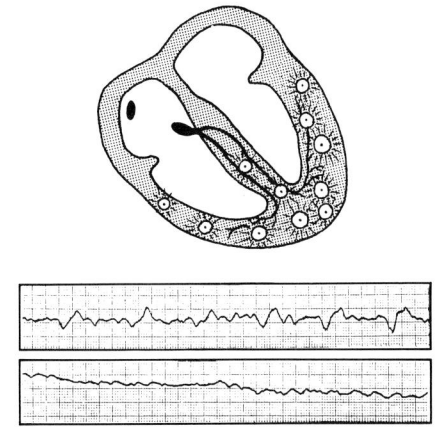

Ventricular Fibrillation. Ventricular fibrillation is the most serious of the cardiac tachyarrhythmias. This condition is characterized by uncoordinated, erratic, and ventricular contractions and no effective contraction of the ventricle chambers occurs (Figure 3.13l). Consequently, lack of cardiac output, if not treated immediately, leads to circulatory arrest and death.

A main cause of ventricular fibrillation is the "R on T phenomenon." During the vulnerable period in the depolarization phase of the cardiac cycle, ventricular cells may respond to an impulse from a ventricular ectopic focus by spontaneous firing, resulting in either ventricular tachycardia or ventricular fibrillation. Thus, when the ectopic focus impulse (QRS) falls on the vulnerable phase of the ECG (T wave apex), a ventricular arrhythmia—the R on T phenomenon—occurs (Figure 3.13m).

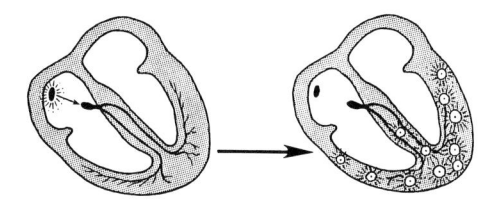

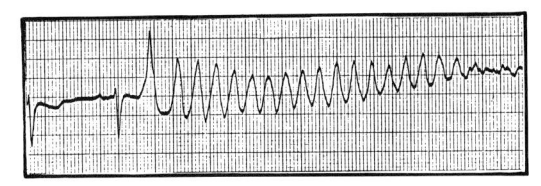

Fig. 3.13m R on T phenomenon.

CONGESTIVE HEART FAILURE (CHF)

Possibly as a consequence of aging, the heart slowly becomes less efficient, a situation somewhat analogous to that of a machine wearing out when operated for too long. When the ventricles lose their ability to pump out sufficient blood to supply the body, congestive heart failure (CHF) occurs.

As indicated previously, the two ventricles eject about 120 ml of blood per beat and that blood is returned to the heart (after passing through the capillaries) by the veins in which blood is forced along by the milking action of the muscles. In a healthy individual, the volume of blood leaving the heart via the arteries equals that the veins return. Should the myocardium (ventricle walls) become less efficient, the tissues receive an inadequate blood supply and a symptom known as hypoxia results. Meanwhile, however, the muscles continue pushing blood along in the veins, but, since the pumping action of the heart is inadequate to eject all the blood returned to it by the veins, a

Fig. 3.13l Ventricular fibrillation.

build-up or congestion occurs in the veins, hence the designation "congestive heart disease."

In CHF, the pressure in the veins elevates; as a result, fluids are forced through the capillaries into the tissues (this accounts for the swollen ankles frequently observed in CHF patients). Increased pressure in the veins leads to pulsation in the larger veins. The heart rate increases as it attempts to pump out more blood and the heart also enlarges. This enlargement occurs as the muscle fibers of the myocardium stretch, which illustrates an axiom of physiology, namely, a muscle under tension (stretched) will contract more forcefully than one which is relaxed (Starling's law). In spite of the heart's efforts to increase its efficiency, the disease progresses and unless treated, the patient's condition worsens.

Congestive heart failure (CHF), a condition where the heart fails to function as an effective pump, does not ordinarily remain limited to one ventricle and may develop parallel in both ventricles. However, the disease is specifically described as either left-sided or right-sided heart failure.

Often brought on by high systemic arterial pressure, left-sided heart failure produces pulmonary (lung) congestion. Hence, a common precipitating factor in left-sided failure is prolonged hypertension. Another is mechanical obstruction or regurgitation of left ventricle blood outflow. In this condition, dilation and hypertrophy of the left ventricle occurs. Breathing difficulty resulting from pulmonary congestion is a common symptom.

Occurring less frequently, primary right-sided failure is usually caused by pulmonary obstruction (similar to that seen in emphysema). Disease characteristics include right ventricle dilation and hypertrophy, venous pressure elevation, liver enlargement, and development of peripheral edema.

Arteriosclerosis (thickening and loss of elasticity) in the coronary vessels is a common cause of CHF due to the progressive inadequacy of oxygen supply to the heart. Other precipitating factors are congenital deformities, rheumatic fever, and syphilis; by adverse effects on the heart valves, these conditions result in obstruction and regurgitation of blood flow.

In the early CHF stages, the body attempts to maintain adequate cardiac output by compensatory mechanisms involving sympathetic stimulation and decreased vagal activity. Specifically, increased sympathetic stimulation promotes peripheral vasoconstriction and release of aldosterone and ADH which leads to salt/water retention by the kidneys. This in turn produces increases in blood volume, venous return, and thus, cardiac output. Eventually, however, the total body fluid overload (expanded blood volume) results in the characteristic signs and symptoms of CHF: increased pressure in peripheral vessels causing fluid movement into tissues which results in peripheral edema; increased left ventricle filling pressure causing elevated left atrial pressure which results in pulmonary congestion (evidenced by orthopnea and shortness of breath).

CORONARY ARTERY DISEASE

The heart, unable to tolerate an oxygen debt, must receive an adequate blood supply at all times. This is accomplished by the coronary arteries which branch from the aorta just as it emerges from the heart. During periods of increased activity, the tissues require additional oxygen, supplied by the blood, and the same is true of the heart. To fulfill this demand for more oxygen, the heart rate increases; consequently, the arteries (including the coronaries) carry more blood to the tissues. Impairment of blood flow in the coronary arteries may result from coronary artery occlusion (heart attack), a quickly fatal condition if the impairment involves one or more of the larger branches of the coronary arteries.

Since the heart cannot tolerate an oxygen debt, any interference with its blood supply causes the affected part to become nonfunctional. Within a few weeks, the nonfunctional part is replaced by scar tissue into which the capillaries of the coronary arteries extend and branch in order to provide oxygen and nourishment. The scar tissue remains nonfunctional, however, and after recovery the patient's ECG shows an abnormality.

If only a minute branch of one of the coronary arteries is occluded, the capillaries in the myocardium can branch and extend sufficiently to nourish the small area affected by the occlusion. In such cases, the patient usually recovers and the ECG ordinarily returns to normal within a few weeks, although a day or so after the occlusion has occurred the ECG indicates some slight abnormalities.

Obviously, if a large branch of the arteries is involved, a large area of the heart becomes nonfunctional; this represents the massive heart attack that is often fatal. More often than not, however, small branches of the coronary arteries are involved and, assuming that proper treatment is initiated, the patient recovers. The term myocardial infarction (MI) is used for the condition in which an occulsion (clot) occurs in a coronary artery, resulting in deprivation of an adequate oxygen supply to the heart.

Heart attack symptoms frequently include severe chest pain that sometimes radiates outward in the arm. Precipitating factors of coronary artery disease include obesity, heavy smoking, high fat diets, and a "high pressure-fast lane" lifestyle. Hereditary traits may also be involved. Although the incidence of heart attacks is higher in men than in women, statistics indicate it is rising at a rather rapid rate in women.

Atherosclerosis represents the deposition in the intima and inner media of large and medium-sized arteries of lipoid material, including cholesterol, a component found in the fat portion of the diet. Atherosclerosis may exist in the coronary arteries of many patients who have recovered from heart attacks; these deposits (atheromas) can obstruct blood flow in the arteries. Partial obstruction of a branch of the coronary arteries reduces the amount of blood supplied to an area of the heart. This condition often produces angina pectoris, an excruciating, grasping type of pain in the chest. Angina attacks, which vary in severity and duration, may be brought on by strenuous activity, emotional factors, and the like. Drugs that dilate coronary vessels and reduce the peripheral resistance are often valuable in correcting angina pectoris.

HYPERTENSION

Hypertension is the condition in which the pressure exerted by the blood on the arterial system is persistently higher than the normal limits. Two clinical values used in determining blood pressure are the systolic blood pressure and the diastolic blood pressure.

Systolic pressure is due mainly to the driving force of the heart; diastolic pressure is the force to which the arterial system is subjected at all times. In healthy young adults at rest, the normal range for systolic pressure is between 110 and 120 mm and for diastolic pressure is between 60 and 70 mm.

Average diastolic pressure increases with age and is usually about 90 mm at age 65 in the male. Uncorrected hypertension carries an increased rate of morbidity and mortality; controlled studies indicate that treatment with antihypertensive drugs lowers this risk. Thus, the dangers of high blood pressure effects on the brain, heart, and kidneys mandate institution of effective control measures (perhaps with antihypertensive drugs) in hypertensive patients.

Normally, blood pressure is controlled by centers in the brain which, in turn, respond to changes in baroreceptors in the arterial system. For example, when the blood pressure rises, the carotid sinus reflex lowers the heart rate and dilates arteriolar smooth muscle by effects on the medullary vagal and vasomotor center, respectively. Lack of oxygen and/or certain drugs may stimulate both the vagus and vasomotor center.

Psychogenic stimuli also affect blood pressure. For instance, epinephrine release by the adrenal medulla in stress results in blood pressure elevation. Blood pressure increase subsequently activates the baroreceptors, which counteracts the blood pressure elevation. This homeostatic mechanism represents an important example of negative feedback control of blood pressure.

Several other factors are involved in the

maintenance of blood pressure within normal limits. Blood volume and viscosity are normally regulated by the kidneys. Resistance of the arterial system to blood flow and the driving force of the heart constitute critical determinants of blood pressure. The following equation represents this important relationship:

$$\frac{\text{Mean arterial}}{\text{pressure}} = \frac{\text{Cardiac}}{\text{Output}} \times \frac{\text{Total Peripheral}}{\text{Resistance}}$$

(Blood Pressure = CO × TPR)

Disease processes can have a profound influence on this relationship. For instance, if the arterial system becomes laden with atherosclerotic deposits, the diameter of the artery is reduced, and since more force is required to push blood through a constricted vessel, the pressure inside the affected artery increases. When the wall of the arteries loses its elasticity and becomes leathery or sclerotic, the progressive condition known as arteriosclerosis ("hardening of the arteries") occurs.

As the blood pressure rises due to increased resistance to flow in the arterioles, a greater work load is placed upon the heart, simply because it must overcome the increased resistance. Consequently, the heart enlarges and the rate increases. Increased pressure to which the arterioles are subjected often causes one or more of them to rupture (just as too much air pressure in a bicycle tire causes a blowout). If the rupture occurs in the arterioles of the heart or the brain, the consequences are serious because neither of these organs can tolerate an oxygen debt. In the heart, a possibly fatal myocardial infarction (MI) ensues; in the brain, a cerebrovascular accident, or stroke, occurs which may be fatal or cause paralysis, the severity of which depends upon the amount of the brain deprived of oxygen as a result of the rupture.

Hypertension occurs in about 20% of the population; no apparent cause can be found in about 90% of these cases. This type of high blood pressure is known as essential hypertension (the word "essential" designates either unknown cause or simply "essential" for that individual). Some suggest that a hereditary abnormality in the arterioles results in the disease; others hold that overactivity of renin, a substance secreted by the kidneys, evokes an exaggerated constrictor effect on the arterioles, thus, precipitating the condition. Prostaglandins and other local autocoids are also implicated in essential hypertension.

Essential hypertension is much more common in young people than first believed. Also, the disease is more prevalent (and occurs earlier) in blacks than in whites. It affects both sexes and is more common in those who lead relatively inactive lives. The disease, which can worsen during emotional crises (suggesting a psychogenic component), occurs more frequently in obese individuals as well as in heavy smokers. Essential hypertension has an insidious onset; thus, the patient has no symptoms to indicate presence of the disease. Appropriately, hypertension is often termed the "silent disease."

INFECTIONS (ENDOCARDITIS; PERICARDITIS)

Bacterial endocarditis is a febrile systemic disease marked by infection of the heart valves with the formation of pathogen-laden fibrin masses called vegetations. This disease, which impairs valve function, may be either acute with an abrupt onset and rapidly progressing course or subacute with an insidious onset and protracted course. Streptococcus viridans commonly causes bacterial endocarditis; staphylococci, also frequently found in endocarditis, are the most frequent cause of pericarditis in children.

Damaged heart valves, such as those that occur after rheumatic fever or in congenital abnormalities, are particularly vulnerable to pathogenic organisms in the bloodstream. If septic emboli enter the bloodstream, they may lodge elsewhere in the body and spread the infection.

DRUGS USED IN THE TREATMENT OF CARDIOVASCULAR DISEASE

A 1983 FDA survey, "Drug Utilization in the U.S.," named cardiovascular drugs as the most frequently dispensed product class, constituting 14% of all prescriptions. Drugs, such as digoxin and disopyramide, that are used to treat serious cardiovascular disease have a relatively narrow therapeutic range. This means that a drug serum concentration just below a certain level (therapeutic range) results in loss of control of the disease, for example, as in certain cardiac arrhythmias. On the other hand, slight increases above the therapeutic dosage range increase the likelihood of toxic effects of the drug. Thus, in the case of many cardiovascular drugs, a drug titration to the individual patient's requirement for control is essential. The pharmacokinetic data of specific products regarding protein binding and free-drug availability become important factors in clinical decisions. Thus, the therapeutic goal of proper dosing with cardiovascular drugs requires careful scrutiny of generic equivalence and individual therapeutic response.

CARDIAC ARRHYTHMIAS

Drug therapy for cardiac arrhythmias is directed toward restoration and maintenance of normal sinus rhythm, suppression and prevention of ectopic rhythms, and controlling the ventricular rate. Antiarrhythmic drugs (Table 3.1) are classified according to their activity on

Table 3.1 ANTIARRHYTHMIC DRUGS.*

Available products	Trade names	Daily dosage range
Amiodarone HCl	Cardarone	Oral, 200–800 mg; slow IV, 5–10 mg/kg; initial bolus of 300–500 mg followed by an infusion of 50 mg/min
Bretylium tosylate	Bretylol	IV or IM 5–10 mg/kg
Disopyramide	Norpace	150 mg q. 6 hrs following an initial loading dose of 300 mg
Encainide	Enkaid	25–35 mg t.i.d.
Flecainide	Tambocor	100 mg b.i.d.
Lidocaine HCl	Xylocaine	Single IV bolus dose of 50–100 mg followed by a continuous IV infusion at a rate of 1–4 mg/min.; IM, 300 mg (approx. 4.3 mg/kg or 2 mg/lb)
Mexiletine	Mexitil	Oral, 400–800 mg; IV, loading dose of 100–250 mg within 4–10 min., followed by an infusion of diminishing concentration
Phenytoin dose, 300–400 mg	Dilantin	Initially, 100 mg t.i.d.; Maintenance
Procainamide HCl	Pronestyl; Promine; Sub-Quin	Initial oral doses of 1 g followed by a maintenance dose of 6 mg/kg/day q. 3 hrs
Propranolol HCl	Inderal	Oral, 10–30 mg t.i.d or q.i.d.; IV, 1–3 mg at a rate of no more than 1 mg/min with careful monitoring
Quinidine gluconate	Quinaglute; Duraquin; others	Oral, 200–300 mg; IM, 600 mg followed by 400 mg repeated as often as every 2 hrs; IV, 300–750 mg at a rate of 1 ml/min of a dilute solution
Quinidine polygalacturonate	Cardioquin	Oral, 275–825 mg for conversion, repeated in 3 or 4 hrs if necessary; Maintenance: 275 mg morning and evening
Quinidine sulfate	Quinora; Cin-Quin; others	200–300 mg t.i.d. or q.i.d.
Tocainide	Tonocard	400 mg q. 8 hrs
Verapamil HCl	Calan; Isoptin	Oral, 80 mg t.i.d. or q.i.d.; slow IV, 5–10 mg over 2 min

* Some cholinergic, anticholinergic, adrenergic, and digitalis glycoside drugs are also used in the treatment of cardiac arrhythmias.

Table 3.2 ELECTROPHYSIOLOGICAL CLASSIFICATION OF ANTIARRHYTHMIC DRUGS.

Type I	Depression of Phase 0 Depolarization
Type I-A	Moderate
	Prolongation of repolarization
	Widening of QRS interval
Type I-B	Weak
	Shortening of repolarization
	Minimal effects on QRS interval
Type I-C	Potent
	Minimal effffect on repolarization
	Prolongation of QRS interval
Type II	Inhibition of Sympathetic Tone by Beta-adrenergic Blockade
	Depression of Phase 4 depolarization
Type III	Prolongation of Repolarization (Phase 3)
Type IV	Blockade of Calcium Channels
	Prolongation of Phases 1 and 2
	Depression of Phase 4 depolarization
Type V	Effects on Central Nervous System
	Electrophysiological mechanisms unclear
Digitalis glycosides	Decrease of Maximal Diastolic Potential and Action Potential Duration
	Increase in the slope of Phase 4 depolarization

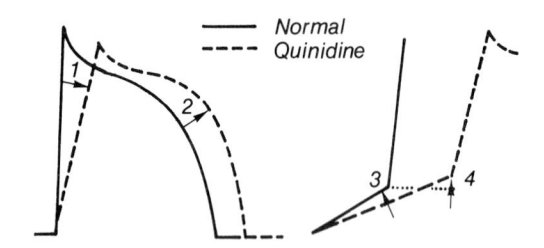

Fig. 3.14 Electrophysical effects of quinidine. (1) Decrease of speed of depolarization. (2) Prolongation of the resting state (plateau) of the refractory period. (3) Decrease in speed of diastolic depolarization. (4) Elevation of the diastolic threshold. (Modified from Nager, F.: Klinische Befunde bei koronarer Herzkrankheit. Schweiz. Med. Wochenschr., 102: 1836, 1972.)

the cardiac action potential or their inherent pharmacologic properties (Table 3.2).

TYPE I ANTIARRHYTHMIC DRUGS

Type I antiarrhythmic drugs depress Phase 0 depolarization.

Quinidine. Quinidine is the dextrostereoisomer of the alkaloid, quinine. The antiarrhythmic effect of quinine was accidentally discovered when malaria patients with pre-existent atrial fibrillation were converted to normal cardiac rhythm following quinine therapy. Quinidine has stronger cardiac effects than those of quinine and is more toxic in clinical doses. Quinidine also possesses other pharmacologic effects similar to quinine, including antimalarial, antipyretic, and oxytocic activities. The alkaloid quinidine may be obtained from various species of Cinchona and their hybrids, from Remijia peduculata Fluckiger (Fam. Rubiaceae), or prepared from quinine.

Mechanism of Action. Quinidine, a classic Type I antiarrhythmic drug, has a moderate effect in depressing Phase 0 depolarization (Figure 3.14). The influx of sodium and the efflux of potassium is inhibited resulting in a decrease in the speed of conduction through the atria, ventricles, and specialized conduction tissue.

Quinidine decreases cardiac cell automaticity by increasing the threshold for diastolic depolarization. The retardation of diastolic depolarization reduces myocardial automaticity.

The excitability threshold for electrical stimuli elevates with quinidine. Thus, the number of extrasystoles decreases and the ability for impulses from these ectopic foci to initiate atrial fibrillation and ventricular tachycardia lessens. The refractory period of the atria and ventricles, as well as the A-V node, is prolonged. The refractory period of the A-V node is defined as the shortest interval between two stimuli originating in the atria which can both be propagated into the ventricles. The prolongation of the refractory period, which usually extends into Phase 4, is the most important determinant in suppressing and interrupting the re-entry phenomenon, a recognized factor in the initiation of arrhythmic activity.

Quinidine has a secondary vagal-blocking effect that has an opposite action on the A-V node excitability when compared to the primary effect of quinidine to decrease excitability. The vagal-blocking effect increases A-V node excitability, as evidenced by a decrease in the refractory period. Additionally, vagal-blocking activity may increase A-V nodal conduction, an opposite effect of the primary action. These secondary vagal-blocking effects present a clinical problem since they tend to antagonize the primary pharmacologic activity as well as aid and abet the aberrant processes being treated with quinidine.

The primary antiarrhythmic actions of quinidine are to prolong the effective refractory period of the atria, ventricles, and A-V node and decrease the excitability of ectopic foci. Depression of excitability, conduction velocity, and contractility result from the inhibition of Phase 0 sodium ion (Na^+) influx and potassium ion (K^+) efflux. Also, quinidine blocks vagal activity and facilitates impulse conduction in the A-V node.

Clinical Indications. Quinidine is indicated for prevention of premature nodal, atrial, or ventricular contractions. Additional indications include maintenance of normal sinus rhythm following spontaneous or electrical conversion of nodal, atrial, or ventricular tachycardia, atrial flutter, and atrial fibrillation.

In patients with atrial fibrillation, the ventricular rate may increase due to the facilitation of A-V conduction by quinidine. Prior administration of a digitalis glycoside is indicated, followed by combined glycoside-quinidine therapy. The glycoside depression of A-V conduction counters the quinidine-induced increase in A-V node conduction due to its vagal-blocking action.

In general, quinidine's therapeutic niche is as a prophylactic drug in the long-term suppression of atrial fibrillation and premature atrial, nodal, and ventricular depolarizations. Quinidine is recommended in the preparation for cardioversion of atrial fibrillation or flutter and for prophylaxis against recurrence of arrhythmias after successful cardioversion.

Adverse Effects/Precautions. Gastrointestinal disturbances, especially diarrhea, are common with quinidine therapy. Diarrhea can be minimized by lowering the dose if an effective clinical response can still be achieved with the reduced dose. Aluminum hydroxide gel may be given with the quinidine dose to offset the gastrointestinal disturbance.

Hypotension occurs frequently with parenteral administration of quinidine but happens rarely with oral use. Quinidine syncope sometimes occurs after the first dose or with subsequent chronic administration, apparently resulting from the induction of a ventricular arrhythmia. Heart block is also possible with quinidine therapy with the widening of the QRS interval indicative of conduction reduction. Paradoxically, tachyarrhythmias may occur with quinidine.

Cinchonism, as reflected in tinnitus aurium, headache, nausea, dizziness, vertigo, lightheadedness, tremor, and disturbed vision, may occur with quinidine therapy. These symptoms can happen after a single dose.

Blood dyscrasias, including thrombocytopenia, are another adverse effect, as is hepatotoxicity which results from quinidine hypersensitivity. Consequently, during long-term quinidine therapy, periodic blood counts and liver function tests are suggested.

Potassium balance is important in quinidine activity. The enhancement in quinidine effect seen with hyperkalemia may increase the incidence of quinidine adverse effects. Hypokalemia, on the other hand, reduces quinidine action.

Procainamide. Procainamide is the amide analog of the local anesthetic, procaine. A Type I antiarrhythmic drug, it displays electrophysiologic effects similar to those of quinidine.

Mechanism of Action. Procainamide depresses the excitability of cardiac muscle to electrical stimulation and slows conduction in the atria, ventricles, and the Bundle of His. Prolongation of the atrial refractory period is more extensive than that of the ventricle. Cardiac output and contractility are usually not affected unless myocardial damage is present. Effects on the cardiac action potential are characteristic of a Type I-A antiarrhythmic drug and result from the inhibition of ion currents mainly during Phase 0 depolarization.

Excessive procainamide dosage is most often reflected in the widening of the QRS complex.

In the absence of any arrhythmia, procainamide may induce heart rate acceleration which suggests an adjunctive anticholinergic action. High doses of procainamide can induce A-V block and ventricular extrasystoles which may precipitate ventricular fibrillation.

Procainamide is converted to a cardioactive metabolite, N-acetylprocainamide. Patients with a more effective inherent acetylating system (N-acetyltransferase) are rapid acetylators and convert a larger percentage of procainamide to N-acetylprocainamide ($>25\%$).

Clinical Indications. Procainamide is used in the treatment of premature ventricular contractions (PVCs) and ventricular tachycardia and in atrial fibrillation and paroxysmal atrial tachycardia (PAT). Some reports indicate the drug is more effective than quinidine in treating ventricular arrhythmias.

Adverse Effects/Precautions. The half-lives of both procainamide and N-acetylprocainamide are prolonged in renal disease and CHF. Thus, if a patient who has concurrrent renal disease or CHF, is a rapid acetylator, and receives a high dose of procainamide, N-acetylprocainamide may accumulate to toxic levels. A reduction in procainamide dosage (30 to 50%) may be necessary in CHF patients due to the reduced renal clearance of procainamide and N-acetylprocainamide. Hence, monitoring plasma levels of both procainamide and N-acetylprocainamide is critical in patients with renal compromise.

Prolonged use of procainamide may lead to a systemic lupus erythematosus-like (SLE-like) syndrome; estimates indicate that approximately 25% of the patients on chronic procainamide therapy develop this syndrome. Maintenance therapy with procainamide often (in 80 to 90% of the patients with 3 to 6 months of therapy) results in the development of a positive antinuclear antibody (ANA) test with or without symptoms of a SLE-like syndrome. After consideration of the patient benefit-to-risk potential, alternate antiarrhythmic drug therapy may be indicated. The SLE-like syndrome is characterized chiefly by fever, polyarthralgia, arthritis, and pleuritic pain. This syndrome is usually reversible upon discontinuation of procainamide therapy.

Oral administration of procainamide may cause gastrointestinal disturbances, blood dyscrasias, and hypersensitivity reactions. Additionally, IV procainamide administration may produce hypotension as a result of peripheral vasodilation.

Disopyramide. Disopyramide, a Type I antiarrhythmic agent, is pharmacologically similar, yet chemically dissimilar, to quinidine and procainamide.

Mechanism of Action. Disopyramide, which markedly resembles quinidine in action, decreases the rate of Phase 4 diastolic depolarization, decreases the Phase 0 slope, prolongs the refractory period (Phases 2 and 3), and lengthens the action potential duration of cardiac cells. Anticholinergic effects, similar to those of quinidine, occur frequently.

Disopyramide lengthens the effective refractory period of the atria and the ventricles. Data on the A-V node are inconclusive, but enhancement of conduction is possible. The negative inotropic effect of disopyramide is more marked than with quinidine or procainamide; this action assumes clinical importance if prior myocardial damage is significant.

Clinical Indications. Disopyramide is used to suppress and prevent premature ventricular contractions and episodic ventricular tachycardia.

Adverse Effects/Precautions. Myocardial depression is a potential serious adverse effect. In CHF, disopyramide may worsen the condition and produce serious hypotension. Other possible adverse cardiac effects are tachycardia and heart block.

Anticholinergic side effects include urinary retention, dry mouth, and blurred vision. Contraindications for its use, due to disopyramide's anticholinergic action, are in urinary retention or glaucoma. A myasthenic crisis may be precipitated in patients with myasthenia gravis as a result of this activity.

Lidocaine. Lidocaine, a Type I-B antiarrhythmic drug, has significant local anesthetic properties. It exhibits poor bioavailability and is therefore restricted to IV administration.

Mechanism of Action. Lidocaine, like the Type I-A drugs (quinidine, procainamide, and disopyramide), suppresses the "fast" sodium current in myocardial cells, thereby decreasing their excitability (Figure 3.15). Lidocaine slows Phase 4 diastolic depolarization, decreases automaticity, and causes a decrease or no change in excitability and membrane responsiveness. The action potential duration and effective refractory period of the ventricles decrease and the ventricular fibrillation threshold elevates. In contrast to the Type I-A antiarrhythmic agents that consistently prolong the QRS interval in higher doses, lidocaine has no effect on the ECG. Lidocaine has no clinically significant effect on sinus node function or atrial, A-V nodal, or ventricular refractory periods. In Purkinje fibers and ventricular muscle, the ratio of effective refractory period to the action potential duration increases, allowing less time during an action potential for an ectopic impulse to generate another action potential.

Lidocaine is converted to at least two cardioactive metabolites, monoethylglycinexylidide (MEGX) and glycinexylidide (GX).

Clinical Indications. Lidocaine is the drug of choice in the acute treatment of premature ventricular complexes. The drug is used in the acute management of ventricular arrhythmias, such as those occurring in relation to acute MI or during cardiac surgery. The most effective dosing of lidocaine is achieved with an IV loading dose followed by maintenance therapy.

Adverse Effects/Precautions. CNS adverse effects of lidocaine include drowsiness or agitation, disorientation, coma, seizures, and paresthesias. Cardiac depression may occur, especially if CHF or liver failure is present or in IV infusions of more than 24 hours' duration.

Tocainide. A Type I-B antiarrhythmic drug, tocainide is a chemical congener of lidocaine. The drug is orally effective, which accounts for its "oral lidocaine" designation.

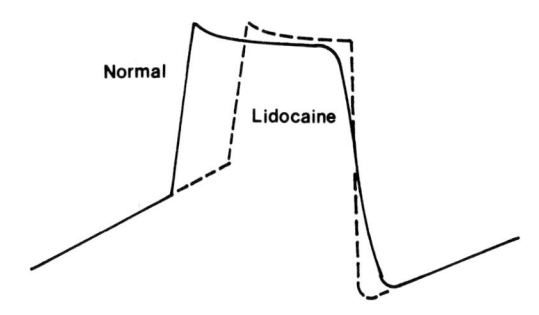

Fig. 3.15 Electrophysical effects of lidocaine. (Modified from Simon, H., and Bloomfield, D.A.: Cardioactive Drugs. Baltimore, Urban and Schwarzenberg, 1983.)

Mechanism of Action. Like lidocaine, tocainide produces dose-dependent decreases in sodium and potassium conductance, thereby decreasing the excitability of myocardial cells. Tocainide shortens the action potential duration and effective refractory period of Purkinje fibers and ventricular muscle. Systolic depolarization (Phase 0) is prolonged as its rate of rise is reduced. Phase 3 shortens, causing an overall lessening of the action potential and the refractory period. Like lidocaine but unlike the Type I-A antiarrhythmic drugs, tocainide does not prolong the PR, QRS, or QT intervals. Theoretically, therefore, tocainide should be useful in the treatment of ventricular arrhythmias associated with a prolonged QT interval.

Clinical Indications. Tocainide suppresses a variety of ventricular arrhythmias, including premature ventricular contractions and ventricular tachycardia. The drug has been effective in preventing, reducing, and abolishing ventricular arrhythmias after a recent MI. Tocainide is indicated in chronic maintenance therapy to prevent (or reduce) complex ventricular arrhythmias and in arrhythmias refractory to other antiarrhythmic agents. Of patients suffering from the latter, 50 to 60% benefit from tocainide therapy; lidocaine response is a useful predictor of tocainide efficacy in this population. Tocainide has been employed as an antiarrhythmic drug in patients with atherosclerotic heart disease, cardiomyopathy, hypertensive heart disease, valvular heart disease, and in patients with no identifiable heart disease other than ventricular arrhythmias.

Patients not benefited by lidocaine therapy are usually unresponsive to tocainide as well. Effective in about 70% of the patients who respond favorably to lidocaine, tocainide is successful in only about 15% of the patients unresponsive to lidocaine.

Adverse Effects/Precautions. Tocainide's most frequent adverse effects involve the gastrointestinal tract and the central nervous system (CNS). Gastrointestinal effects include nausea, vomiting, and anorexia. Tremors, dizziness, lightheadedness, anxiety, paresthesias, and confusion are common CNS adverse reactions to tocainide.

As with other antiarrhythmic drugs, tocainide has the potential to worsen cardiac arrhythmias. The drug should be used with caution in patients with CHF or minimal cardiac reserve, although severe negative inotropic effects that aggravate CHF treated with disopyramide appear to be less likely with tocainide therapy.

Allergic reactions, including fever, arthralgias, and severe erythematosus maculopapular rashes, have been reported. Tocainide use is contraindicated in patients who are hypersensitive to amide local anesthetics such as lidocaine, dibucaine, or carbocaine.

Phenytoin. Although not approved by the FDA as an antiarrhythmic drug, phenytoin is commonly used in the treatment of digitalis-induced arrhythmias. The drug has characteristics similar to those of a Type I-B antiarrhythmic drug.

Mechanism of Action. Phenytoin has a weak depressant effect on Phase 0 depolarization and shortens repolarization in cardiac cells. The drug does not exert a significant action on the QRS interval. The antiarrhythmic action of phenytoin, possibly due to its CNS depressant activity, apparently resides in its membrane-stabilizing effect. Phenytoin reverses digitalis-induced potassium efflux and increases the ratio of extracellular to intracellular sodium from cardiac cells. Ion current alterations, along with slight acceleration of A-V transmission, are probably responsible for a significant proportion of phenytoin's antiarrhythmic activity in reversing digitalis-induced arrhythmias.

Clinical Indications. Phenytoin is used orally or intravenously as an alternate drug in the control of digitalis-induced tachyarrhythmias.

Adverse Effects/Precautions. Ataxia, nystagmus, drowsiness, and coma are CNS effects reported with phenytoin use. Blood dyscrasias may also occur, and rapid IV administration of phenytoin can result in cardiac toxicity.

Mexiletine. Mexiletine, a Type I-B antiarrhythmic drug, resembles lidocaine both chemically and pharmacologically.

Mechanism of Action. In therapeutic doses, mexiletine reduces Phase 0 sodium influx without eliciting an effect on the initiation and conduction of cardiac impulses.

Clinical Indications. Used in the control of ventricular ectopic beats, mexiletine is effective in controlling A-V nodal re-entry tachycardias. It is also used in combination therapy with verapamil or propranolol.

Adverse Effects/Precautions. Side effects, which occur in about 25% of the patients taking mexiletine, manifest mainly in the gastrointestinal tract or CNS. These adverse effects include nausea, vomiting, gastric discomfort, dizziness, visual disturbances, and confusion.

Intraventricular conduction delay or A-V block represents a contraindication for mexiletine use.

Flecainide. Flecainide is a Type I-C antiarrhythmic drug.

Mechanism of Action. Flecainide has a potent effect on Phase 0 depolarization and little effect on repolarization. The QRS interval is prolonged and should be monitored since excessive prolongation may occur.

Clinical Indications. Used in the treatment of symptomatic sustained ventricular tachycardias, the drug is characterized by a long half-life (14 to 20 hours).

Adverse Effects/Precautions. Flecainide's adverse effects, related to the gastrointestinal tract and CNS, include dizziness, blurred vision, tremor, nausea, and vomiting.

Encainide. A Type I-C antiarrhythmic drug, encainide is used as an alternative to traditional drugs in the treatment of symptomatic ventricular arrhythmias.

Mechanism of Action. Encainide blocks Phase 0 depolarization and has minimal effect on repolarization. Encainide slows cardiac conduction, reduces membrane responsiveness, inhibits automaticity in the myocardium, and increases the ratio of the ERP to action potential duration.

Clinical Indications. Used in life-threatening arrhythmias such as non-sustained ventricular tachycardia and premature ventricular complexes, encainide may be especially valuable in refractory, non-sustained ventricular tachycardia and refractory, potentially fatal ventricular arrhythmias.

Adverse Effects/Precautions. Dizziness and blurred vision are the most commonly noted side effects of encainide.

TYPE II ANTIARRHYTHMIC DRUGS

Type II antiarrhythmic drugs produce their effects by inhibiting sympathetic tone by beta-adrenergic blockade.

Propranolol. Classified as a Type II antiarrhythmic drug, propranolol is a beta-adrenergic blocking agent.

Mechanism of Action. The sympathetic nervous system contains two main types of peripheral adrenergic receptors, which are designated as alpha- and beta-adrenergic receptors. The latter have been subdivided into beta$_1$ and beta$_2$ categories depending upon their distribution and the physiologic response induced upon receptor activation.

Beta$_1$-adrenergic receptors are found in the heart and their agonist activity increases heart rate (positive chronotropic effect) and cardiac contractility (positive inotropic activity). Additionally, beta$_1$-adrenergic receptor stimulation produces an acceleration of A-V conduction. Activation of beta$_2$-adrenergic receptors, found in the bronchi and blood vessels, produces bronchodilation and vasodilation.

Type II antiarrhythmic agents are beta-adrenergic blocking drugs of which propranolol is the prototype. Propranolol blocks the effects of beta-adrenergic agonists (such as epinephrine) on receptors in the heart, bronchi, and blood vessels. Beta-adrenergic blockade decreases the rate of sinus node and ectopic pacemaker firing together with a slowing of the A-V conduction rate (Fig. 3.16). Thus, in cardiac arrhythmias associated with increased sympathetic tone, propranolol is beneficial. For example, propranolol controls the ventricular rate in atrial tachycardias by increasing the degree of A-V block and by depressing the impulse rate at the S-A node.

Clinical Indications. Propranolol has been used for both supraventricular and ventricular arrhythmias and as an alternate drug in the control of digitalis-induced tachyarrhythmias. The most effective response is seen in the management of supraventricular arrhythmias. Propranolol is generally not the first choice for

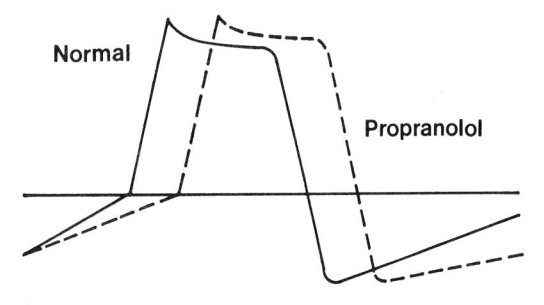

Fig. 3.16 *Electrophysical effects of propranolol.* (Modified from Simon, H., and Bloomfield, D.A.: Cardioactive Drugs. Baltimore, Urban and Schwarzenberg, 1983.)

emergency drug treatment of ventricular arrhythmias. Although several other beta-adrenergic blockers possess antiarrhythmic activity, they have not received FDA approval for this indication.

Adverse Effects/Precautions. Propranolol is potentially dangerous in patients with heart disease, since CHF can be induced in predisposed patients by blocking sympathetic stimulation of the heart. The drug can also cause severe bronchospasm in patients with concurrent asthma or chronic obstructive pulmonary disease (COPD).

Hypotension, acute heart failure, and heart block can occur with propranolol therapy. Sudden withdrawal of propranolol in patients with angina pectoris can precipitate angina attacks, cardiac arrhythmias, or a MI.

TYPE III ANTIARRHYTHMIC DRUGS

Type III antiarrhythmic drugs prolong Phase 3 repolarization.

Bretylium Tosylate. Bretylium, a bromobenzyl quaternary ammonium compound that is classified as a Type III antiarrhythmic drug, inhibits norepinephrine release from adrenergic nerve endings.

Mechanism of Action. The most prominent electrophysiologic effect of bretylium is prolongation of the cardiac action potential duration (and the ERP, see Figure 3.17). Bretylium accumulates in sympathetic ganglia and postganglionic adrenergic neurons where it inhibits norepinephrine release by depressing adrenergic nerve terminal excitability. Thus, the drug induces a chemical sympathectomy-like state. Norepinephrine stores are not depleted by bretylium.

A transient release of norepinephrine often produces a fleeting sympathomimetic effect on the heart (tachycardia) and on peripheral resistance (rise in blood pressure). After the initial sympathomimetic action, bretylium blocks norepinephrine release upon neuron stimulation and exerts effective adrenergic blockade.

Clinical Indications. Used for the prophylaxis and therapy of ventricular fibrillation, bretylium is also employed in the treatment of life-threatening ventricular arrhythmias (such as ventricular tachycardia) when other measures have failed.

Adverse Effects/Precautions. Bretylium administration produces hypotension in about one-half of the patients in a supine position.

Amiodarone. The derivative of a thyroxine analogue, amiodarone possesses Type III antiarrhythmic properties.

Mechanism of Action. Amiodarone's electrophysiologic effects resemble hypothyroidism, and its mode of action evidently involves a depression of thyroxine-dependent metabolic pathways. Cardiac action potential duration increases with a primary slowing effect on the S-A node. Amiodarone suppresses re-entrant conduction pathways.

Clinical Indications. Amiodarone is used in the treatment of life-threatening supraventricular and ventricular arrhythmias in patients resistant to conventional therapy.

Adverse Effects/Precautions. Side effects include nausea, vomiting, and constipation. Reversible corneal deposits are the most serious complication of amiodarone therapy. Clinical evidence of hypo- or hyperthyroidism is unusual.

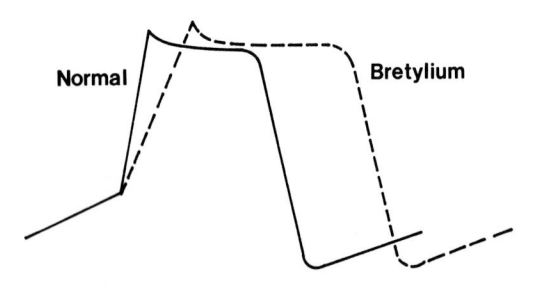

Fig. 3.17 Electrophysical effects of bretylium. (Modified from Simon, H., and Bloomfield, D.A.: Cardioactive Drugs. Baltimore, Urban and Schwarzenberg, 1983.)

TYPE IV ANTIARRHYTHMIC DRUGS

Type IV antiarrhythmic drugs block Ca^{++} channels in the cell membrane.

Verapamil. Classified as a Type IV antiarrhythmic agent, verapamil is a calcium channel blocker that also has a coronary vessel dilating activity.

Mechanism of Action. Verapamil inhibits the calcium ion inward current from the extracellular space in cardiac muscle (Figure 3.18). The antiarrhythmic effect of verapamil can be explained by the calcium antagonist effect since calcium (along with its contribution to cardiac cell transmembrane current) participates as a major factor in myocardial contraction and thus in oxygen consumption by the heart.

Verapamil raises the stimulation threshold, delays the rise of the action potential, and lengthens the refractory period. These effects decrease excitability and ectopic foci formation. Verapamil also prolongs conduction in the atria and A-V node to interrupt re-entry mechanisms. The drug is particularly effective in treating re-entrant tachycardias that involve the A-V node and represent an intranodal re-entry circuit.

Clinical Indications. Primarily used to control supraventricular tachyarrhythmias of various causes, verapamil is also valuable in converting arrhythmias precipitated during cardiac catheterization and anesthesia. When used orally, the drug action is characterized by a high first-pass effect. Thus, lower doses are indicated when the drug is administered parenterally.

Adverse Effects/Precautions. Constipation is the most common side effect of verapamil use. Other frequently encountered adverse effects are nausea, hypotension, bradycardia, heart block, and the worsening of cardiac failure.

Verapamil should be used cautiously or not at all in patients with A-V nodal dysfunction due to this calcium channel blocker's potent A-V nodal depressant activity. Verapamil can increase digoxin levels when these drugs are used

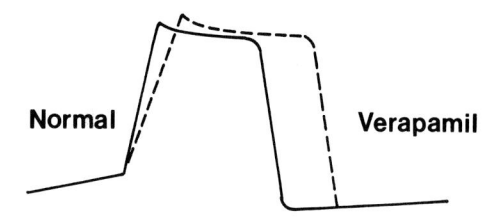

Fig. 3.18 Electrophysical effects of verapamil. (Modified from Simon, H., and Bloomfield, D.A.: Cardioactive Drugs. Baltimore, Urban and Schwarzenberg, 1983.)

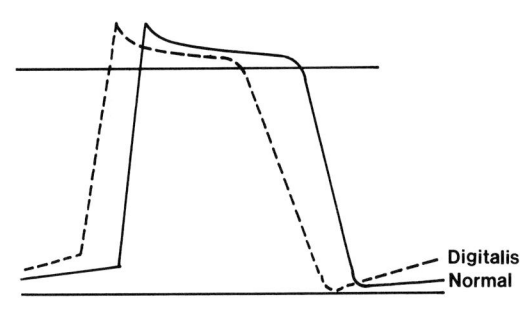

Fig. 3.19 Effects of digitalis on Purkinje fibers. (Modified from Simon, H., and Bloomfield, D.A.: Cardioactive Drugs. Baltimore, Urban and Schwarzenberg, 1983.)

concurrently which necessitates monitoring of plasma digoxin levels.

DIGITALIS GLYCOSIDES

Digitalis glycosides (Table 3.3) have both antiarrhythmic properties and pronounced cardiotonic activity.

Digoxin; Digitoxin. Digoxin is the most widely used digitalis glycoside. The digoxin dosage required in the treatment of arrhythmias is usually considerably higher than that used in CHF.

Mechanism of Action. Digoxin decreases maximal diastolic potential and action potential duration; it also increases the slope of Phase 4 depolarization (diastolic depolarization, see Figure 3.19). Digoxin increases the A-V node refractory period. In paroxysmal supraventricular tachycardia due to A-V nodal re-entry, di-

Table 3.3 CARDIAC GLYCOSIDES

Available products	Trade names	Daily dosage range*
Deslanoside	Cedilanid-D	1.6 mg IV or IM
Digitalis glycosides mixture	Digiglusin	Maintenance: 0.5 – 3 USP digitalis units
Digitalis, powdered (dried leaf)	Digifortis	Initial total loading dose: 1.2 g; Oral, 1 – 2 g; Maintenance: 100 – 200 mg
Digitalis, tincture	—	Initial total loading dose: 10 – 15 ml, oral; Maintenance: 0.75 – 1.5 ml
Digitoxin	Crystodigin; Purodigin	Initial total loading dose: 1.2 – 1.6 mg, IV; Maintenance: 0.05 – 0.3 mg
Digoxin	Lanoxin	Initial total loading dose: 1.0 – 1.5 mg, oral; 0.5 – 1.0 mg IV or IM; Maintenance: 0.125 – 0.025 mg
Gitalin	Gitaligin	Initial total loading dose: 4.0 – 8.0 mg, oral; Maintenance: 0.25 – 1.0 mg

* Maintenance Dosage

goxin prolongs the refractory period and slows the conduction velocity in the anterograde limb of the re-entry circuit, thus making emergence of a tachyarrhythmia less likely.

Digitalis increases vagal activity and decreases sensitivity to catecholamines in the A-V node. These indirect effects of digitalis, mediated by the ANS, combine with its direct effect on A-V conduction to diminish the rate at which atrial impulses are transmitted to the ventricles. Therefore, in atrial tachycardia, atrial flutter, and atrial fibrillation, digitalis decreases the ventricular rate by blocking a significant number of atrial impulses in the A-V node.

Clinical Indications. Digoxin is used to control the ventricular rate in the treatment of atrial flutter and fibrillation. The drug's clinical value in prevention, control, and conversion of supraventricular tachycardias is generally recognized.

Adverse Effects/Precautions. Patients should be carefully monitored for clinical and electrocardiographic evidence of toxicity. Digoxin should be avoided in Wolff-Parkinson-White syndrome since the drug enhances conduction in the accessory pathways, potentiating the arrhythmia.

CONGESTIVE HEART FAILURE

The clinical objective in treating congestive heart failure (CHF) is to return the ineffective, decompensated heart to a functional blood pump. Drugs correct this situation by improving the muscle tone of the dilated, weak heart and by increasing its force of contraction. Cardiac glycosides improve circulation and increase cardiac output, thereby relieving peripheral edema, pulmonary congestion, and other consequences of a failing heart. Diuretic drugs, also used in CHF treatment, are discussed in Chapter 5.

CARDIAC GLYCOSIDES

Cardiac glycosides (Table 3.3) are present in several plants, including Urginea maritima ("sea onion"), Strophanthus gratus, Digitalis purpurea, and Digitalis lanata.

Digitalis glycosides. The digitalis glycosides constitute almost all of the cardiac glycoside preparations used in modern medicine. Glycosides are compounds containing a carbohydrate (sugar) molecule that yield, upon hydrolysis, the sugar and a nonsugar aglycone portion. The aglycone of cardiac glycosides is comprised of a steroid nucleus attached to a lactone ring; the sugar portion is composed of from 1 to 4 molecules of a sugar, digitoxose. Cardiac glycosides of plant origin are usually found in association with saponins. Digitalis glycosides are obtained from the leaves of Digitalis purpurea or Digitalis lanata.

Mechanism of Action. In CHF, digitalis glycosides act to increase the force of systole, slow the heart rate, and inhibit A-V conduction. The positive inotropic action of digitalis is the most dramatic pharmacologic property seen in CHF treatment. The increased force of contraction increases cardiac output and decreases venous pressure, cardiac size, and blood volume. The ultimate benefit of digitalis resides in its action to increase the ability of the heart to pump at any given filling pressure.

The basic biochemical mechanism involved in the positive inotropic response by digitalis is inhibition of membrane-bound sodium-potassium ATPase, which initially slows the Na^+ efflux from the cell. Inhibition of sodium-potassium ATPase reduces the efficiency of the so-called "sodium pump" so that in addition to the elevated intracellular Na^+, an increase in extracellular potassium occurs.

A cellular Na^+-Ca^{++} exchange process involves the transfer of intracellular Ca^{++} for extracellular Na^+ (Figure 3.20). The calcium ion plays a central role in cardiac muscle contraction and in oxygen consumption. Slowing Na^+ efflux and consequent elevated intracellular Na^+ diminishes the exchange of extracellular Na^+ for intracellular Ca^{++}. Higher intracellular Na^+ also probably inhibits Ca^{++} release from the cardiac cell endoplasmic (sarcoplasmic) reticulum to increase Ca^{++} stores. The ultimate result is the increase in the intracellular concentration of free Ca^{++}, necessary for the activation of myofibril-ATPase and the binding of the contractile proteins (Figure 3.21).

The steroid nucleus is the portion of the glycoside molecule that incorporates the receptors in the binding of membrane ATPase. The speci-

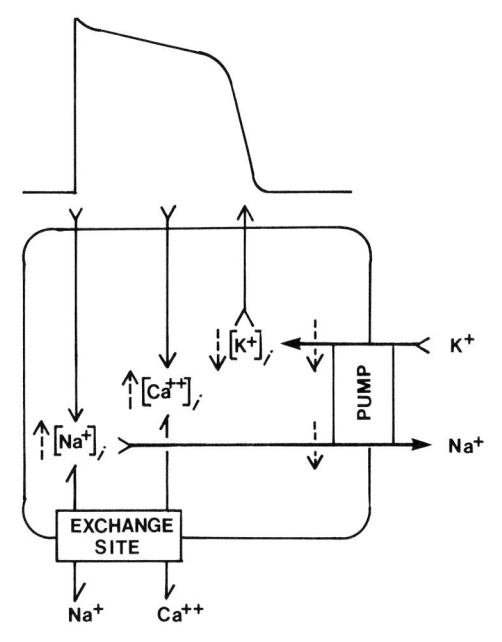

Fig. 3.20 Na^+-Ca^{++} ion exchange process in the cardiac cell. (Modified from Gilman, A.G., et al. (eds.): The Pharmacological Basis of Therapeutics. 7th Ed. New York, Macmillan Publishing Co., Inc., 1985.)

ficity and extent of action of different cardiac glycosides is determined by the relative affinity for this binding site. The lactone ring contains the functional group which combines with the membrane sodium-potassium ATPase (Figure 3.22). Thus, the pharmacologic activity resides in the aglycone portion of the glycoside molecule. The receptor proteins specific for the cardiac glycosides are also the receptors for K^+ molecules.

Certain clinical aspects of digitalis action can be more clearly viewed through examination of this biochemical mechanism. For instance, changes in the intracellular/extracellular ratio of K^+, as well as for Ca^{++}, can influence glycoside action. Competitive binding explains the increased glycoside effect in hypokalemia; specifically, the glycoside binding to the receptor is more likely if less K^+ is present to compete with the binding site. The low potassium states produced by certain diuretics accentuate digitalis action and may lead to toxicity. This concept also explains the benefit of potassium salts in the treatment of digitalis toxicity.

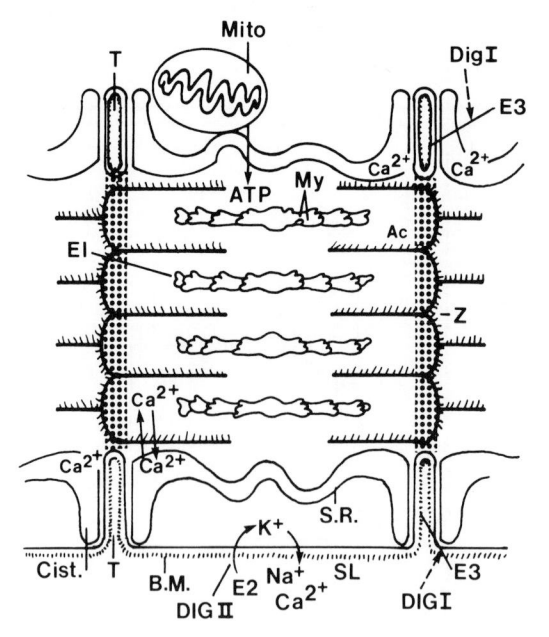

Fig. 3.21 Proposed sites of action of digitalis. SL, sarcolemma; B.M., basement membrane; S.R., sarcoplasmic reticulum or longitudinal tubular system; T, transverse tubular system (T tubules); My, myosin filaments; Ac, actin filaments; Z, Z line; Cist., terminal cisternae of S.R.; Mito, mitochondrion; E1, myosin ATPase; E2, sarcolemmal ATPase (Na "pump"); E3, T-tubular ATPase; DIG I, proposed site of action of digitalis for inotropic effect; DIG II, site for toxic arrhythmic effect. (Modified from DiPalma, J.R.: Basic Pharmacology in Medicine. New York, McGraw-Hill, Inc., 1982.)

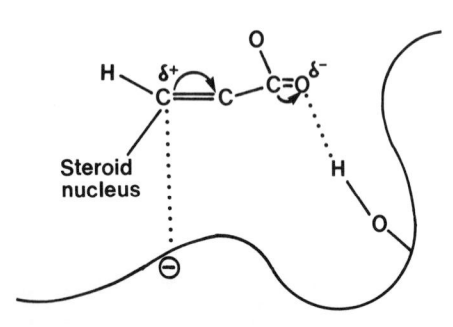

Fig. 3.22 Hypothetical digoxin-ATPase interaction. (Modified from Gringuaz, A.: Drugs. How They Work and Why. St. Louis, C.V. Mosby, 1978.)

Additionally, phenytoin, a drug used in the treatment of digitalis toxicity, also binds to the same receptor site on sodium-potassium ATPase as do cardiac glycosides and potassium.

This could explain the benefit of phenytoin in the treatment of digitalis toxicity since phenytoin would bind to the receptor site in competition with the cardiac glycoside. The phenytoin binding, thus, would reduce cardiac glycoside receptor attachment and decrease glycoside action.

The excitation-contraction coupling process in the sarcomere involves passage of free Ca^{++}, released from its sequestered form in the longitudinal reticulum, into the sarcoplasma (Figure 3.23). The free Ca^{++} apparently binds to troponin, thus releasing the block exerted by the troponin-tropomyosin complex on the actin-myosin reaction. Ca^{++} suppresses blockade of the actin-myosin reaction by the troponin-tropomyosin complex and permits myofibril magnesium ATPase stimulation, reaction of actin with myosin, and effective systole of the myofibrils (Figure 3.24).

The release rate of Ca^{++} sequestered in the sarcoplasmic reticulum increases by elevation of free Ca^{++} in the sarcoplasm. Also, the bound Ca^{++} stores in the sarcoplasmic reticulum (available for release into the sarcoplasm) are elevated when free Ca^{++} is increased. Thus, the rate and amount of Ca^{++} released from the sarcoplasmic reticulum increases in response to an action potential, consequently permitting a more forceful contraction.

Clinically, in CHF, digitalis helps supply deficient free Ca^{++} for myocardial contraction since an aberrant Ca^{++} milieu may be a site of disturbance in the failing heart. In addition to the myofibril ATPase activation and the contractile protein binding, the rise in free Ca^{++} by digitalis increases the synthesis and breakdown of energy-rich phosphates (ATP). The ATP cleavage provides the energy required for transport processes in the myocardial cell. Thus, an extrapolation of events in the ultrastructure of the heart to clinical observations is possible with this excitation-contraction coupling model.

Digitalis' direct effects on the cardiac Purkinje fibers are significant and depend upon the dose and the myocardial disease status. The effects of digitalis on the transmembrane potential indicate a decrease in maximal diastolic potential, an increase in the Phase 4 depolarization slope, and a decrease in action potential duration (Figure 3.19). Delayed afterdepolarization sometimes occurs with digitalis and results in an extra action potential propagation (Figure 3.25).

Digitalis' effects on electrical activity and transmembrane potential of cardiac fibers are ancillary to the aforementioned cardiac contractility mechanisms. The digitalis-induced changes noted in the Purkinje fiber action potential assume importance in determining digitalis toxicity. The enhanced automaticity inherent in the Phase 4 slope increase and the development of afterdepolarizations herald digitalis toxicity. Thus, digitalis can generate ectopic impulses by the enhancement of normal Phase 4 depolarization or the development of delayed afterdepolarization.

The His-Purkinje system is strongly influenced by the sympathetic nervous system

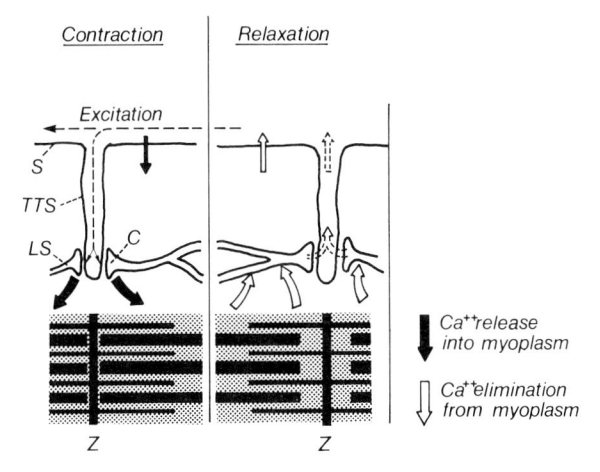

Fig. 3.23 Excitation-contraction coupling process in the myocardial cell. (Modified from Reindell, H., and Roskamm, H.: Herzkrankheiten. Berlin, Springer, 1977.)

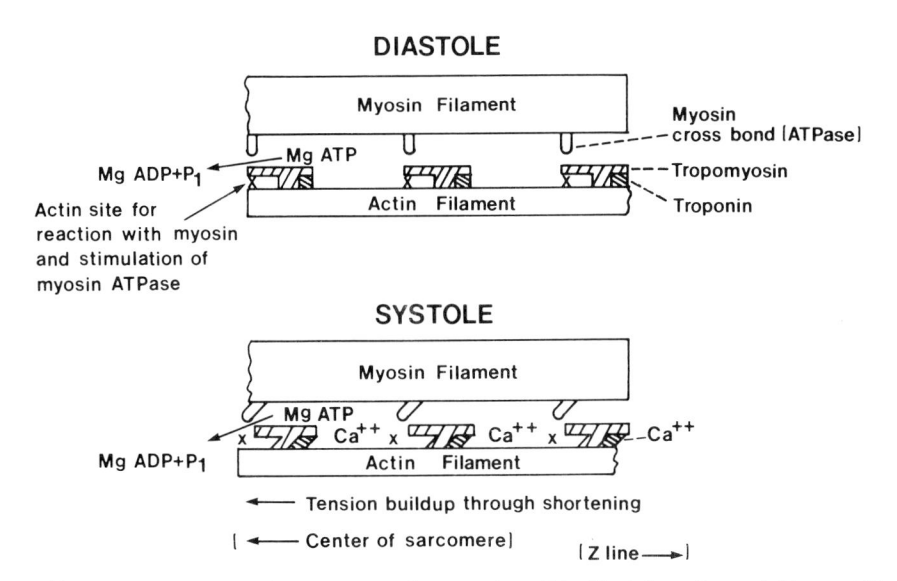

Fig. 3.24 Ca^{++} binding to troponin-tropomyosin complex. (Modified from Katz, A.M., and Hecht, H.H.: Editorial: the early "pump" failure of the ischemic heart. Am J Med, **47**:497, 1969.)

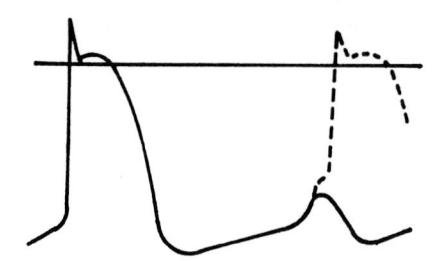

Fig. 3.25 Digitalis-induced delayed afterdepolarization. (Modified from Gilman, A.G., et al., (eds.): The Pharmacological Basis of Therapeutics. 7th Ed. New York, Macmillan Publishing Co., Inc., 1985.)

and is less likely to be sensitive to vagal activity. Thus, the indirect effects of digitalis mediated through the sympathetic nervous system are more likely to influence the specialized ventricular conducting system.

Digitalis decreases the heart rate in the CHF patient but does not significantly affect that of the normal individual. Most of the clinically significant effects on the S-A node impulse generation result from indirect digitalis effects on the ANS. Digitalis, by increasing vagal impulse traffic and by a sympathetic tone reflex reduction, decreases the S-A rate in CHF. Digitalis alters the myocardium's sensitivity to autonomic neurotransmitters and increases the S-A node's sensitivity to the negative chronotropic effect of acetylcholine. It also decreases the S-A and A-V nodes' response to catecholamines and efferent sympathetic impulses.

The ANS largely mediates the effects of digitalis on the A-V node (as with the S-A node). Direct effects of high digitalis doses slow the A-V conduction rate, increase the effective refractory period, and block the A-V node. However, enhanced vagal activity and decreased sensitivity to catecholamines also have a pronounced effect on A-V nodal action potential generation and impulse transmission through the node. Thus, in the A-V node, both the direct and indirect digitalis effects bring about similar changes and block an increased fraction of atrial impulses in the A-V junction.

Digitalis has a pronounced indirect vagal effect on the atria, especially if cardiac disease exists. If the refractory period is significantly reduced due to disease, digitalis improves action potentials and atrial conduction, apparently as a result of acetylcholine release.

Clinical Indications. The most important therapeutic use of digitalis is in the treatment of CHF. Digitalis is effective regardless of whether the CHF is primarily left-sided or right-sided or a combination of both. Cardiac glycosides are most valuable in CHF characterized by enlargement of the heart. Digitalis initiates a beneficial cycle in which increased contractility results in more efficient emptying of the heart chambers; the consequent heart size reduction further enhances the myocardial contractility. These effects are more pronounced in low-output failure than in high-output failure conditions (such as anemia, beri-beri, and thyrotoxicosis).

CHF associated with hypertension and valvular regurgitation often improves with digitalis due to the increased cardiac output and decreased end-diastolic pressure. In chronic CHF, a recognized therapeutic regimen is the concomitant use of potent diuretics to reduce heart size and vasodilators to decrease cardiac work.

Commonly used digitalis products are the pure crystalline glycosides: digoxin and digitoxin. Deslanoside is sometimes used in emergencies because of their rapid onset of action and the quickness at which the peak glycoside effect is reached. More often, parenteral digoxin is used in urgent situations with a later change to oral digoxin for maintenance.

Intestinal absorption of digitoxin is almost complete (95 to 100%), whereas the amount of digoxin absorbed orally is between 70 and 80%. Digitoxin is extensively metabolized by liver enzymes; in contrast, digoxin is essentially unchanged. About ¼ of a given dose of digitoxin enters the enterohepatic circulation, which largely accounts for its persistence in the body. Significant protein-binding occurs with digitoxin, but not with digoxin.

Digoxin has a relatively rapid onset of action and intermediate duration of action which makes it valuable in achieving a fast therapeutic action and in maintaining long-term control with relative stability and safety. Digitoxin, however, has a long elimination half-life, and a stable level can be maintained even if the patient occasionally misses a few doses.

A large loading dose of a digitalis preparation administered over 12 to 24 hours customarily initiates therapy in patients requiring rapid digitalization. After the level of drug in the heart reaches an optimal therapeutic concentration, treatment continues with a much lower daily maintenance dose. This amount of drug replaces the digitalis metabolized and/or excreted since administration of the last dose. A slightly higher dose than that needed to replace the "missing" glycoside results in the glycoside accumulation; over a period of time, this can lead to digitalis toxicity (Figure 3.26).

Rapid digitalization is usually reserved for patients requiring quick control, as in cases of acute pulmonary edema. Slow digitalization, using small daily doses over a period of about a week, is currently employed frequently in place of former rapid loading techniques. Present clinical practice indicates loading digoxin doses that are about ½ of that previously recommended. Also, the fractional doses of the glycoside administered after the loading dose are given at longer intervals. Digitoxin is not administered gradually for slow digitalization, as is done with digoxin, because of digitoxin's long half-life and the small fraction that is eliminated daily.

Adverse Effects/Precautions. Digitalis intoxication, a common adverse reaction, represents a hazardous clinical situation. Digitalis toxicity symptoms include cardiac abnormalities and extracardiac manifestations. The therapeutic dose of digitalis is approximately 50 to 60% of that producing toxic symptoms. Figure 3.27 illustrates the "narrow window" between therapeutic and toxic levels of the cardiac glycosides. Also, many clinical factors can increase the sensitivity to the toxic effects of digitalis; among these are cardiac disease, COPD, decreased renal function, hypokalemia, hypomagnesemia, and hyperkalemia. Advanced age and low thyroid function can also increase the patient's response to digitalis and precipitate toxic reactions. The most frequent cause of digi-

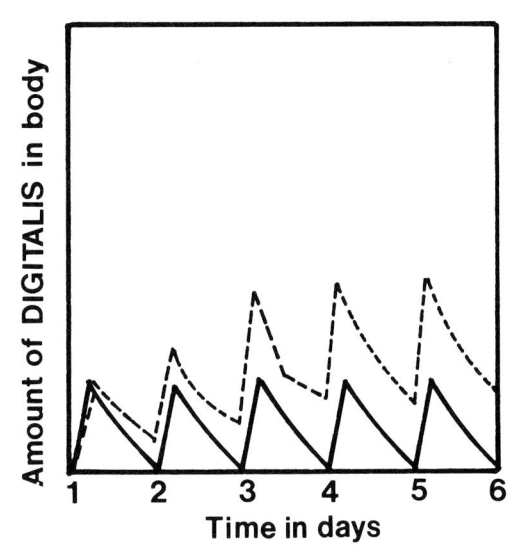

Fig. 3.26 Digitalis accumulation in the body. (Modified from Goth, A.: Medical Pharmacology. 11th Ed. St. Louis, C.V. Mosby, 1984.)

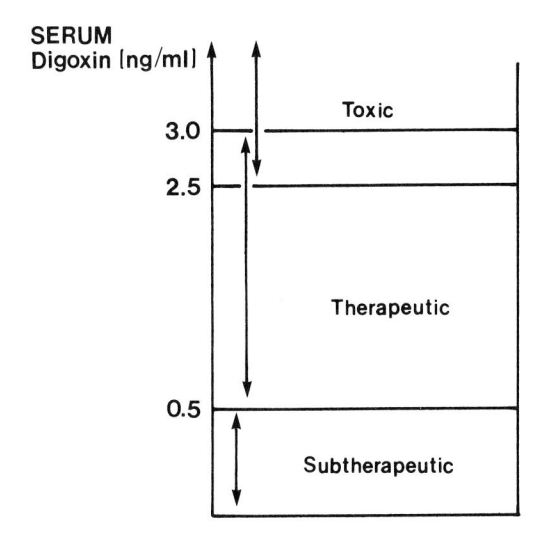

Fig. 3.27 Digitalis safety window. (From Goth, A.: Medical Pharmacology. 11th Ed. St. Louis, C.V. Mosby, 1984.)

talis toxicity is concurrent administration of a potassium-wasting diuretic.

Side effects occur in approximately 20% of the patients taking digitalis. Two-thirds of these patients manifest cardiac rhythm disturbances, while the remainder exhibit gastrointestinal symptoms, neurologic abnormalities, endocrine dysfunction, or allergic reactions.

Multifocal premature ventricular contractions, A-V junctional tachycardia, and paroxysmal atrial tachycardia with block are common cardiac abnormalities in digitalis poisoning. Sinus bradycardia, S-A block, and partial A-V block may also result from digitalis toxicity. Atrial fibrillation, atrial flutter, ventricular tachycardia and fibrillation, and complete A-V block are less likely in glycoside toxicity.

Gastrointestinal disturbances, originating from the CNS, include anorexia, nausea, vomiting, and diarrhea. Neurologic disorders include headache, drowsiness, fatigue, nightmares, hallucinations, depression, and psychoses. Visual disturbances, also due to neurologic involvement, are characterized by chromatopsia; specifically, the patient may report yellow-green lights, the presence of "snowflakes," and double vision. If these visual effects, which signal digitalis overdosage, are not corrected, cardiotoxicity may occur. Gynecomastia is the most prevalent hormone dysfunction reported.

Although the first (and occasionally the only) sign of digitalis toxicity is an abnormal cardiac rate or rhythm, most patients initially complain of signs and symptoms of gastrointestinal upset and CNS stimulation. Headache, anorexia, and nausea are also common symptoms of early digitalis toxicity.

Treatment of digitalis toxicity may simply involve discontinuation of the digitalis. Overdosage symptoms may soon disappear, especially if rapidly eliminated digoxin is involved. Also, upon the cessation of digitalis use, extracardiac adverse effects tend to subside quickly. Digitoxin overdosage usually requires a longer treatment period because of the drug's long half-life.

Oral or intravenous potassium salts are indicated in patients who exhibit PVCs or supraventricular tachycardias (such as PAT). The possibility of PVC occurrence increases with depletion of body potassium and hypokalemia. Caution should be exercised in the administration of potassium salts, especially if given IV, since the possibility of a potassium overdose can result in heart block and cardiac arrest. PVCs are usually treated with lidocaine because of its rapid onset of action and lack of effect on A-V nodal conduction.

Phenytoin is also used as an alternate drug in treating digitalis-induced tachyarrhythmias. Propranolol is sometimes employed if the digitalis-induced arrhythmia originates from a supraventricular ectopic site and there is no sign of A-V block. The ECG must be carefully monitored when any of the various antiarrhythmic drugs are used due to the drug-induced slowing of conduction and the reduction of myocardial contractility.

Digitalis poisoning may also produce bradycardia and heart block. Drug treatment of these conditions involves a "chemical pacemaker," such as atropine. Atropine, which increases the heart rate and reduces the degree of block, acts to block the vagal effects of digitalis on the S-A and A-V nodes. Isoproterenol, a beta-adrenergic agonist, is sometimes used in selected cases to increase heart rate. Since Ca^{++} contributes to digitalis cardiotoxicity, a Ca^{++} chelating agent, such as disodium edetate, has proved successful in digitalis toxicity treatment, especially in cases involving hypercalcemia.

ADRENERGIC AGONIST CARDIAC STIMULANTS

$Beta_1$-adrenergic receptor agonists are clinically useful in producing a positive inotropic cardiac response.

Dobutamine. Dobutamine (Dobutrex^R), a synthetic catecholamine related to isoproterenol, is a $beta_1$-adrenergic receptor agonist.

Mechanism of Action. Dobutamine almost exclusively affects the $beta_1$-adrenergic receptors in the heart. A positive inotropic effect occurs with less tachycardia as compared to standard adrenergic agonists. The cellular mechanism of beta-adrenergic activation involves the elevation of adenosine 3', 5'-monophosphate (cyclic AMP) levels.

Clinical Indications. Dobutamine increases myocardial contractility in the short-term treatment of cardiac decompensation in CHF.

Adverse Effects/Precautions. Cardiac adverse effects such as hypertension, tachycardia, and ectopic beats, may occur with dobutamine therapy.

Dopamine. Dopamine (Intropin^R; Dopastat^R) is an endogenous catecholamine and a precursor of norepinephrine.

Mechanism of Action. Dopamine acts directly as an alpha- and beta-adrenergic receptor agonist. The beta$_1$-adrenergic receptor agonist activity results in a positive inotropic effect on the heart with an increased cardiac output. Dopamine does not increase the myocardial oxygen consumption to the degree of isoproterenol. Elevation of intracellular cyclic AMP levels is characteristic of beta-adrenergic receptor activation and represents the cellular mechanism of action.

Clinical Indications. Dopamine is indicated in the treatment of chronic cardiac decompensation, as in CHF.

Adverse Effects/Precautions. Ectopic beats, tachycardia, and palpitations are cardiac side effects that may occur with dopamine therapy.

BIPYRIDINE CARDIAC STIMULANTS

Amrinone, a cardiac stimulant bipyridine compound, was recently introduced for use in CHF.

Amrinone. Amrinone (Inocor^R) is a synthetic myocardial stimulant.

Mechanism of Action. Amrinone apparently influences myocardial excitation-contraction coupling in producing its positive inotropic effect.

Clinical Indications. Amrinone is used parenterally in the treatment of severe CHF.

Adverse Effects/Precautions. Adverse effects are generally limited to those on the cardiovascular system related to increased positive inotropic effect.

CORONARY HEART DISEASE

Attacks of angina pectoris (stable) are ordinarily transient and of short duration (less than 3 minutes). These painful episodes are often precipitated by physical exertion or emotional stress and commonly terminate when the patient rests. The increased sympathetic activity that usually initiates the attack increases both the heart rate and contractility. Thus, the myocardial oxygen consumption necessarily increases, and pain impulses travel from the oxygen-deficient heart muscle tissue to the brain by way of sympathetic afferent nerve fibers.

Acute coronary insufficiency (unstable angina) is characterized by the presence of chest pain, even during rest. The pain is usually more severe (and longer lasting) than that seen in stable angina.

Antianginal drugs act to correct the temporary imbalance between myocardial oxygen consumption and the deficient oxygen supply available to the heart muscle in times of excessive physical activity or emotional stress. The diseased or sclerotic coronary vessels are unable to deliver sufficient oxygenated blood to heart muscle tissue during these periods; antianginal drugs, by their action on the vascular system, relieve or prevent chest pains precipitated by myocardial ischemia or hypoxia. Thus, by improving the passage of oxygenated blood through the coronary vessels, as well as by reducing the heart's oxygen demand, antianginal drugs effectively counteract the causative painful stimulus in anginal attacks.

ANTIANGINAL DRUGS

Antianginal drugs (Table 3.4) include rapid-acting nitrates to relieve the pain of acute angina and long-acting preparations used for prophylaxis or to decrease the severity of angina pectoris. Other anginal drugs for the prevention of chronic angina include dipyridamole, beta-adrenergic blocking agents, and calcium antagonists.

Nitrates. Examples of organic nitrates, useful as antianginal drugs, include nitroglycerin, isosorbide dinitrate, erythrityl tetranitrate,

Table 3.4 ANTIANGINAL DRUGS

Available products	Trade names	Daily dosage range
Amyl nitrite	Aspirols; Vaporoles	0.18 or 0.3 ml by inhalation
Diltiazem HCl	Cardizem	30 mg q.i.d.
Dipyridamole	Persantine; Pyridamole; others	50 mg t.i.d.
Erythrityl tetranitrate	Cardilate	5–10 mg sublingually
Ethaverine HCl	Ethaquin; Ethatab; others	100–200 mg t.i.d.
Isosorbide dinitrate	Isordil; Sorbitrate	2.5–10 mg sublingually; 5 mg, chewable; 5–30 mg q.i.d., tablets
Nadolol	Corgard	80–320 mg once daily
Nifedipine	Procardia	Oral, 10–20 mg t.i.d.
Nitroglycerin, IV	Nitrol IV; Nitrostat IV; others	Initially, 5 mcg/min via an infusion pump; titrate to the clinical situation
Nitroglycerin, sublingual	Nitrostat	0.2–0.6 mg
Nitroglycerin, sustained release	Ang-O-Span; Nitrostat; Nitro-Bid	2 or 3 times daily at 8–12 hr intervals
Nitroglycerin, topical	Nitro-Bid; Nitrol	25–50 mm q. 8 hrs
Nitroglycerin, transdermal systems	Nitrodisc	See manufacturer's directions
Nitroglycerin, transmucosal	Susadrin	1 mg t.i.d.
Papaverine HCl	Pavabid	100–300 mg, 3 to 5 times daily
Pentaerythritol tetranitrate (P.E.T.N.)	Peritrate; Pentol; others	10 or 20 mg q.i.d.
Propranolol HCl	Inderal	10–30 mg t.i.d. or q.i.d.
Verapamil HCl	Calan; Isoptin	Orally 80 mg t.i.d. or q.i.d.; slow IV 5–10 mg over 2 min

mannitol hexanitrate, pentaerythritol tetranitrate, and trinitrate phosphate. Amyl nitrite is administered by inhalation, and the other nitrates are given either sublingually, transdermally, or orally depending upon the product.

Mechanism of Action. The principal pharmacologic action of nitrates is relaxation of vascular smooth muscle. The nitrate ion acts directly on vascular muscle fibers, and its relaxant action is independent of the innervation to the vessels. Effects on veins are predominant, but a dose-dependent dilation of arterial vessels also occurs. Dilation of the large veins and postcapillary venules causes peripheral pooling of the blood (for example, in the legs) and reduces the return of blood to the right-side of the heart. This action on the veins lowers preload pressure or left ventricular end-diastolic pressure by lessening the amount of blood the heart must pump. Due to arteriole relaxation, afterload pressure (arterial pressure) and systemic vascular resistance are lowered . This effect on the arterioles makes it easier for the left ventricle to eject blood into the aorta.

These vascular responses to the nitrates reduce myocardial oxygen consumption or demand, resulting in a more favorable supply-demand ratio. The nitrates also promote redistribution of coronary circulation along collateral channels to improve oxygen delivery to ischemic myocardium.

Clinical Indications. Nitrates, such as amyl nitrite and nitroglycerin, are used to terminate an acute attack of angina pectoris. Administered sublingually and transdermally, nitroglycerin, because of its fast action and ease of administration, is the drug most frequently used to abort acute angina attacks. Amyl nitrite, a volatile liquid, has a more rapid onset of action, but its use is limited due to the inconvenience of administration (ampule breaking followed by inhalation of a highly odoriferous drug).

Use of rapid-acting nitrates, such as isosorbide dinitrate and erythrityl tetranitrate, accomplish prophylaxis for impending angina attacks. When taken immediately prior to events likely to precipitate an attack, these drugs are effective for prevention as they act almost as quickly as nitroglycerin and have a much longer duration of action. In fact, after the initial vasodilator effects (which begin in 5 minutes), protective vasodilator effects are achieved for at least 2 hours. Transmucosal or sublingual nitroglycerin, sublingual or chewable isosorbide dinitrate, and amyl nitrite are drugs also included in acute angina treatment regimens.

Long-acting nitrates, such as pentaerythritol tetranitrate, are used in the management of angina pectoris. Whether the long-acting nitrates are more effective than placebos in chronic recurrent angina pectoris is a matter of extensive controversy. The FDA lists the nitrates, other than amyl nitrite and nitroglycerin, as being possibly effective for the prophylactic management of angina pectoris. Also, nitroglycerin may be administered by topical, transdermal "patches," transmucosal, or oral sustained release doses for prophylaxis and long-term management of recurrent angina.

Tolerance to the effects of nitroglycerin patches can develop rapidly. Minimal pharmacologic activity is seen after 24 hours and, with continued use, decreased antianginal effects are observed in the first 8 hours (application of a patch every 24 hours). Thus, even moderately high doses of transdermal nitroglycerin appear to be less effective than sublingual nitroglycerin. Although continued use of topical nitroglycerin ointment may result in tolerance development, clinical results are inconclusive with this preparation.

Intravenous nitroglycerin is employed in the control of perioperative hypertension (such as in cardiac bypass procedures). Other uses of IV nitroglycerin include CHF associated with acute MI and production and maintenance of controlled hypotension during surgical procedures.

Adverse Effects/Precautions. Headache, dizziness, and flushing are the most common adverse reactions to nitrate therapy. The vascular nitrate headache is sometimes accompanied by syncope because of the hypotensive action of the nitrate ion. Tachycardia and palpitations are frequent cardiovascular side effects; gastrointestinal symptoms and CNS toxicity have also been reported. Cutaneous reactions (especially with transdermal or topical products) are additional adverse effects.

Tolerance and cross-tolerance occur with the organic nitrates. The condition known as "Monday disease," a term used to describe the illness afflicting factory workers who manufacture explosives (nitroglycerin), illustrates the short-lived nitrate tolerance. Specifically, the tolerance acquired by the workers during the weekdays is lost over the weekend; thus, on Monday, vascular effects of headache, nausea, and other nitrate toxicity symptoms occur. Organic nitrate dependence, after chronic exposure, has resulted in severe myocardial ischemia after only a few days without contact.

Dipyridamole. Dipyridamole, a coronary vasodilator, is chemically unrelated to the nitrates.

Mechanism of Action. Selective dilation of the coronary arteries increases coronary blood flow. Dipyridamole inhibits adenosine deaminase and thereby produces an accumulation of adenosine nucleotides and adenosine, compounds which possess potent vasodilator properties. Phosphodiesterase inhibition also occurs with dipyridamole use, resulting in cyclic AMP accumulation. Elevated cyclic AMP levels are associated with vasodilation.

Clinical Indications. Dipyridamole has been classified by the FDA as "possibly effective" for long-term therapy of chronic angina pectoris.

Adverse Effects/Precautions. Adverse reactions are mild and transient in therapeutic doses. Side effects such as headache, dizziness, flushing, syncope, GI disturbances, and rash disappear upon cessation of dipyridamole therapy. Excessive doses can promote hypotensive episodes.

Beta-adrenergic Receptor Blocking Agents. Propranolol and nadolol are FDA approved for use in angina pectoris.

Mechanism of Action. Beta-adrenergic blockade is advantageous in angina because the sympathetic overactivity characteristic of this condition is detrimental to the patient. Occurring when the oxygen demand of cardiac muscle exceeds the supply of oxygen, angina attacks are often precipitated by exercise, emotional stress, or other factors associated with increased sympathetic (adrenergic) activity in the heart. Beta-adrenergic blocking drugs decrease the oxygen demands of the heart muscle at any given level of effort by blocking the effects of catecholamine-induced increases in heart rate, systolic blood pressure, and cardiac inotropism. Additionally, however, in certain conditions such as CHF, the heart's oxygen requirements may be increased, presenting a clinical problem. The overall effect of the beta-adrenergic blockers on the myocardium is positive and becomes apparent by a delayed onset of pain during exercise and increased work activity.

Clinical Indications. Propranolol and nadolol are indicated as prophylactic drugs in chronic recurrent angina pectoris resultant from coronary atherosclerosis.

Adverse Effects/Precautions. Sympathetic activation is vital in certain clinical situations where sympathetic blockade might prove disastrous. Exacerbation of angina pectoris, MI, and ventricular arrhythmias have occurred after abrupt withdrawal of chronically-administered beta-adrenergic blocking drugs.

Most adverse effects of the beta-adrenergic blockers are minimal and transient. Withdrawal of therapy usually involves side effects exerted on the cardiovascular system or the CNS.

Calcium Channel Blocking Agents. Diltiazem, nifedipine, and oral verapamil have been FDA approved for chronic stable angina and angina pectoris caused by coronary artery spasm.

Mechanism of Action. Two types of membrane channels permit the influx of Ca^{++}. Electromechanical excitation-contraction coupling (in cardiac contraction) involves a potential dependent channel activated by changes in the electrical charge of the cell membrane. Pharmacomechanical coupling involves a second channel that is dependent upon an agonist-receptor interaction (i.e., norepinephrine-receptor) to open Ca^{++} channels (Figure 3.28).

Calcium channel blockers inhibit the movement of Ca^{++} across the cell membrane of vascular smooth muscle, depressing the contractil-

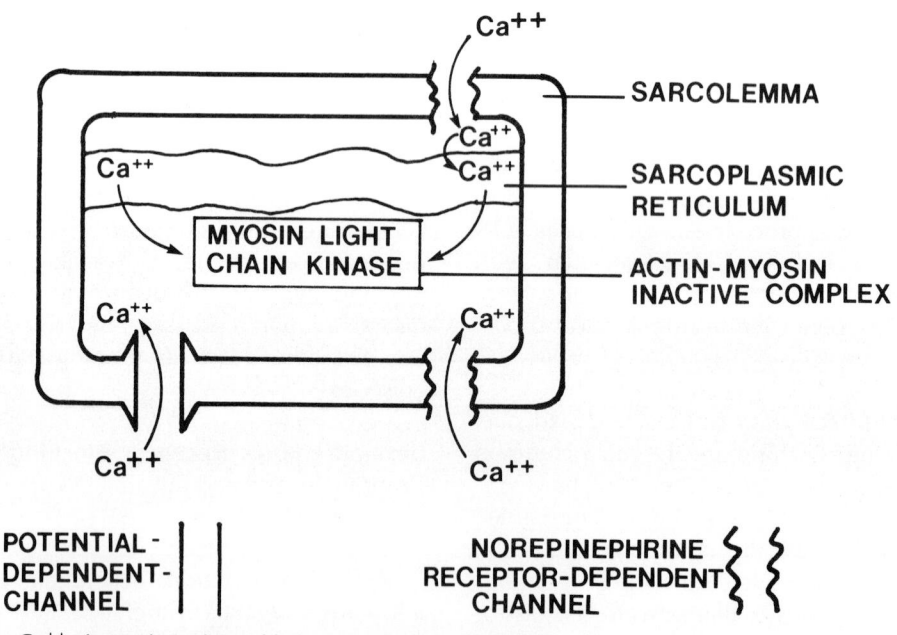

Fig. 3.28 Ca^{++} channels activated in coronary smooth muscle.

ity of smooth muscle (including coronary arteriolar smooth muscle). These agents dilate the coronary arteries and arterioles, thereby inhibiting coronary artery spasm. Calcium channel blockers have different degrees of selectivity in their effects on vascular smooth muscle and myocardial contractility, automaticity, or conduction.

In the smooth muscle cells of coronary and peripheral arteries, Ca^{++} from the surrounding tissue flows through "slow" calcium channels into the cell's interior. This Ca^{++} influx triggers the release of additional Ca^{++} from internal stores in the sarcolemma and sarcoplasmic reticulum. Intracellular Ca^{++} activates calmodulin, a calcium-binding protein, that is involved in coronary and peripheral artery contraction. The activated Ca^{++}-calmodulin complex stimulates a myosin light chain kinase that, in turn, phosphorylates one of the light chains of myosin. This phosphorylated myosin light chain then interacts with actin producing contractions (Figure 3.29).

Verapamil (and other calcium antagonists) blocks the Ca^{++} influx and thus inhibits the contractile mechanism. In this way, coronary artery spasm is countered and better perfusion of the heart occurs from coronary artery dilation.

Clinical Indications. The beneficial effects of calcium antagonists in chronic stable angina result from increased coronary perfusion following systemic and coronary artery dilation. Reduced myocardial contractility also decreases oxygen demand in the heart muscle and contributes to the favorable pharmacologic response.

In variant or unstable angina (Prinzmetal's angina), calcium channel blockers prevent coronary artery spasm. These drugs also inhibit platelet aggregation, thus reducing the endogenous release of thromboxane A_2, a potent vasoconstrictor.

Adverse Effects/Precautions. Cardiovascular side reactions, such as hypotension and bradycardia, may occur. CNS effects (dizziness and fatigue) and constipation are other reactions that frequently disappear spontaneously or after dose reduction.

POST-MYOCARDIAL INFARCTION

In myocardial infarction (MI), which is characterized by persistent chest pain not relieved by rest, the myocardial tissue that is cut off from the blood supply becomes necrotic. The resulting dead tissue (infarct) is eventually replaced by scar tissue in the surviving patient. The usual course of an MI is occlusion of a coronary artery by a blood clot (coronary thrombosis) or by a lipid fragment, from an atherosclerotic artery, that is carried down to a narrower part of the channel. The infarct area becomes electrically aberrant and subject to cardiac arrhythmias. Also, if the infarct area is extensive, the heart's pumping action is compromised and CHF may ensue.

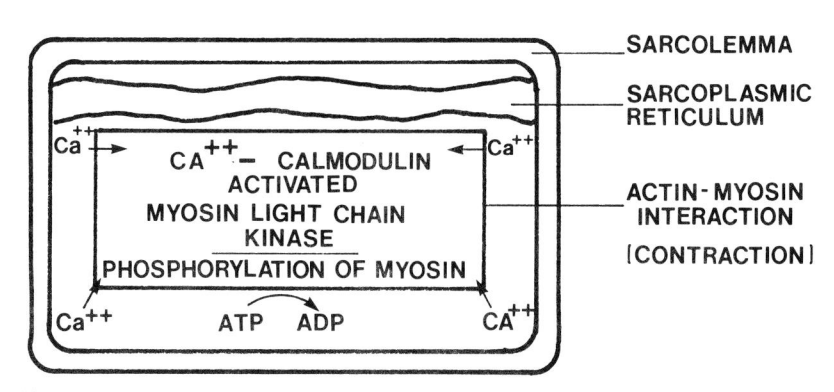

Fig. 3.29 Ca^{++} role in coronary artery smooth muscle contraction.

Beta-adrenergic Blocking Agents. Selected beta-adrenergic receptor blocking drugs are useful in the management of post-myocardial infarction.

Mechanism of Action. In 1982, timolol, a nonselective beta-adrenergic blocker, became the first drug to be indicated for reducing the long-term risk of cardiovascular mortality and reinfarction in stabilized MI survivors. Propranolol and IV metoprolol are now also FDA approved for this clinical situation.

The value of beta-adrenergic blockers lies in their ability to reduce oxygen demand and consumption in a heart impaired by the reduced oxygen supply distal to the MI. This is due to the prevention, via receptor blockade, of catecholamine-induced increased contractility, blood pressure, and heart rate.

Beta-adrenergic blockers may also decrease oxygen demand by the damaged heart by reducing free fatty acid levels, preventing platelet aggregation, and decreasing blood viscosity. They also reduce conduction velocity and increase the refractory period for A-V conduction. These changes in electrical activity elevate the threshold for ventricular fibrillation and help prevent the development of life-threatening ventricular arrhythmias. Arrhythmias apparently are the primary causative factor in sudden death within the first few weeks following infarction.

Clinical Indications. In clinically stable patients who have survived an acute MI, timolol, propranolol, or IV metoprolol is indicated to reduce cardiovascular mortality and risk of reinfarction.

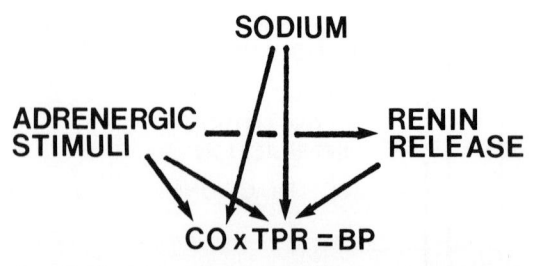

Fig. 3.30 Major determinants of blood pressure. (From Ayerst Laboratories: Update—Hypertension. New York, Ayerst Laboratories, 1977.)

Adverse Effects/Precautions. Beta-drenergic blocking drugs present problems in clinical situations where sympathetic activation is vital (such as CHF and A-V block). Extreme caution must therefore be exercised in these instances. Other adverse reactions are mild and transient, disappearing after cessation of drug therapy.

HYPERTENSION

Major determinants of blood pressure are sodium, adrenergic stimuli, and renin release (Figure 3.30). Antihypertensive drugs (Table 3.5), with different sites of action and pharmacologic mechanisms, have been introduced into therapy to affect these determinants with a resultant fall in elevated blood pressure. An ideal antihypertensive drug would cause a blood pressure reduction of sufficient degree and duration, as well as maintaining a normally functioning cardiovascular system. Homeostatic reflexes should remain viable, and common side effects, such as orthostatic hypotension and excessive reflex tachycardia during exercise, should be minimal. Effectiveness in an oral dosage form is desirable since long-term treatment is required in essential hypertension. Additionally, lack of tolerance development in extended therapy enhances an antihypertensive drug's usefulness.

Antihypertensive drugs are pharmacologically grouped according to the site of their antihypertensive activity. The physiologic control of blood pressure involves a complex interaction of homeostatic mechanisms (Figure 3.31). Thus, the CNS, autonomic ganglia, postsympathetic-ganglionic nerve terminals, vascular smooth muscle, and adrenergic postsynaptic receptor sites represent prime components of blood pressure control amenable to drug action.

DRUGS ACTING ON THE CENTRAL NERVOUS SYSTEM

Some antihypertensive agents lower blood pressure by a central action either on the vasomotor center in the medulla or on higher centers in the hypothalamus. General anesthetics and

Table 3.5 ANTIHYPERTENSIVE DRUGS.*

Available products	Trade names	Daily dosage range
Acebutolol	Sectral	400–800 mg
Alseroxylon	Rauwiloid	2 mg
Atenolol	Tenormin	50 mg once daily
Captopril	Capoten	25 mg t.i.d.
Clonidine HCl	Catapres	0.2–0.8 mg orally in divided doses
Deserpidine	Harmonyl	0.25 mg
Diazoxide, parenteral	Hyperstat IV	300 mg by rapid IV bolus injection
Enalapril	Vasotec	10.4 mg
Guanabenz acetate	Wytensin	4 mg b.i.d.
Guanadrel sulfate	Hylorel	20–75 mg b.i.d.
Guanethidine sulfate	Ismelin	25–75 mg orally
Guanfacine	Tenex	1 mg orally
Hydralazine HCl	Apresoline	40–200 mg orally; 20–40 mg, IV
Labetalol	Normodyne; Trandate	400–800 mg
Methyldopa and Methyldopate HCl	Aldomet	500 mg-2 g orally in divided doses or 250–500 mg q. 6 hrs, IV
Metoprolol tartrate	Lopressor	100–450 mg
Minoxidil	Loniten	10–40 mg
Nadolol	Corgard	80–320 mg once daily
Nitroprusside sodium	Nipride; Nitropress	0.5–10 mcg/kg/min by IV infusion as needed
Pargyline HCl	Eutonyl	25–50 mg
Pindolol	Visken	5 mg t.i.d.
Prazosin HCl	Minipress	6–15 mg in divided doses
Propranolol	Inderal	120–240 mg in divided doses
Rauwolfia derivatives	Raudixin; Hiwolfia; others	200–400 mg in 2 divided doses
Rescinnamine	Moderil	0.25–0.5 mg
Reserpine	Serpasil; Sandril	0.1–0.25 mg
Timolol maleate	Blocadren	20–40 mg
Trimethaphan camsylate	Arfonad	Infused IV at a rate of 1–4 mg/min

* Some diuretic drugs are also used in the treatment of congestive heart failure; see Chapter 5.

barbiturates have a central hypotensive action. A more widely recognized group of central acting antihypertensive drugs are clearly antiadrenergic in nature and include clonidine, guanabenz, guanfacine, and methyldopa.

Clonidine. An imidazole derivative, clonidine acts as an orally effective central antiadrenergic antihypertensive drug.

Mechanism of Action. Clonidine stimulates both alpha$_1$- and alpha$_2$-adrenergic receptors in the lower brain stem and the periphery. The transient blood pressure elevation seen shortly after clonidine administration is due to the activation of peripheral alpha$_1$-adrenergic receptors, resulting in vasoconstriction.

Clonidine's potent alpha-agonist activity in the CNS is responsible for the drug's hypotensive effect. The alpha$_2$-adrenergic agonist action in the CNS results in a presynaptic inhibition of neuronal norepinephrine release and consequently, a decrease in the sympathetic outflow from the brain. Additionally, activation of alpha$_1$-adrenergic (postsynaptic) receptors in certain brain stem nuclei may be associated with inhibition of central sympathetic tone and impulse outflow. These receptor interactions inhibit medullary sympathetic cardioaccelerator and sympathetic vasoconstrictor centers to decrease central sympathetic impulse traffic.

Clonidine may have a peripheral action preventing cardiac stimulation by sympathetic activation. This action is due to a presynaptic inhibitory effect of clonidine, where presynaptic alpha$_2$-adrenergic receptor agonist activity reduces the neuron release of norepinephrine.

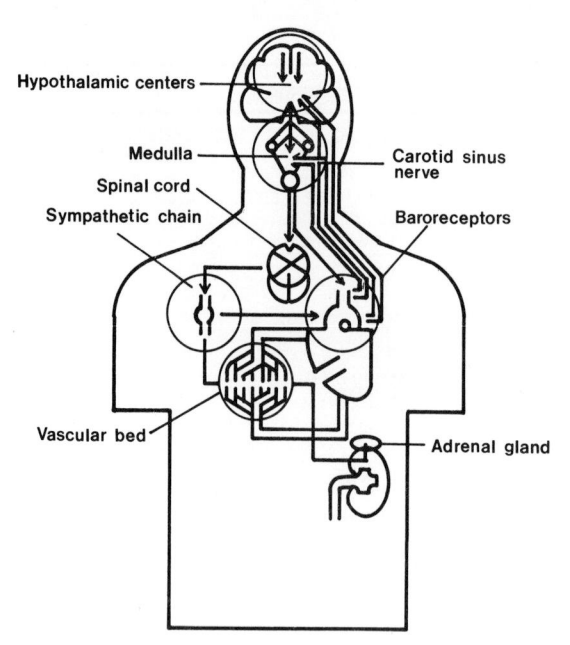

Fig. 3.31 Blood pressure and its control. (Courtesy Boehringer Ingelheim Pharmaceuticals, Inc., Ridgefield, CT.)

Clinical Indications. Clonidine is used in the treatment of mild to moderate essential hypertension. The drug may be combined with a diuretic and/or antihypertensive drugs for optimal control of hypertension.

Adverse Effects/Precautions. Dry mouth, drowsiness, and sedation are common adverse reactions. Tolerance to these effects tends to develop after several weeks of therapy.

A "rebound hypertension" phenomenon may occur with abrupt discontinuation of clonidine therapy. Consequently, patients should discontinue therapy by reducing their clonidine dose over a period of 2 to 4 days in order to avoid a hypertensive reaction.

Guanabenz. Guanabenz, an aminoguanidine derivative, acts as an orally effective central antiadrenergic antihypertensive drug.

Mechanism of Action. Guanabenz is a central alpha$_2$-adrenergic receptor agonist. Activation of central alpha$_2$-adrenergic receptors (presynaptic) decreases medullary sympathetic impulse traffic to the peripheral sympathetic system. The long-term effect of guanabenz therapy relates to decreases in peripheral resistance.

Also, guanabenz induces small decreases in serum cholesterol and total triglycerides. Plasma norepinephrine and renin levels decrease during extended guanabenz therapy, but the significance of these observations is presently unclear.

Clinical Indications. Guanabenz is an effective antihypertensive agent alone or in combination with a thiazide diuretic.

Adverse Effects/Precautions. As with clonidine, common adverse effects are dry mouth, drowsiness, and sedation. Since these side effects may be dose-related, dosage adjustment may diminish their occurrence. "Rebound hypertension" may occur with sudden cessation of guanabenz therapy.

Guanfacine. A central acting oral antihypertensive drug, guanfacine should be administered in once daily doses.

Mechanism of Action. Guanfacine is a central alpha$_2$-adrenergic agonist.

Clinical Indications. Guanfacine is used in the treatment of hypertension.

Adverse Effects/Precautions. Xerostomia, sedation, dizziness, and constipation are adverse reactions to guanfacine therapy. Abrupt cessation of orally active central alpha$_2$-adrenergic agonists may be associated with "rebound hypertension."

Methyldopa. The l-isomer of alpha-methyldopa, methyldopa acts as a central acting antiadrenergic agent.

Mechanism of Action. Methyldopa is biotransformed to alpha-norepinephrine that is probably the active antihypertensive moiety. Alpha-methylnorepinephrine, an alpha$_2$-adrenergic receptor agonist, reduces the sympathetic outflow at the medullary level. The active metabolite may also act as a false-transmitter (in place of epinephrine) by functioning as a fraudulent, impotent adrenergic transmitter. Additionally, methyldopa reduces plasma renin levels, possibly contributing to its antihypertensive activity.

Clinical Indications. Methyldopa is used in the treatment of hypertension. Methyldopate HCl is an injectable methyldopa ester hydrochloride that has been employed for the initiation of therapy in hypertensive crises.

Adverse Effects/Precautions. CNS effects, such as sedation and dizziness, are common adverse reactions. Cardiovascular responses, including bradycardia, prolonged carotid sinus hypersensitivity, and aggravation of angina pectoris, have been reported. If edema or signs of CHF appear, methyldopa therapy should be discontinued.

A positive Coomb's test, hemolytic anemia, and liver disorders may also occur with methyldopa therapy. Since methyldopa is contraindicated in acute hepatic disease or if previous methyldopa therapy has been associated with liver disorders, the drug should be used with caution (or not at all) in patients with impaired liver function.

With IV methyldopate, a paradoxical hypertensive response has been reported.

DRUGS ACTING ON THE AUTONOMIC GANGLIA

The autonomic ganglionic blocking drugs were the first potent antihypertensive drugs introduced into clinical medicine. They have generally been replaced with drugs with less severe and pronounced side reactions.

Ganglionic Blocking Agents. The ganglionic blocking agents include hexamethonium, pentolinium, mecamylamine, and trimethaphan (see Chapter 2).

Mechanism of Action. The ganglionic blocking drugs occupy postsynaptic acetylcholine receptors in autonomic ganglia to prevent the depolarizing action of acetylcholine released from presynaptic nerve endings. Blockade of transmission in sympathetic ganglia produces the hypotensive action, whereas many of the side effects associated with ganglionic blocking drugs are due to inhibitory effects on parasympathetic ganglia.

Clinical Indications. Trimethaphan camsylate is a short acting ganglionic blocking agent administered IV for the production of controlled hypotension during surgery and for the short-term control of blood pressure in hypertensive emergencies. Another indication is in the emergency treatment of pulmonary edema related to pulmonary hypertension in patients with associated essential hypertension.

Mecamylamine is used orally for the management of moderately severe to severe hypertension and in selected cases of malignant hypertension.

Adverse Effects/Precautions. The precipitous blood pressure lowering effect possible with IV trimethaphan may present a clinical emergency. A vasopressor drug may be needed to return the undesirable low blood pressure to normotensive levels.

Common adverse effects that occur with mecamylamine involve the gastrointestinal tract, postural hypotension, and reactions related to the blocking of parasympathetic ganglia, including blurred vision, urinary retention, constipation, and paralytic ileus.

DRUGS ACTING ON POSTGANGLIONIC ADRENERGIC NERVE ENDINGS

Adrenergic neuron blocking drugs may prevent norepinephrine release from or accumulation in postganglionic adrenergic nerve terminals.

Guanadrel. Guanadrel is an orally effective synthetic antihypertensive agent of the adrenergic-neuron blocking class.

Mechanism of Action. Guanadrel inhibits norepinephrine release from adrenergic nerve endings and depletes norepinephrine stores from adrenergic nerve terminals. A hypotensive effect results from the relaxation of vascular smooth muscle and the consequent decrease in total peripheral resistance and venous return. The hypotensive effect is greater in the standing position than in the supine.

Clinical Indications. Guanadrel is used in the treatment of hypertension refractory to thiazide monotherapy.

Adverse Effects/Precautions. Orthostatic hypotension, dizziness, and weakness occur frequently in patients taking guanadrel. To reduce the possibility of vascular collapse during surgery, guanadrel should be discontinued several days before elective surgery.

Guanethidine. Guanethidine, a guanidine derivative, exerts potent and prolonged antihypertensive action.

Mechanism of Action. Guanethidine inhibits norepinephrine release from postganglionic adrenergic nerve endings to exert its antihypertensive action, effectively blocking adrenergic neurons. Guanethidine also depletes norepinephrine stores in adrenergic nerve terminals. An initial transient release of norepinephrine from the adrenergic nerve terminals results in fleeting sympathomimetic action. Postsynaptic adrenergic receptor sites, following guanethidine therapy, are sensitive to exogenous catecholamines. Guanethidine also prevents norepinephrine uptake by adrenergic neurons, thereby allowing for pronounced adrenergic responses.

Clinical Indications. Guanethidine, either alone or in combination, is indicated in moderate and severe hypertension.

Adverse Effects/Precautions. Orthostatic hypotension and syncope are frequent side effects caused by the greater hypotensive effect that occurs with patients in the standing position.

Frequent adverse effects due to unopposed parasympathetic activity include bradycardia and diarrhea. Inhibition of ejaculation is another common reaction to guanethidine. Sodium and fluid retention with edema may mandate using a thiazide diuretic or ceasing guanethidine therapy. Withdrawing guanethidine therapy 2 weeks prior to surgical procedure reduces the possibility of vascular collapse and cardiac arrest during the operation.

Guanethidine effects are cumulative, mandating careful scrutiny of increasing dosage increments. This drug is prone to cause disturbing clinical problems; thus, its use must be monitored carefully.

Rauwolfia Derivatives. The rauwolfia derivatives include the whole root rauwolfia, alseroxylon (an extractive preparation), and the purified alkaloids—reserpine, rescinnamine, and deserpidine.

Mechanism of Action. The antihypertensive effect of the rauwolfia alkaloids is due to depletion of norepinephrine in postganglionic adrenergic nerve endings. The mechanism operant is an inhibition of catecholamine storage in protective presynaptic granules, thereby allowing for extensive metabolism of catecholamines (norepinephrine) by the cytoplasmic monoamine oxidase (MAO).

Clinical Indications. Rauwolfia derivatives are indicated for the treatment of essential hypertension.

Adverse Effects/Precautions. Many side effects are associated with parasympathetic predominance as a result of decreased sympathetic influence. These effects include nasal stuffiness, diarrhea, and hypersecretion in the gastrointestinal tract. CNS adverse effects, characterized by mental depression, melancholia, and nightmares, result from adrenergic inhibition (amine depletion) in the brain.

DRUGS ACTING ON VASCULAR SMOOTH MUSCLE

Blood vessels are actively dilated by a direct relaxant effect on vascular smooth muscle.

Diazoxide. Diazoxide, an emergency antihypertensive agent, is a chemical relative of the thiazide derivatives.

Mechanism of Action. Diazoxide produces rapid and profound dilation of blood vessels. The drug may antagonize Ca^{++} in vascular smooth muscle as it blocks the generation of a Ca^{++}-dependent action potential. Experimentally, diazoxide inhibits barium (Ba^{++})-induced smooth muscle contraction. Arteriolar smooth muscle is preferentially relaxed and arterioles dilate with little effect on veins. In contrast to the thiazide derivatives, diazoxide causes a marked retention of sodium and water.

Clinical Indications. Diazoxide is used intravenously in the emergency treatment of hypertensive crisis.

Adverse Effects/Precautions. Marked hypotensive reactions may occur due to reflex sympathetic stimulation. Rare cases of hyperglycemia have been reported.

Hydralazine. Hydralazine, an effective vasodilator drug, is employed as an antihypertensive agent.

Mechanism of Action. Hydralazine produces peripheral vasodilation by a direct relaxant effect on vascular smooth muscle. The major site of action is the arteriolar smooth muscle, with minimal activity observed on the venous capacitance vessels. Decreased peripheral resistance occurs, as well as reduced arterial blood pressure (Figure 3.32). Reflex tachycardia with increased cardiac output characteristically occurs with this drug. Preferential dilation of arterioles, as compared to veins, minimizes postural hypotension and promotes the increase in cardiac output.

Clinical Indications. Hydralazine is employed, usually in combination with other drugs, in the treatment of hypertension.

Adverse Effects/Precautions. The incidence of side effects is high with hydralazine therapy. Headache, palpitations, anorexia, nausea, vomiting, and diarrhea are commonly observed effects. Also, a drug-induced SLE-like syndrome occurs in 10 to 20% of the patients taking over 400 mg of hydralazine daily. Myo-

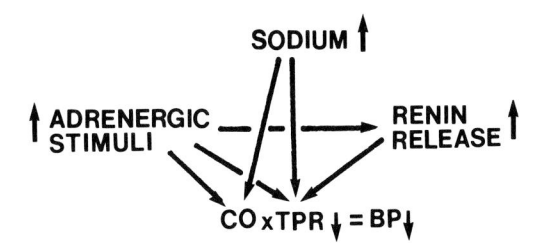

Fig. 3.32 Vasodilator therapy. (Modified from Ayerst Laboratories: Update—Hypertension. New York, Ayerst Laboratories, 1977.)

cardial stimulation associated with hydralazine administration can produce angina attacks.

Consequently, a beta-adrenergic blocker (such as propranolol) is often administered concurrently with hydralazine. The beta-adrenergic blocking drug limits the cardiovascular response, thus often blocking undesirable cardiac stimulation. Also, addition of a beta-adrenergic blocker minimizes the hydralazine dosage requirement because of the additive antihypertensive effects of the combined drugs.

Minoxidil. Minoxidil is an orally effective direct acting vasodilator.

Mechanism of Action. Minoxidil causes direct relaxation of vascular smooth muscle. The resulting peripheral dilation lowers elevated diastolic and systolic pressure by reducing peripheral resistance. The drug apparently blocks Ca^{++} uptake through the muscle cell membrane.

Clinical Indications. Minoxidil is indicated in the treatment of severe hypertension not amenable to other antihypertensive agents. This drug is usually taken in combination with at least two other antihypertensive medications.

Adverse Effects/Precautions. Minoxidil may produce serious cardiac side effects, including myocardial stimulation due to reflex activation of the sympathetic nervous system. Consequently, in susceptible patients, angina pectoris may be exacerbated. Pericardial effusion may also be produced, possibly leading to cardiac tamponade. Fluid retention, often to excessive amounts, is another adverse effect. Minoxidil induces growth and darkening of body hair in about 80% of the patients taking this drug (see Chapter 10).

Nitroprusside. Sodium nitroprusside, a potent direct acting vasodilator, is administered by IV infusion.

Mechanism of Action. Nitroprusside rapidly relaxes both arteriolar and venous smooth muscle. The venous dilation decreases preload to the heart, an action similar to the nitrates. In this light, angina pectoris often improves when nitroprusside is given. This contrasts with drugs that cause arteriolar dilation without venous dilation (i.e. hydralazine, minoxidil, and diazoxide) and that may possibly induce myocardial ischemia as a result of preload maintenance and reflex activation of the sympathetic nervous system.

Clinical Indications. Nitroprusside is used as an emergency antihypertensive agent in hypertensive crisis and as an adjunct in acute MI or CHF.

Adverse Effects/Precautions. Nitroprusside may produce excessive vasodilation and hypotension. Other side effects include nausea, vomiting, sweating, restlessness, and headache. These adverse reactions disappear when the IV infusion is stopped.

Thiazide Derivatives. Thiazide derivatives are diuretic drugs (see Chapter 5) that also relax vascular smooth muscle by a direct effect.

Mechanism of Action. The thiazide derivatives' initial beneficial effect in hypertension relates to diuresis, resulting in altered sodium balance with a consequent reduction in blood volume and a decrease in cardiac output (Figure 3.33). In chronic therapy, however, cardiac output returns to normal and peripheral resistance falls. Expanding the blood volume with dextran does not reverse the blood pressure lowering. Evidently, the decrease in peripheral resistance relates to salt excretion and results in a direct action on arteriolar smooth muscle.

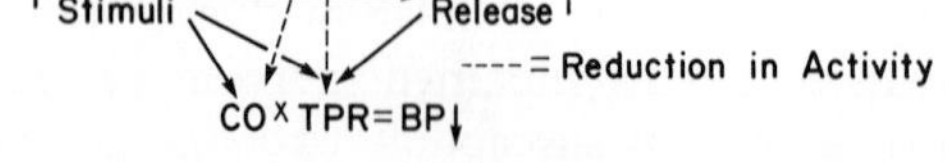

Clinical Indications. Thiazide derivatives are usually the first drugs employed in the control of mild essential hypertension. Thus, they are considered Step 1 drugs; if additional control is required, other antihypertensive drugs are added to the patient's regimen.

Adverse Effects/Precautions. Hypokalemia, hyperglycemia, and hyperuricemia are primary side effects seen with these drugs.

DRUGS THAT ACT AS ADRENERGIC RECEPTOR BLOCKING DRUGS

Adrenergic receptor blocking drugs compete with catecholamines and other adrenergic agonists for adrenergic receptors. Thus, by competitive inhibition, these agents prevent the effects of adrenergic agonists on adrenergic receptors.

ALPHA-ADRENERGIC RECEPTOR BLOCKING DRUGS

Classical alpha-adrenergic receptor drugs, such as phenoxybenzamine and phentolamine, are not routinely used in hypertension therapy (see Chapter 2). Prazosin, a new alpha-adrenergic receptor blocking agent, has a more selective effect on postsynaptic receptors than the classical drugs.

Prazosin. An orally effective antihypertensive drug, prazosin was synthesized as a prototype compound in the search for potential phosphodiesterase inhibitors.

Mechanism of Action. Prazosin blocks postsynaptic alpha$_1$-adrenergic receptors in the blood vessels to elicit its antihypertensive effect. In contrast to other alpha-adrenergic

Fig. 3.33 Diuretic therapy. (Modified from Ayerst Laboratories: Update—Hypertension. New York, Ayerst Laboratories, 1977.)

blockers, like phenoxybenzamine and phentolamine, prazosin has little effect on presynaptic adrenergic receptors.

This drug also inhibits phosphodiesterase, an enzyme that catalyzes the degradation of cyclic AMP. The significance of this biochemical event in the peripheral vasodilation, induced by prazosin, is unclear although elevated cyclic AMP levels are associated with beta-adrenergic receptor activation and vascular smooth muscle relaxation.

Prazosin dilates both arterioles and veins, and unlike the conventional alpha-adrenergic blockers (phenoxybenzamine and phentolamine), the antihypertensive effect is not accompanied by reflex tachycardia.

A decrease in plasma renin activity has been noted with prazosin, in contrast to the direct acting vasodilators that increase renin release. No significant changes in cardiac output, heart rate, or renal blood flow are seen in prazosin therapy.

Clinical Indications. Prazosin is indicated for mild to moderate hypertension. It can also be used as the initial drug or in combination with a diuretic or other antihypertensive agents.

Adverse Effects/Precautions. Prazosin elicits the "first dose" effect of syncope with sudden loss of consciousness in about 1% of the patients given an initial dose of 2 mg or more. This reaction may result from excessive postural hypotension. Tachycardia may precede the syncope which usually occurs 1 to 1.5 hours after the initial dose. A reduction of syncopal episodes is achieved by limiting the initial dose to 1 mg, by subsequently increasing the dosage slowly, and by cautiously adding any additional antihypertensive drugs to the treatment regimen.

Dizziness, drowsiness, headache, weakness, and palpitations are common adverse reactions to prazosin therapy. These side effects usually decrease or disappear with continued prazosin use.

BETA-ADRENERGIC BLOCKING DRUGS

Beta-adrenergic receptor blockade interferes with adrenergic stimuli affecting cardiac function (Figure 3.34).

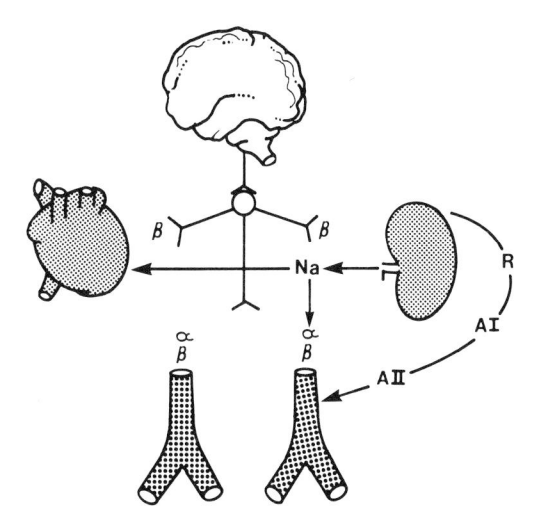

Fig. 3.34 Adrenergic receptors and their relation to physiologic function. (Modified from Ayerst Laboratories: Update—Hypertension. New York, Ayerst Laboratories, 1977.)

Acebutolol. Acebutolol, a beta$_1$-selective blocking drug, has a greater effect on cardiac (beta$_1$-adrenergic) receptors than on the beta$_2$-adrenergic receptors in the bronchi and peripheral blood vessels. However, this cardiac selectivity is dose-dependent; in the doses used to treat hypertension, acebutolol can cause bronchospasm in asthmatic patients.

Having some partial agonist activity, acebutolol may not lower the heart rate as much as beta-adrenergic blockers not possessing intrinsic sympathomimetic action. A membrane-stabilizing action (quinidine-like) is also observed with acebutolol.

Atenolol. Atenolol is a cardioselective beta-adrenergic receptor blocking drug. As with acebutolol, the selectivity is dose-dependent and atenolol may induce bronchospasm in asthmatic patients.

Labetalol. Labetalol is a nonselective beta-adrenergic receptor blocking drug. Additionally, labetalol has postsynaptic alpha-adrenergic blocking activity. This dual action sets it apart from the other drugs in this category.

Metoprolol. Metoprolol is a cardioselective beta-adrenergic receptor blocking drug. As with acebutolol and atenolol, the cardioselectivity depends upon dose, and higher doses block both beta$_1$- and beta$_2$-adrenergic receptor sites.

Oxprenolol.* Oxprenolol is a nonselective beta-adrenergic receptor blocker. The drug also possesses intrinsic sympathomimetic action and a membrane-stabilizing (quinidine-like) activity.

Nadolol. Nadolol is a nonselective beta-adrenergic receptor blocker with a longer half-life as compared to other drugs in this class. It can be administered in a once a day dosage regimen to treat hypertension.

Pindolol. Pindolol is a nonselective beta-adrenergic receptor blocker with intrinsic sympathomimetic activity and a membrane-stabilizing (quinidine-like) action.

Propranolol. Propranolol is a nonselective beta-adrenergic receptor blocker with a marked membrane-stabilizing effect. Propranolol is the most lipophilic of this class of drugs and therefore enters the CNS more readily.

Timolol. Timolol is a nonselective beta-adrenergic receptor blocking drug.

Mechanism of Action. Adrenergic stimuli cause an increased cardiac contractility (positive inotropism), increase heart rate (positive chronotropism), and elevate the cardiac output. Beta-adrenergic receptor blockade has little effect on the normal heart in a patient at rest, but marked responses occur when sympathetic control of the heart is high. All beta-adrenergic receptor blockers reduce the inotropic and chronotropic effects of cardiac sympathetic activity and circulating beta-adrenergic receptor agonists. Thus, in patients exercising or experiencing emotional stress, these drugs effectively block adrenergic receptors reducing the sympathetic predominance.

Beta-adrenergic activation in the kidney results in renin release, subsequent formation of angiotensin I and II, and resultant arteriolar vasoconstriction. Beta-adrenergic receptor blocking drugs reduce the release of renin. Reduction in plasma renin activity (PRA) by beta-adrenergic blockers is more prominent when these levels are elevated.

The antihypertensive activity of beta-adrenergic blockers involves several mechanisms. Decreased cardiac output, inhibition of renin secretion, reduction of plasma volume, and decreased central sympathetic activity apparently contribute to the blood pressure lowering effect of these drugs (Figure 3.35).

Clinical Indications. All of the clinically available beta-adrenergic blocking drugs are FDA approved for the treatment of hypertension. These drugs are used alone as a Step I agent or in combination with other drugs (usually a thiazide diuretic). Beta-adrenergic receptor blocking agents are not indicated in the treatment of hypertensive emergencies.

Adverse Effects/Precautions. Beta-adrenergic blocking drugs depress cardiac contractility and should be used with caution in CHF patients. The respiratory tract and cardiovascular system are particularly susceptible to these drugs because of the prevalence of beta-adrenergic receptors at these sites. Consequently, adverse effects, such as bronchospasm, bradycardia, and heart failure or block, may occur in beta-adrenergic receptor blocker therapy.

Other effects include hyperglycemia or hypoglycemia, CNS depression, and gastrointestinal distress. In general, adverse effects to beta-adrenergic blocker therapy are mild and transient, rarely requiring cessation of treatment.

---

* Although FDA approved for treatment of hypertension, this drug is currently not on the market.

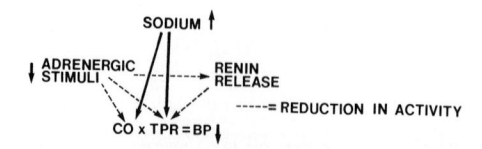

Fig. 3.35 Adrenergic blocking therapy. (Modified from Ayerst Laboratories: Update—Hypertension. New York, Ayerst Laboratories, 1977.)

DRUGS THAT AFFECT THE RENIN-ANGIOTENSIN SYSTEM

Captopril and Enalapril. These drugs interfere with the renin-angiotensin system, reducing peripheral resistance.

Mechanism of Action. Captopril and enalapril compete with angiotensin I converting enzyme (ACE) to prevent the conversion of angiotensin I to angiotensin II. The competitive inhibition of ACE (peptidyl dipeptidase) thus blocks the formation of the potent vasoconstrictor, angiotensin II. The resultant reduction of peripheral arterial resistance lowers blood pressure in hypertensive patients with either no change or an increase in the cardiac output.

Clinical Indications. ACE inhibitors are usually given together with a diuretic or beta-adrenergic receptor blocker and are not considered to be primary agents in the treatment of hypertension. Captopril and enalapril are used in patients refractory to other antihypertensive agents. Captopril has also received FDA approval for the treatment of CHF.

Adverse Effects/Precautions. Adverse effects include headache, skin rashes, dizziness, proteinuria, neutropenia, and excessive hypotension. Increases in serum creatinine and BUN have been reported.

FUTURE ANTIHYPERTENSIVES

Atrial naturetic factor (ANF) is a peptide secreted by the heart cells. Injection of ANF decreases plasma epinephrine levels and it reduces norepinephrine production in isolated pheochromocytoma cells. ANF apparently inhibits catecholamine synthesis by inhibiting dopamine-beta-hydroxylase. Preliminary studies indicate that this hormone-like peptide relaxes the arteries and has naturetic properties.

SPECIAL TREATMENT REGIMEN FOR ANTIHYPERTENSIVE DRUGS

The stepped care treatment presents a progressive rational approach to pharmacotherapy for essential hypertension. Thiazides (or in special cases, a beta-adrenergic blocker) are considered Step 1 antihypertensive drugs. Monotherapy with a thiazide is extended by increasing the dosage gradually. If Step 1 thiazide therapy is unsuccessful, Step 2 involves the addition of an antiadrenergic drug (such as a central adrenergic blocking drug, adrenergic neuron blocking drug, or adrenergic receptor blocking agent) to the treatment regimen. Thiazide therapy is usually continued.

In cases in which a thiazide and an antiadrenergic drug are ineffective in controlling the hypertension, a vasodilator is added to institute "triple-drug" antihypertensive therapy (Figure 3.36). Drugs used in Step 3 include hydralazine and captopril. Step 4 represents the use of additional adrenergic inhibiting agents and increasing the dosage to achieve effective control of the hypertensive state.

ANTI-INFECTIVES

Endocarditis caused by Streptococcus viridans is usually penicillin sensitive and a treatment course with combined penicillin G-streptomycin therapy is advocated in these cases. Enterococcal endocarditis is best treated with two antibiotics, i.e., penicillin G intravenously in combination with an aminoglycoside. Other anti-infectives used to treat endocarditis caused by susceptible organisms include amoxicillin, ampicillin, benzylpenicillin, carbenicillin, ceforanide, cephalothin, cefazolin, cloxacillin, gentamicin, kanamycin, methicillin, phenoxymethylpenicillin, vancomycin, trimethoprim, and sulfamethoxazole. Chapter 7 contains a discussion of the mechanisms of action and related material on these anti-infectives.

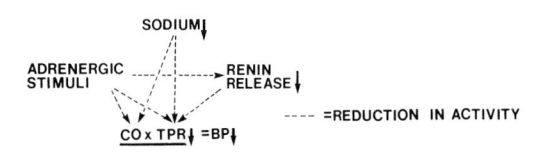

Fig. 3.36 Combination antihypertensive therapy ("Triple Therapy"—vasodilator, diuretic, and adrenergic blocker). (Modified from Ayerst Laboratories: Update—Hypertension. New York, Ayerst Laboratories, 1977.)

DRUG INTERACTIONS

Multiple drug therapy is routine in the management of cardiovascular disease; thus, the likelihood of drug interactions, some which are life-threatening, is increased in such cases. Additionally, cardiovascular disease is common to the elderly, a population in which adverse reactions represent a serious problem.

ANTIARRHYTHMIC DRUGS

AMIODARONE

Oral Anticoagulants. Since amiodarone may reduce oral anticoagulant metabolism, its use should be avoided in patients on oral anticoagulant therapy. If amiodarone is used, patients should be monitored for the hypoprothrombinemic response to oral anticoagulants. Following initiation of amiodarone therapy, the prothrombin time should be monitored for several weeks since the onset of interaction is delayed in some patients.

Digitalis Glycosides. Since both pharmacokinetic and pharmacodynamic interactions may be involved, patients should be observed for indications of altered digoxin response if amiodarone therapy is initiated or discontinued.

DISOPYRAMIDE

Lidocaine. Reports of isolated cases indicate occurrences of impaired intraventricular conduction and ventricular asystole in predisposed patients receiving combined therapy with disopyramide and lidocaine.

Phenytoin Phenytoin may stimulate disopyramide metabolism through microsomal enzyme induction. The reduction of disopyramide plasma levels may decrease pharmacologic activity. Concurrent administration can exert additive cardiodepressant effects.

Quinidine. Since both are Type I antiarrhythmic drugs, concurrent administration of quinidine and disopyramide can result in combined cardiodepressant effects.

Rifampin. As with phenytoin, rifampin stimulates the hepatic metabolism of disopyramide. Thus, if rifampin is initiated or discontinued, monitoring serum disopyramide levels allows early detection of this possible interaction.

LIDOCAINE

Beta-adrenergic Blockers. Beta-adrenergic blockers tend to reduce cardiac output and hepatic blood flow, which reduces hepatic lidocaine metabolism. Beta-adrenergic blockers may inhibit the activity of hepatic microsomal drug metabolizing enzymes. Although the clinical importance of the additive negative inotropic effect of lidocaine and beta blockers is not yet established, concurrent therapy with beta-adrenergic blockers may necessitate lowering lidocaine dosage.

Cimetidine. Known to inhibit hepatic microsomal drug metabolism, cimetidine may reduce hepatic blood flow, as well as alter the distribution and protein binding of lidocaine. Also possible are combined effects of both drugs on cardiac function and mental status. Thus, concurrent administration may result in excessive lidocaine effect, necessitating reductions in lidocaine dosage.

Neuromuscular Blocking Agents. Reports indicate that lidocaine and other antiarrhythmics may enhance neuromuscular blockade of skeletal muscle relaxants by impairing transmission impulses at the motor nerve terminals.

Phenytoin. Excessive cardiac depression may occur if combined therapy with IV diphenylhydantoin and IV lidocaine is initiated.

PROCAINAMIDE

Cholinergics. Having neuromuscular blocking properties, procainamide may antagonize the effect of cholinergic drugs on skeletal muscle.

Cimetidine. Cimetidine may reduce the renal excretion of procainamide and its major metabolic, acetylprocainamide. Indications of enhanced procainamide and acetylprocainamide response in the presence of cimetidine therapy may necessitate reducing the procainamide dose.

QUINIDINE

Digitalis Glycosides. Quinidine raises digoxin levels by inhibiting the renal excretion of digoxin. Serum digoxin levels may be two to three times higher in digitalized patients receiving quinidine (beginning 1 to 3 days after starting quinidine therapy). The drug may produce arrhythmias in digitalized patients and should be used with caution in digitalis intoxication.

Consequently, reduction in digoxin dosage or the administration of an alternate antiarrhythmic drug (other than quinidine) may be indicated in some clinical conditions. Digitalis is indicated for pretreatment before quinidine use in the treatment of atrial flutter or fibrillation. After achieving control, the digitalis glycosides and quinidine are sometimes combined for effective prophylaxis against these arrhythmias.

Oral Antacids. Reports indicate that some oral antacids can increase urinary pH which in turn increases the proportion of un-ionized quinidine. Since this process can lead to increased tubular reabsorption, caution should be exercised in administering antacids to patients on quinidine therapy. Also, monitoring quinidine blood levels as a precautionary measure may allow early detection of this problem.

Aluminum hydroxide apparently does not alter the gastrointestinal absorption of quinidine, but the effect of other antacids on quinidine gastrointestinal absorption is not established.

Oral Anticoagulants. Quinidine may potentiate the anticoagulant effect of warfarin; therefore, caution should be exercised in administering quinidine to patients on oral anticoagulant therapy. Reduction in prothrombin levels and clotting factors occurs with this combination, and the patient receiving both drugs should be monitored for bleeding. Instances of quinidine-induced hypoprothrombinemic hemorrhage have been reported in patients on chronic oral anticoagulant (warfarin) therapy.

Barbiturates. Phenobarbital tends to decrease the pharmacologic effects of quinidine. An enhancement of the hepatic metabolism of quinidine by phenobarbital apparently is the interaction mechanism. Initiation or discontinuation of barbiturate therapy in patients receiving quinidine may require changing the quinidine dose.

Cimetidine. Cimetidine may elevate blood plasma quinidine levels by inhibiting hepatic microsomal enzymes, thus decreasing quinidine metabolism. Successful concurrent administration may require reducing the quinidine dose.

Neuromuscular Blocking Agents. By a curare-like action on the myoneural junction and depression of the muscle action potential, quinidine evidently potentiates both nondepolarizing and depolarizing muscle relaxants. Thus, in the immediate postoperative period when muscle relaxant effects may still be present, quinidine use should be avoided, if possible. Its use in such instances may necessitate respiratory support.

Phenytoin. Since phenytoin may enhance the hepatic metabolism of quinidine, larger than normal quinidine doses may be necessary in the initiation of phenytoin therapy in patients receiving quinidine.

Rifampin. Rifampin apparently reduces quinidine plasma concentration by stimulating the hepatic metabolism of quinidine. Patients receiving rifampin and quinidine concurrently should be observed for reduced quinidine response.

CARDIAC GLYCOSIDES

DIGITALIS

Amiloride. Amiloride may increase renal clearance and reduce nonrenal digoxin clearance. Hence, altered responses to digoxin may occur in patients receiving both digoxin and amiloride. Specifically, amiloride may produce substantial increases in serum digoxin levels in patients with impaired renal excretion of digoxin; on the other hand, decreased serum digoxin levels resulting from an amiloride-induced increase in renal digoxin clearance may develop in patients with impaired extrarenal digoxin excretion.

Oral Antacids. Some antacids may impair gastrointestinal absorption of digoxin, and patients receiving concurrent antacid therapy should be monitored for possible reduced digoxin effect. Spacing the doses (to minimize mixing in the gastrointestinal tract) may reduce the inhibitory effect of antacids on digoxin absorption; also, using digoxin capsules instead of tablets may minimize the interaction.

Barbiturates. Due to induction of hepatic microsomal enzymes, phenobarbital may enhance the metabolism of digitoxin to digoxin. Thus, patients receiving both digitoxin and a barbiturate should be monitored for possible underdigitalization.

Calcium Preparations. Since parenteral calcium may precipitate cardiac arrhythmias in patients receiving digitalis glycosides, administration of parenteral calcium should be avoided. However, high serum calcium levels may be avoided by not giving the calcium rapidly or in large amounts.

Cholestyramine. Cholestyramine apparently binds digitoxin in the gut to interrupt the enterohepatic circulation of digitoxin and shorten its half-life. Since cholestyramine can impair absorption of digoxin and digitoxin, patients receiving digitalis glycosides should be monitored for underdigitalization if cholestyramine is also given. Administering the digitalis product 1.5 to 2 hours before the cholestyramine dose may help reduce this interaction.

Potassium-losing Diuretics. Potassium deficiencies produced by diuretics like furosemide, ethacrynic acid, bumetanide, chlorthalidone, metolazone, and thiazides can result in digitalis toxicity. Another contributing factor may be magnesium deficiency, which can occur after diuretic therapy. Patients on concomitant diuretic-digitalis therapy should be monitored for potassium and magnesium levels; if necessary, replacement potassium therapy should be initiated.

Kaolin-pectin. Patients on digoxin should limit their use of kaolin-pectin, an apparent inhibitor of gastrointestinal absorption of digoxin. If used, kaolin-pectin should be given two hours after digoxin tablets. Administration of digoxin capsules may also reduce the interaction.

Metoclopramide. Metoclopramide increases gastrointestinal motility, possibly decreasing the digoxin effects. Use of rapidly dissolving products or digoxin capsules may minimize the interaction.

Propantheline. An anticholinergic drug, propantheline decreases gastrointestinal motility and may increase gastrointestinal absorption of slowly dissolving brands of digoxin.

Spironolactone. Potential adverse reactions include reduced renal excretion of digoxin, inhibition of the positive inotropic effect of digitalis glycosides, and production of false elevations in plasma digoxin by some methods. Spironolactone may also enhance the metabolism of digitoxin. Use of potassium supplements instead of spironolactone may avoid these problems.

Sympathomimetics. Concomitant use of sympathomimetics and digitalis glycosides can increase the possibility of cardiac arrhythmias since both produce ectopic pacemaker activity. Thus, caution should be exercised in administering sympathomimetics to digitalized patients.

Verapamil. Verapamil apparently inhibits renal excretion of digoxin and chronic treatment increases serum digoxin levels by 50 to 70% during the first week of therapy. Careful monitoring of digoxin serum concentration is advised with concurrent verapamil treatment. Since verapamil and digoxin have additive pharmacodynamic effects, slowed A-V conduction may occur.

ANTIANGINAL DRUGS

BETA-ADRENERGIC BLOCKING DRUGS

Antidiabetic Agents. Effects of beta-adrenergic blocking agents that interact with diabetes therapy include: beta-adrenergic blocker-induced delayed glucose recovery from insulin-induced hypoglycemia; beta-adrenergic blocker-induced hypertension during hypoglycemia; beta-adrenergic blocker-induced inhibition of the tachycardia during hypoglycemia; insulin secretion inhibition; and peripheral circulation impairment. In diabetic patients (especially those predisposed to hypoglycemic episodes), cardioselective agents may prove more beneficial than nonselective beta-adrenergic blockers.

Cimetidine. Cimetidine inhibits the hepatic metabolism of propranolol and some other beta-adrenergic blockers, thereby increasing their blood plasma levels. Thus, an increase in the pharmacologic effect may occur, resulting in reduced pulse rate, sinus bradycardia, and hypotension.

Epinephrine. Epinephrine effects (alpha-adrenergic: vasoconstriction; beta-adrenergic: vasodilation and cardiac stimulation) ordinarily result in mild increases in heart rate and minimal changes in mean arterial pressure. However, when propranolol is used to block epinephrine's beta-adrenergic effects, the alpha-adrenergic effects predominate. This produces hypertension and a reflex increase in vagal tone, resulting in bradycardia. Therefore, epinephrine should be administered with caution to patients receiving propranolol or other nonselective beta-adrenergic blockers.

Rifampin. Rifampin tends to decrease the effects of beta-adrenergic blockers by enhancing the hepatic metabolism of these drugs.

Theophylline. Beta-adrenergic blockers' inhibition of hepatic microsomal drug metabolism may reduce theophylline clearance that occurs after propranolol or metoprolol treatment. Further, beta-adrenergic blockers and theophylline have some antagonistic pharmacologic effects.

Verapamil. In cases of refractory angina pectoris, concurrent use of verapamil and beta-adrenergic blockers may be advantageous. However, if high beta-adrenergic blocker doses are used or if the patient has compromised left ventricular function, patients should be observed for indications of excessive cardiodepresssant effects with administration of this combination.

ORGANIC NITRATES

Ergot Alkaloids. Ergot alkaloids, which may precipitate angina and work against the antianginal effects of nitroglycerin, should be avoided in patients taking nitroglycerin for angina pectoris.

Ethanol. Hypotension may occur after combined use of ethanol and nitroglycerin due to the vasodilation both agents produce. Thus, patients receiving nitroglycerin should use ethanol cautiously.

ANTIHYPERTENSIVE DRUGS

CAPTOPRIL

Indomethacin. Indomethacin's ability to inhibit prostaglandin synthesis is apparently responsible for the inhibition of the antihypertensive response to captopril. Careful monitoring for reduced hypertensive response is beneficial in patients receiving captopril and indomethacin; due to indomethacin's inhibitory action, substituting another antihypertensive drug for captopril may not circumvent the problem.

CLONIDINE

Tricyclic Antidepressants (TCADs). Concomitant use of clonidine and TCADs is not recommended. Also, since TCADs evidently interact with guanethidine, bethanidine, and debrisoquin, they would not be suitable alternatives. Apparently methyldopa is reasonably safe when used with a TCAD, but little is known about the combined use of TCADs with other antihypertensives.

DIAZOXIDE

Thiazides. Since diazoxide competes with the thiazide diuretics for plasma protein binding, caution should be exercised in the concomitant administration of these drugs which has enhanced hyperglycemic activity in several patients.

GUANETHIDINE

Tricyclic Antidepressants (TCADs). TCADs inhibit the update of guanethidine into the adrenergic neuron, inhibiting the antihypertensive effect. Thus, the combination of these drugs should be avoided.

METHYLDOPA

Levodopa. Since this combination may adversely affect response to levodopa, patient reaction, dose of drugs, and other factors need consideration.

Lithium Carbonate. Lithium intoxication may result from concurrent use.

PRAZOSIN

Indomethacin. Indomethacin may inhibit prostaglandin synthesis. Concurrent administration with indomethacin (or other nonsteroidal anti-inflammatory agents) necessitates monitoring for reduced hypotensive response to prazosin (or other antihypertensive agents).

RESERPINE

Monoamine Oxidase Inhibitors (MAOIs). MAOIs cause norepinephrine accumulation in storage sites within the adrenergic neuron. The reserpine-induced release of norepinephrine results in an exaggerated response because of the increased amount of neurotransmitter present at the adrenergic receptor.

Patients receiving MAOI therapy may experience excitation and hypertension if also given reserpine. Therefore, concomitant use of an MAOI and reserpine should be avoided.

SUMMARY

The nature of cardiovascular disease often dictates the heroic treatment of an initial emergency situation. In this case, potent drugs are usually given, often along with other therapeutic measures such as cardioversion, and the medication for each patient is individually titrated to achieve a finely balanced, stable cardiovascular response. The pharmacist, as a member of the health care team, is then responsible to monitor the patient's drug therapy and to assure that the delicate balance achieved in the initial clinical improvement is maintained.

In the pharmacotherapy of cardiovascular disease, certain factors assume clinical significance. First, the pharmacist must exercise extreme caution in dispensing a generic equivalent cardiac drug. The question of "therapeutic" equivalence versus "generic" equivalence is raised extensively with cardiac drugs such as digoxin and disopyramide. The exact drug product and dosage form that the patient receives on the initial prescription must be continued on subsequent refills to guarantee optimal patient care.

Second, the treatment protocol often requires the use of several drugs to control the cardiovascular disease processes. In the treatment of hypertension, for example, multiple drug therapy is common. Certain advantages accrue with this treatment regimen. To illustrate, each antihypertensive drug can be given at a lower dose than required if one were given alone. A routine clinical finding is the reduction of side effects that are often seen with higher doses of individual drugs. Additive synergistic activity due to the different sites and mechanisms of individual antihypertensive drugs also occurs. Additionally, responses to individual agents often interact to counter potential adverse effects. Hydralazine, for example, tends to cause sodium retention leading to edema and a reversal of its antihypertensive activity. Thiazides, routinely included in the therapeutic regimen with hydralazine, favor sodium excretion; thus, fluid retention is considerably reduced with this drug combination.

Third, long-term, often lifetime, therapy with cardiovascular drugs is common since many of the diseases being treated are chronic. The pharmacist must carefully monitor, through patient medication records and consultations, the therapeutic regimen. Thus, factors such as tolerance, adverse effects, and drug interactions must be constantly reviewed. For instance, ingestion of the OTC drug phenylpropanolamine (commonly used as a nasal decongestant or diet aid) by a CHF patient taking digoxin or by another patient taking antihypertensive medication could result in a clinically significant adverse response because of the sympathomimetic nature of phenylpropanolamine.

Patient compliance, another of the pharmacist's concerns, becomes especially difficult to achieve in many cases. Some conditions, such as hypertension, are often essentially symptom free, and the drug treatment may produce noxious side effects. In such instances, the patient may perceive the disease treatment as worse than the disease itself. The pharmacist, by realizing that dosage modification or medication change may affect hypertension control without producing untoward effects in the patient, can help the patient avoid discomfort. This option is clinically preferable because of the long-term effects of untreated hypertension.

Finally, the pharmacist must reemphasize to the patient the importance of nondrug therapeutic measures as an integral part of the treatment mosaic. A weight reduction program and restricted salt intake are often essential in a cardiovascular disease patient. Thus, a holistic approach, including behavioral modification, is indicated in achieving designated therapeutic goals and optimal patient care.

SUGGESTED READINGS

Acebutolol. Med Lett Drugs Ther, 27:58, 1985.
Akera, T., and Brody, T.M.: Myocardial membranes. Regulation and function of the sodium pump. Annu Rev Physiol, 44: 375, 1982.
Bernstein, K.N., and O'Connor, D.T.: Antiadrenergic antihypertensive drugs. Their effect on renal function. Annu Rev Pharmacol Toxicol, 24:105, 1984.
Beyer, K.H., and Peuler, J.D.: Hypertension. Perspectives. Pharmacol Rev, 34:287, 1982.
Cardiac Arrhythmias. Whippany, NJ, Knoll Pharmaceutical Company, 1981.
Chatterjee, K., and Parmley, W.W.: Vasodilator therapy for chronic heart failure. Annu Rev Pharmacol Toxicol, 20: 475, 1980.
Couvin, C., Loutzenhiser, R., and Van Breemen, C.: Mechanisms of calcium antagonist-induced vasodilation. Annu Rev Pharmacol Toxicol, 23:373, 1983.
Davis, R.L.: Beta blockers. Am Col Apoth Profess Pract Newsletter, 5:1, 1984.
Drug use little changed in 1983. Am Col Apoth Newsletter, 43:2, 1985.
Drugs for hypertension. Med Lett Drugs Ther, 29:1, 1987.
Fabiato, A., and Fabiato, F.: Calcium and cardiac excitation-contraction coupling. Annu Rev Physiol, 41:473, 1979.
Farah, A.E., Alousi, A.A., and Schwartz, R.P., Jr.: Positive inotropic agents. Annu Rev Pharmacol Toxicol, 24:275, 1984.
Gilman, A.G., et al. (eds.): The Pharmacological Basis of Therapeutics. 7th Ed. New York, Macmillan Publishing Co., Inc., 1985.
Hanston, P.D.: Drug Interactions. 5th Ed. Philadephia, Lea & Febiger, 1985.
Herbette, L., Messineo, F.C., and Katz, A.M.: The interaction of drugs with the sarcoplasmic reticulum. Annu Rev Pharmacol Toxicol, 22:413, 1982.
Hoffman, B.B., and Lefkowitz, R.J.: Adrenergic receptors in the heart. Annu Rev Physiol, 44:475, 1982.
Hondeghem, L.M., and Katzung, B.G.: Antiarrhythmic agents. The modulated receptor mechanisms of action of sodium and calcium channel-blocking drugs. Annu Rev Pharmacol Toxicol, 24:387, 1984.
Hussar, D.A.: Cardiovascular drug interactions. Wellcome Trends in Hospital Pharmacy, 7:5, 1985.
Johnston, S.M., et al.: Comparison of verapamil and nifedipine in the treatment of variant angina pectoris. Preliminary observations in 10 patients. Am J Cardiol, 47:1295, 1981.
Kastrup, E.K., and Boyd, J.R., (eds.): Drug Facts and Comparisons. Philadephia, J.B. Lippincott Co., 1985.
Labetalol. Univ Colorado Drug Inf Bulletin, 3:2, 1985.
Leon, M.B., et al.: Clinical efficacy of verapamil alone and combined with propranolol in treating patients with chronic stable angina pectoris. Am J Cardiol, 48: 131, 1981.
McDonald, T.F.: The slow inward calcium current in the heart. Annu Rev Physiol, 44:425, 1982.
Nitroglycerin patches. Med Lett Drugs Ther, 26:59, 1984.
Simon, H., and Bloomfield, D.A.: Cardioactive Drugs. A Pharmacologic Basis for Practice. Baltimore, Urban & Schwarzenberg, 1983.
Spear, J.F., and Moore, E.N.: Mechanisms of cardiac arrhythmias. Annu Rev Physiol, 44:485, 1982.
Subramanian, B., et al.: Combined therapy with verapamil and propranolol in chronic stable angina. Am J Cardiol, 49:125, 1982.
Tocainide. W Va Univ Drug Inf Bulletin, 10:1, 1985.
Tocainide for arrhythmias. Med Lett Drugs Ther, 27:9, 1985.

Treatment of cardiac arrhythmias. Med Lett Drugs Ther, 25:21, 1983.

Utt, J.K.: Tocainide. An "oral lidocaine." Am Col Apoth Profess Pract Newsletter, 6:1, 1985.

Vedin, J.A., and Wilhelmsson, C.E.: Beta receptor blocking agents in the secondary prevention of coronary heart disease. Annu Rev Pharmacol Toxicol, 23:29, 1983.

Wilson, H.: Drug therapy for cardiac arrhythmias. Am Druggist, 189:137, 1985.

CHAPTER EXAMINATION

A patient has been taking quinidine sulfate for nearly 6 months to control cardiac arrhythmias. He comes into your pharmacy and complains of "ringing in the ears" and dizziness.

1. The symptoms the patient describes probably represent
   a. an inadequate daily dose of quinidine sulfate
   b. tolerance developing to the drug
   c. cinchonism
   d. none of the above
2. Quinidine sulfate, as an antiarrhythmic drug,
   a. suppresses re-entry mechanisms that may induce arrhythmias
   b. has a membrane-stabilizing effect on myocardial membranes
   c. prolongs the cardiac refractory period
   d. all of the above

A patient with controlled angina pectoris (organic nitrate therapy) has been taking a thiazide-reserpine combination for moderate essential hypertension. The physician changes the antihypertensive medication to a thiazide-reserpine-hydralazine combination. A few days later the patient complains of chest pains.

3. The patient probably
   a. has not taken the new antihypertensive medicine
   b. has stopped taking the organic nitrates
   c. is experiencing the effects of the addition of hydralazine to the therapeutic regimen
   d. none of the above
4. Hydralazine may
   a. produce reflex bradycardia
   b. precipitate angina attacks in previously controlled patients
   c. reduce cardiac output
   d. all of the above
5. An unusual adverse effect seen with hydralazine therapy (usually high doses in chronic therapy) is
   a. a syndrome resembling SLE
   b. CNS depression
   c. gingival hyperplasia
   d. none of the above

A middle-aged male CHF patient has been taking digoxin and hydrochlorothiazide for several years. Extensive public speaking assignments have caused him significant prespeech anxiety. His physician prescribes propranolol to alleviate his anxiety. The patient calls your pharmacy and complains of ankle swelling and shortness of breath.

6. The addition of propranolol may cause
   a. a hypertensive crisis
   b. excessive intracellular potassium loss in the patient
   c. reappearance of CHF symptoms
   d. all of the above
7. Propranolol
   a. is a cardioselective beta-adrenergic receptor blocker
   b. probably enters the CNS to induce both antihypertensive and antianxiety effects
   c. has potent intrinsic sympathomimetic activity
   d. none of the above
8. The physician decides to change the antianxiety medication. The best choice is
   a. a beta-adrenergic receptor blocking drug with a longer half-life
   b. a beta-adrenergic receptor blocking drug with a less lipophilic nature

c. a benzodiazepine derivative, such as diazepam
d. none of the above

9. The patient's ingestion of the digoxin-hydrochlorothiazide combination for several years has probably resulted in
    a. hyperkalemia
    b. marked CNS depression
    c. reduced sensitivity to beta-adrenergic blocking drugs
    d. none of the above

10. The use of propranolol in this clinical situation represents an example of
    a. the varied clinical indications of propranolol therapy
    b. the most popular therapeutic application of propranolol
    c. sympathomimetic synergism
    d. none of the above

11. If the patient additionally exhibited periodic bronchial asthma, propranolol use would be
    a. of additional benefit due to its bronchodilatory properties
    b. contraindicated
    c. irrelevant
    d. none of the above

A patient who is well-titrated on disopyramide wants you to switch to a generic equivalent since he has read that "drugs are drugs" and he wants to save money.

---

12. Disopyramide is a
    a. valuable drug in treating CHF
    b. potent direct acting vasodilator
    c. drug with a similar pharmacologic profile to that of quinidine
    d. none of the above

13. This clinical situation represents an opportunity for the pharmacist
    a. to substitute a generic equivalent without sacrificing safety to the patient
    b. to explain to the patient the difference between "therapeutic" equivalence and "chemical" equivalence
    c. expound on the clinical implications of drug interactions
    d. all of the above

A patient has been taking propranolol for the treatment of essential hypertension. Lately, she has developed a feeling of melancholia and has nightmares and trouble sleeping. She calls and asks you if her medicine could be responsible.

---

14. Propranolol
    a. never causes CNS effects since it doesn't cross the blood brain barrier
    b. routinely stimulates the motor and sensory cerebral cortex
    c. is the beta-adrenergic receptor blocker most likely to enter the brain and cause effects
    d. none of the above

15. Her physician calls and asks you to recommend a longer acting beta-adrenergic blocking drug with less likelihood of CNS effects. A good choice is
    a. nadolol
    b. timolol
    c. metoprolol
    d. diltiazem

16. Congestive heart failure develops in the patient and digoxin is added to the treatment regimen. The beta-adrenergic receptor blocking drugs least likely to aggravate the CHF are
    a. metoprolol and propranolol
    b. acebutomol and pindolol
    c. atenolol and pindolol
    d. oxprenolol and metoprolol

A patient with variant or vasospastic angina is initially treated with verapamil. Control is not effectively achieved requiring an additional drug in the regimen for optimal control of the angina.

---

17. A rational drug to be added to the patient's therapy is
    a. digoxin
    b. procainamide
    c. bretylium
    d. isosorbide dinitrate

18. The patient develops CHF and digitalization is required. Since verapamil is also being used with the digitalis preparation (digoxin), care must be exercised because
    a. the chronic administration of verapamil increases serum digoxin levels
    b. the chronic administration of verapamil decreases serum digoxin levels
    c. reflex tachycardia may induce heart block
    d. convulsions are common with this drug combination
19. In the initial therapy with verapamil, another drug that could have been substituted for verapamil in the monotherapy is
    a. reserpine
    b. guanadrel
    c. diltiazem
    d. clonidine
20. The most common side effect of verapamil therapy is
    a. diarrhea
    b. diplopia (double vision)
    c. xerostomia (dry mouth)
    d. constipation

ANSWER KEY

1. c	11. b
2. d	12. c
3. c	13. b
4. b	14. c
5. a	15. a
6. c	16. b
7. b	17. d
8. c	18. a
9. d	19. c
10. a	20. d

chapter 4

CIRCULATORY/ RETICULOENDOTHELIAL SYSTEM

CHAPTER OBJECTIVES

After studying this chapter, you should be able to:
1. Discuss the basic principles involved in the absorption of iron from the gastrointestinal tract.
2. Define the following: transferrin, ferritin, myoglobin, hemoglobin, reticuloendothelial cells.
3. Name several iron preparations and indicate their advantages.
4. Describe the symptoms of iron overdose.
5. Identify the characteristics of erythrocytes in a patient with iron deficiency anemia.
6. Name several situations in which iron deficiency is likely to occur.
7. Describe the hematologic, neurologic, and clinical characteristics noted in pernicious anemia.
8. Describe the cyanocobalamin molecule.
9. Name several sources of vitamin B_{12}.
10. Discuss Castle's hypothesis regarding pernicious anemia.
11. Outline the preparations, routes of administration, and dosage of vitamin B_{12}.
12. Describe the danger of including folic acid in multiple vitamin preparations.
13. Name the main therapeutic uses of cyanocobalamin.
14. Explain the relationship of cyanocobalamin to pteroylglutamic acid in intermediary metabolism.
15. Describe the reticulocyte response, hemoglobin level, and erythrocyte response in a patient with pernicious anemia after beginning therapy with liver extract preparation (with intrinsic factor).
16. Name several therapeutic uses of pteroylglutamic acid.
17. Describe two megaloblastic anemias that respond to drugs other than vitamin B_{12} and folic acid.
18. Name several natural sources of folic acid.
19. Outline the major steps in fibrin formation.
20. Name several hemostatic substances that are employed therapeutically.
21. Discuss the mechanism of action of the oral anticoagulants and heparin.
22. List several therapeutic uses of vitamin K substances.
23. Compare the route of administration, onset and duration of action, and therapeutic indications for heparin-dicumarol; vitamin K-protamine sulfate; and warfarin-phenindione.
24. Discuss the drug interactions involving oral anticoagulants.
25. Compare the chemical composition of the following lipoproteins: VLDL; LDL; HDL; and IDL.
26. Name several drugs that reduce elevated plasma lipoprotein level and state the specific type of hyperlipoproteinemia influenced by each drug.
27. Discuss the proposed mechanisms of antilipidemic action for clofibrate, colestipol, gemfibrozil, dextrothyroxine, cholestyramine, nicotinic acid, and lovastatin.

209

28. Describe several drug interactions seen with the antilipidemic drugs.
29. Describe the major adverse effects of the antihyperlipidemic drugs.
30. Describe drug therapeutic regimens used in cases of hyperlipidemia.
31. Discuss the cell cycle phases of cellular replication.
32. Describe the mechanism of action of the alkylating agents as cytotoxic drugs.
33. Name several antimetabolites employed as antineoplastic drugs.
34. State the components of several combination antineoplastic regimens and discuss the rationale of a particular multiple drug approach.
35. Discuss the major adverse effects seen with antineoplastic drugs.

INTRODUCTION

Blood and lymph are actually connective tissues in which the intercellular material is fluid and the cells are freely suspended within it. The blood is normally confined to the cardiovascular system consisting of the heart and blood vessels. The lymph is transported in lymph vessels and enters the blood stream via the thoracic duct; together, the blood and lymph systems constitute the circulatory system.

Transport within the body is the chief function of blood. Blood circulates through all tissues of the body and is instrumental for oxygen-carbon dioxide exchange in cells. In addition, by counteracting invading micro-organisms, the blood cells combat infection as part of the body's defense mechanisms. The blood also carries hormones to various tissues and organs where they function as chemical messengers that regulate metabolic activity. The blood also serves as the site of homeostatic processes for water, electrolyte, acid-balance, and temperature regulation.

Blood carries oxygen from the lungs to the tissues and carbon dioxide from the tissues to the lungs (Figure 4.1). It connects and integrates the metabolic activities of the organs by transporting nutrients from the gastrointestinal tract to the liver, intermediary metabolites from one organ to another, and metabolic waste substances to the kidneys and other organs of excretion.

The lymphatic capillaries originate in the tissues as thin-walled, closed-end endothelial tubes. Tissue fluid, protein, and particulate matter (such as cells) enter the tube lumen. The lymphatic capillaries unite to form the lymph nodes. Although found throughout the body, the lymph nodes are located primarily in the neck, at junctions of the limbs with the body trunk, and in the abdomen and thorax along the anterior spinal cord.

Lymphatic ducts carry lymph from the nodes to the main lymphatic vessel (the thoracic duct) which discharges into the subclavian vein. The ducts have endothelial flaps at intervals along their length that act as valves by permitting movement of lymph only away from the tissues. Pressure applied by muscular contraction, pressure pulses from neighboring arteries, and respiratory movements push the lymph to the lymph nodes and then to the thoracic duct.

Lymphoid tissue and lymphocytes identify and react against antigens or high molecular weight "foreign bodies" that enter the organism. This immune response is the lymphoid system's reaction against infectious disease and also represents the bodily defense against neoplastic disease. Immune responses are also implicated in hypersensitivity reactions and several autoimmune disorders.

ANATOMY AND PHYSIOLOGY OF THE CIRCULATORY/ RETICULOENDOTHELIAL SYSTEM

The microscopic cellular components of the blood and lymph perform varied and crucial physiologic functions.

BLOOD

Observation of a drop of blood under the microscope reveals that it contains several different types of cells. The most numerous are the pale red, disc-shaped erythrocytes, while the remainder are the colorless leukocytes (white cells), thrombocytes (blood platelets), monocytes, and lymphocytes. The rest of the blood is fluid which contains protein, certain minerals, sugar (glucose), fat, urea, and water. If a quantity of blood is removed from the body and allowed to stand in a test tube, it quickly separates into two fractions: plasma, a clear, straw yellow fluid; and a semisolid mass (clot) that includes the cells described above.

The erythrocytes are rigid structures which easily rupture; the leukocytes are nonrigid cells that can assume any shape. Leukocytes are considerably larger than the erythrocytes, while the thrombocytes are the smallest of the blood cells. Counting the number of the various cells present in a small quanitity of blood, a relatively easy procedure, is an extremely important diagnostic tool.

ERYTHROCYTES ("RED BLOOD CELLS"; RBCs)

The erythrocytes carry oxygen to the tissues and, as they pass through the capillaries, that oxygen is exchanged for the waste product carbon dioxide. In the capillaries of the lungs, a reversal of that exchange results in the erythrocytes releasing carbon dioxide and taking up oxygen. The transport of oxygen and carbon dioxide by the erythrocyte requires the cellular presence of hemoglobin, a red substance partially composed of iron.

The number of erythrocytes in the blood

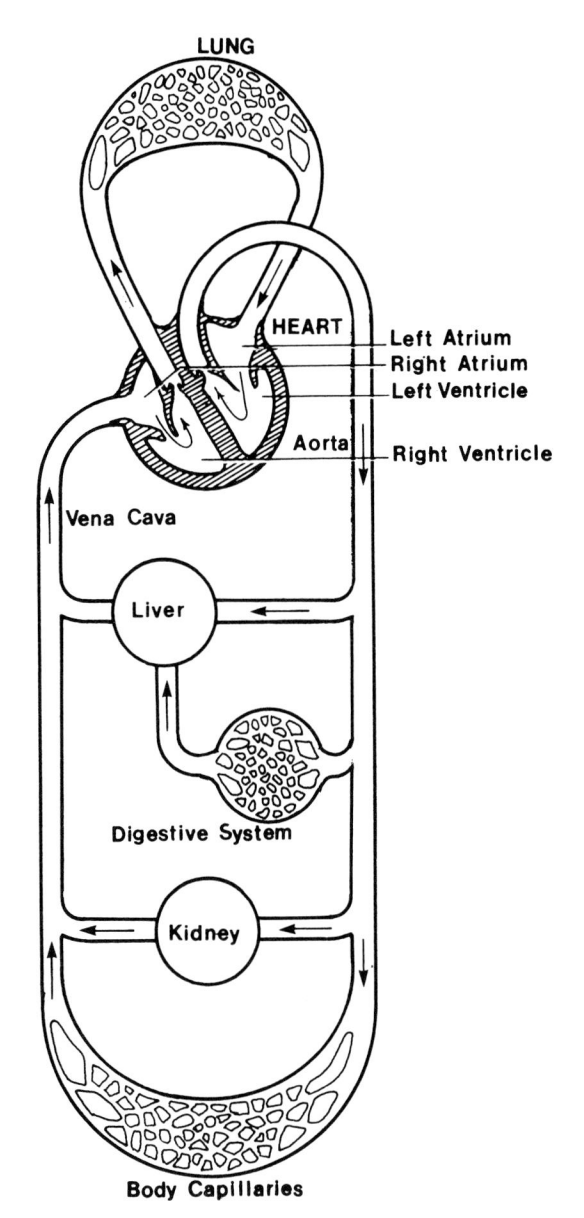

Fig. 4.1 Schematic diagram of the circulatory system. (Adapted from Estes, J.W., and White, P.D.: William Withering and the purple foxglove. Sci Am, 212:110, 1965.)

changes quickly as oxygen demand by the body changes. To illustrate, at sea level the erythrocyte count is about 5.4 million per cubic millimeter (cu mm) of blood, but at an elevation of a mile above sea level (where the amount of oxygen in the atmosphere is less) the count is about

6 million per cu mm. The erythrocyte count is somewhat lower in females than in males, i.e., about 4.7 million per cu mm at sea level. The body contains about 5 L of blood and 10^6 cu mm are in a liter. Thus, an adult male Denverite would have $5 \times 10^6 \times 6,000,000 = 30,000,000,000,000$ (30 trillion) total erythrocytes in his blood.

With strenuous exercise, a person's erythrocyte count increases quickly so as to meet the increased oxygen demand caused by the exercise. Factors other than exercise and altitude that increase the number of erythrocytes are hemorrhage, certain nutritional deficiencies, and emotional states. The increase in the erythrocyte count is often temporary and after the demand by the body that caused the increase has been met, the count returns to a normal value. The life of erythrocytes is about 120 days at which time they begin to fragment. Erythrocytes are slightly larger than some of the capillaries through which they must pass and since their cell wall is rather fragile, rupture occurs. Somewhere between 2 million and 10 million erythrocytes are destroyed each second either by fragmentation or by the spleen and liver as the erythrocytes become less efficient. Fortunately, erythrocyte synthesis occurs very rapidly.

LEUKOCYTES ("WHITE BLOOD CELLS"; WBCs)

Several types of leukocytes are in the blood and these differ as to size, internal structures, and their affinity for certain dyes. Leukocytes consist of granulocytes (eosinophils, basophils, and neutrophils) and nongranulocytes (monocytes and lymphocytes). Blood count tests determine the total number of cells present, the number of each type of cell, and the existence of any abnormalities in color, shape, or size—essential information for accurate disease diagnosis.

Granulocytes exist in the blood in either an immature or a mature form; the immature forms are called bands or stabs (nonsegmented nucleus) and the mature cells are called segs (segmented nucleus). Band forms of neutrophils represent the majority of leukocytes. During acute infection when large numbers of segmented neutrophils are needed, the band population increases. As the infection subsides and recovery occurs, the number of segs increases and the proportion of bands decreases.

Neutrophils are primarily phagocytic; they engulf and digest organisms and products of infection. Eosinophils have a phagocytic action against antigen-antibody complexes and are important in allergic reactions. Besides having a phagocytic role in cleaning up infection debris, monocytes are also the source of macrophages, which are highly phagocytic cells.

Two types of lymphocytes (T lymphocytes and B lymphocytes) function in the immune response. The T lymphocytes originate from stem cells that form in the bone marrow. The stem cells migrate to the thymus gland where they mature. When T lymphocytes are sensitized, they interact with the sensitizing antigen and neutralize it. Certain T lymphocytes (T-helper or T-suppressor cells) may alter the immune response of other lymphocytes.

The B lymphocytes, which also begin as stem cells in the bone marrow, migrate to the lymphoid tissue in the colon, small intestine, and appendix for maturation. After antigen sensitization, the B lymphocytes are converted to plasma cells. These cells secrete immunoglobulins that are critical in antigen-antibody reactions.

The leukocytes constitute one of the body's defenses against certain diseases. They are considerably larger than erythrocytes and are much fewer in number—somewhere between 5,000 and 10,000 per cu mm of blood. While the cell wall of the erythrocyte is rigid and fragile, that of the leukocyte is quite flexible, allowing these cells to change shape. Their prime function is to engulf (phagocytose) bacteria that invade the body, a function they perform by literally pouring themselves around the bacteria. Very soon after the skin is broken, leukocytes migrate to the site of the break in great numbers. The cause for this phenomenon is unclear, but the leukocyctes may respond to chemical changes originating at the place where the skin in broken. In addition to surrounding bacteria, leukocytes also attack other substances foreign to the body, such as wooden splinters or rose thorns that become imbedded under the skin.

When an infection by micro-organisms

reaches threatening proportions, the number of leukocytes possibly increases to 30,000 per cu mm of blood. As these cells battle the infecting micro-organisms, many leukocytes are lost. The pus that is found at the site of the infections contains leukocytes, as well as debris consisting of dead cells and tissue fluids.

THROMBOCYTES

Large numbers of thrombocytes (very small, colorless blood platelets) are also in the blood. About one-half the diameter of an erythrocyte, thrombocytes are present in numbers that range from 140,000 to 350,000 per cu mm of blood. They function in the clotting of blood, a defensive process that provides protection against the loss of vital blood when cuts or other injuries allow blood to escape.

PLASMA LIPIDS

Plasma lipids include free fatty acids and lipoproteins.

Free Fatty Acids. Adipose cells release free fatty acids following the lipolysis of triglycerides in the adipose tissue. A number of hormone influences (including corticotropin, norepinephrine, glucocorticoids) control lipolysis. Prostaglandin E_1, a local autocoid, inhibits, as does insulin, the norepinephrine and corticotropin-induced release of free fatty acids. Plasma free fatty acids are also derived to a limited extent from the digestion of dietary fats.

A small percentage of the plasma free fatty acids are incorporated into lipoproteins. Most of the free fatty acids, however, are bound to plasma albumen. Excess free fatty acids are mainly taken up by the liver where they are esterified and incorporated into lipoproteins. Fatty acids are also extracted from the plasma by adipose cells and esterified to form depot triglycerides.

Lipoproteins. Blood cholesterol and triglycerides are present as an integral part of lipoproteins. Lipoproteins consist of phospholipids, specific proteins, and varying amounts of cholesterol and/or triglycerides (Figure 4.2).

The ratio of lipid to protein determines the densities of the different lipoproteins. The least dense are the chylomicrons that are composed almost entirely of lipids. The chylomicrons are formed in the epithelial cells of the small intestine and are transferred into the lymph from which they enter the blood stream through the thoracic duct. Since their half-life is short (5 to 15 minutes), they disappear from the blood a few hours after fat ingestion.

The liver synthesizes very low density lipoprotein (VLDL). The main role of the VLDLs is to transport triglycerides that constitute just over 50% of their total weight. The half-life of VLDLs in the blood stream is from 6 to 12 hours. Fatty acids from VLDLs and chylomicrons are transferred to depot fat by the action of an adipose tissue lipoprotein lipase. The loss of triglycerides from the lipoproteins also results in the conversion of chylomicrons to VLDLs.

Low density lipoproteins (LDLs) transport cholesterol; a LDL contains about 40 to 50% cholesterol esters or free cholesterol by weight. The blood half-life of LDLs is normally 3 to 4 days.

High density lipoproteins (HDLs) are not associated with any pathophysiology; in fact, they actually contribute to a reduced incidence of cardiovascular disease. HDL activates lipoprotein lipase and delivers cholesterol and other lipids to various tissues. The blood plasma half-life is approximately four days.

THE LYMPHATIC SYSTEM

In addition to the vessels that transport blood, another extensive network carries the fluid called lymph. The lymphatic system includes the lymph capillaries, the lymphatic vessels, lymphatic ducts, and lymph nodes; closely allied with the entire system are the spleen, tonsils, and thymus gland.

Lymph serves a vital purpose because as the blood passes through the capillary beds, some of the blood constituents, principally proteins, leak through the capillary walls into the tissues. The lymph picks up the lost proteins and returns them to the blood stream. Flow of lymph

214 THERAPEUTIC PHARMACOLOGY

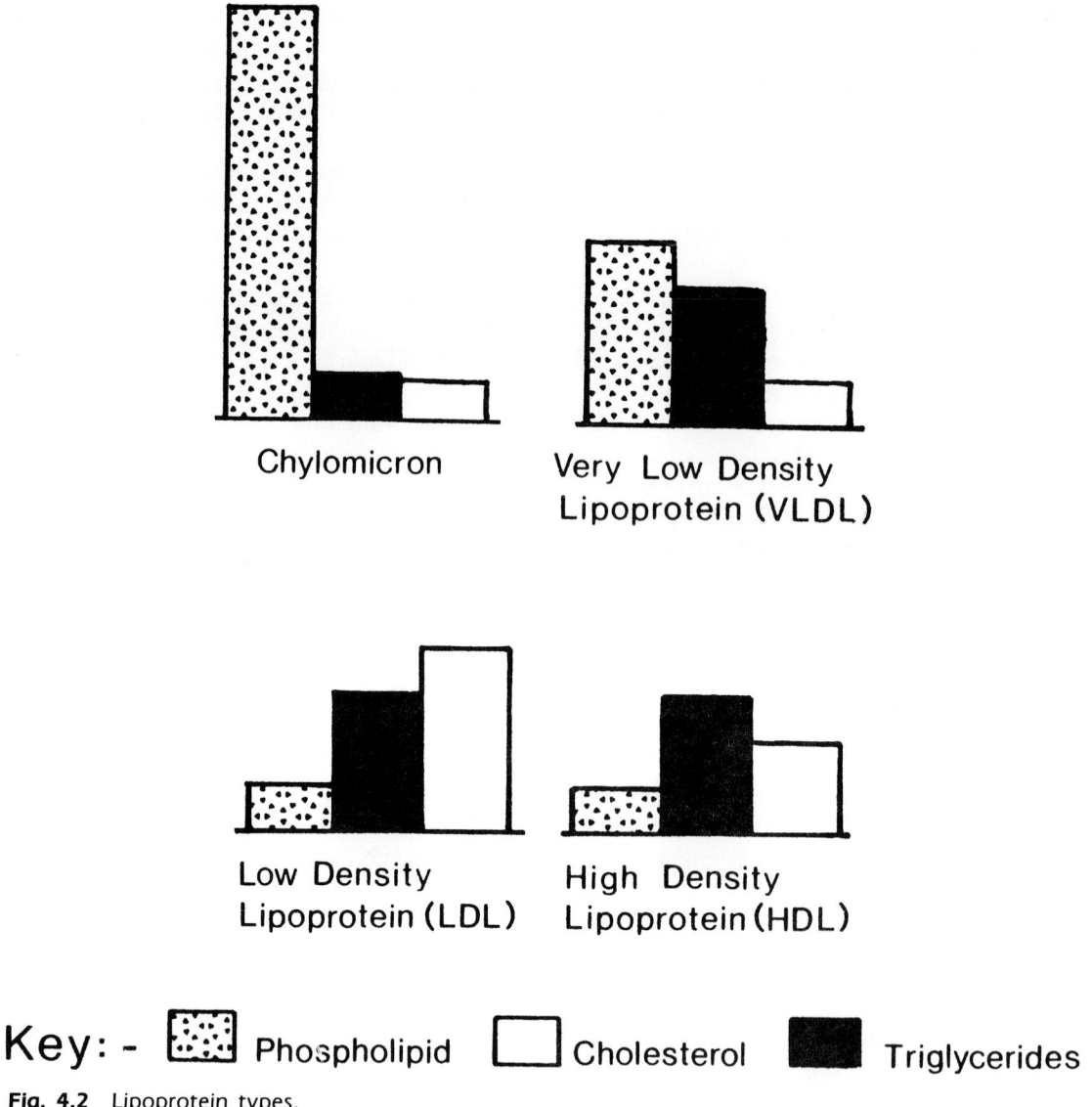

Key: - ▨ Phospholipid ☐ Cholesterol ■ Triglycerides

Fig. 4.2 Lipoprotein types.

occurs slowly due to several factors including the continuous formation of new lymph which forces flow in the lymphatic vessels and the push exerted by arteries whose pulsating action exerts a milking or squeezing motion against the vessels encouraging lymph flow. Some of the leukocyctes are called lymphocytes because they are synthesized by the lymphatic system. Lymphocytes are multipurpose in function in that the body can convert them to other cells and they can also form antibodies that protect against various toxins produced by infectious organisms. Additionally, the lymphatic system makes monocytes, another type of leukocyte.

Although a few decades ago many surgeons advocated tonsillectomy, recent studies indicate the importance of this part of the lymphatic system in the formation of antibodies. Since the tonsils are larger in children than in adults, the tonsils may account for immunity against childhood diseases. Similarly, the thymus gland (located in the upper chest) is large in children but begins to degenerate by the time of puberty making it very small in adults. Thus, this component of the lymphatic system may also help produce immunity against childhood diseases.

THE BLOOD-FORMING ORGANS

Besides the cells (lymphocytes and monocytes) that are synthesized by the lymphatic system, other cells of the blood are produced by the bone marrow, a primary blood-forming organ. Prior to maturity, the bones are filled with a dark red marrow; in the adult, the marrow in the shafts of the long bones of the arms and legs is yellowish or fatty. In the joints and in the flat or irregular bones, however, the marrow remains red; this is the site of the formation of erythrocytes and most of the leukocytes.

In the red marrow, a series of complex processes occur in a stepwise fashion resulting in conversion of primitive cells to completed blood cells. As discussed previously, the transport of oxygen by erythrocytes depends upon the presence of hemoglobin, an iron-containing red pigment. The iron required must be supplied to the body in the diet at an amount of about 15 mg daily; any iron in excess of that needed by the body is excreted, mostly in feces. The body salvages a great deal of the iron liberated when erythrocytes are destroyed.

Although leukocytes are also formed in an orderly stepwise manner from primitive cells, two of the leukocytes found in the blood (lymphocytes and monocytes) are produced by the lymphatic system rather than by the bone marrow.

The thrombocytes (blood platelets) are produced in the marrow in a somewhat different manner in that megakaryocytes, very large cells, fragment to yield the thrombocytes.

ERYTHROCYTE FORMATION

The hemoglobin present in the erythrocytes is a complex protein that contains iron. It is formed in the bone marrow simultaneously with the synthesis of the erythrocytes; in each 100 ml, there are about 15 g of hemoglobin in males—in females, there are about 14 g/100 ml of blood. Hemoglobin carries about 98% of the oxygen present in the blood; the remaining 2% is transported as a solution of oxygen in the blood. Through a series of complex reactions in the liver and then in the bone marrow, iron that is present in the diet is incorporated into a protein that contains a globin (hence the name hemoglobin) and is subsequently introduced into the erythrocyte. In order for bone marrow to utilize iron, trace elements of copper must be present in the diet.

Erythrocytes, in the human, contain no nucleus and have a fragile cell wall. Since they are larger than some of the capillaries they must pass through, many are broken up as they circulate through the tissues. As they rupture, the hemoglobin is released into the blood stream and the liver breaks it down while at the same time salvaging a considerable amount of iron for reuse. This scavenging action of the liver, however, is not 100% efficient with the result that about 1.5 mg of iron are excreted each day, mostly in the feces. Therefore, the human daily diet must include 15 mg of iron to replace that which is lost (10% absorption).

Normal persons have an extremely low iron requirement because only minute amounts are excreted in the feces and urine. A characteristic of iron metabolism is the body's inability to rid itself of excess iron.

The mucosal block phenomenon limits iron absorption in the small intestine (Figure 4.3). Iron is transferred from the intestinal lumen into the mucosal cells in the duodenal and jejunal region. A fraction of this iron is transferred into the blood; the rest remains in the mucosal cells until it is excreted as sloughing of these cells. The absorption of iron into the bloodstream is an active and/or facilitated transport process. Iron present in these mucosal cells inhibits the further absorption of luminal ferrous ion (thus, the term "mucosal barrier" appropriately describes this block). Iron deficiency and increased bone marrow reticulocyte formation increase intestinal absorption of iron; decreased bone marrow activity and iron excess reduce the absorption of iron.

In the event of an iron deficient diet, the bone marrow cannot produce a sufficient amount of

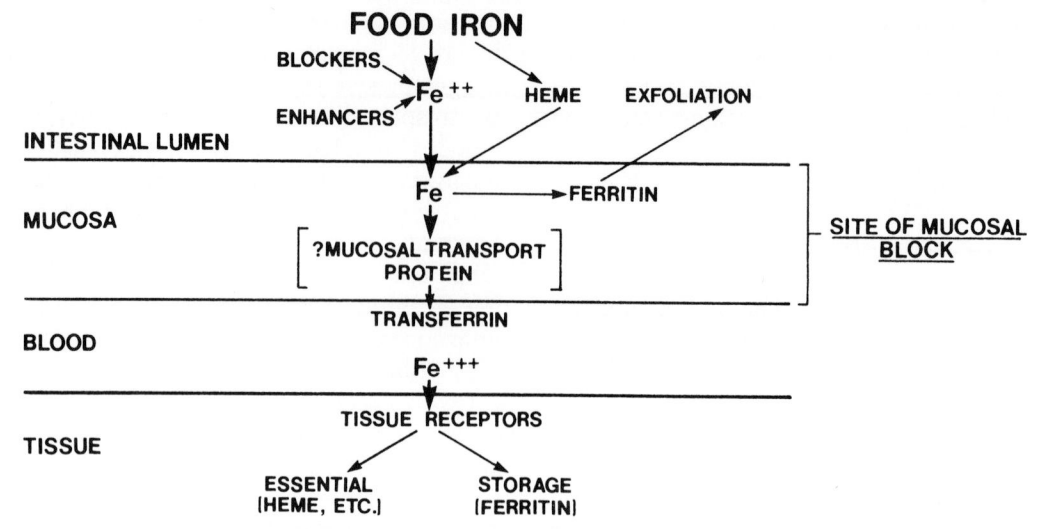

Fig. 4.3 Iron metabolism and mucosal barrier. (From Gilman, A. G., et al. (eds.): The Pharmacological Basis of Therapeutics. 7th Ed. New York, Macmillan Publishing Co., Inc., 1985.)

hemoglobin; this, in turn, means that the blood cannot transport enough oxygen to adequately supply the tissues, resulting in anemia. Treatment consists of furnishing iron to the body via tablets or capsules of iron salts. In iron deficiency anemia, the number of erythrocytes is likely to be within normal limits, but they are pale since the amount of hemoglobin is lower than normal.

More than a century ago, the disease pernicious anemia in which the erythrocytes do not mature in the bone marrow, was first identified. A patient with pernicious anemia has large numbers of immature, abnormal erythrocytes in his blood stream that are incapable of transporting oxygen. Prior to about 1925, pernicious anemia was almost invariably fatal, but scientists discovered that administering liver extracts stimulated the maturation of erythrocytes, thus identifying the state as a deficiency disease.

Subsequent research showed the involvement of two factors: an intrinsic factor present in the inner wall (lining) of the stomach and upper intestinal tract and an extrinsic factor present in the diet. The two factors were thought to be combined by the body to form an "antipernicious anemia" principle which was stored in the liver. Later research indicated that the extrinsic factor was vitamin B_{12} and this "antipernicious anemia" factor was found in the liver. Vitamin B_{12} is the only naturally occurring substance, necessary by the body, that contains cobalt—the generic name for the vitamin is cyanocobalamin. Treatment of pernicious anemia consists of administering adequate amounts of the vitamin. A potent therapeutic agent, vitamin B_{12} in doses of 30 mcg administered initially once every day for 5 to 10 days and then 100 to 200 mcg monthly often controls pernicious anemia.

In the erythrocyte, the protein globin is present as a part of the hemoglobin molecule. The bone marrow also synthesizes globin. The vitamin folic acid is necessary (along with vitamin B_{12}) for that synthesis to occur. Like vitamin B_{12}, (RDA: 3 mcg), folic acid is necessary in the diet, and a deficiency of either of these vitamins could result in anemia. The daily requirement of folic acid in the diet is about 0.4 mg (400 mcg).

Biochemical research indicates that hemoglobin transports oxygen efficiently only when it is properly arranged or "stacked" in the erythrocyte. A peculiar type of anemia, found almost exclusively in the black race, exists in which a large proportion of the erythrocytes are abnormal in shape, as well as in size. Instead of being normal disc-shaped structures, large numbers are crescent or "sickle" shaped, hence the name "sickle cell anemia." No drugs currently exist that are effective in treating this hereditary disease.

BLOOD CLOTTING MECHANISMS

Normally, the blood does not coagulate (clot) in the vascular system because of a balance between anticoagulant and procoagulant principles in the blood. When an injury to a vessel occurs, however, a chain of events begins that overcomes the anticoagulant influence and protects the body against blood loss. Several physiologic mechanisms act together to achieve this hemostasis (the prevention and control of hemorrhage). The integrity of the blood vessels and the fullness of tissues influence resistance to hemorrhage. Also, injury to blood vessels releases chemicals that cause constriction and retard the flow of blood. Thrombocytes (blood platelets) aggregate at injury loci and seal off leaking blood vessels. Finally, blood coagulation that occurs within damaged vessels and wounds prevents further bleeding. Vascular and platelet factors cause hemostasis by co-functioning with a number of blood components (Table 4.1).

Vascular factors are important in the consideration of trauma to tissues. Blood vessels, especially those that are superficial, are readily damaged and the resulting leakage produces black and blue bruise spots (ecchymosis). The extent to which blood flows from an injury site depends upon the type of surrounding tissue. For instance, the periorbital tissue offers little resistance to extravascular blood spread following trauma (as evidenced by the "black eye" after injury around the eye). Additionally, abnormal fragility of blood capillaries, as seen in punctate hemorrhage (petechiae) and ecchymosis, is characteristic of vitamin C deficiency. Thus, vitamin C may assist in the maintenance of capillary integrity and the normal resistance of capillary membranes.

Platelet factors are essential for hemostasis. Appearing within 1 to 2 seconds following damage to the blood vessel endothelium, thrombocytes adhere to the injured surface and form a dense aggregate. This is the first stage of blood clot formation. Platelets perform two main functions in hemostasis: they contribute substances that speed coagulation or constrict vessels and they function in blood clot shrinking (retraction).

Platelet aggregation is stimulated by adenosine diphosphate (ADP) released from the platelets when they come in contact with and adhere to collagen, capillary basement membranes, and subepithelial microfibrils. This reaction initiates blood clot formation in injured vessels.

Platelets are uniquely sensitive to the action of the thrombin enzyme that is formed during blood coagulation. Thrombin stimulates platelet aggregation and initiates morphologic changes in the platelets that eventually lead to their dissolution. These thrombin-induced platelet changes result in clot retraction.

Arachidonic acid, released from platelet phospholipids following injury, is responsible for platelet aggregation. Prostaglandins G_2 and H_2, formed from arachidonic acid, undergo further conversion to thromboxane A_2, a potent stimulator of platelet aggregation. Platelets also release lipoproteins and phospholipids that accelerate the formation of thrombin.

The concluding reactions and final stage in bleeding control occur within the injured vessel and in the wound. Table 4.2 lists the substances involved in blood coagulation; Figure 4.4 outlines the complex mechanisms involved. When a vessel is cut or damaged, the tissues surrounding the damaged area release thromboplastin, a substance that reacts with calcium in the blood to form an activator of prothrombin (another blood constituent).

Within seconds, the activated prothrombin yields thrombin if calcium salts are present. Thrombin causes yet another component of the blood, fibrinogen, to yield fibrin in the form of "threads." These develop a net at the site of the cut or injury that entraps erythrocytes, leukocytes, and thrombocytes to form a clot.

Also, blood clots commonly form in the vessels even in the absence of injury. When this occurs, the condition may be quite serious and sometimes fatal. To illustrate, atherosclerosis represents an accumulation or build up of cholesterol derivative on the lining of the arteries. Normally, the lining (endothelium) is very smooth, facilitating the passage of blood over it.

Table 4.1 BLOOD CLOTTING FACTORS.*

Factor	Name	Description
I	Fibrinogen	Synthesized in the liver. Soluble plasma protein. Precursor of fibrin, the solid strands of filaments that form the structure of the blood clot.
II	Prothrombin	Produced in the liver. Plasma protein. Vitamin K dependent. Precursor of thrombin, the proteolytic enzyme that acts on Factor I to form fibrin.
III	Thromboplastin	Released by injured body tissues. Lipoprotein. Triggers reactions in the extrinsic system that convert Factor II to thrombin.
IV	Calcium	Ions. Necessary for reactions that activate Factor II to produce thrombin and to form fibrin.
V	Proaccelerin	Plasma protein (globulin). Speeds the rate at which Factor II converts to thrombin.
VII	Proconvertin	Produced in the liver. Plasma protein. Vitamin K dependent. Speeds extrinsic system reactions involving Factors III and IX that convert Factor III to thrombin.
VIII	Factor (AHF); Antihemophilic Globulin (AHG)	Plasma protein. Works with Factor IX and a phospholipid released by blood platelets (Factor III) in the intrinsic pathway reactions that activate Factor II. Not present in cases of classic hemophilia (Hemophilia A).
IX	Christmas Factor; (PTC) Plasma Thromboplastin Component	Vitamin K-dependent. Works with Factor VIII and platelet Factor III in the presence of calcium ions in intrinsic pathway reactions that speed the reaction of Factor II to thrombin.
X	Stuart Factor	Produced in the liver in the presence of vitamin K. Plasma factor. Acts in both intrinsic and and extrinsic pathway interactions to produce a prothrombin-converting principle.
XI	Plasma Thromboplastin Antecedent	Plasma globulin. Activated by Factor XII. Helps speed the production of thrombin.
XII	Hageman Factor	Plasma factor. Helps trigger intrinsic system reactions. Activates Factor IX. May participate in inflammatory and clotting reactions.
XIII	Fibrin Stabilizing Factor	Plasma component. When activated by thrombin, makes fibrin stronger and capable of forming the gel that seals breaks in blood vessels.

*From Rodman, M.J., and Smith, D.W.: Pharmacology and Drug Therapy in Nursing. 2nd Ed. Philadelphia, J.B. Lippincott, 1982.

The somewhat rough atherosclerotic deposits, however, obstruct the flow of blood and also act as sites for clot formation. As part of the aging process, the arterial muscle sometimes becomes less elastic; this loss of elasticity coupled with thickening of the endothelium can serve as a site of clot formation.

Since neither the heart nor the brain can tol-

CIRCULATORY/RETICULOENDOTHELIAL SYSTEM

Table 4.2 SUBSTANCES INVOLVED IN BLOOD COAGULATION.*

Numeric designation	Common name	Dependent on vitamin K	Pathway: Intrinsic/	Extrinsic
I	Fibrinogen		+	+
II	Prothrombin	+	+	+
III	Tissue factor			+
IV	Calcium		+	+
V	Proaccelerin		+	+
VII	Proconvertin (SPCA)	+		+
VIII	Antihemophilic factor (AHF)		+	
IX	Christmas factor (PTC)	+	+	
X	Stuart factor	+	+	+
XI	Plasma thromboplastin antecedent (PTA)		+	
XII	Hageman factor		+	
XIII	Fibrin-stabilizing factor		+	+

* From Conley, C.L.: Hemostasis. In Medical Physiology. 14th Ed. Edited by V.B. Mountcastle. St. Louis, C.V. Mosby, 1980.

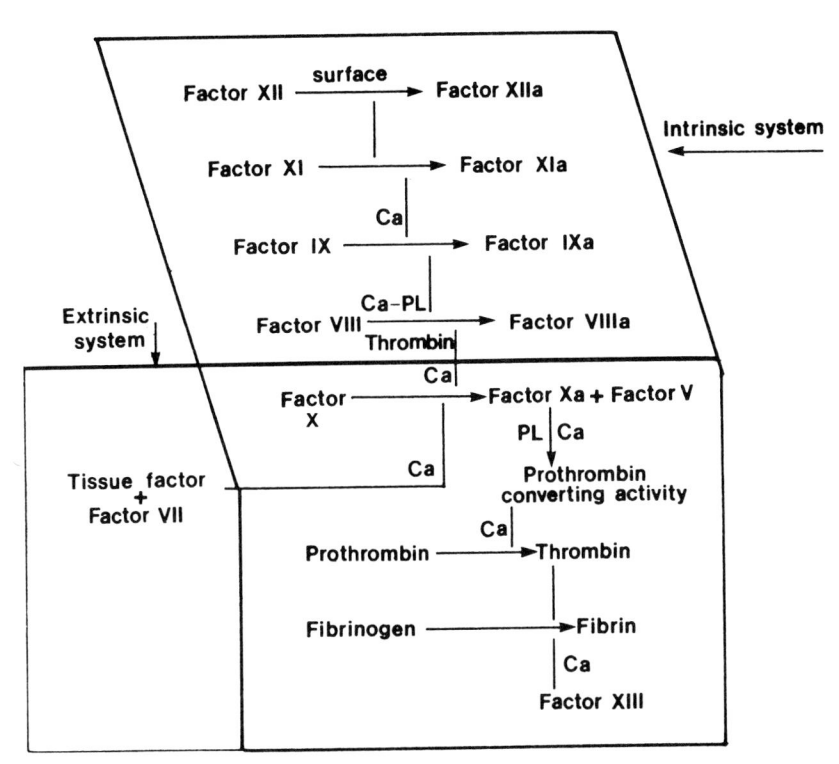

Fig. 4.4 Scheme of blood coagulation. (Modified from Williams, W.J.: Clinical application of our new knowledge of blood coagulation. Res Staff Phys, 15:39, 1969. Medical Pharmacology. 11th Ed. St. Louis, C.V. Mosby, 1984.)

erate an oxygen debt, a clot formed in a vessel supplying either of these organs produces serious consequences. The lining of a vein, for undetermined reasons, sometimes becomes inflamed and a clot may form at the inflammation site. This condition, i.e., phlebitis, is serious because if the clot is dislodged, it travels the venous system to the heart and then to the lungs. A clot attached to the vessel wall is called a "thrombus"; upon dislodgement and subsequent vessel (artery) blockage, it is termed an "embolism."

A number of drugs prolong the clotting process. Heparin can be isolated from various tissues, usually the lungs of cattle; when administered parenterally, it evokes a pronounced anticoagulant effect. Heparin acts by preventing the conversion of prothrombin to thrombin and the conversion of fibrinogen to fibrin. Heparin also inhibits the clumping together of blood platelets.

In 1929, Dam, a scientist in Denmark, showed that chicks fed a certain synthetic diet developed hemorrhage in the intestinal tract. By adding alfalfa to the diet, Dam found that the hemorrhage no longer occurred; he then postulated that alfalfa contained a "Koagulation vitamin" that he named vitamin K. Later studies determined that the liver synthesizes prothrombin only in the presence of adequate amounts of vitamin K. Over 50 years ago, Schofield reported that spoiled sweet clover fed to cattle over a period of a week or so caused hemorrhage under the animals' skin. Investigation revealed that the spoiled sweet clover contained a substance named dicumarol that evokes a powerful anticoagulant effect that reaches its maximum potency after administration for several days. Dicumarol antagonizes vitamin K by interfering with the utilization of the vitamin by the liver. Vitamin K deficiency seldom exists in adults because the bacteria that normally inhabit the adult bowel synthesize vitamin K; newborn infants, however, are sometimes deficient in the vitamin. Aspirin, taken for prolonged periods in fairly high doses, also interferes with vitamin K utilization and thus has an anticoagulant effect.

A rare disorder of blood clotting occurs in those who suffer from hemophilia, an inherited disease. (This condition is somewhat common in members of certain European royal families, possibly due to the wide practice of intermarriage for political reasons that unfortunately led to transmission of the gene responsible for the disease to the offspring.) The blood of these patients is deficient in the antihemophilia factor, necessary for clotting to occur. Without adequate treatment, hemophilic patients may bleed to death from even a very minor cut. Since the antihemophilia factor can be isolated, it is administered to hemophiliacs when they need it.

DISEASES INVOLVING THE BLOOD ELEMENTS AND CLOTTING MECHANISMS

Blood disorders may be either mild, readily reversible deficiencies in blood components or complex malignant neoplastic diseases. Several blood diseases have a genetic basis (e.g., hemophilia and some types of hyperlipoproteinemia), others are diet-related (e.g., iron deficiency anemia), and some are of unknown pathophysiology (e.g., leukemia).

ERYTHROCYTE DISORDERS

Erythrocyte disorders include the various anemias and polycythemia vera.

ANEMIAS

Anemia is a condition in which the concentration of hemoglobin is below the normal for the age and sex of the patient. There is usually a reduction in the number and volume of red blood cells. Whereas a fall of the hemoglobin values to 60% of normal may signal a few symptoms of anemia, a reduction to approximately 40% of normal is always accompanied by severe anemia.

Anemia may result from imperfect nutrition, wasting disease, defective absorption processes, or direct loss of blood. Symptoms of anemia mainly involve the central nervous and cardiovascular systems and include paleness of the skin and mucous membranes, loss of energy, and palpitations.

In severe anemia, symptoms may include faintness, drowsiness, and clouding of consciousness. Neurologic impact is evidenced by giddiness, headache, tinnitis, and paresthesias. The major influence of anemia on the cardiovascular system is an increase in cardiac output to compensate for the deprivation of tissue oxygenation due to a lack of hemoglobin. The diversion of blood from the skin to more vital organs (such as the liver and kidneys) results in pallor, a characteristic of anemia.

Iron Deficiency Anemia. The total amount of iron in the body ranges from 2 to 6 g. Iron in the body is found principally as a component of the hemoglobin molecule. Normal blood contains about 15 g of hemoglobin per 100 ml of blood. While ferritin and transferrin bind significant amounts of iron, the cytochrome enzymes and myoglobin contain only traces of the element. The iron content of blood is about 500 mg/L of blood. Of the total iron present in the body, approximately 80% is found in the hemoglobin of red blood cells (erythrocytes).

Erythrocytes are broken down at a steady rate with a life span of approximately 120 days. Hemoglobin that is released from the erythrocyte degradation is recycled; thus, the daily iron requirement is low. Menstruation and pregnancy increase the daily iron requirement.

Iron requirements vary as adult men and postmenopausal women require only about 10 mg of iron (dietary) to maintain iron stores. Premenopausal females, adolescents, and children require 15 to 20 mg of dietary iron daily. The increased requirement results from menstrual blood loss in adult premenopausal women and from the rapid growth rate with accompanying increases in the total erythrocytes in children and adolescents. Iron deficiency anemia develops far more readily in these high-need groups. When this condition develops in adult men or postmenopausal females (low-need groups), a more serious disorder may be present necessitating a greater degree of concern.

Bleeding ulcers, hemorrhoids, excessive menstruation, and gastrointestinal cancer can result in iron deficiency anemia. Diets not containing any iron (strict vegetarian diets and those with no iron-containing vegetables) eventually lead to iron deficiency anemia. Rarely, in certain ethnic groups, compulsive eating of starch or pica (a perverted appetite marked by a craving for unnatural food or substances) results in anemia.

A common problem in infants and toddlers is milk anemia, a condition in which cow's milk is the primary foodstuff in the diet. Although breast-fed infants receive some iron from their mother's milk, they still require iron supplementation.

The diagnosis of iron deficiency anemia is made, in addition to symptomatology, on the basis of a low erythrocyte count, decreased blood hemoglobin, and particularly low corpuscular volume. Iron deficiency anemia is thus characterized by small erythrocytes (microcytic) and a low hemoglobin (hypochromic) value. The symptoms of iron deficiency anemia (especially the subjective ones) improve rapidly with iron therapy. A standard practice in treating iron deficiency anemia is continuation of iron therapy until the deficient iron stores are replenished to avoid relapse. This situation contrasts sharply with the hemolytic anemias in which iron stores are usually high. Because of the possibility of iron toxicity, a differential diagnosis for anemia is important. This toxicity potential also limits iron's "tonic" use for nonspecific low energy and lassitude.

Pernicious Anemia (Addisonian Anemia). Pernicious anemia, a condition that usually affects adults, results when the gastric mucosa fails to secrete adequate intrinsic factor causing malabsorption of vitamin B_{12}. Until 1926, when liver was introduced as a palliative treatment, pernicious anemia was incurable. Vitamin B_{12} is now recognized as the extrinsic factor in Castle's hypothesis regarding pernicious anemia. The intrinsic factor of Castle's theory is a gastric mucoprotein that is responsible for the absorption of dietary vitamin B_{12}. In the majority of pernicious anemia cases (an autoimmune disease), plasma antibodies direct against intrinsic factor and a fraction of the gastric parietal cells that secrete the intrinsic factor are detectable.

Cyanocobalamin is one of the forms of vitamin B_{12} that was first isolated from the liver. Chemically, cyanocobalamin is characterized by a tetrapyrrole nucleus in which a cobalt atom exists in a keystone position (as does iron in the hemoglobin molecule).

The metabolic functions of vitamin B_{12} include an important role in the synthesis of purine and pyrimidine bases and their incorporation into deoxyribonucleic acid (DNA). Erythropoiesis (formation of red blood cells) requires large amounts since 10 to 20 g of red blood cells are formed daily. A deficiency in vitamin B_{12} results in faulty cell division and inhibition of erythrocyte maturation. The bone marrow contains abnormal cells called megaloblasts (in place of normoblasts); these are precursors of macrocytes instead of functional erythrocytes. Thus, the erythrocyte count is low and the hemoglobin concentration is reduced. However, in this condition, the mean corpuscular hemoglobin concentration (MCHC) is normal, and the mean amount of hemoglobin (MCH) per erythrocyte is higher than normal. The descriptive term macrocytic (large cell) hyperchromic (high hemoglobin) anemia aptly characterizes vitamin B_{12} deficient anemia.

Vitamin B_{12} is also necessary for maintaining nerve cell integrity. A deficiency in this vitamin leads to degeneration of the axons of peripheral nerves and of axons in the pyramidal tracts of the spinal cord.

Folic Acid Deficiency Anemia. Folic acid, first isolated from spinach, is found in leafy green plants (i.e., folia). Chemically, folic acid is pteroylglutamic acid. In plants, folic acid is conjugated with polyglutamate, which is split off by hydrolysis in the intestinal tract. Other good sources of folic acid are liver and kidney.

Intestinal absorption of folic acid is either an active or passive process depending upon the concentration of the vitamin. If the folic acid concentration is low, active energy-requiring mechanisms operate, whereas after ingestion of the pure vitamin, passive diffusion predominates. Folic acid synthesized by micro-organisms in the human intestinal tract contributes to the intake of the vitamin.

Although the daily requirement of folic acid is unknown, the recommended daily intake of 0.4 mg probably provides a multiple safety margin. The biochemical reactions in which folic acid participates are important in the synthesis of DNA. Folic acid primarily assists in the formation of purine and pyrimidine nucleotides. The vitamin folic acid is the precursor of the coenzyme tetrahydrofolate. An important coenzyme in the transfer of single carbon units, tetrahydrofolate has extensive metabolic roles and interactions (Figure 4.5).

Folic acid deficiency damages tissues in which DNA synthesis and turnover are rapid. These sensitive tissues include the hematopoietic tissues, gastrointestinal tract mucosa, and the developing embryo. Requirements for folic acid increase with rapid multiplication of cells (for example, in pregnancy or in neoplastic disease—leukemia). Reserves of folic acid in the body, about 15 mg, sufficiently last for 2 to 4 months before clinical symptoms of deficiency appear.

Although the signs and symptoms of folic acid deficiency anemia resemble those of pernicious anemia, an important difference is the absence of demyelination disease in nerve fibers. A major contrast to pernicious anemia is the absence of neurologic symptoms. Folic acid deficiency anemia patients experience fatigue and lethargy; their gastric mucosa and digestion are usually normal.

Dietary deficiency is a major cause of folic acid deficiency anemia. Alcohol abuse often results in folic acid deficiency, which is probably a consequence of poor diet, increased folic acid utilization, and impaired absorption due to gastrointestinal damage.

Drug-induced folic acid deficiency may also cause this form of anemia. Folic acid reductase inhibition by methotrexate and aminopterin could result in tetrahydrofolate deficiency. Pyrimethamine and trimethoprim also block the conversion of folic acid to tetrahydrofolate by inhibiting the reductase enzymes. Deficiency disorders of this type are treated with folinic acid (leucovorin) since folinic acid circumvents the drug blockade that prevents folic acid utilization. Additionally, certain anticonvulsant drugs (such as phenytoin and primidone) inhibit the liberation of folic acid from the poly-

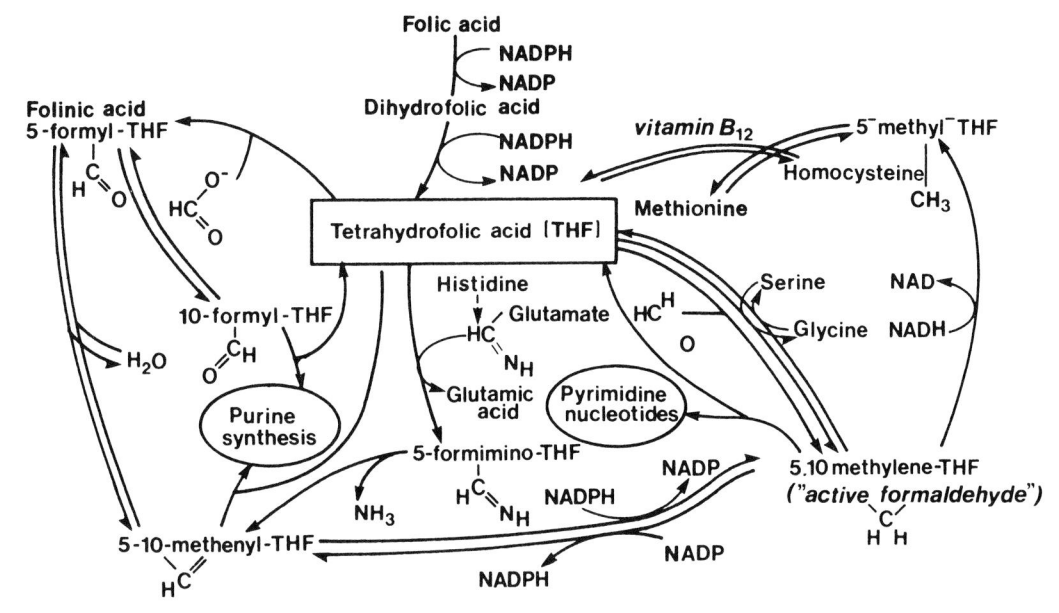

Fig. 4.5 Metabolic roles of THF acid. (From Bowman, W.C., and Rand, M.J.: Textbook of Pharmacology. 2nd Ed. Oxford, Blackwell Scientific Publications, 1980.)

glutamate conjugates in vegetables, resulting in deficient folic acid absorption.

In megaloblastic macrocytic anemia due to folic acid deficiency, daily doses of folic acid rapidly return the blood profile to a normal range. Folic acid is never given alone unless vitamin B_{12} deficiency has been ruled out. The neurologic defects associated with pernicious anemia are not corrected by folic acid. However, the correction of the blood picture together with the general sense of well-being experienced by the patient receiving folic acid may mask the progressive neurologic damage of the disease.

Pyridoxine-responsive Anemia. Pyridoxine is found in significant amounts in yeast, liver, rice, bran, and wheat germ. An impairment in hemoglobin synthesis is characteristic of pyridoxine-responsive anemia.

The active form of pyridoxine, pyridoxal phosphate, is a coenzyme in decarboxylation reactions. In pyridoxine deficiency, the synthesis of protoporphyrin (heme) is impaired and excess iron accumulates in siderotic granules. Normoblasts containing these siderotic granules are called sideroblasts. Siderotic anemia thus involves a derangement in heme synthesis in which iron stores of the reticuloendothelial tissues almost always increase and bone marrow normoblasts contain iron (sideroblasts).

Pyridoxine deficiency may result from a general vitamin deficiency in an inadequate dietary intake or from gastrointestinal malabsorption of the vitamin. Certain antitubercular drugs, such as isoniazid and aminosalicylic acid, may produce pyridoxine deficiency and resultant sideroblastosis after long-term treatment. Cycloserine and pyrazinamide frequently cause sideroblastic anemia.

Polycythemia Vera. An excessive increase in the number of red blood cells characterizes polycythemia vera, a disorder of unknown etiology. Patients with this disease are often cyanotic and have a feeling of tension in the head, a florid complexion, and a tendency toward nosebleed. Hypertension and increased blood viscosity may result in congestive heart failure (CHF). Red cell counts range from 6 to 10 million per cu mm with corresponding elevations in hemoglobin and hematocrit values. A leukemia occurs with a white cell count as high as 80 thousand per cu mm. About ⅓ of the fatalities from polycythemia vera result from thrombotic complications, usually in the brain or heart. Leukemia complications contribute to deaths in about 15% of all polycythemia vera patients.

LEUKOCYTE DISORDERS

The most prevalent diseases involving leukocytes encompass the malignant proliferative diseases. This category includes the lymphomas, leukemias, and dysproteinoses. Hodgkin's disease, initially considered as a form of lymphoma, is characterized by abnormal lymphoid tissue.

LYMPHOMAS

Lymphomas are characterized by proliferation of native cells within lymphoid tissue; these cells include lymphocytes, histiocytes, or reticular stem cells. Although lymphomas, present in lymphoid tissue, may occur anywhere in the body, they usually arise within the lymph nodes. Lymphomas are most common between the ages of 50 and 70 years and form more frequently in men than in women.

Certain conditions apparently increase the risk of lymphoma formation. Among these are renal transplantation, immunosuppressive drug therapy, congenital immune deficiencies, and autoimmune diseases such as systemic lupus erythematosus (SLE).

Lymphoma formation probably involves a dual-stimulus mechanism. An unknown immune stimulus is first required, followed sometime later by a neoplastic change. One hypothesis indicates that the initiating pathogenesis is an interference in the normal negative feedback control of lymphoproliferation.

Patients with lymphomas are otherwise healthy individuals with a painless enlargement of one or more lymph nodes. Lymphomas usually occur in the cervical lymphatic node chain. Hepatosplenomegaly (enlargement of the liver and spleen) occasionally indicates extranodal involvement at this stage. In more advanced cases, fever, weight loss, weakness, and anemia are present. Differentiated lymphocytic lymphoma may represent the tissue expression of chronic lymphocytic leukemia. In fact, a usual progressive course of development of differentiated lymphocytic lymphoma is into chronic lymphocytic leukemia.

Manifestations of advanced widespread lymphoma include diarrhea, pain and pathologic bone involvement, and both peripheral and central nervous system (CNS) involvement.

Burkitt's lymphoma, the first human cancer strongly linked to a specific virus, usually manifests itself as a large maxillary tumor mass. This lymphoma is a common form of cancer found in central African children although sporadic cases occur in other areas, including the United States.

LEUKEMIA

A flooding of the blood and bone marrow with leukocytes characterizes leukemia. White cells, many of which are morphologically immature, are found in the circulating blood. A diffuse replacement of the bone marrow by these cells also occurs. Infiltration of the liver, spleen, and lymph nodes heralds its metastasis. Leukemia, especially devastating to children, causes most of the deaths from white cell disorders.

Leukemia is divided into four main forms: acute, chronic, acute myelogenous, and chronic myelogenous. Minimal spleen enlargement characterizes acute lymphocytic leukemia (ALL). This type of leukemia occurs primarily in children and if untreated is usually fatal within 4 months. Chronic lymphocytic leukemia (CLL) occurs mainly in the elderly; these patients exhibit considerable hepatosplenomegaly, as well as extensive lymph node swelling. Acute myelogenous leukemia (AML) occurs in all ages in a fairly uniform distribution. The accumulation of immature granulocytes morphologically characterizes AML. Also, enlargement of the liver and spleen is not remarkable and swelling of the lymph nodes may be absent. Chronic myelogenous leukemia (CML), characterized by granulocyte involvement, has a strong genetic association. Enlargement of the spleen is a common clinical finding in CML, a disease that occurs primarily in middle-age. In leukemia, the cause of death is usually hemorrhage (often intracranial) or extensive bacterial superinfections.

The peripheral white cell count in acute leukemia is typically between 30,000 to 100,000 cells per cu mm. Acute forms of leukemia usually have a rapid onset with fever, profound weakness, and lethargy. Enlargement of the liver, spleen, and lymph nodes are not always apparent. Joint and bone pain may reflect bone infiltration. Recurrent bleeding and bacterial infection indicate the untreated course of the disease.

Extreme elevations of the circulating white cells are found in the chronic leukemias. White cell counts approximating 1,000,000 cells per cu mm are sometimes noted. Chronic leukemia has a more insidious onset in which the patient usually experiences an extended period of vague feelings of fatigue with concurrent weight loss. Spleen enlargement is sometimes the first clinical indication of chronic leukemias. Anemia, hemorrhages, or recurrent intractable infections are usual late developments of chronic leukemia.

DYSPROTEINOSES

Dysproteinoses (plasma cell dyscrasias) are manifested by the expansion of a single colony of genetically identical cells derived from a single cell of asexual division (clone) that secrete an antibody (immunoglobulin). Serum levels of a single homogeneous immunoglobulin or its fragments increase as a result of this secretion.

These diseases occur most frequently in middle-aged to elderly individuals, especially those exposed to a prolonged antigenic stimulus, such as chronic cholecystitis, tuberculosis, osteomyelitis, or nonspecific pneumonitis. Three major disorders are classified as dysproteinoses: multiple myeloma and its variants, Waldenstrom's macroglobulinemia, and heavy chain disease.

Multiple myeloma, the most frequently occurring of the dysproteinoses, consists of multifocal erosive plasma cell tumors scattered throughout the skeletal system. Two variants of multiple myeloma (solitary myeloma and soft tissue plasmacytoma) may represent early stages of the disease. Solitary myeloma refers to the presence of only a single skeletal lesion. Soft tissue plasmacytoma is a tumor usually appearing in the mouth and nose region. Plasma cell leukemia is a rare form of multiple myeloma in which neoplastic cells flood the circulating system.

Waldenstrom's macroglobulinemia is characterized by a limited infiltration of the bone marrow, spleen, liver, and lymph nodes by precursors of plasma cells. No focal erosive lesions develop in the skeletal system.

Heavy chain disease is a plasma cell dyscrasia that affects mainly the lymphoid tissue of the small intestine and adjacent mesentery.

Multiple myeloma apparently requires a dual stimulus for its development. The first influence is evidently prolonged antigenic exposure. This precedes the oncogenic event leading to neoplastic progression.

Clinical recognition of multiple myeloma usually occurs by patient complaints of bone and joint pain due to the skeletal lesions. This pain may only become a symptom after 10 to 20 years of asymptomatic disease. Frequently associated symptoms include anemia, fatigue, bleeding, and a predisposition to infections. Blood coagulation defects possibly result from an interaction between the myeloma immunoproteins and one of the clotting factors (Factor V or VII or prothrombin). An inability to produce normal gamma globulins evidently increases the incidence of bacterial infections.

The course of multiple myeloma is quite variable. Abnormal gamma globulins are often present for years without myeloma development. Generally, however, a multiple myeloma shows a progressive worsening with development of extensive bone lesions. Progressive cachexia, renal failure, hemorrhage, or infection usually cause death from multiple myeloma.

HODGKIN'S DISEASE

Hodgkin's disease apparently represents an interaction between neoplasia initiation and the body's defensive mechanisms. The disease is characterized by distinctive cells (Reed-Sternberg, R-S) that are present in lymphoid tissue accompanied by a variable leukocytic and connective tissue reaction. Clinically and morphologically, it represents a hybrid symptomatology between chronic infection and malignant tumor.

The clinical picture and progression of Hodgkin's disease resemble that of the lymphomas. Painless enlargement of the affected lymph nodes precedes weight loss, weakness, fever, night sweats, pruritus, and anemia. The overall prognosis is usually better than that of the lymphomas.

ACQUIRED IMMUNE DEFICIENCY SYNDROME (AIDS)

Approximately 35,000 people in the United States developed AIDS during the first 5 years of the present epidemic, circa 1980. Over the next 5 years, the U.S. Public Health Service estimates that more than 235,000 new cases will occur; of this number, most are presently infected with the virus.

The AIDS virus, human immunodeficiency virus (HIV), is transmitted by sexual contact, through contaminated blood or blood platelets, and to children born to infected mothers. Commonly associated with cells (such as infected T lymphocytes or macrophages), the virus is found in blood, semen, vaginal secretions, saliva, sweat, tears, and other body tissues, including brain and skin.

Since the predominant method of AIDS transmission is sexual contact, those persons with multiple sexual partners are at great risk to develop the disease. Homosexual men are statistically a high risk group, as determined in the numbers presently affected by AIDS. The incubation period is as long as 5 years.

In AIDS, host resistance is lost, especially the body's ability to destroy or inactivate injurious influences and to repair the resultant injury. Glomeruli, small blood vessels, and joint tissues are particularly susceptible. AIDS is characterized by a deficiency in "T-helper cells," which are crucial to the body's immune system. Conditions that are moderately or highly associated with the loss of body immunity are present in the clinical disease. These conditions include Kaposi's sarcoma, pneumonia caused by pneumocystis carinii, and other so-called "opportunistic infections."

Neurologic problems are common in AIDS patients, and as many as 3 out of 5 patients are predicted to develop dementia. Recent results suggest that the retrovirus that causes AIDS enters the brain to attack specific areas and cells located there. The virus is found most often in the white cells in the brain and in multinucleated giant cells derived from macrophages. Still another characteristic of AIDS is hepatic involvement with resultant complete liver breakdown.

Screening tests for AIDS virus, which are intended mainly for screening blood donors, are now available. An AIDS vaccine will probably not be available for general use before 1990, but limited testing is in progress. A safe and effective antiviral agent to treat AIDS is not likely to be available for several years.

HEMORRHAGIC DISORDERS

Several factors can cause abnormal hemorrhage; among these are increased fragility of blood vessels, platelet deficiency or dysfunction, and abnormalities in the clotting mechanisms.

Increased fragility of the blood vessels occurs with scurvy (severe vitamin C deficiency) and certain infections such as meningococcemia, infectious endocarditis, rickettsial diseases, and typhoid fever. A vascular fragility-based hemorrhagic diathesis is characterized by spontaneous petechial and ecchymotic spots on the skin and mucous membranes, as well as a positive tourniquet test. A blood scan reveals a normal platelet count, bleeding time, and coagulation time.

Deficiencies of platelets (thrombocytopenia) are important causes of bleeding disorders. Bone marrow suppression for various reasons (idiopathic, myelotoxin, and drugs) results in an excessive hemorrhagic phenomenon. Thrombocytopenia and platelet dysfunction resemble increased capillary fragility and are characterized by petechiae and ecchymoses, as well as easy bruising, nosebleeds, excessive bleeding from minor trauma, and menorrhagia. With these conditions, the tourniquet test is positive and coagulation time is in a normal range. In contrast to excessive vascular fragility, however, the bleeding time is prolonged.

A bleeding disorder based entirely on a derangement in clotting mechanisms differs from vascular or platelet dysfunctions in a number of ways. Petechiae and ecchymoses are usually absent, as is evidence of bleeding from minor trauma. The coagulant time is usually prolonged, whereas the bleeding time range is normal. Massive bleeding may follow surgical procedures, and hemorrhage into joints is characteristic.

Disseminated intravascular coagulation (DIC) is a hemorrhagic diathesis that involves both platelets and the clotting factors. This acute, subacute, or chronic disorder is characterized by intravascular fibrin deposition within arterioles and capillaries with resultant depletion of clotting factors and platelets. DIC most commonly results from activation of either the extrinsic or intrinsic coagulation system. The clinical profile of DIC is paradoxical as a bleeding tendency occurs in the presence of extensive fibrin formation and coagulation. The prognosis of DIC is variable and depends upon the cause and extent of intravascular clotting. In some cases, the DIC is self-limiting; in others, heparin treatment results in prompt improvement. Unfortunately, fatalities often occur within days after the development of the disorder.

HYPERLIPOPROTEINEMIAS

Frederickson classified the various forms into five major types (Types I-V); see Table 4.3.

Type I. An absence of lipoprotein lipase characterizes this rare congenital disorder. The biochemical error (lack of lipoprotein lipase) re-

Table 4.3 TYPES OF HYPERLIPOPROTEINEMIA.*

Type	I	II	III	IV	V
	Familial hyperchylomicroanemia	Familial hypercholesterolanemia	Broad-beta disease	Carbohydrate-induced hyperlipidemia	Mixed hyperlipoproteinemia
Etiology:	Inherited	Type IIA: homozygous; Type IIIB: heterozygous predisposition	Predominantly inherited	Mostly secondary or acquired	Inherited, secondary or acquired
Triglyceride:	Markedly increased	Normal or slightly increased	Slightly to moderately increased	Moderately increased	Moderately increased
Cholesterol:	Normal	Markedly increased	Moderately increased	Slightly increased	Moderately increased
Chylomicrons:	Markedly increased	Normal	Normal	Normal	Markedly increased
VLDL:	Normal	Low or slightly increased	Moderately increased	Very markedly increased	Moderately increased
LDL:	Normal	Moderately increased	Increased and abnormal	Normal	Normal
Relative frequency:	Rare (0.1)**	Common (45–55)**	Uncommon (2–5)**	Common (35–50)**	Fairly common (5–10)**

* From Bowman, W.C., and Rand, M.J.: Textbook of Pharmacology. 2nd Ed. Oxford, Blackwell Scientific Publications, 1980.
** Relative percentage incidence of hyperlipoproteinemia.

sults in an extended prolongation of the half-life of chylomicrons in the circulation.

Yellow chylomicron deposits in the skin (xanthomata) are common in Type I hyperlipoproteinemia. In addition, the liver and spleen are frequently enlarged. A diet with reduced intake of long-chain fatty acids reduces the amount of circulating chylomicrons.

Type II. Two subgroups are in familial Type II hyperlipoproteinemia. Type IIA, the smallest subgroup, is characterized by a specific increase in beta-lipoproteins (LDL). The blood levels of VLDLs (pre-beta-lipoproteins) are usually within a normal range. Elevated blood levels of cholesterol and LDLs are not lowered by a dietary restriction of fat. Type IIB represents a genetically determined predisposition for hyperlipoproteinemia that is reinforced by a high-fat diet, low thyroid activity, high blood pressure, and ischemic heart disease.

Acute myocardial infarction in young adults inevitably occurs in association with either Type IIA or IIB familial hyperlipoproteinemia.

Type III. Elevated circulating levels of VLDLs and LDLs are present in this form of hyperlipoproteinemia, an uncommon familial disorder. Xanthomata, atherosclerosis, and glucose intolerance characterize Type III hyperlipoproteinemia.

Type IV. This common form of hyperlipoproteinemia is found in over 1 in 10 middle-aged males who have a standard North American diet and lifestyle. Type IV hyperlipoproteinemia ordinarily occurs in conjunction with obesity, glucose intolerance, and high blood uric acid levels. In this type of hyperlipoproteinemia, the VLDL is the only lipoprotein class significantly and consistently elevated.

Xanthomata, diabetes mellitus, gouty arthritis, atherosclerosis, ischemic heart disease, and hypertension frequently occur with Type IV hyperlipoproteinemia.

Type V. Type V hyperlipoproteinemia is commonly found as a secondary disorder to diabetes mellitus, pancreatitis, or nephrotic syndrome. This condition may also occur as a reversible disorder in alcohol abuse. Hypertension is present in about 1 in 3 Type V hyperlipoproteinemia patients, and ischemic heart disease occurs in approximately 25% of the patients with this disorder.

DRUGS AFFECTING THE CIRCULATORY/ RETICULOENDOTHELIAL SYSTEM

These drugs range from simple replacement therapy (such as with iron products) to complex combination regimens affecting multiple processes (for example, antineoplastic polytherapy).

DRUGS USED IN THE TREATMENT OF THE ANEMIAS

These drugs (Tables 4.4, 4.5) supply elements that are necessary in the synthesis of hemoglobin and/or erythrocytes.

DRUGS THAT AFFECT IRON DEFICIENCY ANEMIA

Supplying adequate iron corrects the consequences of iron deficiency anemia. Ferrous salts are the most commonly used forms of oral iron.

Table 4.4. IRON-CONTAINING PRODUCTS.

Available products	Trade names	Daily dosage range
Oral:		
Ferrous fumarate	Ircon; Feostat; others	100–325 mg
Ferrous gluconate	Fergon; Simron; Ferralet	same as above
Ferrous sulfate	Mol-Iron; Fer-Iron; others	same as above
Ferrous sulfate exsiccated	Feosol; Fer-In-Sol; others	Dosage is about ⅔ of the above
Parenteral:		
Iron Dextran	Imferon; Feostat; Irodex	See manufacturer's directions

Table 4.5. HEMATOPOIETIC VITAMINS AND RELATED SUBSTANCES.

Available products	Trade names	Daily dosage range
Cyanocobalamin, crystalline	Berubigen; Rubramin; Betalin 12; Redisol; others	Orally, IM, or SC in variable doses
Folic acid	Folvite	IV, orally, IM, or SC, 0.4 mg daily
Hydroxocobalamin, crystalline	AlphaRedisol; Alphamin; Droxomin	IM, 30 mcg/day for 5 days, followed by 100–200 mcg monthly
Leucovorin calcium	Wellcovorin	1 mg daily IM

The ferrous salts of organic acids are evidently less irritating to the gastrointestinal mucosa than are the salts of inorganic acids. Ferric iron chelates may reduce the astringent and irritant effect of orally administered iron. Oral iron preparations often consist of complex mixtures of one or more vitamins (ordinarily vitamin C) and trace metals.

Parenteral iron preparations are available for patients who are intolerant to oral iron products. Patients with defective iron gastrointestinal absorption (or those characteristically unreliable in their patient compliance) may also benefit from parenteral iron administration.

Oral Iron Preparations. Commonly used oral iron supplements are ferrous sulfate, ferrous fumarate, ferrous gluconate, and iron-polysaccharide.

Mechanism of Action. Iron occupies the keystone position in the hemoglobin molecule and adequate amounts of hemoglobin are necessary for effective erythropoiesis and the resultant oxygen-transporting capacity of the blood. Iron also serves a similar function in myoglobin, as well as being a cofactor in cytochrome enzymes.

Clinical Indications. Iron preparations are indicated in the prevention and treatment of iron deficiency conditions that may result from inadequate diet, malabsorption, pregnancy, and/or blood loss.

Adverse Effects/Precautions. Oral iron preparations sometimes produce gastrointestinal irritation, anorexia, nausea, vomiting, constipation, and diarrhea. Taking iron salts often produces stools that appear darker in color or black. Iron-containing liquids may stain teeth.

Early signs of iron overdose are diarrhea, nausea, stomach pain, and emesis (occasionally hematemesis). Late signs of iron poisoning include bluish-colored lips, fingernails, and the palms of hands; drowsiness; pale, clammy skin; unusual tiredness and/or weakness; and a weak and unusually fast heartbeat.

Iron Dextran. Iron dextran, a colloidal preparation, contains a complex of ferric hydroxide with dextran.

Mechanism of Action. Iron dextran must first be phagocytized by reticuloendothelial (RE) cells. Dissociation of the iron dextran by the RE system releases the ferric ion. Transferrin then transports the ferric ion to sites where it is incorporated in hemoglobin. Some of the liberated ferric ion returns to the plasma and becomes available to erythroid marrow. Most of the ferric ion remains trapped within the reticuloendothelial cell where the deposits gradually convert into a utilizable form of iron.

IM administration of iron dextran elevates plasma iron concentration for days (up to two weeks). Of the IM iron dextran dose, 10 to 50% is fixed locally in tissues for many months.

Clinical Indications. Iron dextran is used in the treatment of iron deficiency anemia. Intramuscular or intravenous iron injections are generally recommended only for patients with clinically demonstrable iron deficiency anemia and those in whom oral iron preparations are unsatisfactory.

Adverse Effects/Precautions. Hypersensitivity reactions, including dyspnea, urticaria, fever, and allergic purpura, have been reported. Variable degrees of soreness and irritation at injection sites are frequent patient complaints. Also, fatal anaphylaxis has followed the parenteral use of iron dextran. Patients with iron deficiency anemia and rheumatoid arthritis may have an acute worsening of joint pain and swelling following IV administration of iron dextran.

DRUGS AFFECTING PERNICIOUS ANEMIA

Vitamin B_{12} (see Table 4.5) corrects the neurologic and hematologic manifestations of pernicious anemia.

Cyanocobalamin. Cyanocobalamin is a synthetic form of vitamin B_{12}.

Mechanism of Action. Cyanocobalamin functions in methylation reactions associated with nucleic acid and protein synthesis (Figure 4.6). The metabolic roles of vitamin B_{12} and folic acid are exquisitely interwoven. Vitamin B_{12} contributes to erythropoiesis by activating folic acid coenzymes. For example, a major physiologic role of cyanocobalamin is in the regeneration of tetrahydrofolic acid ($H_4PteGLu_1$) from methyltetrahydrofolic acid ($CH_3H_4PteGLu_1$) by homocysteine transmethylation.

Vitamin B_{12} is both the extrinsic factor and the erythrocyte maturation factor in pernicious anemia etiology. Tissues with the greatest cell turnover, such as those responsible for hematopoiesis, show the most dramatic changes when vitamin B_{12} and folic acid are deficient. By increasing DNA synthesis, vitamin B_{12} and folic acid correct the megaloblastosis seen in pernicious anemia. The nucleic acid pathway affected by vitamin B_{12} is the formation of DNA thymine from deoxyuridylate (dUMP).

A reduction in the rate of the dUMP to thymidylate (dTMP) reaction impairs DNA synthesis and a resultant megaloblastic anemia occurs in patients deficient in either vitamin B_{12} or folic acid. In vitamin B_{12} deficiency, methyltetrahydrofolate ($CH_3H_4PteGLu_1$) is trapped by the lack of vitamin B_{12} to accept the donated methyl group in the dUMP to dTMP reaction.

Intracellular vitamin B_{12} is present as active coenzymes in methyl group interactions. Methylcobalamin is a methyl group donor for the conversion of homocysteine to methionine. This reaction is coupled to the formation of tetrahydrofolate ($H_4PteGlu_1$) from methyltetrahydrofolate ($CH_3H_4PTeGLu_1$). Deoxyadeno-

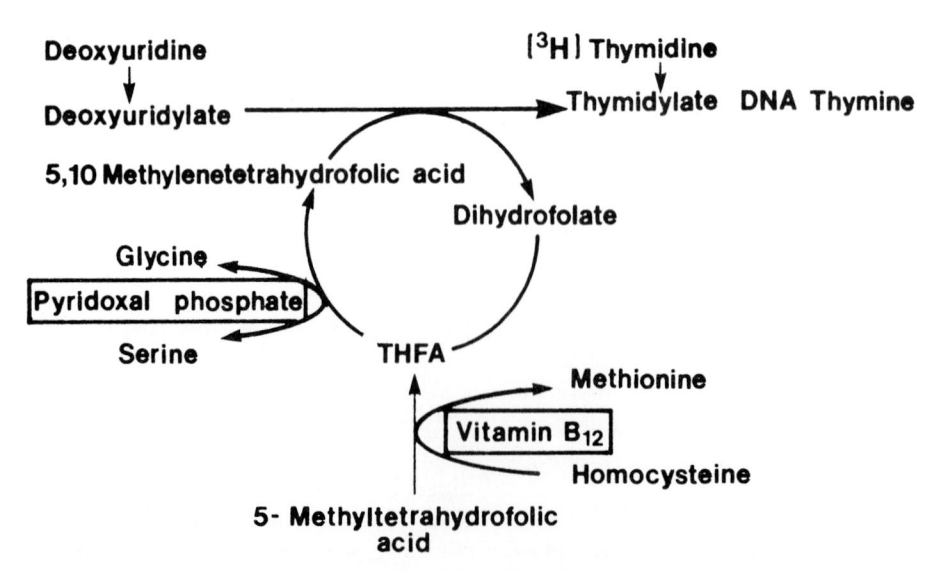

Fig. 4.6 Pathways for DNA thymine synthesis. (Modified from Waxman, S., Corcino, J., and Herbert, V.: Aggravation or initiation of megaloblastosis by amino acids in the diet. JAMA, 214:101, 1970.)

sylcobalamin is a vitamin B_{12} coenzyme in the isomerization of methylmalonyl coenzyme A to succinyl CoA. This important reaction in carbohydrate and lipid metabolism may relate to myelin sheath integrity.

Thus, vitamin B_{12} is required not only for the DNA-dependent cell division, but also for maintenance of neuron integrity. A deficiency of vitamin B_{12} leads to degeneration of peripheral nerve axons and of neuraxons in the spinal cord. This condition is recognized as subacute combined degeneration of the spinal cord. Vitamin B_{12} deficiency that progresses for more than 3 months may produce permanent degenerative lesions of the spinal cord. Neurologic damage could result from a lack of vitamin B_{12} to participate (as a coenzyme) in an isomerase reaction in the conversion of methylmalonyl CoA to succinyl CoA. Failure of this reaction impairs the utilization of fatty acids with an odd number of carbon atoms in the chain. This biochemical lesion may contribute to defective maintenance of the myelin sheath of axons.

Clinical Indications. Cyanocobalamin is indicated for treatment of pernicious anemia due to lack of or inhibition of intrinsic factor. Other of cyanocobalamin's uses include treatment of vitamin B_{12} deficiency resultant from gastrointestinal disease, dysfunction, or surgical procedures; fish tapeworm infestation; gluten enteropathy, sprue, and concurrent folic acid deficiency. Cyanocobalamin also supplies the increased vitamin B_{12} requirements associated with pregnancy, hemorrhage, hemolytic anemia, thyrotoxicosis, malignancy, and hepatic and renal disease.

Adverse Effects/Precautions. Hypersensitivity reactions reported with parenteral vitamin B_{12} include anaphylaxis. Pulmonary edema, itching, and pain at the injection site are additional adverse reactions.

DRUGS AFFECTING FOLIC ACID DEFICIENCY ANEMIA

Folic acid deficiency anemia is treated by replacement and supplementation therapy with folic acid; see Table 4.5.

Folic Acid. Folic acid, pteroylglutamic acid ($PteGlu_1$), functions in the maintenance of normal erythropoiesis and nucleoprotein synthesis.

Mechanism of Action. As indicated by Figure 4.6, folic acid participates in reactions important in DNA synthesis. Folic acid is especially valuable in those tissues in which DNA synthesis and turnover are rapid, such as hematopoietic tissue, gastrointestinal mucosa, and the developing embryo. Folic acid is biotransformed to the active coenzyme form tetrahydrofolic acid ($H_4PteGLu_1$). Tetrahydrofolate acts as a methyl (C_1) acceptor in a number of metabolic interconversions and functions together with vitamin B_{12} in several coupled biochemical reactions.

Methyltetrahydrofolate ($CH_3H_4PteGlu_1$) is a methyl donor in the conversion of homocysteine to methionine. Vitamin B_{12} acts as a cofactor in this reaction with the consequent formation of intermediate methylcobalamin. The conversion of serine to glycine requires tetrahydrofolate ($H_4PteGLu_1$) as an acceptor of a methylene group from serine. Pyridoxal phosphate is required as a cofactor in this reaction. The resultant formation of 5,10 methylenetetrahydrofolic acid (5,10 $CH_2H_4PteGLu_1$) supplies the coenzyme for the synthesis of thymidylate (dTMP).

Methyltetrahydrofolate ($CH_3H_4PteGLu_1$) donates a methyl group to deoxyuridylate (dUMP) for the synthesis of dTMP, an important step in DNA synthesis. Tetrahydrofolate ($H_4PteGLu_1$) functions in histidine metabolism by accepting a formimino-group in the conversion of formiminoglutamic acid to glutamic acid.

Purine nucleotide synthesis requires folic acid for anabolic reactions in purine ring formation. 5,10 $CH_2H_4PteGLu_1$ adds formyl groups to important intermediates in the formation of the purine ring structure. Finally, utilization or generation of formate occurs by the reversible reaction of $H_4PteGLu_1$ with 10-$CHOHH_4PteGLu_1$ (Figure 4.5).

Clinical Indications. Folic acid is used in the treatment of megaloblastic anemias due to a deficiency of folic acid as seen in sprue, anemias of nutritional origin, pregnancy, infancy, or childhood. Requirements of folic acid may arise in liver cirrhosis, hemolytic anemia, and oral contraceptive use.

Adverse Effects/Precautions. Although no side effects are associated with folic acid use, allergic sensitization has been reported. Large doses of folic acid may cause yellow discoloration of the urine.

Folic acid should not be given until the diagnosis of pernicious anemia has been ruled out, since folic acid corrects the hematologic manifestations and masks pernicious anemia while allowing neurologic damage to progress.

DRUGS ALTERING BLOOD COAGULATION

Drugs may act to promote blood clotting in cases where excessive bleeding or its potential are clinical concerns. Conversely, anticoagulants are valuable drugs which prevent potential intravascular clotting; see Table 4.6.

DRUGS THAT PROMOTE BLOOD COAGULATION

Vitamin K is necessary for prothrombin formation by the liver, and its deficiency results in hemorrhagic manifestations.

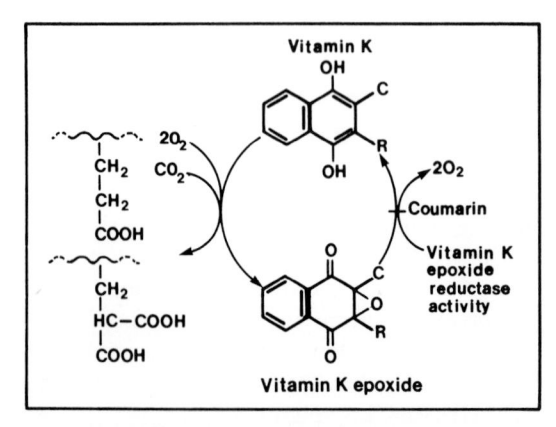

Fig. 4.7 Mechanisms of coumarin action. (Modified from Walsh, P.N.: Oral anticoagulant therapy. Hosp Prac, 18(1):101, 1983.) Drawing by Nancy Lou Gahan Makris.

Vitamin K Substances. 1, 4 naphthoquinones (Figure 4.7), such as phytonadione, have vitamin K activity. Phytonadione (vitamin K) and menadione (vitamin K_3) are lipid-soluble synthetic analogs of vitamin K. Menadiol sodium diphosphate (vitamin K_4) is a water-soluble derivative that is biotransformed to menadione. In contrast with menadione and menadiol sodium diphosphate, phytonadione has a more rapid and prolonged effect.

Mechanism of Action. Vitamin K promotes the hepatic synthesis of active prothrombin (Factor II), proconvertin (Factor VII), plasma thromboplastin component (Factor IX), and Stuart factor (Factor X). The active form of vitamin K is apparently the reduced vitamin K hydroquinone, which is transformed in the presence of oxygen, carbon dioxide, and carboxylase to vitamin K epoxide. In a coupled concurrent reaction, the formation of blood factor precursor proteins occurs (Figure 4.7). These proteins are gamma-carboxylated derivatives of glutamic acid residues. The formation of the new amino acid residues (gamma carboxyglutamic acid moieties) allows the protein to bind Ca^{++} and in turn to be bound to a phospholipid surface. Both actions are necessary for blood clot formation.

Clinical Indications. Vitamin K is useful in coagulation disorders related to defective formation of Factors II (prothrombin), VII, IX, and X when caused by vitamin K deficiency or interference with vitamin K activity. Oral dosage forms (phytonadione and menadiol sodium diphosphate) are indicated in hypoprothrombinemia secondary to obstructive jaundice and biliary fistulae. Bile salts are administered concurrently with phytonadione to aid effective absorption; menadiol sodium is apparently effective alone.

Other clinical uses for oral vitamin K preparations include secondary hypoprothrombinemia due to salicylates and antibacterial therapy. Oral anticoagulant (warfarin, dicumarol)-induced prothrombin deficiency is amenable to oral vitamin K therapy.

Parenteral vitamin K helps correct hypoprothrombinemia resultant from clinical situations that limit the absorption or synthesis of vitamin K. These conditions include obstructive jaundice, biliary fistulas, sprue, ulcerative colitis, celiac disease, intestinal resection, pancreatic fibrosis, regional enteritis, antibacterial therapy, and other drug-induced hypoprothrombinemia due to interference with vitamin K metabolism. Hemorrhagic disease of the newborn also responds to phytonadione.

Adverse Effects/Precautions. Severe reactions, possibly fatal, have occurred immediately following the IV administration of phytonadione. These responses resemble hypersensitivity/anaphylaxis reactions and have been reported even after dilution of the solution to avoid rapid infusion and in patients receiving vitamin K for the first time. Accordingly, IV injection of phytonadione should be restricted to conditions where other routes are not feasible and the serious risk is justifiable.

Adverse allergic reactions include rash and urticaria. Gastric upset, nausea, vomiting, and headache are additional problems associated with oral vitamin K preparations. Following parenteral administration of vitamin K, some newborn infants have experienced hyperbilirubinemia. Also, reports of erythrocyte hemolysis have followed menadione and menadiol sodium diphosphate therapy in persons with G-6-PD deficiency.

DRUGS THAT PROMOTE HEMOSTASIS

A hemostatic drug (Table 4.6) checks the flow of blood via either systemic or local mechanisms.

Aminocaproic Acid. A synthetic compound related to lysine, aminocaproic acid decreases the fibrinolysis of blood clots.

Table 4.6. HEMOSTATIC AGENTS.

Available products	Trade names	Daily dosage range
Drugs That Promote Blood Coagulation:		
Menadiol sodium diphosphate	Synkayvite	Orally, 5–10 mg; parenterally, 5–15 mg
Menadione (K_3)	Menadione	5–10 mg
Menadione sodium bisulfite	Hykinone	0.5–10 mg parenterally
Phytonadione (K_1)	AquaMEPHYTON; Konakion	2.5–25 mg
Vitamin K_5	Synkamin	2–5 mg
Drugs That Promote Hemostasis:		
Absorbable gelatin sponge	Gelfoam	Topical
Absorbable gelatin film, sterile	Gelfilm	Topical
Absorbable gelatin powder, sterile	Gelfoam	Topical
Aminocaproic acid	Amicar	5 g orally or IV, followed by 1–1.25 g hourly
Carbazochrome salicylate	Adrenosem Salicylate	Postoperatively (if also used preoperatively): 5 mg q. 2 hrs IM or orally
Microfibrillar collagen hemostat	Avitene	Apply dry to bleeding area
Negatol	Negatan	Use topically in solutions
Oxidized cellulose	Novocell; Oxycel; Surgicel	Lay on bleeding sites
Thrombin, topical	Thrombinar; Thrombostat	Solution of 100 units/ml
Antihemophilic products:		
Antihemophilic Factor (Factor VIII; AHF)	Factorate; Hemofil; Koate; Profilate	10–30 ml IV
Anti-inhibitor Coagulant Complex	Autoplex; Feiba Immuno	25–100 Factor VIII correctional units/kg by IV infusion
Factor IX complex, human	Konyne; Proplex; Profilnine	20 ml IV (500 units)

Mechanism of Action. Aminocaproic acid reduces the activity of plasminogen activator substances by competitive inhibition; this systemic action decreases fibrinolysis (Figure 4.8). Antiplasmin activity by aminocaproic acid also contributes to the inhibition of fibrinolysis.

Clinical Indications. Aminocaproic acid is indicated in the treatment of severe hemorrhage due to systemic hyperfibrinolysis or urinary fibrinolysis. Secondary hyperfibrinolysis is a compensatory mechanism that follows widespread intravascular clotting, such as premature detachment of a normally implanted placenta or cardiac bypass surgical procedures. The exact indications for aminocaproic acid depend upon the patient response to other therapy, such as transfusion and heparin.

Adverse Effects/Precautions. Patients with upper urinary tract bleeding may experience intrarenal obstruction when receiving aminocaproic acid therapy. Also, patients with disseminated intravascular clotting (DIC) may form a potentially fatal thrombus. Aminocaproic acid should not be administered in the presence of DIC without concomitant heparin.

Adverse reactions include nausea, diarrhea, hypotension, malaise, and myopathy.

Carbazochrome Salicylate. Carbazochrome salicylate is a complex of carbazochrome (an oxidation product of epinephrine) with sodium salicylate.

Mechanism of Action. Carbazochrome apparently decreases excessive capillary permeability to inhibit vessel blood oozing. It is ineffective against massive hemorrhage or bleeding from large vessels. Carbazochrome does not affect any of the blood components connected with the clotting mechanisms.

Clinical Indications. Carbazochrome is used prophylactically and therapeutically in conditions characterized by increased capillary permeability and associated capillary oozing.

Adverse Effects/Precautions. IM injection of carbazochrome sometimes produces a stinging sensation.

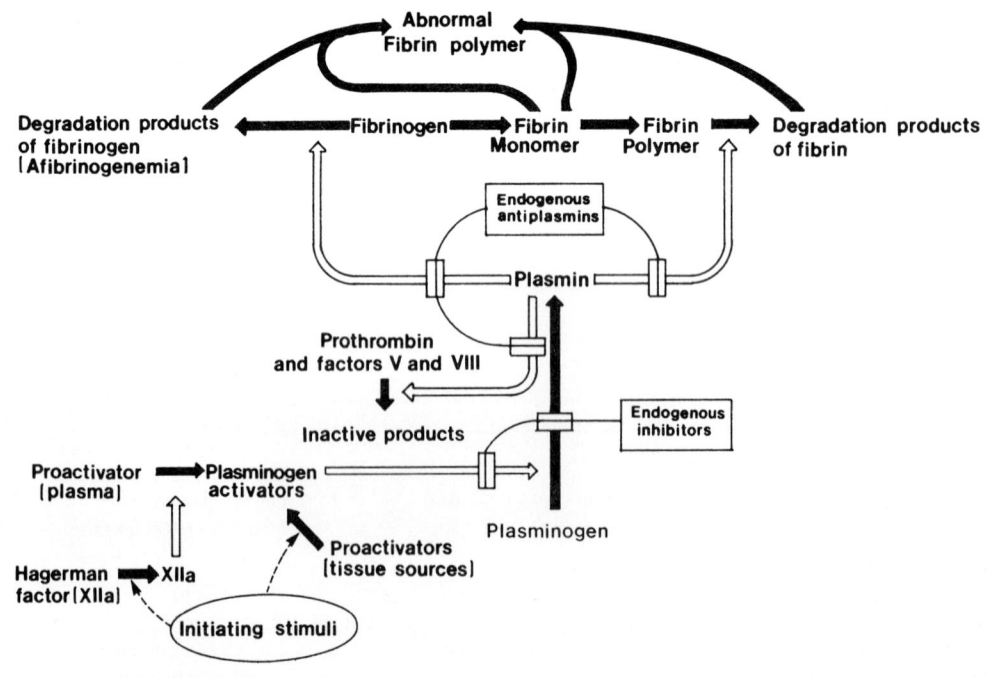

Fig. 4.8 Fibrinolytic system. (From Bowman, W.C., and Rand, M.J.: Textbook of Pharmacology. 2nd Ed. Oxford, Blackwell Scientific Publications, 1980.)

CIRCULATORY/RETICULOENDOTHELIAL SYSTEM

Thrombin. Commercially available thrombin is from bovine sources.

Mechanism of Action. Thrombin, a blood enzyme derived from Factor II (prothrombin), converts fibrinogen to fibrin resulting in blood clot production.

Clinical Indications. Applied topically, thrombin aids in hemostasis when there is capillary oozing. Thrombin is used in operative procedures and to shorten the duration of bleeding from puncture sites in heparinized patients. In some surgical procedures, thrombin solutions are used in conjunction with absorbable gelatin sponges for hemostasis.

Adverse Effects/Precautions. Thrombin should never be injected (particularly intravenously) because of the danger of thrombosis and death. Since thrombin is an antigenic substance, allergic reactions are possible.

Microfibrillar Collagen Hemostat. Microfibrillar collagen hemostat (MCH) is an absorbable hemostatic drug. MCH is prepared as a dry, sterile, fibrous, water insoluble, partial hydrochloric acid salt of purified bovine corium collagen.

Mechanism of Action. MCH, in contact with a bleeding surface, attracts platelets (thrombocytes) which adhere to the fibrils. The platelets undergo the release phenomenon and stimulate platelet aggregation. Thrombic formation in the interstitial fibrous mass ensues.

Clinical Indications. MCH is used in surgical procedures as an adjunct to hemostasis when bleeding control by ligature or other conventional means is ineffective or impractical.

Adverse Effects/Precautions. The most serious adverse reaction with MCH is potentiation of infection, including abscess formation, hematoma, wound dehiscence, and mediastinitis. MCH use in dental extraction sockets may produce postoperative pain in a dental alveolus or "dry socket."

Negatol. A high molecular weight colloidal condensation, negatol is obtained by the reaction of metacresol sulfonic acid with formaldehyde.

Mechanism of Action. Negatol has a coagulant effect on protein substances, is effective in precipitating cervical mucus, and controls minor bleeding from the vagina, cervix, and vulvae.

Clinical Indications. Negatol is employed as an astringent and hemostatic.

Adverse Effects/Precautions. Slight irritation in the perivaginal region may occur. Contact of the negatol solution with the eyes should be avoided.

Absorbable Gelatin Sponge. Absorbable gelatin sponge is a sterile, pliable surgical sponge prepared from purified gelatin solution.

Mechanism of Action. Absorbable gelatin sponge is capable of absorbing and holding many times its weight of whole blood.

Clinical Indications. Used in surgical procedures, absorbable gelatin sponge serves as an adjunct to hemostasis when control of bleeding by conventional means is not feasible. Specific clinical applications are in oral and dental surgery and for insertion into the prostatic cavity during open prostatic surgery. The sponge is ordinarily absorbed within 4 to 6 weeks; if the sponge is applied to a bleeding area, liquefication occurs within 2 to 5 days.

Adverse Effects/Precautions. The sponge may act as a nucleus of infection and abscess formation.

Absorbable Gelatin Film, Sterile. Absorbable gelatin film has the appearance and texture of cellophane. When moistened, the film converts to a rubbery consistency that can be cut and molded for the individual situation.

Mechanism of Action. Absorbable gelatin film absorbs and holds blood.

Clinical Indications. Absorbable gelatin film is used as a dural substitute in neurosurgery, in the repair of pleural defects in thoracic surgery, and in ocular glaucoma filtration operations. Absorption occurs in 1 to 6 months, depending upon the application site.

Adverse Effects/Precautions. The film should not be implanted in grossly contaminated or infected surgical wounds.

Absorbable Gelatin Powder, Sterile. Gelatin powder is applied locally to produce hemostatic and tissue-stimulating effects.

Mechanism of Action. Absorbable gelatin powder is hemostatic and promotes granulation tissue growth and the healing of ulcers.

Clinical Indications. Absorbable gelatin powder is especially useful to promote hemostasis and in the treatment of chronic leg ulcers and decubitus ulcers.

Adverse Effects/Precautions. The powdered ulcer may become a locus for infection and abscess.

Oxidized Cellulose. Oxidized cellulose, an absorbable hemostatic agent, is prepared from cellulose by a special process that converts it into polyanhydroglucuronic acid (cellulosic acid).

Mechanism of Action. Oxidized cellulose provides hemostatic action and swells upon contact with blood. It forms an artificially produced clot within a few minutes.

Clinical Indications. Oxidized cellulose is used as an adjunct in the control of capillary, venous, and small arterial hemorrhage. Special oxidized cellulous pellets are available for hemostatic use in oral and dental surgery.

Adverse Effects/Precautions. Adverse reactions include fluid encapsulation and foreign body reactions, with or without infection.

ANTIHEMOPHILIC PRODUCTS

These drugs include blood replacement factors for the management of hemophilia.

Antihemophilic Factor (Factor VIII, AHF). Antihemophilic factor (AHF), a protein found in normal blood plasma, is necessary for blood clot formation.

Mechanism of Action. AHF supplies the missing factor in hemophilic plasma (Hemophilia A, classical hemophilia) necessary for blood coagulation. AHF is required in the intrinsic pathway for the transformation of Factor II (prothrombin) to thrombin.

Clinical Indications. AHF is clinically useful in the treatment of classical hemophilia (Hemophilia A) that is characterized by a demonstrated deficiency of Factor VIII. AHF temporarily supplies the missing clotting factor needed to correct or prevent bleeding episodes.

Adverse Effects/Precautions. Allergic reactions have resulted from AHF administration.

Anti-Inhibitor Coagulant Complex. Anti-Inhibitor Coagulant Complex, prepared from pooled human plasma, contains variable amounts of activated and precursor clotting factors in concentrated form.

Mechanism of Action. About 10% of all hemophiliacs have circulating inhibitors to Factor VIII. The Anti-Inhibitor Coagulant Complex counteracts the Factor VIII inhibition in these patients.

Clinical Indications. Anti-Inhibitor Coagulant Complex is indicated for hemophilia patients with Factor VIII inhibitors who are bleeding or must undergo surgery.

Adverse Effects/Precautions. Hypersensitivity reactions, such as fever, chills, rashes, and anaphylactoid reactions, have accompanied use of this product.

Factor IX Complex, Human. The human Factor IX complex (plasma thromboplastin component) consists of stable dried purified plasma fractions.

Mechanism of Action. Factor IX Complex contains vitamin K-dependent Factors II, VII, IX, X.

Clinical Indications. Factor IX Complex is indicated via IV administration in the treatment of Factor IX deficiency (Hemophilia B, Christmas disease).

Adverse Effects/Precautions. Adverse reactions include thrombosis or disseminated intravascular coagulation.

ANTICOAGULANTS

Orally effective anticoagulants that interfere with vitamin K metabolism include the coumarins and indanediones (Table 4.7). The 1920s discovery of the hemorrhagic properties of spoiled sweet clover eventually led to the identification of bishydroxycoumarin (dicumarol) as the causative agent. Also noted was a drastic reduction in plasma prothrombin produced by the hemorrhagic effects of this coumarin derivative.

Several congeners of dicumarol were found to decrease blood clotting; the most useful of these was warfarin (acronym for the patent holder — Wisconsin *Alumni Research Foundation* — and the cou*marin*-related suffix). Due to its toxicity, warfarin was initially used as a rat poison (rodenticide); in the mid-1950s, the coumarins were introduced into medicine. Today, the coumarins are valuable in treating clotting disorders.

Dicumarol. Prepared synthetically, dicumarol (bishydroxycoumarin) is used as an anticoagulant drug.

Mechanism of Action. Dicumarol interferes with the hepatic synthesis of vitamin K-dependent clotting factors. The formation of prothrombin (Factor II), proconvertin (Factor VII), Christmas factor (Factor IX), and the Stuart factor (Factor X) is inhibited by dicumarol.

The vitamin K sensitive step in the synthesis of these four clotting factors is the carboxylation of ten or more glutamic acid residues at the amino-terminal of a precursor protein with the resultant formation of gamma-carboxyglutamate. Thus, in the case of prothrombin formation, descarboxyprothrombin (precursor) converts to prothrombin by the carboxylation of at least ten glutamate residues to gamma-carboxyglutamate. This carboxylation reaction couples to a conversion of vitamin KH_2 to vitamin K epoxide.

Dicumarol blocks the regeneration of vitamin

Table 4.7. ANTICOAGULANT DRUGS.

Available products	Trade names	Daily dosage range
Heparin sodium injection	Lipo-Hepin; Liquaemin Sodium	Adjust dosage according to coagulation test results
Coumarin derivatives:		
Dicumarol	Dicumarol; Dicumarol Pulvules	Individualize dosage
Phenprocoumon	Liquamar	0.75 – 6 mg
Warfarin sodium	Coumadin Sodium; Panwarfin; Coufarin	Maintenance dose: 2 – 10 mg
Warfarin potassium sodium	Athrombin-K	Same as for salt; Initial daily range: 40 – 60 mg
Indandione derivatives:		
Anisindione	Miradon	Maintenance dose: 25 – 250 mg daily
Phenindione	Hedulin	Maintenance dose: 50 – 150 mg daily

KH$_2$, an epoxide reductase and reduced nicotinamide adenine dinucleotide (NAD) dependent reaction (Figure 4.7). Thus, the specific step in vitamin K metabolism inhibited by dicumarol and coumarin-type drugs is the reduction of vitamin K epoxide to vitamin KH$_2$. Maximal antithrombotic effects are not realized until all four factors are depleted.

The clinical extension of the inhibitory effect on fibrin formation is for the prophylaxis of venous thrombi since fibrin thrombi occur primarily in the venous system. Dosage with a vitamin K antagonist is adjusted for each patient depending upon the results of the one-stage prothrombin time. The therapeutic goal is adjustment of the prothrombin time to approximately 2 to 2.5 times normal. The normal range for one stage prothrombin time is between 12 to 14 seconds so that a value between 24 to 30 seconds becomes a clinical objective. A value of 35 seconds indicates excessive dosage of the vitamin K antagonist.

Clinical Indications. Dicumarol is indicated for the prophylaxis and treatment of venous thrombosis. Additional uses are in the treatment of atrial fibrillation with embolization, prophylaxis and treatment of pulmonary embolism, and as an adjunct in the treatment of coronary occlusion. Dicumarol activity varies as the drug is incompletely and slowly absorbed by oral administration and the plasma half-life is dose dependent.

Adverse Effects/Precautions. Although diarrhea and bloating of the stomach with gas are frequent side effects, bleeding is the primary adverse effect of oral anticoagulant therapy. Early signs of excessive dicumarol dosage include bleeding from the gums following tooth brushing, unexplained bruises or purplish skin spots, nosebleed, and heavy or unexpected menstrual bleeding.

Phenprocoumon. A long plasma half-life characterizes this oral anticoagulant.

Mechanism of Action. Phenprocoumon interferes with the synthesis of vitamin K clotting factors in the liver. Specifically, phenprocoumon blocks regeneration of vitamin KH$_2$ from vitamin K epoxide, thus inhibiting the hepatic synthesis of prothrombin (Factor II), proconvertin (Factor VII), Christmas factor (Factor IX), and the Stuart factor (Factor X).

Clinical Indications. Phenprocoumon is used as a hypoprothrombinemic agent in the prophylaxis and treatment of venous thrombosis. Other uses include treatment of atrial fibrillation with embolization, prophylaxis and treatment of pulmonary embolism, and as an adjunct in the treatment of coronary occlusion.

Adverse Effects/Precautions. Nausea, diarrhea, and dermatitis have been reported with phenprocoumon therapy.

Warfarin. A coumarin-derivative, warfarin is available commercially as the racemic potassium and sodium salts.

Mechanism of Action. Warfarin, an antivitamin K oral anticoagulant, blocks the reduction of vitamin K epoxide to vitamin KH$_2$. Vitamin KH$_2$ regeneration is important in vitamin K metabolism since its interconversion to vitamin K epoxide links to the hepatic synthesis for active plasma clotting factors. Thus, a depletion of the clotting factors II, VII, IX, and X occurs.

Warfarin's anticoagulant effects depend upon the half-lives of the affected factors; the first effects are noted on the factor with the shortest half-life—Factor VII. Maximum antithrombotic effect is not apparent for several days until the other factors are depleted and the drug achieves steady state kinetics. Prothrombin (Factor II) has the longest half-life (60 hours) and is the last sensitive clotting factor to be depleted.

Clinical Indications. Warfarin is indicated for the prophylaxis and treatment of venous thrombosis. Other uses include treatment of atrial fibrillation with embolization, prophylaxis and treatment of pulmonary embolism, and as an adjunct in the treatment of coronary occlusion.

Adverse Effects/Precautions. Adverse effects other than hemorrhage are uncommon.

Indanediones. Since coumarins are preferred therapeutic agents as oral anticoagulants, indanediones (anisindione and phenindione) have limited therapeutic use. Anisindione, more toxic than the coumarins, is rarely used therapeutically. The indanediones, particularly phenindione, have a greater incidence of severe adverse reactions that include cutaneous, hepatic, and hematologic effects.

Heparin. Heparin is a naturally occurring straight chain heteroglycan that contains glucuronic acid and glucosamine units. First isolated from liver, heparin is highly acidic and commercial preparations are available as the sodium salt.

Mechanism of Action. Heparin prevents blood coagulation at a number of sites. Although not an effective anticoagulant per se, heparin combines with and activates a plasma cofactor (alpha-2 globulin) to alter prothrombin formation. The alpha-2 globulin cofactor is designated as antithrombin III and possesses a proteinase inhibiting action. Antithrombin III participates as part of an intrinsic defense mechanism against thrombosis. Heparin binds to antithrombin III and speeds its combination with thrombin to form an inactive complex that prevents the conversion of fibrinogen to fibrin. Heparin, in combination with antithrombin III, also inhibits the conversion of prothrombin to thrombin.

Antithrombin III not only neutralizes thrombin but also binds and inhibits several activated clotting factors, including II, IX, X, XI, XII, XIII, and kallikrein. The principal rate-limiting step in the blood clotting reaction sequence is the activation of Factor X. Low doses of heparin neutralize the activated Factor X and form the basis for low dose heparin prophylaxis. Heparin cofactor II, distinct from antithrombin III, forms a complex with thrombin to inactivate it.

Clinical Indications. Employed in the prophylaxis and treatment of venous thrombosis, heparin is also used in the treatment of pulmonary embolism, peripheral arterial embolism, and atrial fibrillation with embolization.

Heparin is used in the diagnosis and treatment of acute and chronic consumptive coagulopathies (such as DIC). A low dose heparin regimen is employed to prevent postoperative deep venous thrombosis in high risk patients.

Other clinical indications of heparin are in the prevention of clotting in heart and arterial surgery, as well as in dialysis, blood sampling, and blood transfusions. Heparin is also used for prevention of cerebral thrombosis in poststroke situations and as an adjunct in the treatment of coronary occlusion with acute myocardial infarction.

Adverse Effects/Precautions. The major complication of heparin therapy is hemorrhage. Heparin causes a temporary mild thrombocytopenia in about ¼ of patients; a severe thrombocytopenia rarely develops.

Heparin should not be administered intramuscularly because of the danger of hematoma formation.

HEPARIN ANTAGONIST

Protamine, a physiologic antagonist, effectively counters heparin overdose.

Protamine Sulfate. Protamines are low molecular weight proteins, rich in arginine, and consequently strongly basic. They are found in the sperm or mature testes of fish in the family Salmonidae.

Mechanism of Action. Protamine sulfate, if administered alone, has an anticoagulant effect. However, when administered in the presence of heparin, protamine sulfate (due to its strongly basic nature) forms a stable complex that reduces the anticoagulant activity of both drugs. The heparin inactivating effect is immediate and lasts for about 2 hours.

Clinical Indications. Protamine sulfate is effective in the treatment of heparin overdosage.

Adverse Effects/Precautions. A sudden hypotensive reaction, bradycardia, and dyspnea, followed by anaphylaxis and hypertension, have been reported after protamine sulfate administration. The possibility of fatal anaphylaxis-like reactions require immediate resuscitation measures.

ANTITHROMBOTIC DRUGS

Drugs in this category suppress thrombocyte (platelet) function and thereby reduce platelet aggregation. Antithrombotic drugs are used primarily for arterial thrombotic disease.

Acetylsalicylic Acid (Aspirin). Aspirin has several therapeutic applications, including prophylaxis in clotting disorders, such as in coronary artery disease.

Mechanism of Action. Aspirin inhibits the release of ADP and the formation of prostaglandins and thromboxane A_2. Acetylation of cyclooxygenase by aspirin inhibits the enzyme and thereby decreases the formation of factors that support platelet aggregation. The platelet effects of aspirin are irreversible and thus last for the life of the platelet (several days), even though aspirin is usually excreted a few hours after ingestion. Low dose aspirin is potentially more effective than high doses because larger doses inhibit cyclooxygenase in arterial walls, decreasing prostacyclin synthesis. Prostacyclin (PGI_2), a potent endogenous vasodilator, inhibits platelet aggregation.

Clinical Indications. The FDA has approved a single aspirin dose of 324 mg (5 grains) daily for prophylaxis in acute myocardial infarction in men with unstable angina.

Adverse Effects/Precautions. Low doses (one standard tablet daily) of aspirin rarely produce any adverse effects, unless the patient is allergic to the drug.

Dipyridamole. Dipyridamole may alter platelet function by interfering with phosphodiesterase function. The intracellular concentration of adenosine 3', 5'-monophosphate (cyclic AMP) consequently increases and platelet aggregation decreases. Dipyridamole, in combination with warfarin, is currently recommended for primary prophylaxis of thromboemboli in patients with prosthetic heart valves.

Sulfinpyrazone. Sulfinpyrazone, used primarily as a uricosuric drug, inhibits several platelet functions. This drug reduces prostaglandin synthesis and hampers platelet release and adherence to subendothelial cells. To date, sulfinpyrazone has not received FDA approval for its antithrombotic activity.

THROMBOLYTIC DRUGS

Drugs that promote dissolution of thrombi (such as streptokinase and urokinase) are administered in hospitals where diagnostic and monitoring techniques are available.

Streptokinase and Urokinase. Streptokinase (Kabikinase^R) and urokinase (Abbokinase^R) are proteins that increase fibrinolytic activity.

Mechanism of Action. Streptokinase and urokinase stimulate the activation of endogenous plasminogen to plasmin (fibrinolysin), a proteolytic enzyme that inactivates fibrin (Figure 4.8).

Clinical Indications. Streptokinase and urokinase are employed in pulmonary emboli and coronary artery thrombosis to lyze the emboli in these disorders. Streptokinase is also used in deep vein thrombosis. Since these drugs can profoundly alter hemostasis, extreme caution and expertise are required in their clinical application in thromboembolic disease.

Adverse Effects/Precautions. Bleeding (minor and/or hemorrhage) and allergic reactions may occur with thrombolytic protein therapy.

HEMORRHEOLOGIC AGENTS

The hemorrheologic agent, pentoxifylline, increases red blood cell deformity to improve blood flow to the peripheral vasculature and to promote oxygenation of tissues. Vasodilation is apparently not a component of the drug's beneficial activity in promoting microcirculation.

Pentoxifylline (Trental^R). A substituted xanthine derivative, pentoxifylline lowers blood viscosity and improves erythrocyte flexibility.

Mechanism of Action. Pentoxifylline apparently improves capillary blood flow by increasing erythrocyte flexibility and improving the flow properties of blood by decreasing its viscosity. Decreased platelet aggregation occurs as a result of elevated platelet cyclic AMP due to phosphodiesterase inhibition.

Additionally, fibrinogen levels in the blood decrease due to increased fibrinolytic activity. Hemorrheologic activity increases blood flow to the affected microcirculation in patients with peripheral vascular disease, thus providing an enhanced oxygenation of peripheral tissues.

Clinical Indications. Pentoxyfylline, used for intermittent claudication due to chronic occlusive arterial disease, is also effective in treating diabetic angiopathies. Further clinical studies may determine the drug's efficacy in Alzheimer's disease and prevention of transient ischemic attacks.

Adverse Effects/Precautions. Commonly reported side effects are gastrointestinal, including nausea and vomiting. These reactions occur less frequently with sustained release tablets, as compared to the capsule dosage form. Other reported side effects include dizziness, lightheadedness, headache, hypotension, flushing, and chest pain.

DRUGS USED TO TREAT HYPERLIPIDEMIAS

The elevation of serum cholesterol, triglycerides, or both is characteristic of hyperlipidemia. Certain drugs lower the elevated blood lipids to within a normal range. Oftentimes, a specificity for lowering a particular type of blood lipids is noted with the antilipidemic drugs; see Table 4.8.

CHOLESTEROL-LOWERING DRUGS

Agents included in hypercholesterolemia include binding resins and the d-isomer of a thyroid hormone.

Cholestyramine. Cholestyramine is the chloride salt of a basic anion exchange resin.

Mechanism of Action. Cholestyramine sequesters bile acids in the intestines to form an insoluble complex that is excreted in the feces. Increased fecal loss of bile acids speeds the oxidation of cholesterol. Since bile acids suppress the enzymatic hydroxylation of cholesterol to bile acids, their removal increases cholesterol oxidation.

The stimulated oxidation of cholesterol to

Table 4.8. ANTIHYPERLIPIDEMIC DRUGS.

Available products	Trade names	Daily dosage range
Cholesterol-lowering drugs:		
Cholestyramine	Questran	4 g t.i.d. or q.i.d.
Colestipol	Colestid	15–30 g in 2–4 divided doses
Dextrothyroxine sodium	Choloxin	1–2 mg initially; increase gradually to 4–8 mg daily
Probucol	Lorelco	500 mg b.i.d. with morning and evening meals
Triglyceride-lowering drugs:		
Clofibrate	Atromid-S	2 g daily in divided doses
Gemfibrozil	Lopid	900–1500 mg
Nicotinic acid	Nicotinic Acid	1–2 g with or following meals

bile acids decreases LDL and serum cholesterol levels. Plasma cholesterol levels fall due to increased clearance of cholesterol-rich lipoproteins (LDL) from the plasma. The increased LDL-cholesterol uptake from plasma is due to an increase in hepatic LDL receptors that results from liver compensatory mechanisms after the fecal bile acid loss.

Clinical Indications. Cholestyramine is used, in addition to dietary restrictions, for the reduction of elevated serum cholesterol in patients with elevated LDL (primary hypercholesterolemia). Cholestyramine is recommended as an adjunct in Type IIA hyperlipoproteinemic patients with a significant risk of coronary artery disease who have not responded to diet and other measures, such as weight reduction, exercise, and adequate control of diabetes mellitus.

Adverse Effects/Precautions. Constipation is the most frequent adverse effect. Abdominal pain and distension, gastrointestinal bleeding, nausea, vomiting, and diarrhea are additional side effects of cholestyramine use. Oil-soluble vitamin deficiencies are possible, but infrequent. An increased bleeding tendency may indicate vitamin K deficiency.

Colestipol. Colestipol, an anion exchange resin, is utilized for its plasma cholesterol-lowering properties.

Mechanism of Action. Colestipol binds bile acids in the intestinal tract, largely increasing fecal excretion of bile acids and cholesterol. A fecal loss in bile acids and cholesterol results in compensatory increases in hepatic LDL receptors. A resultant fall in plasma LDL-cholesterol due to increased uptake by the liver cells occurs.

Clinical Indications. Colestipol is used as adjunctive therapy for the reduction of serum cholesterol in patients with Type IIA hyperlipoproteinemia (elevated LDL).

Adverse Effects/Precautions. Constipation is the most frequently reported adverse effect. Less common gastrointestinal complaints include abdominal pain, gastrointestinal bleeding, nausea, vomiting, and diarrhea. Chronic use of colestipol could result in an oil-soluble vitamin deficiency, perhaps evidenced as bleeding episodes due to lack of vitamin K.

Probucol. A cholesterol-lowering agent, probucol causes moderate reductions in plasma LDL-cholesterol.

Mechanism of Action. Probucol lowers serum cholesterol and decreases plasma LDL by speeding the rate of LDL catabolism and by inhibiting cholesterol synthesis. It usually also causes a substantial lowering of HDL-cholesterol.

Clinical Indications. Probucol reduces elevated serum cholesterol in patients who have primary hypercholesterolemia (elevated LDL) and are unresponsive to other measures, such as diet, weight reduction, and control of diabetes mellitus.

Adverse Effects/Precautions. Gastrointestinal effects, such as diarrhea, are common with probucol therapy. Prolongation of the QT interval of the ECG occurs in some patients.

Dextrothyroxine. Dextrothyroxine, the optical isomer of naturally occurring l-thyroxine, lowers plasma LDL in about 1 in 5 patients exhibiting hypercholesterolemia.

Mechanism of Action. Dextrothyroxine increases the synthesis of LDL receptors in liver cells. Consequently, increased removal of excess LDL from the plasma occurs and levels tend to return to the normal range.

Dextrothyroxine also increases the hepatic catabolism and excretion of cholesterol via biliary excretion. Elevated triglycerides may also be reduced by dextrothyroxine.

Clinical Indications. Dextrothyroxine is used as an adjunct to diet and other measures for reducing elevated serum cholesterol (LDL) in euthyroid patients with no known cardiac pathophysiology.

Adverse Effects/Precautions. Although effects related to increased metabolic rate are frequently reported, cardiovascular effects (such as angina pectoris and arrhythmias) are also possible. Nervousness and insomnia are examples of adverse CNS effects.

Lovastatin (Mevinolin^R). Useful in the treatment of hypercholesterolemia, lovastatin has reduced total and LDL cholesterol levels by 30 to 40% in some patients. Lovastatin apparently acts as an antihypercholesteremic agent by blocking mevalonate conversion, which inhibits cholesterol synthesis. For optimal efficacy, patients receiving lovastatin are strongly encouraged to maintain low cholesterol diets.

TRIGLYCERIDE-LOWERING DRUGS THAT LOWER CHOLESTEROL LEVELS

These agents, effective in certain forms of hyperlipoproteinemias, often lower cholesterol levels in addition to their effect on triglycerides.

Clofibrate. Clofibrate is the ethyl ester of chlorophenoxyisobutyric acid. After absorption, it is rapidly hydrolyzed to chlorophenoxyisobutyrate, the active antilipidemic moeity.

Mechanism of Action. Clofibrate lowers plasma triglycerides by 20 to 50% and cholesterol by 15 to 30% in most patients. Enhanced antilipidemic activity occurs when both plasma triglycerides and cholesterol are elevated. If triglyceride blood levels are in the normal range, cholesterol reduction is minimal.

The most marked effect of clofibrate is on serum triglyceride levels and VLDL, and the drug is most useful in hyperlipoproteinemia III. Types IV and V hyperlipoproteinemia usually respond to the drug, but Type II is commonly unresponsive.

An accelerated catabolism of VLDL to LDL probably accounts for the mechanisms of clofibrate activity on serum triglyceride levels. Additionally, hepatic synthesis of VLDL decreases.

Clofibrate inhibits cholesterol synthesis at two points: one site prior to mevalonic acid formation and one site after mevalonic acid synthesis. Androsterone, a natural hormone, is displaced from albumen by clofibrate (this action may contribute to the drug's antilipidemic action). Androsterone, in free form, lowers the plasma concentration of beta-lipoproteins.

Clinical Indications. Clofibrate is used to treat Type III hyperlipoproteinemia that does not adequately respond to diet. Patients with high serum triglyceride levels (as in Types IV and V hyperlipoproteinemia) may also respond to clofibrate therapy.

Adverse Effects/Precautions. Nausea is a common adverse effect. The drug should only be used as indicated due to potential increased risks of malignancy and cholelithiasis.

Nicotinic Acid. Nicotinic acid, a B vitamin, is used in high doses (100 times the MDR) in the treatment of hyperlipidemia.

Mechanism of Action. Nicotinic acid reduces serum triglyceride levels. A decreased hepatic synthesis of VLDL and triglycerides probably results from a decreased supply of free fatty acids to the liver. This occurs as a result of a reduction in lipolysis and release of free fatty acids from adipose cells. Since LDL is a product of VLDL catabolism, less LDL is consequently formed.

Nicotinic acid enters adipose tissue and inhibits the release of free fatty acids from adipose cells. A marked reduction in the plasma concentration of free fatty acids then occurs. Nicotinic acid decreases the elevation of cyclic AMP in response to lipolytic stimuli (although adenyl cyclase is not inhibited).

Clinical Indications. Nicotinic acid is indicated as adjunctive therapy with diet and weight control measures in patients having elevated serum triglyceride and cholesterol levels.

Adverse Effects/Precautions. Cutaneous flushing commonly occurs after nicotinic acid ingestion. Transient itching, tingling, and headache are other reactions, which usually cease with continued therapy.

Gemfibrozil. Gemfibrozil is useful as an adjunct to diet and weight reduction in the treatment of hyperlipidemia.

Mechanism of Action. Serum triglycerides are preferentially decreased by gemfibrozil with a variable reduction in total serum cholesterol. The VLDL fraction is reduced with the greatest regularity; the LDL decrease occurs less frequently. Also, the HDL fraction may actually increase with gemfibrozil therapy.

Gemfibrozil inhibits peripheral lipolysis, reducing the hepatic extraction of free fatty acids. These effects lower hepatic triglyceride production.

Clinical Indications. Gemfibrozil is used in patients having severe Type IV hyperlipidemia and significant risk of coronary artery disease, abdominal pain, or pancreatitis. Generally, gemfibrozil is employed when other measures such as weight reduction, exercise, or adequate control of diabetes mellitus have proved unsuccessful.

Adverse Effects/Precautions. Abdominal pain, diarrhea, and nausea are frequent reactions to gemfibrozil therapy.

Table 4.9. ANTICANCER DRUGS.

Available products	Trade names
Alkylating agents:	
Busulfan	Myleran
Carmustine	BiCNU
Chlorambucil	Leukeran
Cisplatin	Platinol
Cyclophosphamide	Cytoxan; Neosar
Lomustine	CeeNU
Mechlorethamine HCl	Mustargen
Melphalan	Alkeran
Pipbroman	Vercyte
Streptozocin	Zanosar
Triethylenethiophosphoramide	Thiotepa
Uracil mustard	Uracil Mustard
Antimetabolites:	
Cytarabine	Cytosar-U
Floxuridine and Fluorouracil	FUDR; Adrucil
Mercaptopurine	Purinethol
Methotrexate	Folex; Mexate
Thioguanine	Thioguanine
Anticancer drugs from natural sources:	
Bleomycin sulfate	Blenoxane
Daunorubicin	Cerubidine
Doxorubicin HCl	Adriamycin
Mitomycin	Mutamycin
Plicamycin	Mithracin
Inhibitors of cell mitosis:	
Etoposide	VePesid
Vinblastine sulfate	Velban
Vincristine sulfate	Oncovin
Miscellaneous synthetic anticancer drugs:	
Asparaginase	Elspar
Dacarbazine	DTIC-Dome
Hydroxyurea	Hydrea
Mitotane	Lysodren
Prednisone	Meticorten; Deltasone; others
Procarbazine	Matulane
Sodium phosphate P32	Sodium Phosphate P32

DRUGS USED IN THE CHEMOTHERAPY OF HEMATOLOGIC MALIGNANCIES

The early detection and treatment of the hematologic malignancies (acute lymphatic leukemia, myelogenous leukemia, and Hodgkin's disease) now result in greatly increased survival rates. For instance, the survival rate for Hodgkin's disease now approaches 75%.

The current emphasis in cancer chemotherapy is on combination therapy (see Tables 4.9 and 4.10), which are based in part on the cell cycle phase affected by the drug. The parts of the cell cycle are G_1, S, G_2, and M stages (Figure 4.9). The G_1 stage, sometimes called the presynthesis gap, is a resting stage and ends with a sudden increase in RNA synthesis. A marked increase in DNA occurs during the S phase, a period of genetic replication.

This replication ceases when the cells begin the G_2 phase, also termed the postsynthesis gap, that ends with the mitotic process. Mitosis, the process whereby division of the nucleus produces two new nuclei each with the same number of chromosomes as the parent nucleus, occurs during the M phase. The entire process is continual although the division into separate stages classically represents cellular reproduction.

Table 4.10 CHEMOTHERAPY OF HEMATOLOGIC MALIGNANCIES.*

Neoplastic malignancy type	Preferred treatment program(s)	Secondary drugs active against the disease
Acute lymphocytic (lymphoblastic leukemia (ALL)	**Remission Induction** Prednisone and vincristine **CNS prophylaxis** Methotrexate (intrathecal) (plus cranial irradiation) **Remission Maintenance** Mercaptopurine (daily) Methotrexate and cyclophosphamide intermittently	Daunorubicin Asparaginase Cytarabine Doxorubicin 5-Azacytidine Thioguanine
Acute myelocytic (myelogenous myeloid or granulocytic leukemia (AML)	**Remission Induction** Cytarabine and thioguanine or Cytarabine and daunorubicin **Remission Maintenance** (same as above or cytarabine combinations with the listed secondary drugs)	Doxorubicin Mercaptopurine Vincristine Azacytidine Carmustine Cyclophosphamide Prednisone Hydroxyurea Methotrexate Asparaginase
Chronic lymphocytic leukemia	Chlorambucil alone or combined with prednisone	Cyclophosphamide Triethylenemelamine Uracil mustard
Chronic myelocytic leukemia	Busulfan	Mercaptopurine Dibromomannitol Hydroxyurea Pipbroman Melphalan
Multiple myeloma (plasma cell myeloma)	Melphalan and prednisone or cyclophosphamide and prednisone	Carmustine Lomustine Vincristine Cytarabine Procarbazine Chlorambucil Doxorubicin
Polycythemia vera	Busulfan and chlorambucil	Radioactive phosphorus (P32) Cyclophosphamide Melphalan Pipobroman Dibromomannitol
Mycosis fungoides	Mechlorethamine (systemically and topically)	Methotrexate Cyclophosphamide Procarbazine Carmustine Bleomycin Doxorubicin
Burkitt's tumor or lymphoma	Cyclophosphamide	Methotrexate Cytarabine Carmustine Vincristine Ifosfamide
Hodgkin's disease	MOPP combination mechlorethamine vincristine procarbazine prednisone	ABVD combination doxorubicin bleomycin vinblastine dacarbazine
Non-Hodgkin's lymphomas	Under investigation	Under investigation

* Modified from Rodman, M.J., and Smith, D.W.: Pharmacology and Drug Therapy in Nursing. 2nd Ed. Philadelphia, J.B. Lippincott, 1982.

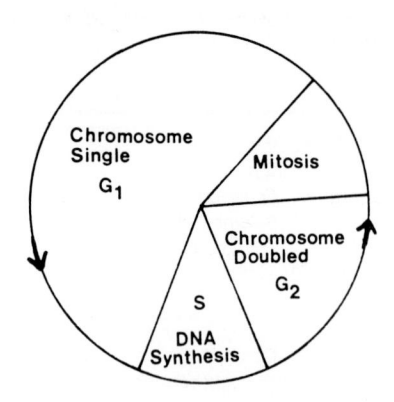

Fig. 4.9 The cell cycle. (From Nora, J.J., and Fraser, F.C., eds.: Medical Genetics. 2nd Ed. Philadelphia, Lea & Febiger, 1981.)

ALKYLATING AGENTS

Alkylating agents form reactive carbonium ions that react with cellular components. Cross-linking and abnormal base pairing in DNA occurs in all cells but especially in rapidly dividing cancer cells.

Mechlorethamine. Mechlorethamine, also known as nitrogen mustard, possesses potent cytotoxic properties.

Mechanism of Action. Mechlorethamine is a cell cycle nonphase-specific antineoplastic drug. Thus, mechlorethamine is effective in malignancies where a high proportion of the cells are in a "resting" state, such as chronic leukemia, Hodgkin's disease, and multiple myeloma. Mechlorethamine forms carbonium ions that cause cross-linking and abnormal base pairing in DNA.

In a freshly prepared form, mechlorethamine is injected intravenously. The drug's vesicant properties necessitate special care to prevent leakage into surrounding tissue or exposure to the skin or eyes.

Clinical Indications. Mechlorethamine is used, in combination with other antineoplastic drugs, in the treatment of hematologic malignancies such as Hodgkin's disease, lymphosarcoma, chronic myelocytic or chronic lymphocytic leukemia, and polycythemia vera.

Adverse Effects/Precautions. Painful inflammation results if extravasation of mechlorethamine into subcutaneous tissues occurs. Local toxicity includes thrombosis and thrombophlebitis; nausea and vomiting are frequent systemic adverse effects. Hematologic abnormalities (such as thrombocytopenia) are often transient; however, bleeding and petechial hemorrhage are possible. Immunosuppression occurs with mechlorethamine therapy and its use is contraindicated in the presence of known infectious disease.

Chlorambucil. Chlorambucil is a bifunctional alkylating agent of the nitrogen mustard type.

Mechanism of Action. Chlorambucil forms reactive carbonium ions that produce cross-linking and abnormal base pairs in DNA.

Clinical Indications. Chlorambucil is used in the treatment of lymphocytic leukemia and malignant lymphomas, including lymphosarcoma, follicular lymphoma, and Hodgkin's disease.

Adverse Effects/Precautions. Bone marrow depression and hyperuricemia are the major adverse reactions to chlorambucil. This drug is probably mutagenic and teratogenic in humans. Chlorambucil is relatively free of gastrointestinal side effects, but it affects fertility.

Mephalan. Mephalan (phenylalanine mustard) is a highly reactive bifunctional alkylating agent.

Mechanism of Action. Mephalan forms carbonium ions that interact with DNA to produce a cytotoxic effect. Cross-linking and abnormal base pairs occur in DNA where an alkyl radical replaces hydrogen atoms. Mephalan also interacts with sulfhydryl, phosphate, and amine groups to elicit a cytotoxic action on both dividing and resting cells.

The phenylalanine "carrier concept" was originally based upon the observation that certain malignant cells tended to take up phenylalanine preferentially.

Clinical Indications. Mephalan is most useful in the treatment of multiple myeloma.

Adverse Effects/Precautions. Acute, non-lymphatic leukemia has followed mephalan chemotherapy and mephalan is potentially mutagenic and teratogenic in humans. High doses cause nausea and vomiting; other dose-related adverse reactions are hematologic abnormalities (anemia, neutropenia, and thrombocytopenia).

Cyclophosphamide. Cyclophosphamide, a synthetic antineoplastic agent, converts to a metabolite that is the active alkylating moiety.

Mechanism of Action. Cyclophosphamide is biotransformed to phosphoramide that transfers alkyl groups to cellular constituents, thereby inducing cytotoxic activity. Cyclophosphamide does not cause tissue irritation (as is the case with the nitrogen mustards like mechlorethamine) and may be administered orally, as well as intravenously.

Clinical Indications. Cyclophosphamide is used in the treatment of malignant lymphomas, such as Hodgkin's disease, nodular or diffuse lymphomas, and Burkitt's lymphoma.

Adverse Effects/Precautions. Alopecia is a frequent complication of cyclophosphamide therapy. Like the other nitrogen mustards, cyclophosphamide causes nausea and vomiting. Bone marrow depression (leukopenia) occurs with this drug, but anemia and thrombocytopenia are seen less frequently than with the other nitrogen mustards. A serious complication of cyclophosphamide therapy is sterile inflammation of the urinary bladder, a condition attributed to irritation by active metabolites of cyclophosphamide.

Uracil Mustard. A polyfunctional alkylating agent, uracil mustard is employed as an antineoplastic drug.

Mechanism of Action. Uracil mustard alkylates DNA in normal and neoplastic cells. The cytotoxic action occurs in all phases of cell division, including the resting phase.

Clinical Indications. Clinical applications for uracil mustard include chronic lymphocytic leukemia, non-Hodgkin's lymphomas, and chronic myelogenous leukemia.

Adverse Effects/Precautions. Hematologic, gastrointestinal, and dermatologic adverse reactions characterize uracil mustard therapy.

Carmustine (BCNU). A significant quality of the nitrosourea compound carmustine is its ability to enter the CNS.

Mechanism of Action. Active metabolites apparently account for carmustine action. The drug alkylates cellular DNA and RNA. Additionally, carmustine inhibits several enzymes by carbamoylation of their amino acids.

Clinical Indications. Carmustine, in combination with prednisone, is employed in multiple myeloma. Carmustine is also effective as secondary therapy in Hodgkin's disease and non-Hodgkin's lymphomas.

Adverse Effects/Precautions. A serious reaction to carmustine is delayed bone marrow toxicity. Gastrointestinal side effects, including nausea and vomiting, are dose-related and may occur shortly after IV therapy with carmustine.

Lomustine (CCNU). Lomustine, a nitrosourea alkylating compound, crosses the blood brain barrier.

Mechanism of Action. Lomustine acts as an alkylating agent to inactivate DNA. Several other key cellular enzymatic processes are inhibited by lomustine.

Clinical Indications. Lomustine is used as a secondary drug in treating Hodgkin's disease.

Adverse Effects/Precautions. Although gastrointestinal and hematologic toxicity are noted with lomustine therapy, delayed bone marrow suppression is a major adverse reaction to this drug.

Busulfan. Busulfan is an alkylsulfonate polyfunctional alkylating agent.

Mechanism of Action. The cytotoxic effect of busulfan is primarily against granulocytic cells; its specific toxicity is on immature malignant bone marrow cells. Busulfan apparently interacts mainly with cellular thiol groups with a minimal cross-linking of nucleoproteins. As with the other alkylating agents, busulfan is nonspecific in cell-phase cytotoxicity and affects resting as well as rapidly dividing cells.

Clinical Indications. Busulfan is indicated for the palliative treatment of chronic myelogenous leukemia. Ninety percent of adult patients with previously untreated chronic myelogenous leukemia exhibit hematologic remission following busulfan therapy.

Adverse Effects/Precautions. Hematologic toxicity requires determination of weekly blood counts to detect early changes in blood cells before hemorrhage or pancytopenia occurs. A rare but important complication of busulfan therapy is pulmonary fibrosis with alveolar exudates that can interfere with breathing.

Pipbroman. An orally effective antineoplastic agent, pipbroman is especially valuable in the treatment of polycythemia vera.

Mechanism of Action. Pipbroman has multiple mechanisms of cytotoxic action, including the alkylation of cellular macroproteins.

Clinical Indications. Pipbroman is useful in the treatment of polycythemia vera and in chronic granulocytic leukemia that is refractory to bulsulfan.

Adverse Effects/Precautions. Adverse reactions to pipbroman are nausea, vomiting, abdominal cramping, diarrhea, and skin rash.

ANTIMETABOLITES

Antimetabolites bear a chemical resemblance to substances that are necessary for proper cell division and reproduction. The antimetabolite structure, however, inhibits the role of the critical metabolite moiety. Thus, they function as fraudulent molecules to block enzymatic reactions important in the growth and development of both normal and malignant cells. Structural analogs (antimetabolites) of the essential metabolites are taken up by normal and neoplastic cells and substitute for them. Antimetabolites are most effective against rapidly dividing cells and so are especially cytotoxic to neoplastic cells. Examples of this class of antineoplastic agents include antimetabolites of folic acid, purine bases, and pyrimidine bases.

Methotrexate. Methotrexate, an analog of the B-complex vitamin folic acid, was the first drug determined to be an effective antineoplastic agent against leukemia.

Mechanism of Action. Folic acid from dietary sources converts to tetrahydrofolic acid, an active intermediate in DNA formation, by the enzyme dihydrofolate reductase. Methotrexate is a competitive, practically irreversible, inhibitor of dihydrofolate reductase and acts to prevent the formation of tetrahydrofolate acid, thus inhibiting DNA formation. Cellular replication is blocked, especially in actively proliferating tissues, such as malignant cells, bone marrow, fetal cells, dermal epithelium, buccal and intestinal mucosa, and cells of the urinary bladder. Since cellular division is more pronounced in malignant tissue, methotrexate usually impairs growth without significant irreversible damage to normal cells.

Clinical Indications. Methotrexate, used in the treatment of acute lymphocytic leukemia, is especially effective in the palliation of acute lymphoblastic (stem-cell) leukemia in children.

Adverse Effects/Precautions. Methotrexate may produce severe bone marrow depression, anemia, leukopenia, thrombocytopenia, and hemorrhage. Leucovorin or folinic acid reverses the immediate effects of toxic doses of methotrexate. Folinic acid supplies a tetrahydrofolate derivative that can "rescue" the bone marrow, intestinal mucosa, and other normal tissue from the adverse effects of methotrexate. Leucovorin "rescue" is now clinically applied when high doses of methotrexate kill previously resistant cancer cells.

Methotrexate is probably hepatotoxic, particularly in high doses or upon prolonged therapy. Diarrhea and ulcerative stomatitis are frequent adverse reactions to methotrexate.

Mercaptopurine. A purine analog, mercaptopurine interferes with DNA synthesis.

Mechanism of Action. Mercaptopurine competes with hypoxanthine and guanine (purine bases) for the enzyme hypoxanthine-guanine phosphoribosyltransferase. Through this reaction, mercaptopurine is converted to thioinosinic acid, a fraudulent intracellular nucleotide, that inhibits several inosinic acid reactions important in DNA synthesis. Thioinosinic acid (TIMP) is methylated to 6-methylthioinosinic acid (MTIMP); both metabolites (TIMP and MTIMP) inhibit purine nucleotide synthesis.

Clinical Indications. Mercaptopurine is used in the treatment of acute lymphocytic leukemia in children and in some adults with acute and chronic myelogenous leukemia.

Adverse Effects/Precautions. A consistent dose-related effect of mercaptopurine therapy is bone marrow depression. Hepatotoxicity may occur and liver necrosis accounts for deaths. Uncommon reactions to therapeutic doses include nausea, vomiting, oral lesions, and gastrointestinal ulceration. Hyperuricemia produced by the rapid leukemia cell lysis may require concurrent use of prophylactic allopurinol.

Thioguanine. Thioguanine is an analog of the purine base guanine.

Mechanism of Action. Thioguanine competes with hypoxanthine and guanine for hypoxanthine-guanine phosphoribosyltransferase. Biotransformation of thioguanine to 6-thioguanylic acid via this reaction results in an interference at multiple sites in the biosynthesis pathway of guanine nucleotides. Additionally, thioguanine hampers the synthesis of purines due to the drug's ability to inhibit glutamine-5-phosphoribosylpyrophosphate aminotransferase. Finally, the incorporation of thioguanine nucleotides into both RNA and DNA produces nonfunctional altered nucleic acids that do not effectively participate in cell division processes.

Clinical Indications. Thioguanine is employed for remission, induction, and maintenance therapy for acute leukemia. Thioguanine is used as a secondary drug to busulfan in the treatment of chronic myelogenous leukemia.

Adverse Effects/Precautions. Bone marrow suppression and hepatotoxicity are major adverse reactions to thioguanine therapy. Nausea, vomiting, and stomatitis may also occur, especially in high doses. Hyperuricemia is often a complication due to rapid cell lysis accompanying the antineoplastic effects on leukemic cells.

Cytarabine (Cytosine Arabinoside). Cytarabine, a synthetic nucleoside, differs from the naturally occurring nucleosides (i.e., cytidine and deoxycytidine) that are required for nucleic acid synthesis by having arabinose in the nucleoside structure as the sugar moiety instead of ribose or deoxyribose.

Mechanism of Action. Cytarabine exhibits cell phase cytotoxicity, primarily affecting cells undergoing DNA synthesis (S-phase), and blocks the progression of cells from the G_1 phase to the S-phase (Figure 4.9). By inhibiting DNA polymerase, cytarabine apparently induces cell-killing effects.

Studies report the incorporation of cytarabine into both DNA and RNA. Maximal beneficial effects with cytarabine in hematologic malignancies are seen in combination therapy with other antineoplastic drugs.

Clinical Indications. Cytarabine, alone or in combination with other antineoplastic drugs, is employed in the induction and remission of acute myelocytic leukemia (AML) of both children and adults. Acute lymphocytic leukemia (ALL) and chronic myelocytic leukemia may also respond to cytarabine therapy.

Adverse Effects/Precautions. A major toxicity noted with cytarabine therapy is bone marrow depression, as evidenced by leukopenia, thrombocytopenia, and anemia. Other reactions include nausea, vomiting, diarrhea, abdominal pain, stomatitis, and liver toxicity.

A reported "cytarabine syndrome" occurs within 6 to 12 hours following administration of the drug; fever, myalgia, bone pain, recurrent chest pain, maculopapular rash, and malaise characterize this reaction.

INHIBITORS OF CELL MITOSIS

Naturally occurring plant alkaloids constitute the members of this antineoplastic drug class.

Vinblastine. Vinblastine is an alkaloid extracted from Vinca rosea Linn. (periwinkle).

Mechanism of Action. The antimitotic effect of vinblastine is characterized by the production of atypical mitotic figures. Vinblastine interferes with the metabolic pathways of amino acids leading from glutamic acid to the tricarboxylic acid (citric acid) cycle and urea. Vinblastine induces an effect on the cellular energy transformations necessary for mitosis and reportedly interferes with nucleic acid synthesis.

Clinical Indications. Malignancies frequently responsive to vinblastine include generalized Hodgkin's disease, lymphocytic lymphoma, and histocytic lymphoma.

Adverse Effects/Precautions. Leukopenia is usually the dose-limiting factor. The incidence of other adverse reactions is dose-related; these effects usually persist no longer than a day following initiation of vinblastine therapy. Commonly reported adverse reactions are gastrointestinal effects, including nausea and vomiting. Neurologic effects (such as numbness, paresthesias, and peripheral neuritis) may also occur.

Vincristine. Vincristine, a frequently employed antineoplastic drug, is an alkaloid obtained from Vinca rosea Linn. (periwinkle).

Mechanism of Action. Vincristine arrests cell division or the metaphase stage of mitosis. Vincristine acts predominantly on rapidly proliferating cells.

Clinical Indications. Vincristine is used in acute leukemia and Hodgkin's disease.

Adverse Effects/Precautions. Adverse reactions to vincristine therapy are usually dose-related and reversible. Leukopenia, neuritic pain, constipation, and ataxia are frequent, but are usually of short duration (about 1 week) and tend to disappear with continued vincristine treatment. Additional adverse reactions, such as hair loss, paresthesia, and neuromuscular difficulties, are more persistent and last for prolonged periods.

A syndrome of inappropriate antidiuretic hormone secretion (SIADH) occurs rarely with vincristine use. High urinary sodium excretion in the presence of hyponatremia characterizes this condition.

ANTIBIOTICS

Certain antibiotics find clinical application in antineoplastic chemotherapy regimens.

Bleomycin. Bleomycin is a mixture of glycopeptide antibiotics that are isolated from a strain Streptomyces verticillus.

Mechanism of Action. Bleomycin inhibits DNA synthesis with ancillary inhibitory effects on RNA and protein synthesis. Bleomycin is cell phase specific with the greatest cytotoxic activity noted in the G_2 and M phases (Figure 4.9).

Clinical Indications. Bleomycin is used, either singly or in combination with other neoplastic agents, for the palliative treatment of lymphomas, such as Hodgkin's disease and lymphosarcoma.

Adverse Effects/Precautions. The major toxic effect of bleomycin therapy is pulmonary fibrosis; this condition occurs most frequently as pneumonitis in elderly patients. Adverse reactions involving the integument and mucous membranes (erythema, hyperkeratosis, alopecia, stomatitis) occur in a high percentage of patients (50%). About 1% of the patients receiving bleomycin experience an idiosyncratic reaction consisting of hypotension, mental confusion, fever, chills, and wheezing.

Doxorubicin. Doxorubicin is an anthracycline antibiotic isolated from cultures of Streptomyces peucetius var. caesius.

Mechanism of Action. Doxorubicin binds to DNA and inhibits nucleic acid biosynthesis in eliciting its cytotoxic action. Rapid cell penetration, extensive chromatin binding, and rapid inhibition of mitotic activity characterize doxorubicin action.

Clinical Indications. Doxorubicin is effective in eliciting remission in acute lymphoblastic leukemia, acute myeloblastic leukemia, and Hodgkin's and non-Hodgkin's lymphomas.

Adverse Effects/Precautions. Myocardial toxicity with delayed CHF is possible with higher dosage levels of doxorubicin. Tissue necrosis results if extravasation occurs during administration of the drug. Impaired hepatic function requires dosage reduction, and hyperuricemia and discolored red urine may necessitate precautionary patient advice. Myelosuppression, usually evidenced as leukocyte reduction, occurs in a high percentage of patients (60 to 84%). Doxorubicin is contraindicated in malignant melanoma, kidney carcinoma, large bowel carcinoma, and brain tumors.

Daunorubicin. Daunorubicin is an anthracycline antibiotic isolated from Streptomyces coeruleorubidus.

Mechanism of Action. By intercalating between the DNA double helix, daunorubicin elicits a cytotoxic action.

Clinical Indications. Daunorubicin induces remission in acute nonlymphocytic leukemia of adults.

Adverse Effects/Precautions. Cardiac toxicity and bone marrow suppression represent major adverse reactions to daunorubicin therapy. Daunorubicin should be given by rapid IV infusion and should never be administered by IM or SC injection. Hepatic and renal dysfunction can enhance daunorubicin toxicity.

MISCELLANEOUS ANTINEOPLASTIC DRUGS

Some neoplastic diseases are effectively managed by agents that are not routinely used in cancer chemotherapy.

Hydroxyurea. Hydroxyurea is an especially valuable antineoplastic drug because of its effectiveness against hematologic malignancies refractory to standard chemotherapy.

Mechanism of Action. Hydroxyurea inhibits DNA synthesis without significant interference with RNA synthesis or protein formation. The incorporation of thymidine into DNA is reduced by hydroxyurea.

Clinical Indications. Cases of chronic myelocytic leukemia that are refractory to prior antineoplastic chemotherapy sometimes respond favorably to hydroxyurea.

Adverse Effects/Precautions. Frequent adverse reactions relate to bone marrow suppression and include leukopenia, anemia, and occasionally thrombocytopenia.

Procarbazine. Procarbazine, a synthetic hydrazine monoamine oxidase inhibitor, was initially recognized for its hematopoietic toxicity.

Mechanism of Action. Procarbazine inhibits DNA, RNA, and protein synthesis. Cross-resistance to procarbazine does not apparently exist with other antineoplastic therapy, including radiotherapy and steroids.

Clinical Indications. Procarbazine is useful in generalized Hodgkin's disease and cases resistant to other forms of therapy. Currently, procarbazine is a component of an effective combination (MOPP) regimen used in the treatment of Hodgkin's disease. Another of its clinical applications is as an adjunct to standard cancer therapy.

Adverse Effects/Precautions. Frequent adverse reactions to procarbazine include leukopenia, anemia, thrombocytopenia, nausea, and vomiting.

Prednisone. A synthetic adrenocorticoid-type, prednisone is often used as adjunctive therapy in antineoplastic chemotherapy.

Mechanism of Action. Prednisone has lympholytic activity and suppresses mitosis in lymphocytes.

Clinical Indications. Prednisone is used as an adjunct in the management of leukemia and lymphomas in adults and in acute childhood leukemia. A drug in the MOPP combination that is especially effective in treating advanced Hodgkin's disease, prednisone also prevents complications (such as fever) in some forms of cancer.

Adverse Effects/Precautions. Reported adverse reactions to glucocorticoid (prednisone) therapy include fluid and electrolyte imbalance, endocrine dysfunction, musculoskeletal disorders, cardiovascular problems, and gastrointestinal toxicity.

Asparaginase. Asparaginase is an enzyme isolated from Escherichia coli.

Mechanism of Action. Malignant cells, especially those present in lymphocytic leukemia, depend upon exogenous asparagine for survival. Asparaginase hydrolyzes asparagine and thus deprives the tumor cell of the required amino acid (asparagine) necessary for cellular protein synthesis. The inhibitory activity is most pronounced in the post-mitotic phase of the cell cycle (Figure 4.9). Normal cells, in contrast to malignant cells, ordinarily synthesize asparagine rendering them less sensitive to the action of asparaginase. Consequently, asparaginase has minimal adverse effects on bone marrow and mucosal or hair follicle cells.

Clinical Indications. Asparaginase is used, primarily in combination with other antineoplastics, to induce remission in acute lymphocytic leukemia in children.

Adverse Effects/Precautions. A hospital setting is recommended for asparaginase administration due to the unpredictability of adverse reactions to the drug. For example, frequent hypersensitivity reactions range from mild skin eruptions to potentially fatal anaphylaxis. Since these reactions may occur during the primary phase of therapy, skin-testing for asparaginase sensitivity is recommended before each course of asparaginase therapy.

Hepatic toxicity also occurs frequently with this enzyme. Asparaginase-induced hepatic damage may increase the toxicity of other antineoplastics, such as vincristine. Pancreatic toxicity has resulted in deaths from hemorrhagic pancreatitis.

Sodium Phosphate P32. Sodium phosphate P32 is a radioactive isotope used to treat certain hematologic malignancies.

Mechanism of Action. Metabolic and proliferative cellular processes require phosphorus. Radioactive phosphorus concentrates in rapidly dividing malignant cells and disrupts the cellular reproductive machinery.

Clinical Indications. Radioactive phosphorus (sodium phosphate P32) is indicated in the treatment of polycythemia vera, chronic myelocytic leukemia, and chronic lymphocytic leukemia.

Adverse Effects/Precautions. Although adverse effects have not been reported, overdosage may produce serious effects on the hematopoietic system.

DRUG INTERACTIONS

Because of the possibility of hemorrhage, adverse drug reactions involving anticoagulants represent a life-threatening problem of multiple drug therapy. On the other hand, positive drug interactions of multiple drug therapy often save many lives, as in the case of leukemia therapy.

DRUGS AFFECTING THE ANEMIAS

Iron Preparations.

Antacids. Concomitant administration with iron preparations may decrease the absorption of iron.

Chloramphenicol. By delaying both iron clearance from plasma and iron incorporation into red blood cells, chloramphenicol may inhibit the response to iron therapy in patients with iron-deficiency anemia.

Oral Tetracyclines. Oral iron preparations interfere with oral tetracycline absorption; thus, these products should not be taken within 2 hours of each other.

Penicillamine. Ferrous sulfate decreases the gastrointestinal absorption of penicillamine, possibly decreasing its effectiveness.

Folic Acid.

Phenytoin. Administering folic acid with phenytoin may increase the frequency of seizures and decrease serum phenytoin levels.

Pyrimethamine. Due to possible inhibition of the antimicrobial effect, administration of folic acid is discouraged in patients receiving pyrimethamine for malaria or toxoplasmosis.

Vitamin B_{12}.

Aminoglycosides. Oral neomycin may decrease the gastrointestinal absorption of vitamin B_{12}. Colchicine administration apparently increases neomycin-induced malabsorption of vitamin B_{12}.

Aminosalicyclic Acid. Aminosalicyclic acid causes malabsorption of vitamin B_{12}.

Chloramphenicol. Reduction of the therapeutic effectiveness of vitamin B_{12} possibly results from interference with erythrocyte maturation.

DRUGS PROMOTING HEMOSTASIS

Aminocaproic Acid.

Oral Contraceptives. Concomitant administration may increase clotting factors and lead to a hypercoagulable state.

Carbazochrome.

Antihistamines. Since antihistamines tend to inhibit the effectiveness of carbazochrome, their use should be discontinued 48 hours prior to initiation of carbazochrome therapy.

ORAL ANTICOAGULANTS

Warfarin; Dicumarol.

Anabolic Steroids. Concurrent use may promote excessive anticoagulant effect.

Antidiabetics. Although tolbutamide may initially enhance the anticoagulant effect of dicumarol, continued therapy with both drugs may decrease plasma levels and the anticoagulant effect of dicumarol.

Barbiturates. Barbiturates induce hepatic microsomal enzymes, increasing the metabolism of coumarin anticoagulants. Whereas barbiturates may decrease gastrointestinal absorption of dicumarol, warfarin absorption is not significantly affected.

Cimetidine. Concurrent administration is discouraged due to inhibition of the hepatic metabolism of the oral anticoagulant.

Clofibrate. By mechanisms not established, clofibrate apparently enhances the effect of warfarin on vitamin K-dependent clotting factor synthesis and/or it may affect the turnover of vitamin K.

Dextrothyroxine. Initiation or discontinuation of dextrothyroxine therapy in a patient stabilized on an oral anticoagulant usually necessitates a change in the maintenance anticoagulant dose.

Disulfiram. Disulfiram evidently increases the hypoprothrombinemic effect and plasma levels of warfarin.

Glutethimide. By inducing hepatic microsomal enzymes, glutethimide apparently increases the metabolism of oral anticoagulants.

Phenylbutazone. Phenylbutazone apparently inhibits the metabolism of warfarin therapy, displaces warfarin from plasma protein binding sites, produces gastrointestinal ulceration, and impairs platelet function. Thus, concomitant use of phenylbutazone with oral anticoagulants is strongly discouraged. The same caution also applies to oxyphenbutazone therapy with oral anticoagulants.

Rifampin. By inducing hepatic microsomal enzymes, rifampin evidently stimulates the metabolism of warfarin, necessitating readjustment of anticoagulant dosage.

Salicylates. Concurrent use is discouraged due to potential reduction of plasma prothrombin levels, displacement of coumarin anticoagulants from plasma protein binding, gastrointestinal bleeding, and impairment of primary hemostasis.

Sulfinpyrazone. Reports of substantial increases in the hypoprothrombinemic response to warfarin have followed sulfinpyrazone therapy.

Sulfonamides. Sulfonamides may impair the hepatic mechanism of oral anticoagulants.

Thyroid Preparations. Thyroid hormones may increase catabolism of vitamin K-dependent clotting factors. Hypothyroidism patients are ordinarily warfarin-resistant and require larger doses of warfarin to achieve effective anticoagulation levels.

PARENTERAL ANTICOAGULANTS

Heparin.

Oral Anticoagulants. Heparin evidently prolongs the prothrombin time in patients receiving oral anticoagulants.

Salicylates and Other Drugs That Affect Platelet Aggregation. By inhibiting platelet aggregation, aspirin impairs a hemostatic mechanism needed for bleeding prevention in patients receiving heparin.

Diazepam. Heparin may increase plasma levels of diazepam.

ANTILIPIDEMIC DRUGS

Cholestyramine.

Acetaminophen. Cholestyramine inhibits the gastrointestinal absorption of acetaminophen.

Corticosteroids. Separate doses of these drugs are recommended to prevent the cholestyramine from inhibiting the gastrointestinal absorption of hydrocortisone.

Digitalis. By binding digitoxin in the gut, cholestyramine interrupts the enterohepatic circulation of digitoxin and shortens its half-life.

Oral Anticoagulants. Possible binding in the gut caused by cholestyramine may result in both impaired absorption and interference with enterohepatic circulation of anticoagulants.

Thyroid Hormones. By binding both thyroxine and triiodothyronine in the intestine, cholestyramine impairs the absorption of these thyroid hormones.

Clofibrate.

Antidiabetics. Clofibrate may increase the hypoglycemic effect of sulfonylureas. Thus, monitoring for hypoglycemia in patients on concomitant therapy is advisable.

Furosemide. Clofibrate and furosemide apparently compete for plasma albumin binding sites.

Oral Anticoagulants. By mechanisms not established, clofibrate evidently enhances the effect of warfarin on vitamin K-dependent clotting factor synthesis and/or affects the turnover of vitamin K.

Colestipol.

Digitalis. By apparently binding digitalis glycosides in the gut, colestipol impairs their initial absorption and enterohepatic circulation.

Thiazide Diuretics. Colestipol apparently inhibits the gastrointestinal absorption of chlorothiazide.

ANTINEOPLASTIC DRUGS

Carmustine.

Cimetidine. Excessive bone marrow suppression may follow concurrent administration of carmustine or other myelosuppressive drugs and cimetidine.

Cyclophosphamide.

Allopurinol. Concurrent administration may produce bone marrow depression.

Barbiturates. Barbiturates may promote the conversion of cyclophosphamide to active alkylating metabolites.

Corticosteroids. Concurrent administration may result in altered cyclophosphamide effect.

ANTIMETABOLITES

Mercaptopurine.

Allopurinol. Concurrent administration necessitates reducing the mercaptopurine dose to ⅓ to ¼ the usual dose to avoid delayed catabolism of mercaptopurine and possible severe toxicity.

Methotrexate.

Salicylates. Salicylates apparently block the renal tubular secretion that methotrexate undergoes. Also, salicylates displace methotrexate from plasma protein binding.

Vaccinations. Since methotrexate impairs the immunologic response to smallpox vaccine resulting in generalized vaccinia, live vaccines should be avoided in patients receiving agents with immunosuppressive activity such as methotrexate.

ANTIBIOTICS

Doxorubicin.

Barbiturates. Barbituarates increase the plasma clearance of doxorubicin.

MISCELLANEOUS ANTINEOPLASTIC DRUGS

Procarbazine.

Ethanol. Concurrent use is discouraged because of a disulfiram-like reaction and possible CNS depression.

Sympathomimetics. Procarbazine has monoamine oxidase inhibiting activity.

SUMMARY

Drug therapy for blood disorders is sometimes the first avenue of treatment, such as in certain neoplastic diseases; othertimes, drug therapy is used only after other therapeutic measures (such as diet, weight control, or exercise) have not proved beneficial, as in the treatment of hyperlipidemia. For decades, replacement therapy (employed in the treatment of iron deficiency anemia) has successfully reversed the disease process. This established therapy regimen contrasts sharply with the experimental stages of drug treatment for acquired immune deficiency disease (AIDS).

The urgency in the search for an antiviral drug for AIDS contrasts markedly with the subdued conjecture that surrounds the benefit of lowering elevated blood lipoproteins to prevent atherosclerosis. Additional therapeutic options in treating blood disorders have emerged because of accelerated research in molecular biology, particularly nucleic acid metabolism. Combination antineoplastic drug therapy attains a rational base as the intricacies of cellular reproductive machinery are better elucidated. This understanding has produced chemotherapy cures in certain neoplastic diseases that were previously amenable only to surgery or radiation therapy. The future in drug treatment of blood disorders appears hopeful as chemical arrows to specific metabolic targets ("magic bullets") are developed and refined.

SUGGESTED READINGS

Barnes, D.M.: Grim projections for AIDS epidemic. Science, 232:1589, 1986.
Cancer Chemotherapy. Med Lett Drugs Ther, 25:1, 1983.
Das, K.C., and Herbert, V.: Vitamin B_{12}-folate interrelationship. Clin Haematol, 5:697, 1976.
DeVita, V.T., and Schein, P.S.: The use of drugs in combination for the treatment of cancer. N Engl J Med, 288:998, 1973.
Ferguson, G.G.: Pathophysiology. Mechanisms and Expressions. Philadelphia, W.B. Saunders Co., 1984.
Finch, C.A., and Huebers, H.: Perspectives in iron metabolism. N Engl J Med, 306:1520, 1983.
Frishman, W.H.: Antiplatelet therapy in coronary artery disease. Hosp Pract, 17:73, 1982.
Gilman, A.G., et al. (eds.): The Pharmacological Basis of Therapeutics. 7th Ed. New York, Macmillan Publishing Co., Inc., 1985.
Hamilton, P.J., Stalker, A.L., and Douglas, A.S.: Disseminated intravascular coagulation. A review. J Clin Pathol, 31:609, 1978.
Hamor, G.H.: Mandrake, periwinkle, and cancer. California Pharmacist, May 1985, 46.
Hanston, P.D.: Drug Interactions. 5th Ed. Philadelphia, Lea & Febiger, 1985.
Herbert, V.: Folic acid and vitamin B_{12}. In Modern Nutrition in Health and Disease. 5th Ed. Edited by R.S. Goodhart and M.E. Shils. Philadelphia, Lea & Febiger, 1973.
Howard, P.: Pharmacotherapy of hyperlipidemia. Pharmacy Times, 52:112, 1986.
Jaques, L.B.: Heparins. Anionic polyelectrolyte drugs. Pharmacol Rev, 31:99, 1980.
Kastrup, E.K., and Boyd, J.R. (eds.): Drug Facts and Comparisons. Philadelphia, J.B. Lippincott Co., 1985.
Mustard, J.F., and Packham, M.A.: Factors influencing platelet function. Adhesion, release, aggregation. Pharmacol Rev, 22:97, 1970.
Perutz, M.F.: Hemoglobin structure and respiratory transport. Sci Am, 239:68, 1978.
Poirier, T.I.: AIDS. Where do we stand today? US Pharmacist, 11:52, 1986.
Reynolds, E.H.: Neurological aspects of folate and vitamin B_{12} metabolism. Clin Haematol, 5:661, 1976.
Robbins, S.L., and Angell, M.: Basic Pathology. 2nd Ed. Philadelphia, W.B. Saunders Co., 1976.
Savin, M.A.: A practical approach to the treatment of iron deficiency. Ration Drug Ther, 11:1, 1977.
Sharma, G.V.R.K., et al.: Thrombolytic therapy. N Engl J Med, 306:1268, 1982.
Tanne, J.H.: Fighting AIDS. On the front lines against the plague. New York, 20:22, 1987.
Vega, G.L., and Grundy, S.M.: Treatment of primary moderate hypercholesterolemia with lovastatin (Mevinolin) and colestipol. JAMA, 257:33, 1987.
Walsh, P.N.: Oral anticoagulant therapy. Hosp Pract, 18:101, 1982.
Weintraub, M., and Evans, P.: Pentoxifylline. A new medication for intermittent claudication. Hospital Formulary, 19:117, 1984.

CHAPTER EXAMINATION

In a recent annual physical examination, a blood screen revealed hyperlipidemia in an overweight middle-aged man with a family medical history of coronary heart disease. The patient enjoys several beers after work and has a penchant for fast food hamburgers and fries. Also, according to his cultural heritage, a good breakfast makes for a good day, so fried eggs, bacon, ham, or sausage, and hash browns are a regular menu.

1. The appropriate initial treatment regimen for this patient is
   a. none, since no evidence indicates that hyperlipidemia contributes to coronary heart disease
   b. diet and weight control
   c. gemfibrozil
   d. probucol
2. The patient blood screen also indicated hypercholesterolemia. The best drug treatment for this condition is
   a. clofibrate
   b. dicumarol
   c. cholestyramine
   d. small doses of aspirin each day

3. Since both cholesterol and triglyceride levels are elevated, an appropriate *single* agent therapy is
   a. niacin
   b. colestipol
   c. probucol
   d. gemfibrozil
4. When both cholesterol and triglyceride levels are elevated, an appropriate *combination* therapy is
   a. cholestyramine and colestipol
   b. levothyroxine and neomycin
   c. clofibrate and gemfibrozil
   d. colestipol and gemfibrozil
5. Colestipol
   a. elevates LDL by speeding the catabolism of VLDL
   b. binds bile acids in the gastrointestinal tract
   c. effectively lowers HDL
   d. none of the above

An elderly patient has taken chloral hydrate for periodic insomnia for several years. Due to stress factors, this patient has used the drug regularly on his physician's advice. After venous thrombosis developed in the patient, the physician prescribed warfarin and phenylbutazone.

---

6. Warfarin is an oral anticoagulant that
   a. inhibits the regeneration of reduced vitamin K from vitamin K epoxide
   b. activates antithrombin III
   c. is minimally bound by plasma proteins
   d. converts to an active metabolite that is responsible for the anticoagulant effect
7. A drug similar to warfarin in mechanism of action and therapeutic application is
   a. heparin
   b. protamine sulfate
   c. dicumarol
   d. folic acid
8. When given concurrently with warfarin, phenylbutazone
   a. decreases the anticoagulant activity of warfarin
   b. increases the anticoagulant activity of warfarin which produces a clinically significant drug interaction
   c. loses its anti-inflammatory activity, especially if chloral hydrate is also administered
   d. does not alter the anticoagulant response

Iron deficiency anemia is diagnosed in a young mother who complains of fatigue and "tired blood." She has recently experienced excessive menstrual periods and has been on a "high protein," low carbohydrate diet.

---

9. The diet regimen may have resulted in
   a. insufficient dietary folic acid and vitamin B_{12}, resulting in the anemia
   b. diversion of iron to keratin stores
   c. insufficient dietary iron in this particular patient
   d. all of the above
10. The iron requirement for adequate hemoglobin and RBC formation increases in excessive menstruation and
    a. pregnancy
    b. always necessitates parenteral iron therapy
    c. is best supplied by ferric salts
    d. always represents a clinical emergency
11. Ferrous salts, such as ferrous sulfate,
    a. supply the keystone of the cyanocobalamin molecule
    b. correct hypochromic microcytic anemia in iron deficient patients
    c. are inactivated by gastric hydrochloric acid
    d. are inferior to ferric salts with respect to gastrointestinal absorption
12. Excessive accidental ingestion of iron tablets by this patient's toddler
    a. can break the child's intestinal mucosal barrier to iron absorption and flood the system with ferritin
    b. is usually treated with the antidote desoxferamine
    c. may cause gastrointestinal bleeding and hypotension
    d. all of the above

THERAPEUTIC PHARMACOLOGY

Pernicious anemia is diagnosed in a patient exhibiting achlorhydria and muscle-wasting. Megaloblastic hyperchromic erythrocytes are also noted.

13. The major biochemical lesion characteristic of pernicious anemia is
    a. defective folic acid synthesis
    b. excessive hepatic vitamin B_{12} catabolism
    c. deficient formation and release of intrinsic factor from the gastric mucosa
    d. a diversion of iron from reticuloendothelial tissues to adipose cells
14. Recommended initial therapy for severe pernicious anemia includes
    a. parenteral vitamin B_{12} (cyanocobalamin)
    b. oral folinic acid (leucovorin)
    c. oral folic acid
    d. ferrous sulfate tablets
15. Folic acid administration
    a. worsens the hematologic abnormalities of pernicious anemia
    b. corrects the hematologic picture, but allows neurologic abnormalities to proceed
    c. stimulates synthesis of the hepatic extrinsic pattern
    d. activates the intrinsic factor

MOPP (**m**echlorethamine, vincristine [**o**ncovin], **p**robarbazine, **p**rednisone) is the therapeutic regimen for a middle-aged, male, Hodgkin's disease patient.

16. This combination
    a. is not indicated in the treatment of Hodgkin's disease
    b. utilizes only alkylating agents as cytotoxic drugs
    c. has produced complete remissions in advanced stages of Hodgkin's disease
    d. is routinely used for psoriasis
17. Vincristine
    a. is an alkaloid isolated from Vinca rosea Linn. (periwinkle)
    b. arrests cell division in metaphase
    c. may produce a syndrome of inappropriate antidiuretic hormone secretion (SIADH)
    d. all of the above
18. Procarbazine
    a. is a purine antagonist
    b. inhibits DNA, RNA, and protein synthesis
    c. and methotrexate are folic acid metabolites
    d. is a pyrimidine antagonist
19. Prednisone
    a. has lympholytic properties, inhibits mitosis in lymphocytes, and prevents complications (such as fever) seen in Hodgkin's disease
    b. occurs naturally as an adrenocorticoid
    c. favors sodium excretion
    d. inhibits asparagine hydrolysis
20. Mechlorethamine
    a. is a nonphase-specific cell cycle antineoplastic drug
    b. is never administered intravenously due to its toxicity
    c. never produces immunosuppression
    d. all of the above

ANSWER KEY

1.	b	11.	b
2.	c	12.	d
3.	a	13.	c
4.	d	14.	a
5.	b	15.	b
6.	a	16.	c
7.	c	17.	d
8.	b	18.	b
9.	c	19.	a
10.	a	20.	a

chapter 5

RENAL SYSTEM*

CHAPTER OBJECTIVES

After studying this chapter, you should be able to:
1. Describe the gross anatomy of the kidney.
2. Identify the parts of a nephron and list three processes that take place within this functional unit of the kidney.
3. Name five major functions of the kidney.
4. Outline the different pharmacologic classes of diuretics.
5. Discuss the main therapeutic indications for diuretic use.
6. Explain the proposed mechanism(s) of action for six widely used diuretics.
7. Describe changes in electrolyte patterns (i.e., Na^+, Cl^-, K^+) seen with diuretic therapy.
8. List four factors of importance in the clinical selection of a diuretic.
9. Give three examples of drug interactions involving diuretics.
10. Describe the mechanisms whereby uricosuric drugs, such as probenecid and sulfinpyrazone, influence the urinary excretion of uric acid.

---

* This chapter has been modified, with revisions and additions, from THE RATIONAL USE OF DIURETICS by Glenn Appelt. Reprinted by permission of University Learning Systems, Inc., Boca Raton, FL, Copyright 1984.

INTRODUCTION

Renal system functions include the maintenance of water and electrolyte balance. If salt intake is excessive or various disease processes are present, the body responds by retaining fluid, that is, it becomes edematous. In this case, dietary restriction of salt or other measures, such as the use of diuretics, may be necessary to rid the body of this unwanted fluid. By a direct action on the kidney, diuretics treat edema by increasing the amount of urine excreted.

How important are diuretics today? Results of a 1982 National Center for Health Statistics survey indicated that nearly 3,000 physicians named the diuretic furosemide as the top drug used in their practices. Overall, this drug was mentioned more than other widely prescribed drugs in the antibiotic, tranquilizer, or analgesic classifications. In the same survey, another diuretic (combination of triamterene and hydrochlorothiazide) placed seventh in number of mentions. Additionally, the 1985 tabulation of the "Top 200 Most Often Prescribed Drugs" in the United States included both of these diuretics in the top eight drugs considering both new and refill prescriptions; the combination triamterene and hydrochlorothiazide was the most prescribed drug product of all categories.

To understand how diuretics work, one must appreciate the basic physiologic mechanisms working in kidney function. Consider a city water purification system (Figure 5.1a). Now, recall the manner in which the body rids itself of waste substances in the urine (Figure 5.1b). The exquisite complexity of the kidney would surpass the most intricate and efficient purification system ever devised by a sanitary engineer. The filtering system in a city water supply may cover acres, but the body's "filtering system" is contained in two bean-shaped organs weighing about 0.24 kg each. These organs are found, one on each side, behind the abdominal cavity.

Under normal circumstances, about ¼ of the blood pumped by each heart beat passes through the kidneys and the entire blood volume passes through the kidneys about 15 times a day. Of the approximately 1,600 L of blood that flow through the kidney every 24 hours, only 1/1,000 is converted to urine. To prevent the body from being poisoned by accumulated wastes from its own metabolism, the kidney rids the body of these substances. By processes to be discussed later, the kidneys regulate fluid and electrolyte balance and keep the body's acid-base balance within the narrow limits necessary for life.

Filtration, the transport processes of reabsorption and secretion (of certain substances), and excretion are carried out by the functional unit of the kidney, the nephron. Approximately one million nephrons are in each kidney, which if stretched end-to-end would measure over 80 km. Such a large functional capacity may explain, in part, how an individual is able to survive (and indeed, thrive) with only one healthy kidney.

Sodium chloride, or common salt, is one of the important substances reabsorbed. Both sodium (Na^+) and chloride (Cl^-) function in countless reactions in the body. Of the 1 kg of salt which passes through the kidneys daily, approximately 0.01 kg is excreted in the urine. This example of electrolyte conservation is an important kidney function.

Diuretics increase the urine flow by blocking reabsorption of sodium, chloride, bicarbonate, and water. This is the basis for their effectiveness in treating certain clinical conditions such as cardiac edema. Other edematous conditions in which diuretics are used are liver cirrhosis, the nephrotic syndrome, and, in some cases, the edema of pregnancy. Specialized uses for the diuretics include glaucoma to reduce intraocu-

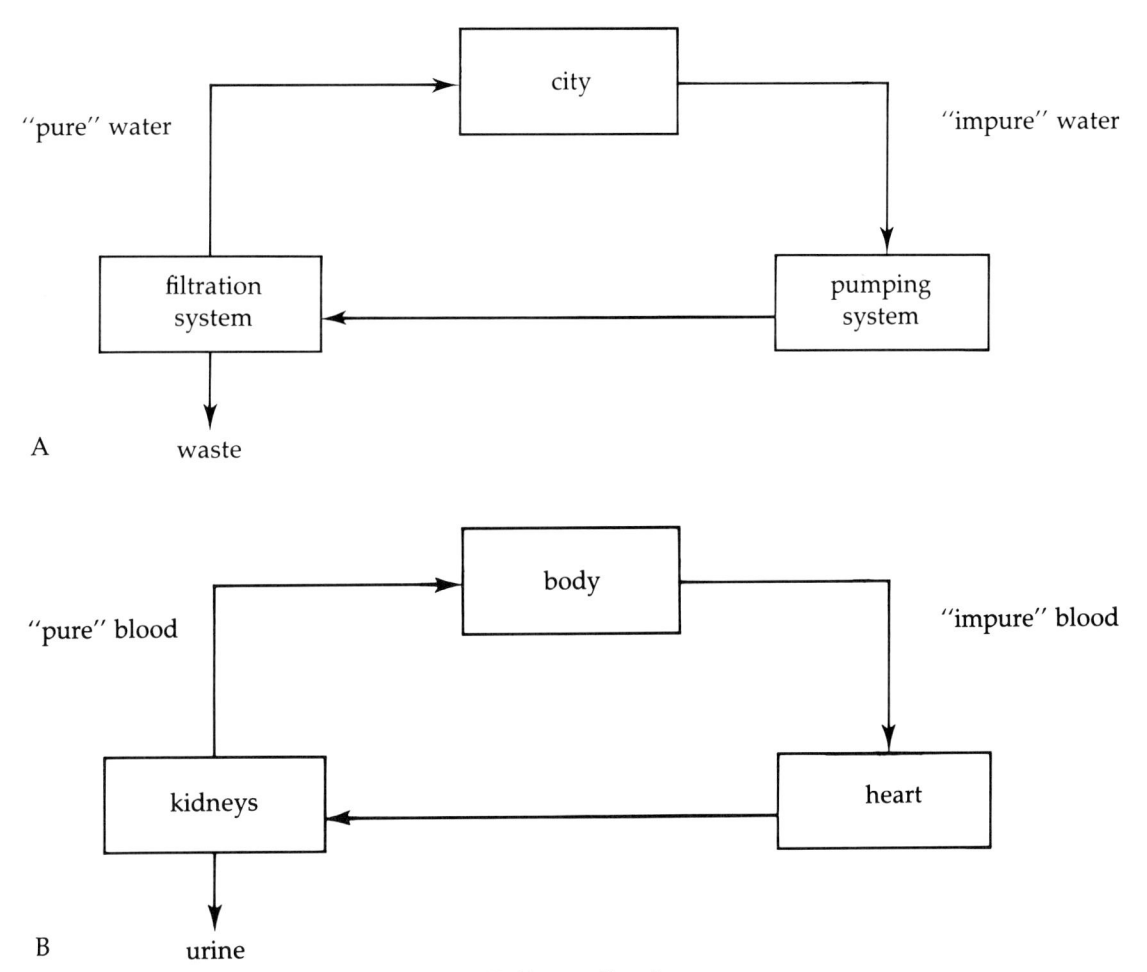

Fig. 5.1 **A,** City water purification system. **B,** Human filtration system.

lar pressure and hypertension by reducing blood volume. The recent discovery that thiazide diuretics increase the thickness and mineral content of bone may herald a new use for these drugs in preventing osteoporosis in elderly patients. The usefulness of diuretics in these dissimilar conditions is based upon the rearrangement of water and electrolyte patterns in body tissues. The use of diuretics in other conditions, such as obesity, is not warranted since only water weight is temporarily lost from the body and fat cells are not affected.

An important point to remember in therapy with diuretics is that their effectiveness depends upon functionally active kidneys. If the kidneys are impaired, diuretic therapy may be viewed as an attempt to force a diseased organ to perform more work. In that instance, the diuretic is of little value and may actually do harm. Conditions such as congestive heart failure (CHF), in which the retention of water is not directly associated with impaired kidney function, are effectively treated with diuretics.

Diuretics may sometimes worsen conditions for which they are generally indicated. For instance, CHF patients may be made worse by diuretics if the lowered blood volume and the decreased cardiac output are too pronounced.

Problems encountered in diuretic therapy include electrolyte disturbances caused by the diuresis and the specific nature of the individual drug. Potassium loss (K^+) produced by a diuretic can enhance the possibility of digitalis toxicity in CHF patients. Certain diuretics, such

262 THERAPEUTIC PHARMACOLOGY

as the thiazide derivatives, can cause a diabetic reaction or precipitate a gout attack due to a specific drug activity.

Several classes of diuretics differ in the sites and mechanisms whereby diuresis is produced. For over three decades, the organic mercurials were the mainstay of diuretic therapy. In the 1950s, carbonic anhydrase inhibitors (such as acetazolamide) and thiazide derivatives (like chlorothiazide) entered the therapeutic arena. More recently, "loop diuretics" or "high ceiling diuretics" (furosemide and ethacrynic acid) have become available. This new class of diuretics is effective orally and is also valuable when the kidney blood flow and filtration rate are greatly reduced in certain disease states. Additionally, diuretics such as spironolactone and triamterene tend to retain potassium (K$^+$) in the body and hence reduce some of the problems associated with potassium loss.

The rational use of diuretics implies an appropriate choice of drug and dosage regimen for different clinical situations. For instance, when initial rapid mobilization of edema fluid is war-

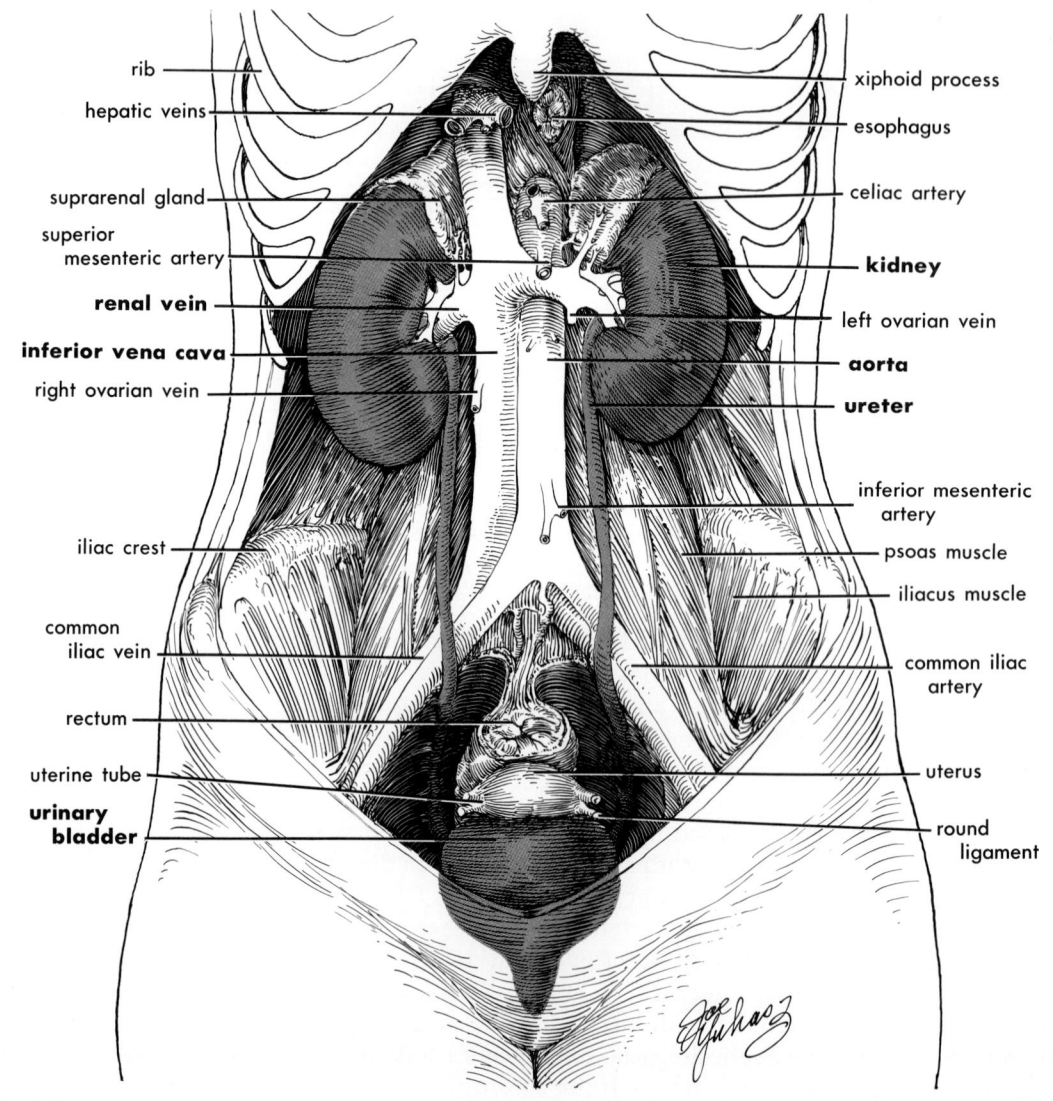

Fig. 5.2 Anterior view of posterior abdominal wall with the peritoneum removed showing kidneys, ureters, and related organs. (From Crouch, J.E.: Essential Human Anatomy. Phildelphia, Lea & Febiger, 1985.)

ranted, the diuretic potency is a prime factor as well as the probable necessity of adjusting the dosage often as the patient's status changes. In the chronic management of edema, the choice of diuretic is based upon a long-term constant therapeutic regimen. Also, since the mechanism of diuretic activity differs, the best choice may be a combination of drugs (such as triamterene and hydrochlorothiazide).

Another class of drugs inhibits renal tubular absorption of organic compounds (such as uric acid) which results in an increased urinary excretion of these substances. Since probenecid and sulfinpyrazone promote uric acid elimination, these drugs are known as uricosuric agents.

ANATOMY AND PHYSIOLOGY OF THE KIDNEY

Figure 5.2 shows the structural relationship of the kidneys, ureters, bladder, and urethra. The two human kidneys consist of an outer rind of tissue called the cortex and an inner portion known as the medulla (Figure 5.3). Each human kidney contains about one million nephrons that form complex loops from the cortex into the medulla.

Since urine is derived from blood, all the substances found in urine have first been present in blood. A unique, intimate association exists between the kidney (renal) blood vessels and the nephron. Exchanges of solutes and water take place almost exclusively between blood capillaries and nephrons. The following introduction to the anatomic and physiologic characteristics of the kidney is divided into a description of the blood circuit and the tubular urine circuit.

BLOOD CIRCUIT

As shown in Figures 5.3 and 5.4, blood flows into the kidney from the renal artery, a short vessel leading from the aorta. The blood supply then penetrates the cuplike structure of Bowman's capsule by way of the afferent arteriole, a vessel that branches from the renal artery. In Bowman's capsule, the afferent arteriole transforms into a capillary tuft known as the glomerulus. At this site, blood filtration occurs with the resulting plasma ultrafiltrate entering the lumen of the nephron. In the normal kidney, only 1% of this filtrate passes from the body as urine, whereas the rest is absorbed into the bloodstream along the tubules of the nephron. The glomerular blood capillaries reunite as the

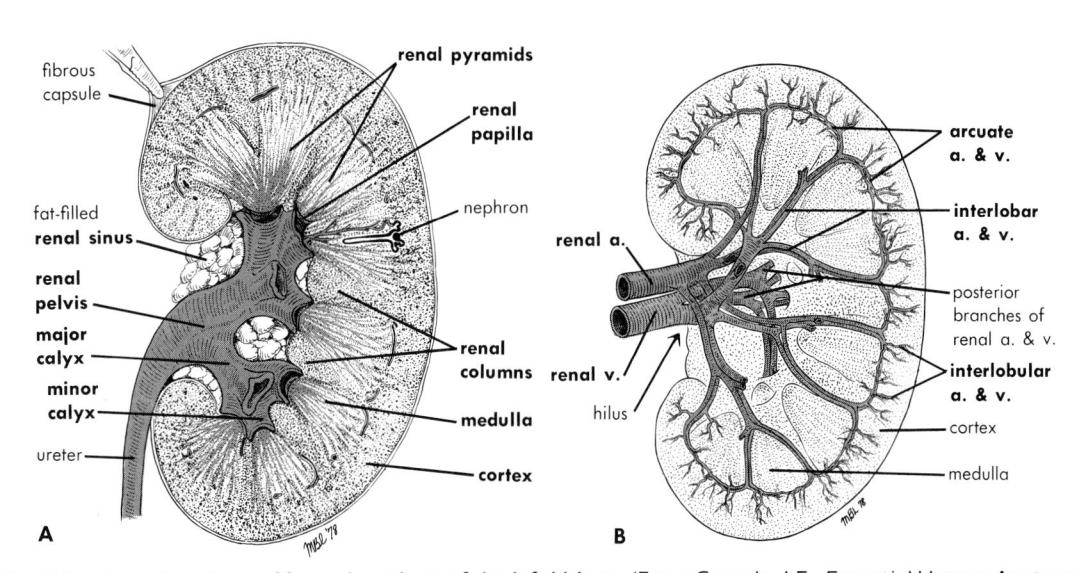

Fig. 5.3 Anterior views of frontal sections of the left kidney. (From Crouch, J.E.: Essential Human Anatomy. Philadelphia, Lea & Febiger, 1985.)

efferent arteriole as the blood leaves the glomerulus. The efferent renal arteriole then divides into many small capillaries to form a dense capillary bed in close proximity to the renal tubules and the loop of Henle. This intimate blood-nephron relationship allows for extensive solute and water reabsorption back into the blood. These capillaries then unite to form the renal vein that delivers the blood back to the systemic circulation via the posterior vena cava.

TUBULAR URINE CIRCUIT

Three distinct processes important for urine formation in the nephron are glomerular filtration, tubular reabsorption, and tubular secretion. These events occur at different sites along the nephron (Figure 5.4).

GLOMERULAR FILTRATION

Much as one would envision the function of filter paper in a physical separation process, the basement membrane of the capillary tuft allows for preferential passage of water and solutes (glomerular filtrate) into the lumen of the nephron. The blood pressure forces small molecules through pores in the basement membrane into the nephron. Due to their large molecular size, proteins are not allowed to enter the nephron (under normal circumstances). Thus, at Bowman's capsule, an essentially protein-free "ultrafiltrate" of plasma is formed at about 120 ml/minute (170,000 ml/day); this is measured as the glomerular filtrate rate (GFR). Of this extraordinary volume of filtrate, over 99% is normally reabsorbed at various sites along the nephron. Analysis of this filtrate shows that it has essentially the same concentration of dissolved substances (glucose, urea, salts, amino acids, etc.) as blood plasma.

The glomerular filtration rate is increased when the plasma volume is expanded and/or systemic blood pressure is elevated. Reduction in the glomerular filtration rate is seen with a decreased systemic blood pressure or when the renal afferent arteriole is constricted or obstructed. Filtration rate can also be reduced by such renal diseases as glomerulitis or glomerulonephritis.

TUBULAR REABSORPTION AND TUBULAR SECRETION

Selective reabsorption to conserve water and dissolved substances is an important function of the renal tubules. After filtration at the glomerulus, as described above, the filtrate follows a course through the proximal convoluted tubule, the descending limb of the loop of Henle, the distal convoluted tubule, and finally into the collecting tubule. Through this circuit and by various control mechanisms, the filtrate is made more concentrated by the reabsorption of water; the modified filtrate (urine) finally voided contains a much higher concentration of dissolved substances than the initial glomerular filtrate.

Sodium reabsorption as NaCl is of utmost importance in kidney function and of paramount interest in considering the mechanism of action of diuretics. This process relates to water reabsorption; water usually moves from one compartment to another in response to the active transport of ions, such as sodium. That is, sodium is actively moved across cell barriers (involves energy), and water follows passively. This activity takes place to varying degrees at the proximal convoluted tubule, the ascending limb of the loop of Henle, the distal convoluted tubule, and the collecting tubule.

It is important, at this point, to consider the osmolarity (concentration of osmotically active solute in solution) of the tubular fluid and the osmotic changes that take place in its journey through the nephron. Along with osmotic changes in the tubular fluid, alteration in the osmolarity of the interstitial tissue surrounding the nephron occurs and is of significance in the mechanism of urine formation. Figure 5.5 illustrates changes that ensue in response to the renal mechanisms for water control and osmolarity regulation.

About 60 to 70% of the filtered sodium and water is reabsorbed in the proximal convoluted tubule, but, because water follows passively, the concentration of sodium leaving the proxi-

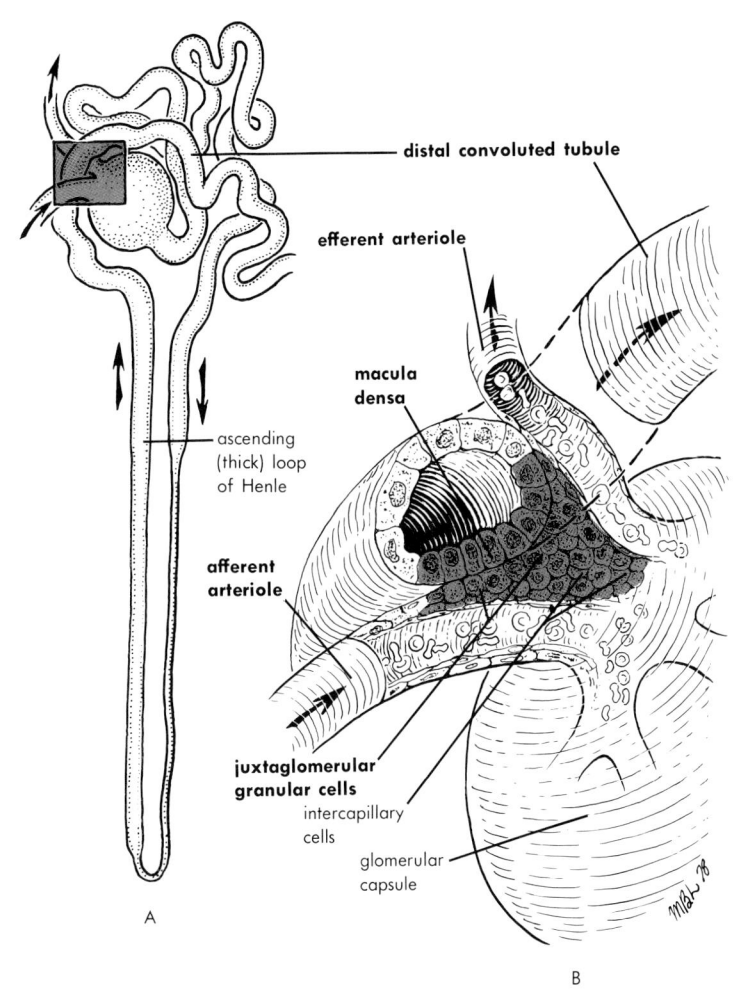

Fig. 5.4 Juxtaglomerular mechanism. **A**, Nephron, showing location of mechanism. **B**, Enlargement of area indicated in **A**. (From Crouch, J.E.: Essential Human Anatomy. Philadelphia, Lea & Febiger, 1985.)

mal convoluted tubule remains about the same as the blood plasma. The proximal tubule cells utilize an active reabsorption process for sodium reabsorption with chloride and water reabsorption following passively. Additionally, a "backleak" mechanism between the cells and lumen of the proximal tubule is important in regulating the net sodium reabsorption.

Since the sodium and chloride reabsorption that occurs in the proximal tubule involves the concurrent reabsorption of water along the osmotic gradient, there is no change in the sodium concentration, or osmolarity, in the tubular fluid. The tubular fluid is thus isotonic when it leaves the proximal tubule. Tubular reabsorption in the proximal tubule accounts for about $2/3$ of the fluid filtered at the glomerulus. The approximately $1/3$ remaining isotonic tubular fluid flows down into the descending limb of the loop of Henle that traverses deep into the renal medulla. The descending limb appears to be impermeable to sodium; no significant sodium reabsorption occurs at this site.

The tubular fluid becomes more concentrated as it nears the "hairpin" curve due to water being drawn from the tubular lumen in the tissue fluids of the hypertonic medulla. The high osmotic pressure in the interstitial tissue of

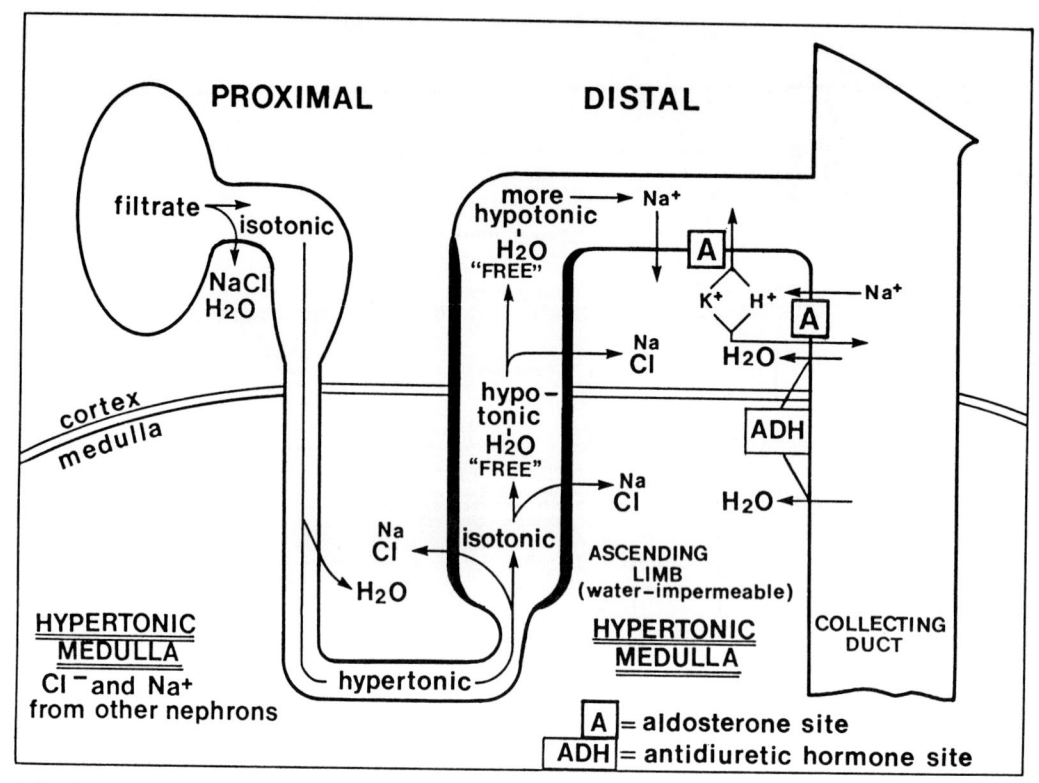

Fig. 5.5 Salt and water transport in the kidney. (From Bricker, N.S. (ed.): The Sea Within Us. San Juan, G.D. Searle & Company, 1975.)

the renal medulla results from the deposition of chloride and sodium after extraction from the tubular filtrate as it flows through the ascending limb of the loop of Henle. Thus, the tubular fluid is hypertonic as it "rounds the bend" upward toward the renal cortex.

The ascending limb of the loop of Henle is water impermeable. At this site, there is active reabsorption of the chloride ion (Cl^-), and the sodium ion (Na^+) follows passively (as NaCl). The chloride pump mechanism, although not as widely distributed in the body as the sodium pumps, is instrumental in the dilution of the tubular urine as it ascends the loop of Henle and enters the distal convoluted tubule. The active chloride pump normally accounts for about 30% of the sodium chloride reabsorption. The chloride pump mechanism actively extracts chloride from the tubular fluid and deposits it into the surrounding medullary tissue. Positive sodium follows negative chloride along the electrochemical gradient, thereby creating a high osmotic pressure in the interstitial tissues of the renal medulla. Water does not osmotically follow the chloride and sodium ions because the cells in the ascending limb of the loop of Henle are impermeable to water. Thus, free water generation occurs as water is separated from sodium and chloride. The tubular fluid then becomes more hypotonic as it ascends toward the distal tubule.

The distal tubule and collecting duct reabsorb most of the remaining sodium and chloride ions. The main mechanism at these sites involves the active reabsorption of sodium that is partially under the influence of the adrenal hormone, aldosterone, and is coupled to the secretion of potassium ions and hydrogen ions (Figure 5.5). Therefore, the secretion of potassium and hydrogen ions depends upon the presence of sodium in this segment. The aldosterone augments potassium and hydrogen ion excretion secondary to a primary effect upon sodium reabsorption. The collecting duct carries the filtrate from an area of low sodium concentration to one of greater sodium concentration in the medulla and ultimately the renal pelvic area. Since the collecting ducts are permeable to water, a more concentrated urine is formed as water leaves the tubular filtrate by passive osmosis. This description of urine production is known as the countercurrent-multiplier model (Figure 5.5). The voiding of either dilute or concentrated urine is dependent upon whether a deficiency or an excess of water is present in the body at that time. The pituitary gland reacts to changes in the amount of body water by releasing the antidiuretic hormone, ADH (vasopressin). Thus, a multiplicity of complex factors interact to determine the volume and concentration of excreted urine.

Depending upon the amount of antidiuretic hormone (ADH) that is present, the distal tubule and collecting duct have varying degrees of "watertightness" (Figure 5.6). In the absence of ADH, the hypotonic tubular fluid is excreted as such since the cells of the distal tubule and collecting duct are water impermeable. If ADH levels increase, the free water present is exposed to the high osmotic pressure of the interstitial tissue of the renal medulla. Varying amounts of water then flow out of the distal tubule and collecting duct into the medulla, resulting in the excretion of a concentrated urine.

FACTORS INFLUENCING DIURESIS

Renal control of water involves several factors. The effective delivery of glomerular filtrate to the ascending limb of the loop of Henle and the consequent separation of water from sodium and chloride at this site are of paramount interest. Additionally, the influence of the ADH on the distal tubule and collecting duct allows for controlled water reabsorption. A defect in any of these processes may compromise or alter water regulation by the kidney. For instance, a severe reduction in effective arterial blood volume may result in the delivery of an inadequate amount of filtrate to the ascending limb of the loop of Henle.

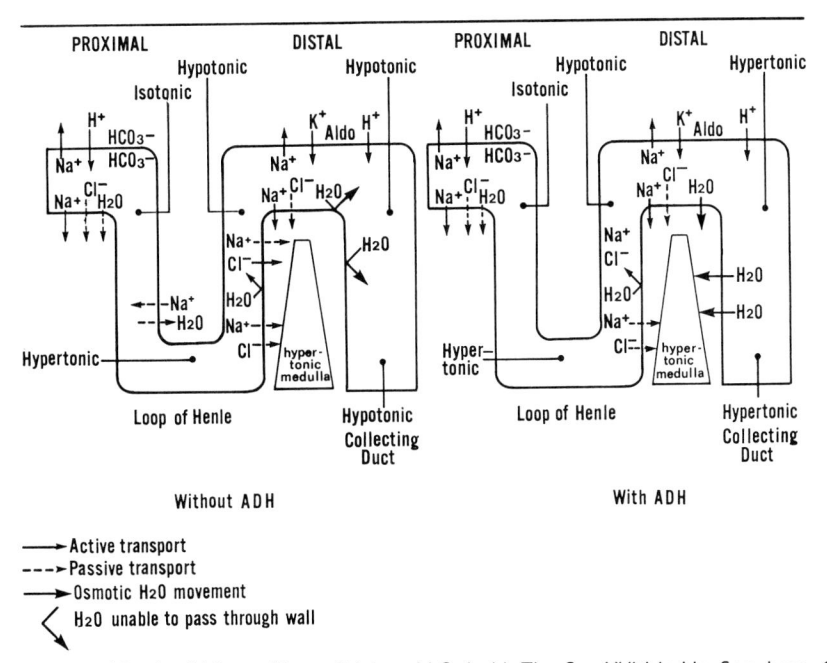

Fig. 5.6 Water control in the kidney. (From Bricker, N.S. (ed.): The Sea Within Us. San Juan, G.D. Searle & Company, 1975.)

Separation of water from sodium and chloride in the ascending limb can be disrupted by the inhibition of reabsorption of chloride and sodium. Diuretics, such as furosemide and ethacrynic acid, impair the active chloride pump reabsorption mechanism working at this site. Hence, salt and water are not separated and a diuretic effect results.

Vasopressin (ADH), released from the posterior pituitary, influences water reabsorption from the distal tubule and collecting duct. The ADH amount released from the posterior pituitary reflects a reaction to the osmotic needs of the body. Specialized nerve cells that are sensitive to osmotic changes in body fluids are located in or near the hypothalamic region of the brain. These nerve cells are called osmoreceptors and have a marked influence on ADH secretion.

Osmoreceptors relay impulses to specific cell nuclei in the hypothalamus that synthesize and secrete ADH. After ADH synthesis by these cells, the hormone is secreted into nerve axons and is carried to the posterior pituitary for storage. Upon appropriate stimulation, it is released into the bloodstream. The osmoreceptors respond to a water load or the dilution of the osmotic concentration of body fluid by relaying inhibitory impulses to the hypothalamic nuclei that synthesize and secrete ADH. This reduces ADH release and the distal tubule becomes essentially watertight and the excessive water is excreted. Additionally, factors unrelated to osmotic change influence ADH release. The left atrium, aortic arch, and carotid arteries contain receptors sensitive to volume changes. A severe volume defect stimulates ADH release independent of osmotic influence. Finally, stresses such as anxiety and severe pain can also take precedence over osmotic factors and stimulate ADH release.

FUNCTIONS OF THE KIDNEY

The normal kidney performs five major tasks: excretion of waste and maintenance of acid-base balance, water balance, electrolyte balance, and renin secretion.

EXCRETION OF WASTE

The kidney filters and excretes waste products, particularly those nitrogenous materials formed in protein metabolism such as urea and creatinine. In addition, acids and bases, water, and drug metabolites may be filtered into the urine and excreted. Large molecules such as blood cells, plasma proteins, and lipids are ordinarily retained in the capillary vessel and do not undergo glomerular filtration.

ACID-BASE BALANCE

A second function is the maintenance of acid-base balance by the ability of the kidney to alter urinary pH and thereby affect systemic pH. This is accomplished by selectively varying the amount of hydrogen ion secreted and sodium ion reabsorbed, mainly through the carbonic anhydrase system. The kidney also allows for the excretion of water formed from the catabolism of carbonic acid, thereby aiding in the operation of the carbonic acid-bicarbonate system (Figure 5.7). The kidneys serve an important regulatory role in acid-base homeostasis by restoring to the blood the bicarbonate (HCO_3^-) ions used in the initial buffering of hydrogen ions produced in metabolism. The kidney must reabsorb all of the filtered bicarbonate (HCO_3^-) because its loss in the urine results in metabolic acidosis and death within a few hours. Additionally, the kidney must regenerate bicarbonate used up in the buffering of metabolic hydrogen ions.

In the renal tubular cell, water is split to form hydrogen ion (H^+) and hydroxide ion (OH^-), as shown in Figure 5.7a. The hydrogen ion is transported across the tubular cell membrane into the tubular lumen. In a bicarbonate ion (HCO_3^-) reclamation process, carbonic acid (H_2CO_3) is then formed from the reaction of the hydrogen ion and the filtered bicarbonate ion. Carbonic acid then dissociates into carbon dioxide (CO_2) and water (H_2O). The carbon dioxide diffuses into the tubular cell where it combines with the hydroxide ion formed initially from the splitting of water. This reaction is under the influence of the enzyme carbonic anhydrase. Hence, bicarbonate ion is moved into the peritubular capillaries and joins the total pool of extracellular fluid bicarbonate ion. In this case, the filtered bicarbonate ion disappears and is replaced by the intracellular bicarbonate ion in a reclamation process. Some filtered bicarbonate ion is apparently reabsorbed as such.

In addition to the reclamation of bicarbonate ion, newly synthesized bicarbonate ion may also occur in the tubular cell. In reactions (Figures 5.7b and 5.7c), the hydroxide ion formed from the splitting of water combines with carbon dioxide from extracellular fluid to represent newly synthesized bicarbonate ion. In this case, the hydrogen ion in the tubular lumen had previously combined with nonbicarbonate buffers, monohydrogen phosphate ion (HPO_4^-), shown in Figure 5.7b, and ammonia (NH_3), represented in Figure 5.7c. Thus, the fate of hydrogen ion in the tubular lumen determines whether either filtered bicarbonate ion is reclaimed by the body or tubular synthesis of new bicarbonate ion occurs.

WATER BALANCE

A third kidney function is to maintain water balance so that the body can adjust to variations in water intake along with changing environmental conditions. As discussed previously, the ADH action on the distal tubule and collecting duct is largely responsible for regulating water balance.

ELECTROLYTE BALANCE

A fourth role of the kidney is the maintenance of electrolyte balance within the various fluid compartments of the body. Important ions, including potassium (K^+), sodium (Na^+), chloride (Cl^-), and bicarbonate (HCO_3^-), are contained in the fluid compartments bathed in a water medium. Water, which comprises over ½ of the body weight, is distributed between two major compartments. Water may exist inside the cells (intracellular) or outside the cells (extracellular).

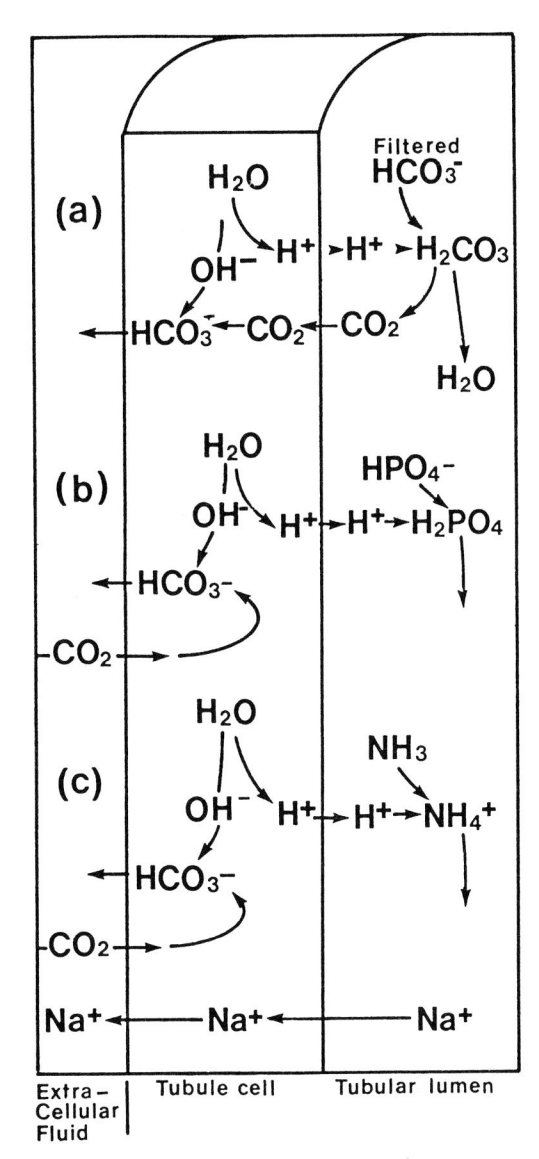

Fig. 5.7 Kidney carbonic acid - bicarbonate reactions: renal handling of bicarbonate reclamation and regeneration. (From Bricker, N.S. (ed.): The Sea Within Us. San Juan, G.D. Searle & Company, 1975.)

Extracellular fluid is further subdivided into the intravascular fluid (blood serum) and the fluid outside the vascular system (interstitial fluid).

Certain ions are characterized by having a particular distribution in the fluid compartments of the body. Potassium (K^+) is primarily an intracellular ion and is present in a high concentration (160 meq/L of cell water) inside the cell. This high potassium concentration is critical in constituting an osmotic force to maintain the cell's optimal water content. Outside the cell, the concentration of potassium is only 4 to 5 meq/L which is very low compared to the intracellular concentration. Obviously, the low potassium concentration does not contribute significantly to the osmotic force of extracellular fluid. Nevertheless, the extracellular potassium levels are critical for proper functioning of cardiac and skeletal muscle. Both high and low potassium serum levels cause abnormalities in cardiac and skeletal muscle.

Maintenance of serum potassium within narrow limits is critical for normal cardiac conduction. Additionally, the ultimate factor in maintaining intracellular potassium is the extracellular or serum potassium levels. The continued loss of potassium from the serum eventually leads to intracellular deficits and clinical problems. Both a normal potassium gradient across cell membranes and sufficient stores of intracellular potassium depend upon a normal serum potassium level.

Since food is rich in potassium, the problem of maintaining potassium balance is one of disposal rather than of conservation. The kidney regulates potassium excretion practically independent of the GFR and the amount of potassium filtered at the glomerulus. About 70% of the potassium filtered is reabsorbed in the proximal tubule and a further 20% is reabsorbed in the loop of Henle. Therefore, under normal circumstances, only about 5 to 10% of the filtered potassium arrives at the distal tubule. Aldosterone plays a primary role in affecting potassium secretion and sodium reabsorption (Figure 5.5). The reabsorption of sodium leaves negatively charged ions such as chloride, sulfate, and phosphate behind in the tubular fluid. These ions constitute an electrochemical force that draws potassium (and hydrogen) back into the tubular lumen. This mechanism requires adequate amounts of sodium to be delivered to the distal tubule as well as the presence of aldosterone to activate sodium reabsorption and potassium secretion in the distal tubule and collecting duct. These two factors (distal tubule sodium delivery and aldosterone) function in a reciprocal manner to maintain a stable potassium secretion.

High serum potassium levels stimulate the release of aldosterone from the renal cortex, which promotes further potassium secretion in the distal tubule and collecting duct. Another influence on potassium secretion, other than aldosterone secretion and distal sodium delivery, is the concentration of intracellular potassium. Thus, a high intracellular potassium level in the distal tubular cells encourages potassium secretion.

RENIN SECRETION

The kidney also has an enzyme secretory function that relates to aldosterone release. Renin, an enzyme synthesized, stored, and released by cells in close proximity to the glomerulus, acts to promote the formation of angiotensin in the blood. Angiotensin, in turn, causes smooth muscle constriction and is a powerful vasopressor thought to play a role in blood pressure control. Additionally, angiotensin activates the synthesis of aldosterone in the adrenal cortex (Figure 5.8). As previously seen, aldosterone promotes sodium retention and potassium secretion.

An example of this system's function is represented when the effective arterial blood volume is reduced. If this situation occurs, as in a low-salt diet, the renin-angiotensin-aldosterone system is stimulated, thereby augmenting the sodium-potassium exchange in the distal tubule and collecting duct. A low effective arterial blood volume increases sodium reabsorption via the renin-angiotensin-aldosterone system, but the concurrent distal tubule delivery of sodium is reduced due to the increased sodium reabsorption in the proximal tubule that results from the decreased effective arterial blood volume. Thus, these homeostatic processes prevent a severe disruption of electrolyte balance.

Conversely, when the effective arterial blood volume is expanded, aldosterone levels are reduced due to an inhibitory effect on the renin system. The preceding examples illustrate the importance of the renin-angiotensin-aldoster-

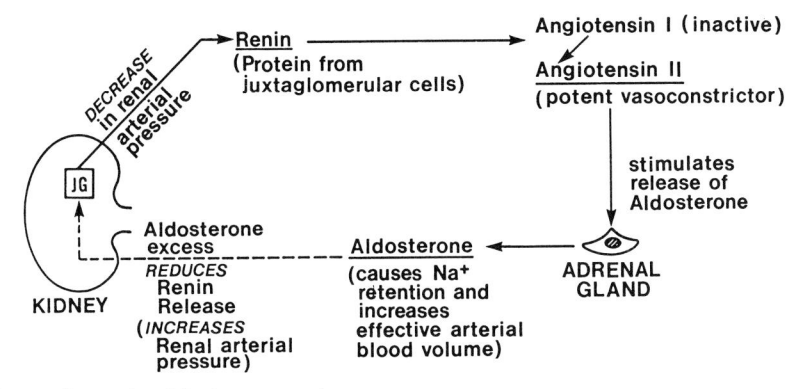

Fig. 5.8 Renin-angiotensin-aldosterone system.

one system in the regulation of electrolyte and water balance.

DISEASES TREATED WITH DIURETIC DRUGS

Edema is a common characteristic of several diseases amenable to diuretic therapy. However, some conditions, such as hypertension, are nonedematous.

EDEMATOUS CONDITIONS

A major therapeutic use of diuretic drugs is in the management of edema. Edema represents a clinical problem in several conditions including congestive heart failure, hepatic cirrhosis, and renal disease.

CONGESTIVE HEART FAILURE

Congestive heart failure (CHF) is a condition where the heart fails to function as an effective pump. Although specifically described as left-sided heart failure or right-sided heart failure, congestive heart failure does not usually remain limited to one ventricle and may develop parallel in both ventricles. See Chapter 3 for a discussion of CHF pathophysiology.

Although diuretics are often associated with CHF edema reduction, they are sometimes not needed in initial CHF treatment. Bedrest and a salt-restricted diet may sufficiently relieve edema. Also, a return to normal cardiac function in CHF conditions by the use of a cardiotonic drug can increase urine volume and relieve edema. Further, if the response to digitalis and salt restriction is sufficient, no diuretic is indicated. Diuretics, however, are a valuable addition to the regimen if initial methods without a diuretic are unsuccessful.

Beneficial effects of diuretics in CHF relate to both a reduction in pulmonary venous pressure during exercise and to a decrease in cardiac size, cardiac output, and systemic and pulmonary arterial pressure, consequently decreasing cardiac work.

A major factor in the selection of an appropriate diuretic in CHF is clinical urgency. When acute pulmonary edema is present, parenteral administration of a potent loop diuretic (like furosemide) is indicated. In a chronic situation where prevention of recurrent edema is a therapeutic objective, an oral thiazide-type diuretic (such as hydrochlorothiazide) is a probable drug of choice. This diuretic should be administered orally in the smallest effective dose and at the longest intervals appropriate to achieve the clinical goal.

If potassium depletion is suspected as a clinical problem, a combination of a thiazide with a potassium-sparing diuretic (like triamterene) is preferable. Some diuretics, such as those in the osmotic diuretic class (e.g., mannitol), are not ordinarily employed for reduction of edema associated with CHF.

Heart failure patients can be made worse by diuretics if the decrease in blood volume and cardiac output is the predominant clinical profile. Symptoms in these patients include malaise, listlessness, postural hypotension, and mental confusion. In such cases, the loss of excessive edema fluid presents a serious clinical situation.

In summary, by reducing the blood volume and thereby improving heart function, diuretics are useful adjunctive drugs in CHF treatment. Their use must be considered in the light of digitalis therapy, dietary salt restriction, and other measures. Additionally, the possibility of clinical problems associated with diuretic therapy must be recognized.

LIVER CIRRHOSIS

Fluid retention, evident as ascites, is a characteristic complication of hepatic cirrhosis and portal hypertension. Enormous quantities of extracellular fluid may accumulate in cirrhotic ascites with the volume reaching 30 to 40 L. This amount could represent as much as 50 to 70% of a patient's body weight.

If the abdomen is severely distended, the ascitic fluid should be removed to alleviate respiratory distress, as well as to prevent development of further complications. On the other hand, the amount of abdominal fluid that accumulates may be small and require no specific treatment other than attempts to improve liver function.

Gross abdominal distention in cirrhosis may serve a useful function. The tension present tends to oppose further losses from the vascular compartment. In the case of cirrhosis, sodium and water retention does not initiate hypertension, cardiac dilation, and pulmonary congestion because of the excess fluid segregation into the ascitic sac. Diuretics, in these cases, should be used with caution since a brisk diuretic effect can remove vascular support, resulting in possible vascular instability and collapse. The therapeutic goal in these situations is not to render the patient edema free, but to dispose of enough fluid to gain comfort for the patient.

Excessive aldosterone release from the adrenal cortex or a defective ability of the liver to inactivate aldosterone may play a role in the salt and water retention that occurs in hepatic cirrhosis. Thus, if diuretic therapy is indicated, spironolactone (an aldosterone antagonist) is often a drug of choice since it inhibits the effect of excessive aldosterone. Other diuretics, such as hydrochlorothiazide or furosemide, may also be used. Frequent monitoring of electrolytes is essential to follow the response to diuretic therapy.

A severe complication of the excessive use of diuretics in treating liver ascites is the precipitation of hepatic coma. Thiazide and loop diuretics promote ammonia movement from the gastrointestinal tract into the blood stream and ultimately into the brain.

RENAL DISEASE

Three types of edema distinguished in renal disease are amenable to diuretic therapy. These are the edema of the nephrotic syndrome, the edema of acute glomerulonephritis, and the edema of hypertensive renal disease subsequent to CHF.

The nephrotic syndrome is characterized by accumulating fluid that has leaked into the interstitial spaces as a result of hypoalbumenuria. Thus, a decreased colloid osmotic pressure allows for the transport of salt and water from the capillaries to the interstitial space. The plasma volume reduction that occurs stimulates aldosterone secretion and sets into play a vicious cycle of salt and water retention. A glucocorticoid, prednisone, is the drug of choice in treating this condition. However, salt and water retention that may occur with glucocorticoid therapy requires the addition of a diuretic such as hydrochlorothiazide or furosemide to the regimen. Also, the aldosterone antagonist spironolactone may be useful for patients who develop secondary hyperaldosteronism (due to decreased plasma volume).

In acute glomerulonephritis, the edema results from the failure of kidney excretory function. The consequent salt and water retention manifests into a greatly expanded blood volume, including arterial blood volume. Also, an increase in plasma volume is possibly the primary factor in edema formation. These conditions result in cardiac dilation, pulmonary congestion, and high venous pressure. Removal of the edema is therefore a critical therapeutic goal for correction of the circulatory disorder and diuretic therapy is indicated. A potent diuretic, such as furosemide, has proved successful in treating this form of edema.

In addition to the previously discussed edematous conditions related to renal disease, acute renal failure may be prevented by using an osmotic diuretic, such as mannitol. The maintenance of adequate fluid in the nephrons is the protective mechanism involved.

PREMENSTRUAL EDEMA

High levels of aldosterone may contribute to the excessive sodium retention that occurs in premenstrual edema. Symptoms such as breast fullness, headache, and vague feelings of restlessness have often been relieved by diuretic therapy. Specifically, thiazide derivatives and an OTC diuretic, pamabrom, have been advocated as beneficial in treating premenstrual syndrome (PMS). Although diuretics can reduce the edema associated with PMS, any effect on the patient's emotional tension sometimes present in this condition remains conjectural.

EDEMA OF PREGNANCY

The edema of pregnancy may relate to hormone changes that occur during pregnancy. The output of androgen, hydrocortisone, and aldosterone progressively increases during pregnancy. However, in the serious toxemia of pregnancy (preeclampsia or eclampsia), diuretics have not been shown to favorably affect hypertension or prevent eclampsia convulsions and other complications of this condition. Thiazide derivatives have been recommended for this purpose, but general consensus for this treatment strategy has not yet been reached.

DRUG-INDUCED EDEMA

Steroid hormones such as hydrocortisone (and other glucocorticoids), estrogens, and adrenal androgens produce a positive sodium balance and contribute to edema formation. Indeed, administration of hydrocortisone and other steroids precipitates acute attacks of CHF and pulmonary edema in some patients with impaired cardiac, hepatic, or renal function. Diuretics, such as hydrochlorothiazide or furosemide, are sometimes used in conjunction with a glucocorticoid in the treatment of the nephrotic syndrome to prevent drug-induced edema.

NONEDEMATOUS CONDITIONS

Diuretics are also valuable drugs in the treatment of certain nonedematous conditions. These include hypertension, electrolyte imbalance, and bromide intoxication.

HYPERTENSION

A major use of diuretics is in the management of hypertension. The precise mechanisms involved in the lowering of blood pressure and the maintenance of the hypotensive effect during long-term therapy have not been documented. However, a reduction in extracellular and plasma volume is apparently a primary factor in lowering elevated blood pressure. With diuretic therapy, the intravascular volume decreases and consequently reduces cardiac output. As diuretic therapy is continued, the blood volume returns to normal, yet this readjustment is not accompanied by a reversal of the early decrease in blood pressure.

The total peripheral resistance remains lower despite the return of the cardiac output and plasma volume to pretreatment levels. This phenomenon is explained by a loss of sodium from the blood vessel walls resulting in decreased sympathetic reactivity. Thus, diuretics appear to reduce the responsiveness of the blood vessels to sympathetic nerve impulses and to circulating catecholamines.

The thiazide derivatives are the diuretics most often used to treat hypertension. Loop diuretics, like furosemide and ethacrynic acid, may be preferable in treating patients who have concurrent kidney disease. Oftentimes, diuretics are combined with other antihypertensives to increase the effective hypotensive action. One explanation is that the diuretics prevent a compensatory rise in plasma volume that would be initiated by the other vasodilator drug. This mechanism involves activation of the renin-angiotensin-aldosterone system when the other vasodilator drug reduces peripheral resistance and arterial pressure. Thus, by preventing an increase in plasma volume, and subsequently peripheral resistance and blood pressure, diuretics allow for the continued effectiveness of the other antihypertensive drug.

An additional advantage to a diuretic-vasodilator antihypertensive combination, such as guanethidine-hydrochlorothiazide, is that a lower dosage of the nondiuretic drug may be clinically effective. This means that dose-related noncirculatory side effects of the nondiuretic drug are generally less likely to occur.

ELECTROLYTE IMBALANCE

Diuretics, such as thiazide derivatives and furosemide, promote potassium excretion. Thus, these agents are recommended in the treatment of hyperkalemia and respiratory acidosis.

BROMIDE INTOXICATION

Although bromides have been replaced by more suitable sedatives, they are still available as therapeutic agents. In bromide overdose, any diuretic that favors chloride excretion helps rid the body of bromide. Since the kidney fails to distinguish between bromide and chloride ion, the bromide ion is excreted in the urine.

DISORDERS TREATED WITH URICOSURIC DRUGS

Elevated levels of blood uric acid characterize gouty arthritis. An increase in uric acid elimination theoretically reduces the incidence of urate deposition in joints.

GOUT

Uricosuric agents increase the urinary excretion of uric acid. In gouty arthritis, a hyperuricemia exists that contributes to the formation of urate crystals in the joints (usually of the great toes, ankles, knees, and shoulders). These deposits, resulting in arthritis, may occur concurrently in one or several joints. Drugs, such as probenecid and sulfinpyrazone, that favor the urinary excretion of uric acid are beneficial in chronic cases of gouty arthritis.

Allopurinol, a xanthine oxidase inhibitor, is currently a mainstay in the treatment of gout patients. Its mechanism of action does not involve renal transport processes, but rather depends upon decreasing the amount of endogenous uric acid synthesized (see Chapter 10).

DRUGS AFFECTING THE RENAL SYSTEM

Drugs acting on the renal system are primarily diuretics. Uricosuric drugs are also useful clinically.

DIURETIC DRUGS

The discussion of this class of drugs is arranged according to mechanisms of diuretic action.

OSMOTIC DIURETICS

Osmotic diuretics (Table 5.1) are considered to be pharmacologically inert by conventional definition. Their action is due primarily to an increase in the amount of osmotically active solute in the glomerular filtrate and tubular fluid.

Mechanism of Action. Osmotic diuretics are freely filtered at the glomerulus and are not significantly reabsorbed as they travel in the tubular fluid through the nephrons. Any significant increase in the concentration of osmotically active particles in the glomerular filtrate is accompanied by the retention of an equivalent amount of water in the tubular lumen which increases the volume of urine excreted. This type of diuresis occurs in untreated diabetes mellitus where high amounts of glucose spill from the blood into the tubular fluid, resulting in a large volume of urine excretion.

Table 5.1 OSMOTIC DIURETICS.

Available products	Trade names	Daily dosage range
Mannitol	Osmitrol	Varies according to clinical situation
Urea	Ureaphil	1–1.5 g/kg in a 30% solution by slow IV infusion
Glycerin	Glyrol; Osmoglyn	1–1.5 g/kg, 1–1.5 hrs prior to surgery
Isosorbide	Ismotic	1–3 g/kg

Table 5.2 CARBONIC ANHYDRASE INHIBITORS.

Available products	Trade names	Daily dosage range
Acetazolamide	Diamox; AK-Zol	250–375 mg once daily for 1 or 2 days, alternate with a day of rest
Dichlorphenamide	Daranide	25–50 mg, 1 to 3 times daily: Indicated for glaucoma
Methazolamide	Neptazane	50–100 mg b.i.d. or t.i.d.: Indicated for glaucoma

Clinical Indications. Mannitol, the most widely used drug in this diuretic class that also includes glycerin, isosorbide, and urea will be discussed as the osmotic diuretic prototype.

Mannitol maintains urine volume even in the presence of decreased glomerular filtration rate (GFR). Since mannitol is filtered at the glomerulus regardless of a reduced GFR, the unreabsorbed mannitol is excreted along with water. Therefore, urine volume can be maintained even in the presence of compromised renal function. An important indication for mannitol is in the prevention of acute renal failure in such clinically distinct situations as cardiovascular operations, severe traumatic injury, operations with severely jaundiced patients, and the management of hemolytic transfusion reactions.

Since mannitol is not absorbed well when taken orally, it must be given intravenously for effective diuresis. Mannitol's duration of action is 2 to 3 hours, depending upon the dose and the volume/duration of IV infusion.

Adverse Effects/Precautions. Common side effects include headache, nausea, and vomiting. Osmotic diuretics are usually contraindicated in CHF because they further increase the volume of both plasma and extracellular fluid. In CHF manifested by cardiac decompensation, further expansion of fluid in the plasma and extracellular compartments may present a serious clinical problem.

Urea is more irritating to tissues than mannitol, and necrosis can result if leakage occurs around the injection site. Urea should not be infused in the superficial and deep veins of the lower extremities in elderly patients since thrombosis may occur.

CARBONIC ANHYDRASE INHIBITORS

Drugs in this classification are unique in that they exert their effort by enzyme inhibition (Table 5.2).

Mechanism of Action. The enzyme carbonic anhydrase catalyzes the following reaction in renal tubules as indicated.

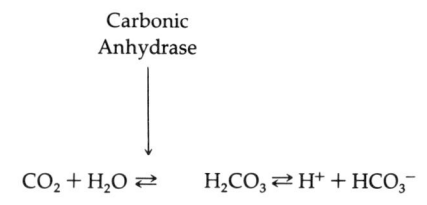

$$CO_2 + H_2O \overset{\text{Carbonic Anhydrase}}{\rightleftarrows} H_2CO_3 \rightleftarrows H^+ + HCO_3^-$$

As shown, carbonic acid (H_2CO_3) then dissociates to form hydrogen ion (H^+) and bicarbonate ion (HCO_3^-). The hydrogen ion and bicarbonate ion so formed in the tubular cell are significant in several renal conservation mechanisms. The hydrogen ion formed is secreted by the tubular cell into the lumen in exchange for the sodium ion (Na^+). The hydrogen ion-sodium ion coupled exchange mechanism is important in the reabsorption of sodium ion back into the body.

```
LUMEN    TUBULAR CELL    INTERSTITIUM
 H⁺    ←      H⁺
 Na⁺   →      Na⁺       →     Na⁺
              HCO₃⁻     →     HCO₃⁻
```

The bicarbonate ion generated is reabsorbed along with the sodium ion, thereby maintaining the plasma bicarbonate concentration. An additional coupled potassium ion (K^+)-sodium ion (Na^+) exchange mechanism is operant in the renal tubular cells as indicated:

```
  LUMEN      TUBULAR CELL
   K⁺    ←       K⁺
   Na⁺   →       Na⁺
   H⁺    ←       H⁺
```

The availability of hydrogen ion in the tubular cell determines the extent of the potassium ion-sodium ion exchange. If the level of hydrogen ion in the tubular cell decreases, more potassium ion is excreted via this coupled exchange mechanism. Thus, inhibition of the enzyme carbonic anhydrase blocks hydrogen ion secretion by the renal tubule. Consequently, an alkaline urine and increases in the urinary concentration of bicarbonate, sodium, and potassium occur with a prompt increase in the urine volume since water follows passively. The urinary concentration of chloride ion decreases and plasma chloride levels elevate. These effects are most pronounced in the distal tubule although an action on the proximal tubule cannot be excluded.

Clinical Indications. The most common application of carbonic anhydrase inhibitors in current medical practice is the reduction of intraocular pressure in glaucoma. Carbonic anhydrase is present in intraocular structures, including the ciliary processes, and a facilitory role has been proposed in the synthesis of aqueous humor. Thus, a carbonic anhydrase inhibitor like acetazolamide decreases the intraocular pressure in glaucoma patients since the rate of aqueous humor formation is reduced. Additionally, the use of acetazolamide in combination with anticonvulsants in grand mal and petit mal seizures may relate to the presence of carbonic anhydrase in the brain; however, the exact role of carbonic anhydrase in the brain is unknown. An increase in local carbon dioxide (CO_2) tension resulting from inhibition of brain carbonic anhydrase may relate to the protective effect of carbonic anhydrase inhibitors in petit mal and grand mal seizures. Also, since metabolic acidosis diminishes epileptic seizures, the systemic acidosis produced by the action of acetazolamide on the kidney may be a related factor.

Carbonic anhydrase inhibitors are rarely used in current medicine as primary diuretics. Their clinical usefulness is limited to combination or alternate use with other diuretics and in treating edema that is refractory to other diuretics.

Adverse Effects/Precautions. Severe adverse reactions are infrequent. With large doses of acetazolamide, drowsiness and reversible paresthesias have occurred. Hypersensitivity reactions are rare and consist of fever, skin reactions, bone-marrow depression, and sulfonamide-like renal damage.

In hepatic cirrhosis, disorientation has been reported, probably related to an increased blood ammonia level as a result of the induced alkaline urine. In addition, because of the drug-induced urine alkalinity, the action of methenamine as a urinary antiseptic is reduced.

THIAZIDE DERIVATIVES (BENZOTHIADIAZIDES)

The thiazide derivatives, as represented by hydrochlorothiazide, were synthesized as a result of studies on carbonic anhydrase inhibitors. It was finally demonstrated, however, that the thiazides have a direct action on the renal tubular reabsorption of sodium and chloride that is independent of any effects on carbonic anhydrase.

Mechanism of Action. The thiazides (Table 5.3) act as diuretics by increasing urinary excretion of sodium, chloride, and water. The diuretic mechanism involves inhibition of sodium reabsorption in the early distal tubules. There is also an elevation in the urinary outflow of potassium by increasing potassium excretion in the distal tubule. Conversely, an antidiuretic

Table 5.3 THIAZIDE DERIVATIVES AND ANALOGS.

Available products	Trade names	Daily dosage range
Bendroflumethiazide	Naturetin	2.5–5 mg
Benzthiazide	Aquatag; Exna; others	50–150 mg
Chlorothiazide	Diuril; Diachlor	0.5–2 g once or twice daily, orally or IV
Chlorthalidone	Hygroton; Hylidone	50–200 mg 3 times weekly
Cyclothiazide	Anhydron; Fluidil	1 or 2 mg
Hydrochlorothiazide	Esidrix; HydroDiuril; Oretic; others	25–200 mg
Hydroflumethiazide	Diucardin; Saluron	25–200 mg
Indapamide	Lozol	2.5 mg
Metolazone	Diulo; Zaroxolyn	5–20 mg
Methyclothiazide	Enduron; Ethon; Aquatensen	2.5–10 mg
Polythiazide	Renese	1–4 mg
Quinethazone	Hydromox	50–100 mg
Trichlormethiazide	Methahydrin; Naqua; others	4 mg

effect occurs in patients with diabetes insipidus, the mechanism of which is not well understood.

Because thiazides favor urinary chloride ion (Cl^-) excretion rather than increasing bicarbonate ion (HCO_3^-) outflow, little alteration of urinary pH occurs and no significant systemic alkalosis or acidosis is produced.

The thiazide derivatives have additional effects upon the kidneys. They act to decrease the glomerular filtration rate (GFR), which could be hazardous to patients with decreased renal reserve. They decrease the renal excretion of calcium and increase the urinary outflow of magnesium. The tubular secretion of urate is decreased, consequently elevating plasma uric acid. This latter effect is clinically significant in gouty arthritis patients since elevated plasma levels of uric acid may precipitate acute attacks.

Additionally, thiazides increase the renal excretion of bromide and iodide. The kidney does not differentiate between chloride ion and the other halide ions, bromide and iodide, in excretion mechanisms. Thus, the increased chloride excretion that occurs with the thiazides also removes bromide and iodide ions from the body. The thiazides may therefore be useful drugs in the treatment of bromide or iodide intoxication.

Clinical Indications. All of the thiazides are rapidly absorbed from the gastrointestinal tract and diuresis usually occurs within an hour. The thiazides are drugs of choice in treating the edema associated with mild to moderate CHF. They are also used to treat edema resulting from chronic renal or hepatic disease. Additionally, the thiazides, especially hydrochlorothiazide, are drugs of choice in the drug management of mild hypertension.

Other less common uses are in the treatment of diabetes insipidus and the management of hypercalciuria associated with recurrent renal calcium stones. A proposed application for thiazide diuretics relates to the alteration of calcium excretion by the kidney; recent studies suggest that thiazides may help prevent osteoporosis in the elderly.

Several analogs of the thiazides, including chlorthalidone, quinethazone, and metolazone, are employed as diuretics (Table 5.3). Although not chemically identified as thiazides, these drugs possess essentially the same pharmacologic properies as thiazide derivatives.

Some practical factors warrant consideration during therapy with the thiazides. The lowest effective dose should be utilized in order to lessen the possibility of electrolyte imbalance. A single daily dose in the morning is preferred if the clinical objective can be achieved with this regimen. Patients with a greater risk to develop hypokalemia should be monitored accordingly. Also, the thiazides cross the placental barrier and appear in breast milk necessitating appropriate precautions in pregnant or nursing females.

Adverse Effects/Precautions. Adverse reactions reported involve the gastrointestinal tract, such as anorexia and gastric irritation; the CNS, reflected by dizziness, vertigo, and paresthesias; blood dyscrasias like leukopenia and agranulocytosis; and hypersensitivity reactions, including purpura, photosensitivity, rash, and fever.

Clinical problems often relate to hypokalemia, especially if other drugs that increase potassium loss from the body, such as digoxin, are taken concurrently. Symptoms of hypokalemia include muscular weakness or fatigue and changes in heart function. Potassium supplementation or the continuation of a thiazide with a potassium-sparing diuretic often correct this clinical problem and maintain potassium balance. However, since thiazide therapy does not automatically guarantee a decrease in serum a potassium-sparing diuretic often corrects this clinical problem and maintains potassium bal-

The plasma uric acid is frequently elevated with thiazide therapy. Consequently, drug-induced hyperuricema may precipitate acute gouty arthritis.

Hyperglycemia produced by the thiazides may intensify the symptoms of diabetes mellitus. This disturbance in carbohydrate metabolism is fairly common and relates to inhibition of insulin release by the pancreas and/or blockade of the peripheral utilization of glucose.

Finally, patients with borderline renal and/or hepatic insufficiency may become worse with thiazide therapy. For example, patients with liver cirrhosis may become comatose from excessive depletion of fluids and electrolytes following extended thiazide therapy. Azotemia, reflected by an elevated NPN or BUN, may occur in severe renal disease.

LOOP DIURETICS

Named for their prominent activity on the ascending limb of the loop of Henle, these agents are known as "high ceiling" diuretics (Table 5.4). These drugs, which include furosemide, ethacrynic acid, and bumetanide, routinely produce a prompt diuresis with far greater urine volume than that seen with other diuretics.

Mechanism of Action. Inhibition of active chloride transport in the ascending limb of the loop of Henle is the major mechanism of action. Like the thiazides, their action is largely independent of exchanges in the acid-base balance in the body. Multiple sites of activity on tubular reabsorption are responsible for the magnitude of the inhibition of electrolyte reabsorption that occurs with these drugs. In addition to the ascending limb of the loop of Henle, the proximal renal tubule and, to a lesser degree, the distal tubule and collecting duct are affected by the high ceiling diuretics. Potassium excretion increases by an effect on the distal tubule. Magnesium and calcium excretion also increase.

Clinical Indications. Loop diuretics are readily absorbed from the gastrointestinal tract and undergo significant binding to plasma proteins. Thus, a drug interaction may occur when these drugs are taken concurrently with other highly protein-bound drugs, such as warfarin or clofibrate.

The loop diuretics' duration of action is from 2 to 4 hours, which is relatively short especially when compared with some of the longer acting thiazides. This short duration of action contributes to their safe use in life threatening situations such as pulmonary edema where their potency and promptness of action is of the essence.

The loop diuretics are effective in relieving the edema of CHF, as well as that of renal or

Table 5.4. LOOP DIURETICS.

Available products	Trade names	Daily dosage range
Bumetanide	Bumex	0.5–2 mg orally; 0.5–1 mg IV or IM
Ethacrynic Acid	Edecrin	50–200 mg orally; 0.5–1 mg/kg IV
Furosemide	Lasix	20–80 mg orally; 20–40 mg IV or IM

hepatic origin. Although the oral use of these drugs is generally preferred, the IV or IM administration of these drugs for a prompt diuresis in acute pulmonary edema may be a clinical necessity. In the presence of nephrosis or chronic renal failure, large doses of furosemide may be necessary to achieve the therapeutic goal. Decreased hepatic function slows the metabolism of furosemide and reduced renal function prolongs the duration of furosemide action.

Although the loop diuretics have essentially the same effects on electrolyte patterns as the thiazides, they tend to have a more pronounced diuretic effect. Their potency allows use of the loop diuretics in patients who have not responded to thiazides. Furosemide has a broader dose response curve than ethacrynic acid and allows for a more stable adjustment upward in dosage to fit the individual clinical requirement of the patient. Due to their potency and prompt action, the loop diuretics have been established as important mainstays in current diuretic therapy.

Adverse Effects/Precautions. Clinical experience with furosemide and ethacrynic acid has identified fluid and electrolyte imbalance, especially hypokalemia, as the major problem associated with their use. Metabolic alkalosis may happen when mobilization of edema fluid is too rapid and contraction of extracellular fluid volume occurs. Adverse effects reported for these drugs include gastrointestinal disturbances and temporary reduction or loss of hearing. Compared to ethacrynic acid, furosemide is less ototoxic, produces fewer gastrointestinal side effects, and is apparently less likely to cause metabolic alkalosis.

The pronounced effects of loop diuretics on electrolyte reabsorption and secretion may require more careful monitoring than with the thiazides.

POTASSIUM-SPARING DIURETICS

Certain diuretics available for clinical use do not cause the compensatory increase in potassium excretion that occurs with the thiazides and loop diuretics. The potassium is therefore "spared" or retained in the body.

Mechanism of Action. The potassium-sparing drugs act by inhibiting the exchange of sodium for potassium in the distal tubule. One mechanism may involve antagonism of the hormone aldosterone. Aldosterone increases sodium retention and potassium excretion by its action on the distal tubule. Therefore, an agent that acts as an aldosterone antagonist produces saluretic and antikaluretic effects. Spironolactone is the only drug marketed that blocks the sodium-potassium exchange mechanism by acting as an aldosterone antagonist. An active metabolite of spironolactone, canrenone, is largely responsible for the diuretic response.

Rather than an indirect effect on the distal tubule, a drug can also act directly to block the sodium-potassium exchange mechanism. Triamterene and amiloride are direct-acting potassium-sparing diuretics available for this therapeutic use (Table 5.5).

Clinical Indications. The potassium-sparing diuretics are valuable in preventing the potassium loss that may accompany therapy with the thiazides and loop diuretics. Consequently, a combination of hydrochlorothiazide with a potassium-sparing diuretic (triamterene) has achieved much therapeutic popularity.

The clinical characteristics of spironolactone therapy differ in some ways from the direct acting potassium-sparing diuretics. Spironolactone is most effective in conditions of increased aldosterone activity, resulting in enhanced so-

Table 5.5. POTASSIUM-SPARING DIURETICS.

Available products	Trade names	Daily dosage range
Amiloride HCl	Midamor	5–10 mg
Spironolactone	Aldactone; Alatone	25–200 mg orally
Triamterene	Dyrenium	100 mg b.i.d. after meals

dium reabsorption and increased potassium excretion. Hepatic cirrhosis and high renin hypertension are examples of conditions where spironolactone is especially effective in blocking the effects of aldosterone on the distal tubule. Spironolactone has a slow onset of activity compared to the prompt action of triamterene and amiloride on the sodium-potassium exchange mechanism. The action of spironolactone is sustained and this long duration of action is often useful in clinical practice. Since spironolactone is chemically related to progesterone, progestational effects such as gynecomastia may occur with its use. The direct acting potassium-sparing diuretics are effective regardless of the aldosterone plasma levels and therefore may produce more predictable diuresis.

A major value of the potassium-sparing diuretics is their rational combination with the thiazide derivatives. It is not surprising that the combination of a thiazide with each of the three potassium-sparing diuretics has resulted in several widely prescribed products including hydrochlorothiazide-triamterene, hydrochlorothiazide-spironolactone, and hydrochlorothiazide-amiloride. Indeed, the potassium-sparing diuretics have established a niche in diuretic therapy.

Adverse Effects/Precautions. The most serious toxic effect associated with the potassium-sparing diuretics is hyperkalemia. Common minor reactions are gynecomastia, androgen-like side effects, and gastrointestinal distress such as nausea and vomiting. Megaloblastic anemia has occurred in patients with alcoholic cirrhosis after triamterene treatment.

Table 5.6. URICOSURIC DRUGS.

Available products	Trade names	Daily dosage range
Probenecid	Benemid; Probalan	1 g
Sulfinpyrazone	Anturane	400–800 mg in 2 divided doses

MISCELLANEOUS DIURETICS

Organomercurials. Before the introduction of the newer diuretics in the 1950s, the organomercurials reliably produced prompt and predictable diuresis. Problems associated with their use include renal toxicity and, in general, the need for parenteral administration. Only one of these compounds, mersalyl and theophylline, is still marketed today. Although important from a historical standpoint, the organomercurials are rarely used diuretic drugs.

Xanthines. Of the many groups of diuretics available for clinical use, only the xanthines are derived from natural sources. Caffeine (tea and coffee) is a weak diuretic, whereas theobromine (chocolate and cocoa) possesses an intermediate diuretic effect. A synthetic xanthine derivative, aminophylline, has limited clinical utility as a diuretic in modern medicine. When used, xanthine derivatives are indicated in the treatment of edema associated with CHF.

The xanthines deserve mention since they are the only diuretics that may actually increase glomerular filtration rate (GFR). Since reduced glomerular filtration is usually basic to cardiac edema, this may be a beneficial, as well as a unique, activity. However, the xanthines' clinical use is limited since they are not as effective as the newer oral diuretics; they tend to produce gastrointestinal irritation; and, when given intravenously, they are extremely toxic.

URICOSURIC DRUGS

Uricosuric drugs (Table 5.6) are sometimes indicated in the management of gouty arthritis although allopurinol is the medication ordinarily prescribed for this disorder.

Probenecid. A lipid-soluble carboxylic acid, probenecid is completely reabsorbed by renal tubule carrier mechanisms in an acid urine. In an alkaline urine, however, net tubular secretion of probenecid occurs.

In fact, probenecid was developed in an effort to find compounds to inhibit the tubular secretion of penicillin when the antibiotic was in short supply. The basis for the drug's benefit in gouty arthritis, however, resides in its ability to reduce hyperuricemia by inhibiting the tubular reabsorption of uric acid.

Mechanism of Action. Uric acid is transported by carrier-mediated mechanisms in the renal tubule. Depending upon dosage, probenecid either decreases or increases the urinary excretion of uric acid. This paradoxical effect results from a difference in sensitivity to the drug on secretory and reabsorption processes for uric acid.

Probenecid's uricosuric action depends upon its ability to inhibit the tubular reabsorption of uric acid. The miscible urate pool is thereby reduced, which in turn retards urate deposition and promotes resorption of urate deposits.

Clinical Indications. Probenecid is indicated to reduce the hyperuricemia in chronic gout and gouty arthritis.

Adverse Effects/Precautions. Headache and gastrointestinal distress are common reactions to probenecid. Acute gout attacks and urate kidney stone episodes have occurred following probenecid therapy. Since urates tend to precipitate out in an acid urine, liberal fluid intake with a urinary alkalinization agent (such as sodium bicarbonate) is recommended.

Sulfinpyrazone. Sulfinpyrazone, a pyrazolone derivative with potent uricosuric effects, also elicits antithrombotic and platelet inhibitory activity.

Mechanism of Action. This drug inhibits the tubular reabsorption of uric acid.

Clinical Indications. Sulfinpyrazone is used in the treatment of gouty arthritis and intermittent gouty arthritis. Its potency renders it effective in many cases of gouty arthritis that are refractory to probenecid therapy.

Adverse Effects/Precautions. Gastrointestinal disturbances are the most frequently noted adverse effects with sulfinpyrazone. Consequently, its use is contraindicated in patients with active peptic ulcer or gastritis. This drug should be administered with milk, food, or antacids.

SPECIAL ASPECTS OF ELECTROLYTE PATTERNS SEEN IN DIURETIC THERAPY

Electrolyte imbalance is sometimes an important factor in diuretic therapy.

HYPOKALEMIA

Diuretics, such as the thiazides and loop diuretics, can produce hypokalemia in clinical usage. The hypokalemia may be prolonged if careful monitoring of serum potassium is not done with intense diuretic therapy. Over an extended period, hypokalemia can lead to actual muscle necrosis (rhabdomyolysis). If serum potassium is low, the arterioles fail to dilate during exercise. Additionally, when intracellular potassium is depleted, glycogen stores are depressed, resulting in insufficient energy for the muscles. These mechanisms may facilitate rhabdomyolysis.

Depletion of intracellular potassium also alters carbohydrate metabolism, resulting in a glucose tolerance curve resembling that which occurs in diabetes mellitus. This metabolic effect can be reversed in nondiabetic patients by the administration of potassium.

Depletion of total body potassium often leads to the development and maintenance of an alkalosis due to the effects on the kidney. A probable cause is the stimulation of ammoniagenesis, followed by an increase in H^+ secreted and HCO_3^- reabsorbed. Potassium depletion also produces polyuria due to an effect on the urine concentration mechanisms in the kidney.

Changes in the ECG and cardiac arrhythmias are symptomatic of severe hypokalemia. Another sign of extreme potassium depletion is respiratory muscle weakness. In these cases, intravenous potassium replacement may be necessary.

Serum potassium is ordinarily used to determine the status of intracellular and total body potassium. As a guideline in potassium replacement therapy, a drop in serum potassium from 4 to 3 meq/L represents a loss of approximately 150 meq of potassium. Each further drop of 1 meq of serum potassium represents an additional deficit of 300 meq.

HYPERKALEMIA

Potassium-sparing diuretics may produce hyperkalemia. For this reason, spironolactone use with direct acting potassium-sparing diuretics should be approached cautiously. Also, if potassium supplements are administered inadvertently with a potassium-sparing diuretic, potassium intoxication may occur. A high serum potassium level is even more dangerous than hypokalemia with disturbances in heart conduction being the primary clinical sign. A serum level of over 6.5 meq/L presents an immediate threat for cardiac arrhythmias.

HYPONATREMIA

Because of their impressive potency, loop diuretics can lower serum sodium levels if used excessively. This occurrence is rare, however, as compared to the possibility of hypokalemia.

HYPERCHLOREMIA

Carbonic anhydrase inhibitors, such as acetazolamide, elevate serum chloride (Cl^-). Since bicarbonate ion (HCO_3^-) excretion is increased with carbonic anhydrase inhibitors, hyperchloremic acidosis may occur.

FACTORS INVOLVED IN THE CLINICAL SELECTION OF A SUITABLE DIURETIC

In a clinical situation, the nature, cause, and amount of fluid or electrolyte to be removed determine the specific diuretic therapy. Correction of the primary cause is always a therapeutic goal, but even as this is being accomplished, a diuretic may be indicated to relieve the fluid accumulation. The disease condition determines the specific preferred diuretic. For instance, edema from CHF would probably be effectively treated with a thiazide or loop diuretic. In a case characterized by increased aldosterone activity, such as liver cirrhosis, spironolactone may be the diuretic of choice.

Clinical urgency and preferred route of administration are also major factors in the selection of an appropriate diuretic. In acute pulmonary edema, parenteral administration of a potent loop diuretic may be indicated, whereas in the edema of cirrhosis, a low salt diet, bedrest, and an oral diuretic may be a long-term treatment plan since this is not an immediate life-threatening urgency.

Concurrent diseases, especially those associated with the geriatric population, are also a consideration in diuretic choice. Liver or kidney disease could alter the choice and dosage of a diuretic. Patients with gout or diabetes mellitus may have clinical difficulties if treated with thiazides or furosemide because of the hyperuricemia and decreased glucose tolerance seen with these diuretics.

The specific toxicity of certain diuretics for selected physiologic processes is also an important consideration. Loop diuretics may cause ototoxicity and elderly patients are more susceptible to this effect, especially when other ototoxic drugs, such as aminoglycoside antibiotics, are used.

The setting in which the diuretic therapy is instituted also determines the diuretic choice. If diet and behavior can be managed effectively, a low salt diet combined with sufficient bedrest may allow for the use of a mild diuretic.

The refractory or resistant nature of some edemas presents a special clinical problem. The heroic use of an organomercurial or a potent loop diuretic, such as ethacrynic acid, may be indicated for cases unresponsive to the more frequently used diuretics.

Finally, there are special clinical situations where the particular therapeutic goal necessitates an osmotic diuretic given intravenously. The use of mannitol to rid the body of excess fluid in general or intracranial surgery is such an example.

DRUG INTERACTIONS

Drug interactions involving diuretic drugs often relate to electrolyte imbalance. Sometimes, as in the case of severe hypokalemia, the situation is potentially life-threatening. Additionally, diuretics may reduce the therapeutic benefit of certain drugs, such as oral anticoagulants and oral hypoglycemic drugs.

Osmotic Diuretics. Clinically significant drug interactions with the osmotic diuretics are rarely encountered due to their pharmacologically inert properties.

Carbonic Anhydrase Inhibitors.

Methenamine. Carbonic anhydrase inhibitors, such as acetazolamide, reduce the urinary antiseptic activity of methenamine by inducing urine alkalinity.

Thiazide Derivatives (Benzothiadiazides).

Digitalis Preparations. Cardiovascular agents (mainly digoxin) and diuretics (such as the thiazides and loop diuretics) are often given concurrently to the CHF patient to increase cardiac contractility and to remove accumulated fluid. The potassium deficiency that may be produced by diuretics predisposes the patient to digitalis toxicity. The introduction of the potent loop diuretics that possess a significant kaliuretic activity has made this drug interaction more likely in digitalis-diuretic therapy. Magnesium deficiency which can occur following diuretic therapy may also be implicated in the increased possibility of digitalis toxicity.

Consequently, the potassium and magnesium serum levels in patients undergoing digitalis-diuretic therapy should be closely monitored. Replacement therapy (with a potassium supplement) should be instituted as needed. Because individual patient reactions vary, routine potassium supplementation (without serum electrolyte information) is not indicated and may, in fact, be harmful as hyperkalemia may develop.

Oral Anticoagulants. Thiazides may inhibit the oral anticoagulant activity of drugs such as warfarin. Mechanisms proposed include a concentration of the clotting factors due to a decrease in plasma water and an increase in clotting factor synthesis by the liver due to an improvement of hepatic congestion and, hence, liver function.

Although thiazides probably have minor effects on the hypoprothrombinemic activity of oral anticoagulants, patients on chronic oral anticoagulant therapy might be monitored for an increase in anticoagulant requirement if diuretics are added to the patient's regimen.

Oral Hypoglycemics. Thiazides tend to elevate blood sugar in diabetic and prediabetic patients. These diabetogenic effects relate to insulin release inhibition and potassium depletion. Thus, thiazides may inhibit the oral hypoglycemic effects of drugs such as chlorpropamide and tolbutamide. In patients who are well controlled with an oral hypoglycemic agent, one must be alert to any change in diabetic control if thiazide therapy is instituted.

Additionally, an increased hyponatremic activity sometimes occurs if thiazides are combined with chlorpropamide. This activity is not noted with the other hypoglycemic drugs.

Trimethoprim and Sulfamethoxazole. In elderly patients (especially those with CHF), the concurrent use of diuretics (primarily thiazides) and a trimethoprim-sulfamethoxazole combination produces a risk of thrombopenia with purpura.

Lithium Carbonate. Long-term thiazide therapy results in reduced lithium clearance that manifests in elevated serum lithium levels and the possibility of lithium toxicity. A compensatory increase in tubular reabsorption of sodium after prolonged thiazide therapy has been proposed as a mechanism since lithium reabsorption is concurrently increased as sodium reabsorption occurs.

Curare-type Muscle Relaxants. Thiazides may increase the skeletal muscle relaxant activity of tubocurarine and gallamine. This effect may be due to thiazide-induced potassium deficiency.

Colestipol. Colestipol may inhibit the gastrointestinal absorption of thiazides. Therefore, if colestipol and a thiazide are both prescribed, the doses should be separated as far apart as possible.

Corticosteroids. Potassium-depleting diuretics, such as the thiazides, taken with corticosteroids may result in excessive potassium loss from the body. Patients receiving both a potassium-depleting diuretic and a corticosteroid should be monitored for potassium balance.

Loop Diuretics.

Cephaloridine. Furosemide (and perhaps other loop diuretics) may enhance the nephrotoxicity of cephaloridine by an unknown mechanism. Cephaloridine should probably be avoided if the combined use of furosemide and a cephalosporin is necessary.

Clofibrate. Furosemide and clofibrate may compete for plasma albumen binding sites. In patients with hypoalbuminemia, caution should be exercised as increases in the free levels of both furosemide and clofibrate have occurred.

Corticosteroids. The mechanism and clinical result are the same as those of the thiazide derivatives.

Lithium Carbonate. The resultant sodium depletion of sustained furosemide therapy decreases lithium excretion. If a patient is also on a salt-restricted diet, the lithium excretion is further impaired. Caution must be exercised if a patients with hypoalbumiremia, caution should be exercised as increases in the free levels of both furosemide and clofibrate have occurred.

Aminoglycoside Antibiotics. The combination of furosemide or ethacrynic acid with other potentially ototoxic drugs increases the possibility of drug-induced deafness (transient or permanent). If a diuretic is indicated, a drug from another class, like the thiazides, is indicated.

Chloral Hydrate. The combination of chloral hydrate and furosemide in some patients may cause vasodilation and flushing, tachycardia, hypotension or hypertension, and sweating. This reaction has been attributed to the displacement of thyroxine from albumen binding sites by both furosemide and chloral hydrate.

Indomethacin. In some patients, coadministration of indomethacin with furosemide has reduced the diuretic effect of furosemide. This effect has been attributed to the inhibition of prostaglandin synthesis by indomethacin.

Digitalis Preparations. Since the loop diuretics have a profound potassium-depleting activity, the possibility of digitalis toxicity is present with concurrent use of digitalis and potassium-losing diuretics. The same guidelines as those indicated with the thiazides should be followed.

Potassium-sparing Diuretics. The hyperkalemia that sometimes occurs with triamterene and other potassium-sparing diuretics is further increased with potassium supplements. Thus, the possibility of clinical toxicity is greatly enhanced if a potassium supplement is inadvertently given to patients taking a potassium-sparing diuretic.

UROCOSURIC DRUGS

Probenecid.

Aspirin. Aspirin antagonizes probenecid's uricosuric effect.

Miscellaneous Drugs. By inhibiting renal excretion, probenecid may increase the plasma levels of the following drugs: aminosalicylic acid (PAS), clofibrate, dapsone, indomethacin, methotrexate, naproxen, pantothenic acid, rifampin, sulfonamides, and sulfonylureas. Patients should be monitored for drug toxicity if probenecid is taken concurrently with these agents.

Sulfinpyrazone.

Aspirin. Aspirin antagonizes the uricosuric effect of sulfinpyrazone.

Coumarin-type Anticoagulants. Sulfinpyrazone may displace coumarin from albumen binding sites, thereby enhancing anticoagulant activity.

Sulfonamides and Sulfonylurea Hypoglycemic Agents. Sulfinpyrazone potentiates the action of sulfadiazine and sulfisoxazole. Since the activity of the sulfonylurea hypoglycemic agents and insulin may be acccentuated by sulfinpyrazone, caution must be exercised with concurrent use.

SUMMARY

Drugs that act on the renal system are important in the treatment of several serious diseases. Rational use of diuretics requires a proper choice of drug to fit the individual clinical condition. For instance, provided that renal function is normal, a thiazide derivative is a drug of choice; whereas in renal failure, a loop diuretic (perhaps in high doses) is indicated. If elevated serum aldosterone is an edema characteristic, as in nephrotic syndrome and cirrhosis ascites, spironolactone should be used in conjunction with thiazides. Intravenous injection of a loop diuretic (such as furosemide) is often indicated in the management of acute pulmonary edema and, in some cases, is used with diazoxide or sodium nitroprusside to treat acute hypertensive crisis. The importance of diuretics in treating mild to moderate hypertension is well known. A diuretic alone, in appropriate doses, sometimes sufficiently controls mild hypertension. Used in combination with another antihypertensive drug, a diuretic often increases the action of the other drug and prevents the development of resistance that may occur if the nondiuretic antihypertensive drug produces plasma volume expansion. Diuretics are not a substitute for dietary sodium restriction in patients with CHF, nephrotic syndrome, cirrhosis with ascites, or renal failure. Instead, these drugs make edema control possible with a less severe dietary restriction of sodium.

Knowledge and interpretation of physical signs occurring during diuretic treatment increase the effectiveness of patient care. Symptoms of improvement with diuretics, such as the loss of "pitting edema" or the reduction of gross abdominal distention in ascites, are obvious to the healthcare clinician and the patient. Additional positive indicators may include cessation of both breathing problems and coughing. By noting these "improvements" to the patient as examples of effective diuretic therapy, the pharmacist reinforces medication compliance. Conversely, the clinical practitioner should also be aware of symptoms related to diuretic-induced rapid mobilization and loss of fluid and/or electrolyte imbalance. Determining the exact nature of the problem(s) encountered with diuretic therapy requires pharmacologic expertise, as well as clinical experience. For instance, hearing difficulty may indicate a serious ototoxicity problem sometimes observed during loop diuretic therapy.

Since diuresis is limited by reduced extracellular fluid volume and low sodium serum levels, the diuretic effect diminishes and the degree of diuresis is considerably less than that seen during initial therapy. Should a patient become refractory to a diuretic, several options are available. Alternatives include increasing the diuretic dose; changing from a "moderate" diuretic (like a thiazide) to a more "potent" diuretic (such as furosemide); or adding an additional diuretic to the regimen.

Knowledge of the multiple sites and mechanisms of diuretic action allows the clinician to better treat the individual patient. For example, therapy with a potassium-sparing diuretic may require a choice between an aldosterone antagonist (spironolactone) or a distal acting Na^+-K^+ exchange inhibitor (triamterene), depending upon the etiology of the disease. Secondary aldosteronism, as in liver ascites, is better controlled with spironolactone as compared to triamterene. On the other hand, if potassium depletion unrelated to aldosterone levels occurs, triamterene is a drug of choice. The same rationale applies when considering a spironolactone-thiazide combination compared to a triamterene-thiazide combination.

Knowledge of the potency and the onset-duration of diuretic activity results in improved treatment monitoring. If a single daily diuretic dose is prescribed, a morning dose is preferable to bedtime administration. Also, if a potent diuretic is expected to produce a marked increase in urine flow, the patient should be alerted to anticipate frequent and demanding urinary urgency. The value of diuretics in certain clinical conditions, such as CHF and hypertension, must be tempered by the potential for danger in others, as in the use of a potent diuretic when kidney function is severely depressed (anuria).

Uricosuric drugs are also valuable therapeutic agents that act upon the renal system. These agents, together with the diuretics, constitute the major classes of drugs that exert pharmacologic effects on the renal system.

SUGGESTED READINGS

Brater, D.C.: Pharmacodynamic considerations in the use of diuretics. Annu Rev Pharmacol Toxicol, 23:45, 1983.
Bricker, N.S. (ed.): The Sea Within Us. A Clinical Guide to Fluid and Electrolyte Balances. San Juan, G.D. Searle & Co., 1975.
Bumetanide (Bumex). A new "loop" diuretic. Med Lett Drugs Ther, 25:61, 1983.
Davis, R.L.: Significant new drugs of 1983. Am Col Apoth Profess Pract Newsletter, 5:1, 1984.
Dennis, V.W., Stead, W.W., and Myers, J.L.: Renal handling of phosphate and calcium. Annu Rev Physiol, 41:257, 1979.
Diuretics may help prevent osteoporosis. Wellcome Trends in Hospital Pharmacy, 6:3, 1984.
Doctors list drugs used, prescribed in practice. Drug Store News, July 1982, 33.
Earley, L.E.: Diuretics. N Engl J Med, 276:1023, 1967.
Frazier, H.S., and Yager, H.: Drug therapy. The clinical use of diuretics. N Engl J Med, 288:246, 1973.
Giebisch, G., and Stanton, B.: Potassium transport in the nephron. Annu Rev Physiol 41:241, 1979.
Gifford, R.W., Jr.: A guide to the practical use of diuretics. JAMA, 235:1890, 1976.
Gilman, A.G., et al. (eds.): The Pharmacological Basis of Therapeutics. 7th Ed. New York, Macmillan Publishing Co., Inc., 1985.
Hansten, P.D.: Drug Interactions. 5th Ed. Philadelphia, Lea & Febiger, 1985.

Indapamide (Lozol). A new antihypertensive agent and diuretic. Med Lett Drugs Ther, 26:17, 1984.
Jacobson, H.R., and Kokko, J.P.: Diuretics. Sites and mechanisms of action. Annu Rev Pharmacol, 16:201, 1976.
Kastrup, E.K., and Boyd, J.R. (eds.): Drug Facts and Comparisons. Philadelphia, J.B. Lippincott Co., 1985.
Modell, W.: Drugs of Choice, 1984–85. St. Louis, C.V. Mosby Co., 1984.
Reidenberg, M.M., and Drayer, D.E.: Drug therapy in renal failure. Annu Rev Pharmacol Toxicol, 20:45, 1980.
Reyes, E., and Appelt, G.D.: Pharmacological aspects of concurrent administration of furosemide and skeletal muscle relaxants. J Pharm Sci, 61:562, 1972.
The top 200 prescription drugs of 1985. Am Druggist, 193:18, February 1986.
Torrett, J.: Sympathetic control of renin release. Annu Rev Pharmacol Toxicol, 22:167, 1982.
Vidt, D.G.: Diuretics. Use and misuse. Postgraduate Medicine, 59:143, 1976.

CHAPTER EXAMINATION

A patient has been taking hydrochlorothiazide and a potassium supplement for over a year. On Monday, her physician changes the thiazide preparation to another diuretic, triamterene. While in your pharmacy to pick up the triamterene, she asks for a refill of the potassium supplement. You question this and call her physician who refuses to approve the refill.

1. In this case, continued use of a potassium supplement may have resulted in
   a. hypokalemia
   b. nephrotic syndrome
   c. potassium intoxication
   d. decreased absorption of triamterene
2. Hydrochlorothiazide therapy was probably producing
   a. hyperchloremia
   b. hypokalemia
   c. hypoglycemia
   d. hypouricemia
3. Another factor responsible for the medication change (hydrochlorothiazide to triamterene) could be that the patient has
   a. diabetes mellitus
   b. primary hyperaldosteronism
   c. diabetes insipidus
   d. shown a fall in blood urea nitrogen (BUN)

A middle-aged female has been taking bendroflumethiazide for several weeks. Her physician orders a blood chemistry for her.

4. Azotemia (an occasional occurrence in thiazide therapy) would be detected by
   a. a rise in either blood urea nitrogen (BUN) or nonprotein nitrogen (NPN)
   b. a metabolic acidosis
   c. hyperkalemia
   d. hyperuricemia
5. Thiazides act as diuretics by
   a. inhibiting the tubular reabsorption of sodium, chloride, bicarbonate and water in the descending limb of the loop of Henle
   b. increasing the glomerular filtration rate (GFR)
   c. increasing tubular secretion of sodium in the distal tubule
   d. inhibiting sodium reabsorption in the cortical portion of the ascending limb of the loop of Henle and in the distal tubule
6. Changes in the blood profile with thiazide therapy include
   a. hypokalemia
   b. hyperuricemia
   c. hyperglycemia
   d. all of the above

A patient has impaired renal function and has been taking ethacrynic acid for hepatic edema. She develops a resistant infection, is hospitalized, and is given gentamicin IM.

7. Ethacrynic acid
   a. is a "loop" diuretic
   b. has clinical application in edema treatment that resembles bumetanide and furosemide
   c. acts on the ascending limb of the loop of Henle
   d. all of the above
8. A drug toxicity reaction that has been noted in clinical situations similar to that seen with this patient is
   a. glaucoma
   b. pulmonary edema
   c. ototoxicity
   d. ascites
9. Another drug choice for hepatic edema if aldosterone levels are elevated is
   a. spironolactone-hydrochlorothiazide combination
   b. triamterene
   c. amiloride
   d. triamterene-hydrochlorothiazide combination

Chlorthalidone is prescribed for a 52-year-old male patient. This patient has had several episodes of gout and a family history of diabetes mellitus.

10. Pharmacologically, chlorthalidone resembles
    a. hydrochlorothiazide
    b. furosemide
    c. mannitol
    d. aminophylline
11. Chlorthalidone can produce
    a. hyperuricemia and hyperglycemia
    b. hyperuricemia and hypoglycemia
    c. hypouricemia
    d. hypoglycemia
12. A history of gout is not an absolute contraindication to the use of chlorthalidone although
    a. a gout medication such as allopurinol or probenecid should probably be added to the regimen
    b. diuretic-induced hyperuricemia may precipitate gout in certain patients with a hereditary predisposition
    c. the hyperuricemia may be persistent and not intermittent
    d. all of the above
13. Diabetes mellitus is not a contraindication to the use of chlorthalidone, although rarely
    a. larger doses of insulin or an oral hypoglycemic agent are required
    b. smaller doses of insulin or an oral hypoglycemic agent are required
    c. a distal tubular diuretic, such as triamterene, should replace chlorthalidone
    d. a and c

A female patient has been taking furosemide and digoxin to treat CHF for an extended period. Dietary potassium supplementation is also a part of her drug treatment regimen. Recently she has complained of muscle cramps and being tired.

14. A potential drug interaction exists between furosemide and digoxin that
    a. may result in symptoms similar to those described by this patient
    b. could produce cardiac arrhythmias
    c. has never proved to be clinically significant
    d. a and b
15. A potassium supplement product
    a. should always be prescribed when a patient is taking a diuretic and digoxin
    b. may be required in this case
    c. is definitely contraindicated in this case
    d. should be "automatically" prescribed for this patient
16. Determination of this patient's serum potassium and digoxin levels
    a. is advisable before adding a potassium supplement to her therapeutic regimen
    b. would not give any valuable information for her future medication.
    c. is unnecessary because sodium serum levels are always the determinant in assessing digoxin toxicity
    d. gives valuable information relating to metabolic alkalosis
17. Furosemide is deleted from this patient's therapeutic regimen and a triamterene-hydrochlorothiazide combination is prescribed. This suggests that her symptoms were due to
    a. hyperkalemia
    b. hyponatremia
    c. hypokalemia
    d. secondary hyperaldosteronism

A patient has cirrhosis with ascites and is initially treated with spironolactone. A revised drug regimen includes a spironolactone-hydrochlorothiazide combination.

18. A probable explanation for the initial use of spironolactone was the presence of
    a. secondary aldosteronism
    b. hyperkalemia
    c. metabolic acidosis
    d. glaucoma
19. A thiazide added to this patient's therapeutic regimen
    a. lessens the possibility of hypokalemia
    b. lessens the possibility of hyponatremia
    c. lessens the possibility of hyperkalemia
    d. blocks renin release from the kidney
20. Spironolactone acts on the distal renal tubule. Two other diuretics that act at this site are
    a. mannitol and urea
    b. amiloride and triamterene
    c. ethacrynic acid and furosemide
    d. bumetanide and triamterene

ANSWER KEY

1. c	11. a
2. b	12. d
3. a	13. d
4. a	14. d
5. d	15. b
6. d	16. a
7. d	17. c
8. c	18. a
9. a	19. c
10. a	20. b

chapter 6

ENDOCRINE SYSTEM

CHAPTER OBJECTIVES

After studying this chapter, you should be able to:
1. List five examples of endocrine glands that are functional in humans.
2. Define hormone.
3. Designate the target organ(s) and predominant effects of the following: ACTH, somatostatin, FSH, P-RIH, TSH, somatotropin, LH, danazol, HCG, and cosyntropin.
4. Describe the relationship of the endocrine system to the nervous system as an information-integrating network.
5. Outline two major biochemical mechanisms whereby hormones elicit effects on target cells.
6. Explain the importance of receptor specificity in hormonal effects induced by the accumulation of intracellular cyclic AMP.
7. Differentiate between the several forms of RNA affected by human growth hormone and explain their relevance to increased protein synthesis in cell nuclei.
8. Describe the hypothalamus-pituitary relationship with respect to hormone release.
9. Discuss several factors that influence the synthesis and release of "tropic" hormones.
10. List six hormones released by the adenohypophysis.
11. Describe the clinical characteristics observed with hypopituitary activity in infants and adults.
12. Compare acromegaly to gigantism.
13. Name the major therapeutic/clinical indications for: human growth hormone, thyrotropin, ACTH gel, and menotropins.
14. Name two hormones secreted by the neurohypophysis.
15. Describe the manner in which oxytocin and vasopressin are synthesized, transported, and stored via the hypothalamus-pituitary interrelationship.
16. Describe the biosynthesis of the thyroid hormones.
17. Name four thyroid preparations used in the treatment of hypothyroidism.
18. List the main clinical symptoms of thyrotoxicosis.
19. Define or identify the following: thyroglobulin, thyroid-binding globulin, iodinium ion, Graves' disease, and Gull's disease.
20. Discuss the consequences of congenital hypothyroidism.
21. Identify three clinically significant drug interactions that occur with the thyroid hormones.
22. Describe three mechanisms of action of antithyroid agents.
23. Outline the site(s) of action of antithyroid drugs such as methimazole.
24. Describe the interrelationship between parathyroid hormone (PTH) and calcitonin.
25. Discuss the treatment of hypoparathyroidism.
26. Name the principal glucocorticoids of the adrenal cortex and describe their effects on the inflammatory process.
27. List the untoward reactions that occur with extended use of the adrenal glucocorticoids.
28. Discuss the therapeutic uses of fludrocortisone.
29. Illustrate the cyclic relationship between estrogen/FSH and progesterone/LH in the female menstrual period.
30. Describe the types of oral contraceptives and discuss the side effects associated with these products.

31. Discuss the potential hazards of androgenic-anabolic steroid use.
32. Describe the major biochemical lesions seen in diabetes mellitus.
33. Discuss the mechanisms whereby insulin corrects the metabolic abnormalities of diabetes mellitus.
34. Compare the second generation oral hypoglycemic agents (such as glyburide) to the first generation oral hypoglycemic drugs (like tolbutamide).
35. List three clinically significant drug interactions that occur with the oral hypoglycemic agents.

INTRODUCTION

The endocrine system, an elaborate and complex integrating system, permits the body to maintain a relatively constant internal milieu or homeostasis, as well as allowing bodily adjustments to environmental stimuli. Perhaps more correctly termed the neuroendocrine system because of the central nervous system (CNS) influence over endocrine function, this constantly adjusting network is necessary for life (Figure 6.1).

Endocrine glands form a finite structural component in the neuroendocrine system; examples of these glands include the pituitary, thyroid, and adrenal glands (Figure 6.2). Endocrine (from the Greek "within" and "secretion") refers to the system of glands or other structures that synthesize substances which are secreted into the circulation. Synthesis and release of these substances (or hormones) does not necessarily take place at the same site. Hormones (from the Greek verb "hormaein," meaning to set in motion) are defined as chemical substances produced endogenously by endocrine glands.

Hormones exert effects on target tissues by three main mechanisms (Figure 6.3). Two of these hormone mechanisms of information transfer involve hormone-cell membrane receptor interactions; the third represents an initial intracellular hormone-cytoplasmic receptor protein binding.

Hormones react with specific receptors in target cell membranes to set in motion reactions that culminate in a physiologic response. Thus, the anterior pituitary hormones, such as adrenocorticotropic hormone (ACTH) and thyrotropin (TSH), interact with membrane receptors in close proximity to adenyl cyclase sites (Figure 6.4). Activation of adenyl cyclase results from a hormone-cell receptor complex influence and elevates intracellular levels of adenosine 3', 5'-monophosphate (cyclic AMP). The cyclic AMP then functions as a "second messenger" to affect various biochemical reactions such as phosphorylation. This produces a physiologic response corresponding to the role of the target structures in bodily function.

Insulin receptors on target cells are also membrane-bound entities. The interaction of insulin with these receptors facilitates glucose transfer into muscle, fat, and, to some degree, hepatic cells. The post-receptor cellular events following the insulin-receptor combination, along with increased intracellular glucose utilization, contribute to insulin's activity in cor-

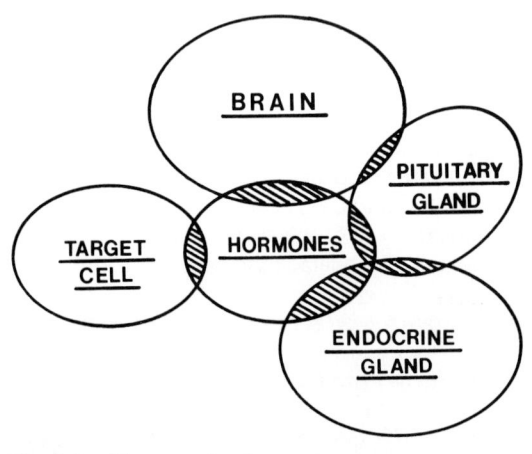

Fig. 6.1 Neuroendocrine system.

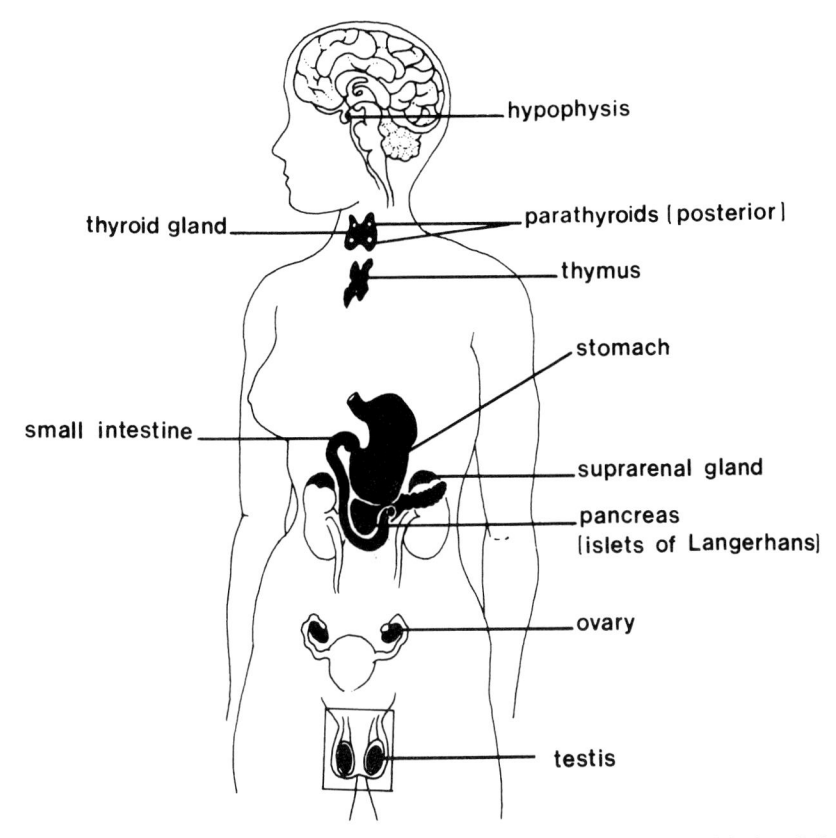

Fig. 6.2 Endocrine glands. (From Crouch, J.E.: Essential Human Anatomy. Philadelphia, Lea & Febiger, 1982.)

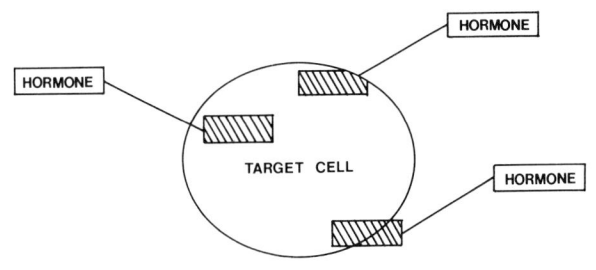

Fig. 6.3 Sites of hormone action on target cells.

recting the metabolic abnormalities seen in diabetes mellitus.

The third hormone mechanism is represented by the actions of steroid hormones on target tissues. Steroids gain access to intracellular sites and combine with protein cytosol receptors, resisting any cellular membrane binding (Figure 6.5). After the hormone-cytoplasmic receptor protein complex is formed, it is then translocated to the cell nucleus, where hormonal effects on protein synthesis occur.

Table 6.1 indicates the mechanism involved in the individual hormone action, as well as the primary stimulus for hormone secretion.

An important concept is that of interrelationships among the endocrine glands (Figure 6.6A). The information transferred among hormonal systems includes factors regulating

292 THERAPEUTIC PHARMACOLOGY

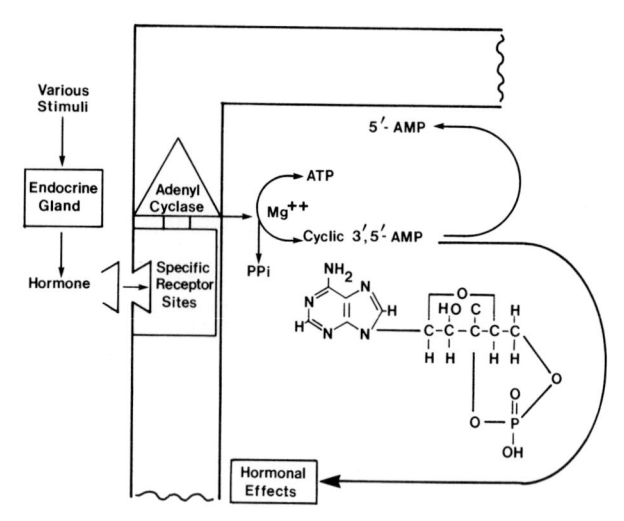

Fig. 6.4 Role of adenyl cyclase in the conversion of ATP to cyclic AMP. (Modified from Meyers, F.H., Jawetz, E., and Goldfein, A.: Review of Medical Pharmacology. 4th Ed. Los Altos, CA, Lange Medical Publications, 1974.)

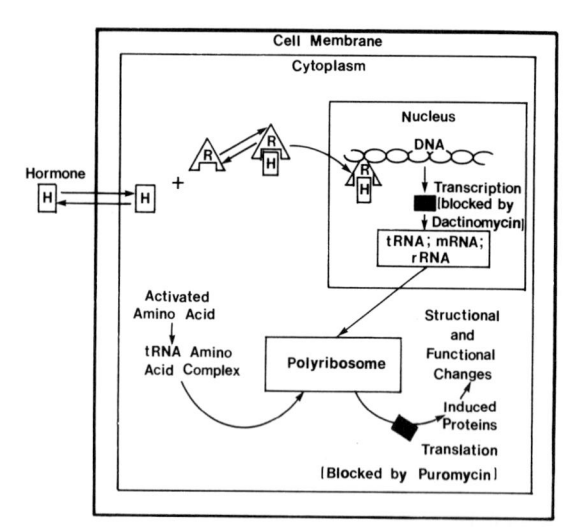

Fig. 6.5 Mechanism of steroid hormone action on protein synthesis. (Modified from Meyers, F.H., Jawetz, E., and Goldfein, A.: Review of Medical Pharmacology. 4th Ed. Los Altos, CA, Lange Medical Publications, 1974.)

gland maintenance and activation as well as negative feedback.

Another way to visualize the importance of these interrelationships to the well-being of the whole organism would be to see them as successful international trade interrelationships in a world of harmony (Figure 6.6B). Suppose a fantasy universe of "Hormonia" exists, which consists of individual countries (endocrine glands and target organs) that require particular imports to produce specific exports. The Recipient Country (peripheral endocrine gland) accepts an import ("tropic" hormone) from a Source Country (anterior pituitary) and manufactures a product for export (hormone), which is released to target countries for their use (response). Manufacturing a product (hormone) from an import is needed for the maintenance and "wellness" of the Recipient Country.

Often, only one particular import (e.g., TSH) is needed by a specific country (e.g., thyroid); if another import (e.g., ACTH) is not required, it is rejected by the country. One country's (e.g., thyroid) rejection of an import is another country's (e.g., adrenal) acceptance; thus, an analogy exists, which reflects specificity of "tropic" hormones to individual target organs. Additionally, excess exports by a Recipient Country (thyroxine/thyroid) require the Source Country to shut off supplying the necessary product (anterior pituitary/TSH) because of the "flooding of the market" phenomenon. Thus, the trade concept of supply and demand is analo-

Table 6.1. HORMONE RELEASE FACTORS AND BIOCHEMICAL MECHANISMS OF HORMONE ACTIVITY.

Hormone	Primary stimulus	Biochem. mech.
Parathormone	blood ionized calcium	cyclic AMP
Calcitonin	blood ionized calcium	cyclic AMP
Insulin	glucose	membrane glucose transport
Glucagon	glucose	cyclic AMP
Adrenal Corticoids: hydrocortisone, aldosterone, desoxycorticosterone	ACTH	protein synthesis
Androgens	gonadotropins	protein synthesis
Estrogens	gonadotropins	protein synthesis
Thyroxin	TSH	protein synthesis
Vasopressin	plasma osmolarity and extracellular volume	cyclic AMP
Oxytocin	undetermined	possibly prostaglandin release
Epinephrine	sympathetic nerve stimulation	cyclic AMP
Somatotropin	GH-RH	somatomedins; increased protein synthesis
Prolactin	P-RIH (negative control)	protein synthesis

gous to physiologic negative feedback mechanisms. A successfully integrated neuroendocrine system which achieves physiologic harmony is comparable to a finely tuned trade interrelationship between countries in the thriving and successful universe, Hormonia.

ANATOMY AND PHYSIOLOGY OF THE ENDOCRINE SYSTEM

The endocrine system is composed of several hormone-releasing structures, many of which are under neural influence. A neuroendocrine designation is applicable and appropriate for certain relationships, such as the hypothalamus-pituitary pathways. Additionally, hormone transport from endocrine gland to target tissue involves the bloodstream. Neural influence on target cell response is sometimes significant.

PITUITARY GLAND

The pituitary gland, a small pea-sized structure suspended from the base of the brain by a thin stalk, weighs only about 0.5 to 0.6 g in adult males and is slightly larger in females. The gland is situated in a special protected hollow at the base of the skull called the sella turcica ("Turk's Saddle"). Its anatomic name, hypophysis, is derived from a Greek word meaning "offshoot," which accurately designates its relationship to the brain. The pituitary gland's importance was largely unrecognized until this century. In fact, the name "pituitary" was derived from the Latin word for "mucus," since the gland's function was originally considered to be mere provision of moisture for the nasal membrane.

The pituitary gland is composed of three discrete anatomically fused structures: the anterior, posterior, and intermediate lobes. These three lobes differ in embryonic origin, as well as histologically and functionally.

The anterior lobe, or adenohypophysis, is formed from an outpocketing of the developing mouth from which it later becomes detached. It is composed of glandular secretory tissue represented by cells which biosynthesize and secrete specific hormones that maintain and stimulate several target glands and structures, including the thyroid and adrenal glands (Figure 6.7). Chemical mediators, formed in the hypothalamus and known as releasing hormones, regulate the secretion of the adenohypophyseal hormones.

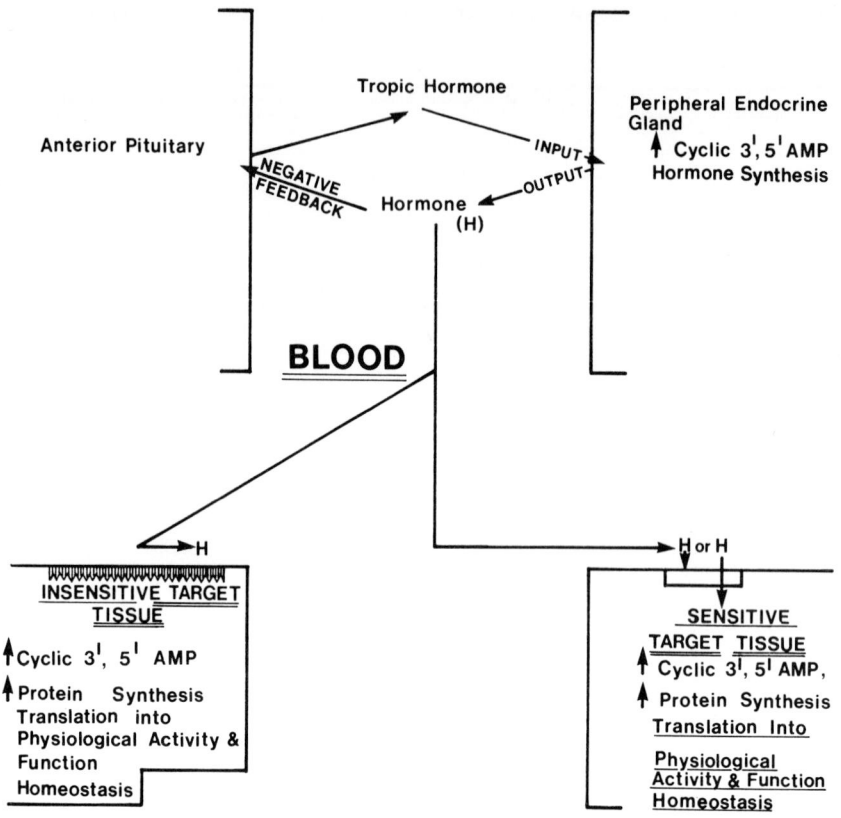

Fig. 6.6 A, Human hormone interrelationships.

The posterior lobe, or neurohypophysis, is formed as an outgrowth of the brain to which it remains attached. The neurohypophysis, then, is an extension of the nervous system derived from the thalamic floor. A special nerve tract extends fibers from cell bodies in the supraoptic and paraventricular nuclei into the hypophyseal lobe (Figure 6.7). These nerve fibers carry oxytocin and vasopressin, hormones of the supraoptic and paraventricular nuclei, to the neurohypophysis. Thus, the posterior pituitary hormones (oxytocin, vasopressin) are actually produced in the hypothalamus and are transported to the neurohypophysis where they are stored for later release by appropriate stimuli.

The intermediate lobe produces and secretes melanocyte-stimulating hormones (alpha-MSH and beta-MSH) that stimulate melanin synthesis. The role of these hormones in human skin pigmentation is uncertain.

HYPOTHALAMIC-ADENOHYPOPHYSEAL RELATIONSHIP

Neuroendocrine transducers are neurons found in the median eminence of the hypothalamus. Specific releasing hormones (RH) or release-inhibiting hormones (R-IH) are secreted from these neurons into the hypophyseal portal system (Figure 6.8). Monoaminergic influences that either favor or inhibit neuroendocrine transducers impinge on these neurons at the hypothalamic level. Therefore, monoaminergic neuron influence from higher centers controls the secretion of RH or R-IH.

Some releasing hormones that have been identified are corticotropin-releasing hormone (C-RH or ACTH-RH), follicle stimulating hormone and luteinizing hormone releasing hormone (FSH-LH/RH), thyrotropin releasing factor (T-RH), and growth hormone releasing

ENDOCRINE SYSTEM **295**

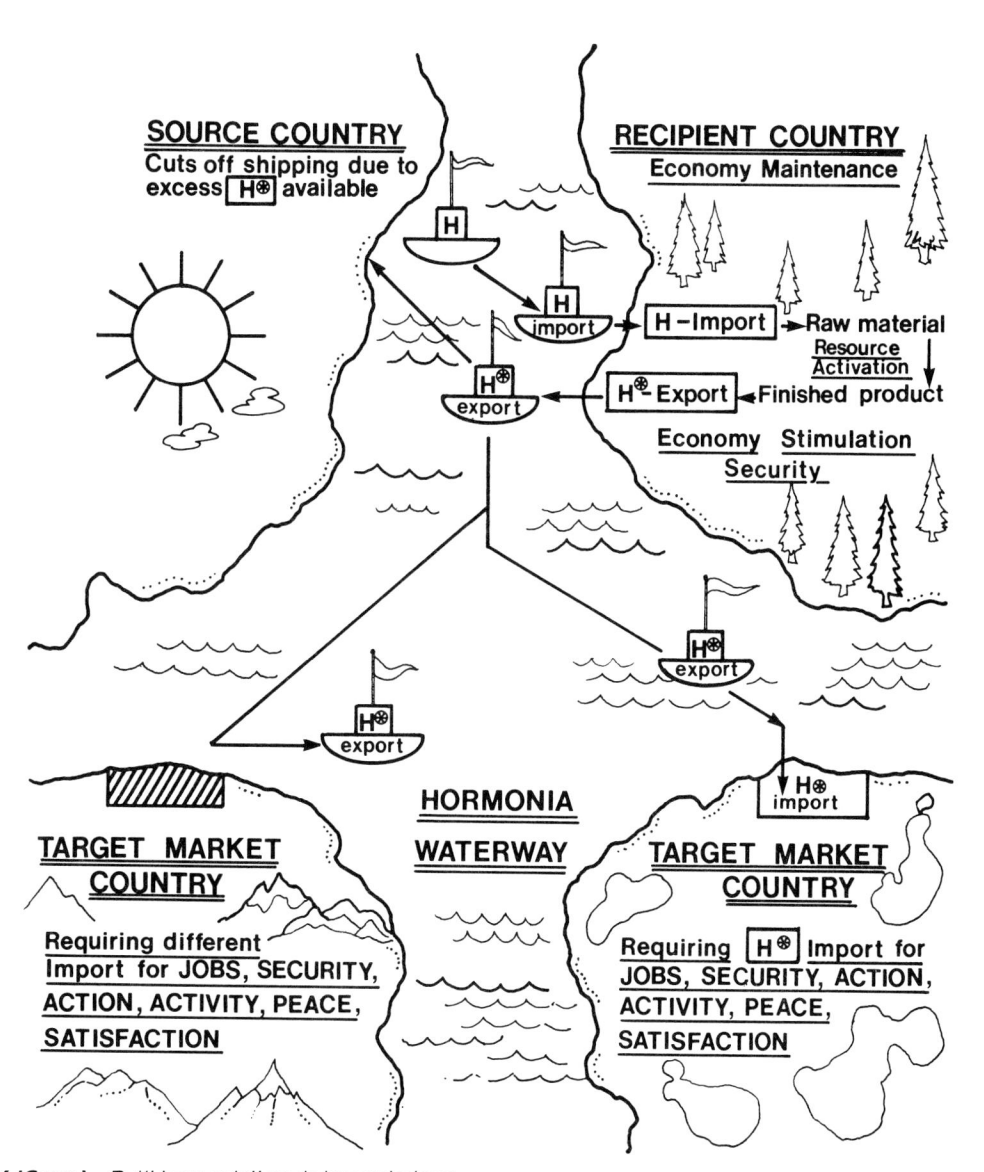

Fig. 6.6 (Cont.) *B*, "Hormonia" trade interrelations.

hormone (GH-RH). Also identified are prolactin release inhibitory hormone (P-RIH) and growth hormone release inhibitory hormone (GH-RIH). The adenyl cyclase-cyclic AMP system mediates the secretion of the releasing hormones by the monoamines.

Examples of dopaminergic influence on P-RIH illustrate clinical expression of basic neurophysiology. Theoretically, activation of hypothalamic dopaminergic receptors promotes secretion of prolactin release inhibitory hormone (P-RIH) and thereby reduces the prolactin secretion from the adenohypophysis. Galactorrhea, associated with increased prolactin secretion, can be successfully treated with a dopamine agonist such as bromocriptine. Conversely, central dopamine antagonists (blockers) like haloperidol or phenothiazine derivatives may induce galactorrhea in some patients.

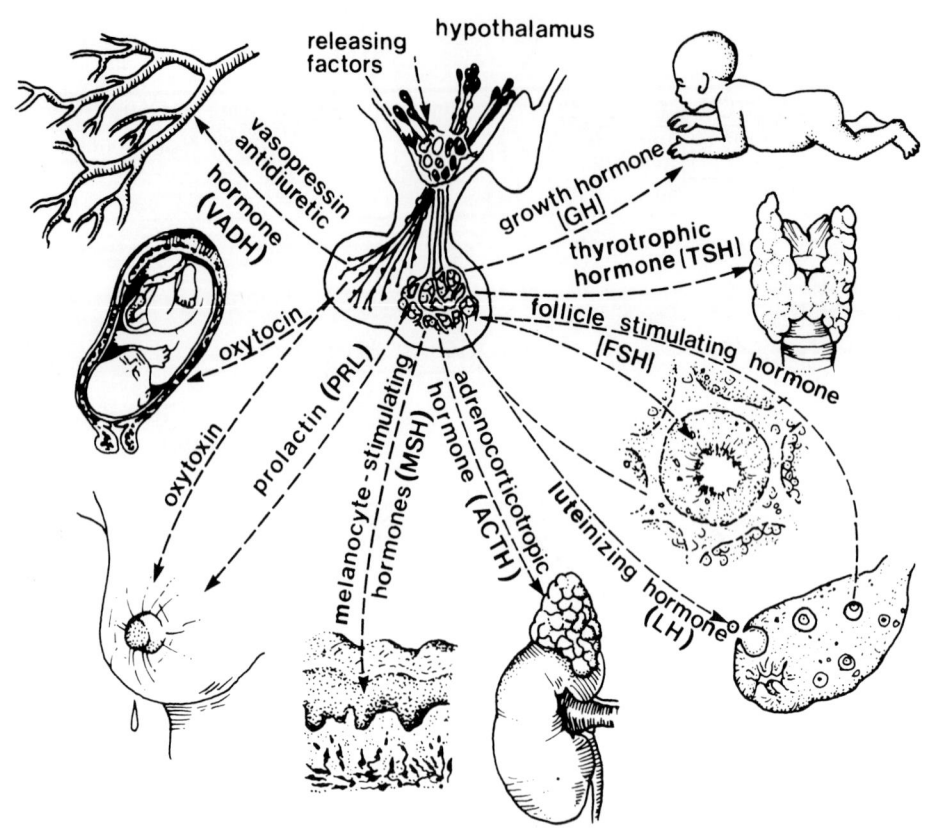

Fig. 6.7 Structural and functional relationships of the hypophysis to the hypothalamus and to other endocrine glands and other tissues. (From Crouch, J.E.: Essential Human Anatomy. Philadelphia, Lea & Febiger, 1982.)

The adenohypophysis has a vascular portal system flowing from the hypothalamus that allows for the transport of the hypothalamic releasing hormones to the adenohypophyseal secretory cells. This unique communication between the hypothalamus and adenohypophysis through a specialized vascular system is known as the hypophyseal portal system. The portal blood vessels are derived from the hypophyseal artery which ends in the median eminence of the ventral hypothalamus in a network of capillary loops called the primary plexus. The primary plexus then drains into vessels that supply blood to the adenohypophyseal capillaries (Figure 6.8). Thus, the hypophyseal portal system begins (primary plexus) and ends (anterior pituitary) in capillaries.

ADENOHYPOPHYSEAL HORMONES

The adenohypophyseal hormones have a sustaining trophic effect on target endocrine glands providing for their maintenance, as well as stimulating their hormonal secretion. Important influences include the gonadotropins in reproduction, normal growth and development control by growth hormone and thyrotropin, and energy metabolism regulation by adrenal corticoids and thyroxin. In vertebrates, at least ten recognized adenohypophyseal hormones are present. Of these, six are of primary importance: growth hormone (GH), thyroid stimulating hormone (TSH), adrenal cortical stimulating hormone (ACTH), follicle stimulating hormone (FSH), luteinizing hormone (LH), and prolactin (Pr); Table 6.2 summarizes their functions.

Some adenohypophyseal hormones accomplish information transfer by activating the membrane-bound adenyl cyclase on target cells. Intracellular reactions, representative of specific target cell function, are then set in motion following the elevation of cyclic AMP. For instance, ACTH stimulates adrenal steroidogenesis by activating the desmolase reaction, thereby promoting cholesterol conversion to the immediate adrenocorticoid precursor, pregnenolone. In this manner, adrenocorticoid synthesis and secretion are stimulated with the resultant effects on end-structure activity (i.e., cortisol on glucose metabolism).

Many hormones of the peripheral endocrine glands, as well as the stimulatory and inhibitory hormones of hypothalamic origin, influence adenohypophyseal hormone secretion. Feedback mechanisms dependent upon the peripheral organ hormones' blood concentration control adenohypophyseal hormone secretion. In this manner, high blood levels of corticosteroids secreted by the adrenal cortex inhibit ACTH release by the adenohypophysis. These feedback mechanisms function by decreasing the secretion of hypothalamic releasing hormones and the release of ACTH by the adenohypophysis.

NEUROHYPOPHYSEAL HORMONES

Oxytocin and vasopressin are small polypeptide hormones stored and secreted by the posterior pituitary. Oxytocin is formed primarily in the paraventricular nuclei of the hypothalamus, whereas the vasopressin biosynthesis occurs in the hypothalamic supraoptic nuclei. Oxytocin and vasopressin are then transported from the hypothalamus along neuron axons that supply the neurohypophysis for storage in the pituitary nerve endings. Appropriate stimuli cause the hormone release from the neurohypophyseal nerve endings where they are absorbed into adjacent capillaries.

Oxytocin stimulates uterine contraction during delivery and causes milk let-down. Uterine oxytocin activity is conditioned by the levels of estrogen and progesterone present. Additionally, certain ions such as calcium, magnesium, and potassium influence oxytocin activity.

Oxytocin binding sites are located on myometrial cell membranes. The oxytocin binding to the membrane receptors elicits an increased frequency and force of contraction in the uterine musculature. The mechanism for translation of the receptor binding to physiologic response is unknown, but prostaglandin release is apparently involved. The uterine sensitivity to oxytocin increases gradually during pregnancy and the hormone may function in the onset of labor.

In the mammary glands, nipple stimulation by the newborn causes oxytocin release. Oxytocin then produces mammary gland smooth muscle contraction and milk ejection.

Vasopressin (ADH) has pronounced antidiuretic activity by acting on the renal tubular epithelium to promote marked tubular water reabsorption. The adenyl cyclase-cyclic 3', 5'

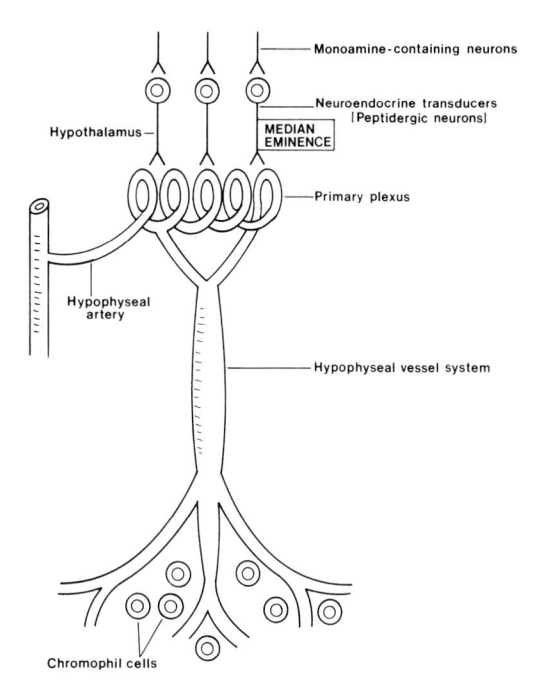

Fig. 6.8 Adenohypophysis portal system. (Modified from Bowman, W.C., and Rand, M.J.: Textbook of Pharmacology. 2nd Ed. Oxford, Blackwell Scientific Publications, 1980.)

Table 6.2. ADENOHYPOPHYSEAL HORMONES.

Hormone	Principal function
GH	Stimulates growth and development—increases protein synthesis; increases blood glucose concentration; mobilizes free fatty acids from adipose tissue
TSH	Stimulates the thyroid gland—maintains the thyroid gland; stimulates the synthesis and release of thyroid hormones
ACTH	Stimulates the adrenal cortex—maintains the adrenal cortex and stimulates the synthesis of adrenocortical hormones, especially hydrocortisone (cortisol)
FSH	Stimulates the growth of ovarian follicles and seminiferous tubules of testes—stimulates the growth of the ovum in the female and the sperm in the male; acts with LH to stimulate estrogen release
LH	Stimulates conversion of ovarian follicles into corpus luteum; stimulates secretion of sex hormones by ovaries and testes—stimulates development of the corpus luteum and acts with FSH to cause progesterone release; stimulates testosterone release in the male
Pr	Stimulates mammary glands to secrete milk—promotes mammary development and lactation

AMP system of the renal medulla is activated by vasopressin and represents the mechanism of hormone activity translation at this site. Vascular smooth muscle contraction is also a prominent action of vasopressin.

Vasopressin release control is partially mediated through hypothalamic osmoreceptors. Dehydration leads to increased vasopressin secretion, whereas hydration reduces its release.

THYROID GLAND

Located in front of and lateral to the trachea and lower larnyx, the thyroid gland is the largest of the endocrine glands weighing about 30 g. The thyroid gland consists of two lobes connected by a central isthmus. Additionally, a pyramidal structure rising upward between the two lobes is present in most glands. The blood supply to the thyroid is rich with the vessels to the thyroid branching from the aortic arch, the common carotid arteries, and the subclavian arteries. The extensive vascular endowment of the thyroid gland caused some early observers to ascribe a shunt function for the gland for blood traveling to the brain.

Thyroid activity is controlled by the thyroid stimulating hormone (TSH) that the adenohypophysis secretes. Synthesis of the thyroid hormones, triiodothyronine (T_3) and thyroxin (T_4), takes place in follicular cells that constitute a major portion of the lobes.

Iodine represents an integral part of thyroid hormones. Circulating iodide must first be "trapped" by gaining entry to intracellular sites in the thyroid tissue. Iodide is then oxidized by a cytoplasmic peroxidase system to a form of iodine (probably iodinium ion, I^+) that can be incorporated into tyrosyl residues of thyroglobulin to form either monoidotyrosyl or diiodotyrosyl entities; this is known as the iodination reaction. When a monoiodotyrosyl residue and diiodotyrosyl residue "couple," formation of triiodothyronine (T_3) results. The "coupling" of two diiodothyronine residues yields tetraiodothyronine or thyroxine (T_4). The "coupling" mechanism depends upon the same peroxidase system functional in the iodination reaction. Thyroglobulin functions as the matrix for T_3 and T_4 formation as in the iodination reactions. Most T_3 is formed from T_4 peripherally.

Calcitonin is another thyroid hormone secreted by the parafollicular or C cells of the thyroid gland. It functions along with parathyroid hormone and vitamin D in calcium homeostasis. The parafollicular cells release calcitonin in response to elevated plasma calcium. Calcitonin functions in an inverse fashion to parathyroid hormone (parathormone, PTH) in that when blood calcium increases, PTH levels decrease and calcitonin release increases; conversely, when blood calcium decreases, an increase in PTH secretion and a decrease in calcitonin occurs. Calcitonin stores are generally large and can be released for several hours without new hormone synthesis.

The major site of calcitonin activity is the bone where inhibition of resorption occurs. This effect relates to adenyl cyclase stimulation and the consequent elevation of cyclic AMP levels.

PARATHYROID GLANDS

The parathyroid glands, usually four in number and weighing 25 to 40 mg each, are embedded like small cultured pearls on the back and lateral surfaces of the thyroid gland. The blood supply to the glands is generous because of the rich vascular endowment of the thyroid gland. Parathormone (PTH) is the major hormone secreted by the glandular cells of these glands. A single chain polypeptide with a molecular weight of approximately 9,500, PTH is synthesized from a prehormone form and is stored within secretory granules prior to its release into the circulation. Since its turnover in the parathyroids is rapid and very little is stored there, most of the PTH is freshly synthesized prior to secretion.

The parathyroids' intimate anatomic arrangement with the thyroid gland does not ensure any commonality of endocrine function. The iodine-containing hormones secreted from the thyroid gland act independently of any interaction with PTH; however, the thyroid hormone calcitonin has an antagonist relationship with the parathyroid hormone.

The primary stimulus for PTH secretion is a low blood concentration of ionized calcium that translates into a "low-calcium trigger" to the parathyroid glands' secretory cells. If this "trigger" operates for prolonged periods and PTH secretion is sustained, hypertrophy and hyperplasia of the parathyroid glands occur. Conversely, in the presence of high ionized calcium, PTH secretion decreases and gland hypoplasia is possible. The relationship between calcium and PTH secretion represents a classical feedback system in that a fall in serum calcium stimulates PTH secretion while an elevation in serum calcium inhibits its release.

PTH's primary function is to regulate calcium and phosphate metabolism. Calcium mobilization from the bones into the bloodstream and the inhibition of renal tubular reabsorption of phosphate are two prominent PTH effects. Thus, bone is the most important source of calcium responsible for the plasma calcium elevation seen with PTH.

Effects of PTH on intestinal calcium absorption and renal tubular calcium reabsorption are of secondary importance compared to the effects on bone resorption. Bone phosphate resorption also occurs with PTH, but the increased plasma phosphate tends to fall because of the additional PTH effect on the renal tubule to inhibit phosphate reabsorption.

PTH indirectly affects the gastrointestinal tract to increase intestinal absorption of calcium and phosphate. An enhancement of calcium and phosphate intestinal absorption depends upon the renal conversion of calcifediol to calcitriol that occurs with PTH. Calcitriol apparently inhibits PTH release, although this effect may result from increased calcium blood levels.

ADRENAL GLANDS

The adrenal glands, two small triangular-shaped structures (each weighing about 3 to 5 g), are located on the upper surfaces and immediately in front of each kidney. The adrenals are embedded in fat and, like the kidney, lie behind the peritoneum; they have a richer blood supply than any other organ of similar size, with the possible exception of the thyroid gland.

The adrenal gland consists of two parts, each with separate endocrine functions. The outer part, known as the cortex, surrounds an inner medulla. The cortex and medulla differ from each other histologically and physiologically.

The adrenal cortex produces three types of hormones: glucocorticoids, mineralocorticoids, and sex steroids. Represented by the prototype hydrocortisone, the glucocorticoids affect carbohydrate, protein, and fat metabolism. Mineralocorticoids, such as aldosterone, regulate water and salt balances. The sex hormones secreted by the adrenal cortex serve as auxillary sources to the gonadal steroid hormone secretions.

The medulla, intimately involved with the sympathetic nervous system, secretes two hormones: epinephrine (adrenaline) and norepinephrine (noradrenaline). Epinephrine is an emergency hormone vital in allowing an individual to meet emergencies and respond to sudden danger. The "flight or fight" reaction initiated by an epinephrine "rush" enables one to react and cope with imminent danger. Epinephrine increases alertness, elevates blood glucose for quick energy, dilates the pupils for better vision (especially in a dim-light situation), and constricts the surface blood vessels allowing for increased blood shunt to the muscles. Epinephrine also stimulates the anterior pituitary to produce and secrete ACTH which in turn stimulates the adrenal cortex. Upon stimulation of ACTH, the glucocorticoids released from the adrenal cortex promote formation of glucose from proteins (gluconeogenesis) and replenish the liver and muscle glucose stores expended in the "flight or fight" reactions. Thus, the ability to react to prolonged stress depends upon a functional hypothalamus-pituitary-adrenal relationship.

GONADS

The gonads or gamete-secreting glands consist of the ovaries in females and the testicles in males.

OVARIES

The female gonads are two ovoid bodies called ovaries that develop behind the posterior abdominal peritoneum and migrate to a permanent niche on the lateral walls of the pelvis. Walnut-sized, the ovaries lie lateral to the uterus and are attached loosely to the posterior side of the broad ligament of the uterus by a short fold of tissue. The ovary has other ligament support from additional attachments to the uterus and the pelvic wall. Thus, the ovaries are held loosely by ligaments allowing for displacement, such as might occur during pregnancy.

Each human ovary contains approximately 400,000 primordial follicles, which constitute the bulk of ovarian tissue. The ovaries participate in a complex cyclic hormonal phenomenon that repeats every 28 days beginning at puberty and continuing until the fourth or fifth decade of life. The oviducts or fallopian tubes originate from the upper part of the uterus and terminate in open ends with fringelike projections near the ovary. Upon ovulation, ripened ova enter these tubes and thereby are conveyed to the uterine cavity. The oviduct is the usual site where fertilization of an ovum by a male sperm occurs.

The dual functions of the ovaries are provision of the ova or egg cells and secretion of the hormones, estrogens and progesterone. The estrogens (female sex hormones) favor development of the secondary feminine sex characteristics of breast growth, pubic and axillary hair, maturation of the genital tract, and contouring of the female figure. Progesterone is the hormone secreted by the corpus luteum after ovulation occurs.

The menstrual cycle, initiated by the onset of puberty, is a precise and complex phenomenon. The anterior pituitary sparks the initiating hormonal stimulus by releasing follicle-stimulating hormone (FSH). FSH stimulates several primary follicles that begin to grow during the cycle; only one of these primary follicles reaches maturity and releases its ovum.

The one "super follicle" (graafian follicle) continues to mature and the ovum it contains expands several times the size of the immature ovum in each of the primordial follicles. As this follicular growth proceeds, small amounts of another anterior pituitary hormone, luteinizing hormone (LH), are continually supplied to the ovary. The graafian follicle assumes an endocrine function as estrogens are biosynthesized and secreted during this growth period. Luteinizing hormone (LH), but probably not FSH, influences the estrogen release and causes ovulation of the graafian follicle that matured under the influence of FSH. At the time of ovulation, both the LH and FSH blood levels peak. The ruptured graafian follicle fills with blood and becomes another endocrine structure called the corpus luteum which produces and secretes progesterone and small amounts of estrogens. This transformation of the ruptured follicle into a corpus luteum is under the influence of LH. Progesterone, often called the hormone of the corpus luteum, supports the preparation of the uterine lining (the endometrium) for reception of a fertilized ovum.

Some estrogen production also continues as long as the corpus luteum functions as an endocrine structure. At the end of the cycle if fertilization hasn't occurred, the endometrium that has been building since the initial FSH impetus to follicle growth breaks off and menstruation begins. The next cycle starts when FSH again activates another immature primordial follicle and it begins to grow. An explanation of why one of the follicles begins to mature and develop into the graafian follicle has yet to be determined.

If the ovum is fertilized and implantation occurs (usually about a week after fertilization), the chorion of the placenta produces human chorionic gonadotropin (HCG) which maintains the functional activity of the corpus luteum. The HCG levels increase for several weeks and then decrease for the remainder of the pregnancy. After the second or third month of pregnancy, the placenta begins to secrete estrogen and progesterone and the corpus luteum becomes obsolete as an endocrine structure. The secretion of large amounts of estrogen and progesterone by the placenta continues until the time of birth.

TESTES

The testes are oval, walnut-shaped structures suspended within the scrotum, an external skin-covered pouch located below the symphysis pubis and in front of the anus. The tubules of the testes are responsible for spermatozoa production, whereas interstitial cells (Leydig cells) produce and secrete the male hormone testosterone.

The testes biosynthesize and secrete the androgens or male sex hormones. Testosterone is the main androgen produced by the testes. Although relatively high in male infants at birth, concentrations of testosterone fall to low prepubertal levels within several months after birth. At the time of male puberty, undefined stimuli increase the amounts of luteinizing hormone (LH) and follicle stimulating hormone (FSH) released from the anterior pituitary. A characteristic cyclic pattern of gonadotropin secretion synchronized with the sleep cycle initially occurs after the start of puberty. The progression of puberty reveals sleep cycle gonadotropin bursts extending into the waking hours. At this stage of young male development, the hypothalamus and anterior pituitary become less sensitive to testosterone negative feedback. LH and FSH are both responsible for the increase in testicular growth, spermatogenesis, and steroidogenesis. The actions of the gonadotropins (as in the female) are mediated through the adenyl cyclase-cyclic AMP system.

LH is also known as interstitial cell-stimulating hormone (ICSH). ICSH interacts with the interstital cells (Leydig cells) of the testes to effect synthesis of androgens from acetate and cholesterol. The adenyl cyclase-cyclic AMP "second messenger" mechanism, set in motion by ICSH, stimulates testosterone production. The male secondary sex characteristics (i.e., penis development, pubic and axillary hair growth, increased muscle mass, voice changes, beard growth, and other signs of maleness) depend upon the increasing amounts of testosterone. Concurrently, tubular germ cells develop into spermatozoa. As the spermatozoa mature, they are stored in sacs called the seminal vesicles located on either side of the prostate gland. Under the influence of testosterone, the prostate gland provides fluid to nurture and sustain the viable spermatozoa. This seminal fluid is discharged just prior to the male climax or orgasm.

PANCREAS

The pancreas, about 14 cm long, stretches like a small bunch of grapes along the lower border of the stomach. At one end it is attached to the duodenum. A distinguishing feature of the pancreas is its dual status as both an endocrine and an exocrine gland. The endocrine portion of the pancreas is the islets of Langerhans, which number between 1 to 2 million and comprise about 1 to 2% of the total pancreas mass. The islets are scattered throughout the pancreas, although the highest concentration occurs in the head of the pancreas. The islets are highly vascular and each cell appears to have direct capillary contact. Autonomic innervation consists of both vagal and sympathetic fibers.

Cells of the pancreatic islets have a common embryologic heritage with the endocrine cells of the gastrointestinal tract.

The islets are composed of a mixture of three cell types. Over 75% of the islets consists of beta cells, which contain insulin granules. Alpha cells, the source of glucagon, are the largest cells, comprising about 20% of a typical islet. The remaining 5%, called delta cells, contain granules considerably smaller than those of the alpha or beta cells. The delta cell granules, which contain somatostatin, are interposed between the alpha and beta cells, resulting in contact with both types.

Insulin is secreted by the islet beta cells; it consists of two chains of polypeptides called the A and B chains. These chains are joined by two disulfide bonds; the A chain contains an additional disulfide bridge.

Proinsulin is the immediate precursor in the biosynthesis of insulin. A single chain polypeptide, proinsulin yields insulin and a biologically inactive fragment known as C-peptide.

Glucose is the most important stimulus to insulin release, although various amino acids, beta-adrenergic agonists (isoproterenol), and glucagon are among the other agents that promote insulin secretion. Alpha-adrenergic agents, such as epinephrine and norepinephrine, inhibit insulin release.

Insulin facilitates the transfer of glucose into cells by interacting with a membrane receptor on target tissues such as muscle, fat, and liver cells. This lowers blood glucose by exposing glucose to mitochondrial oxidative processes and also promotes the conversion of intracellular glucose into glycogen stores. Insulin also reduces fatty acid mobilization and inhibits amino acid conversion into glucose (gluconeogenesis) by blocking protein catabolic processes.

Glucagon is secreted by the islet's alpha cells and is a physiologic antagonist to insulin. A single chain polypeptide, it is released from the pancreas in a prohormone form. Glucagon produces hyperglycemia, glycogenolysis, and ketogenesis by activating cell membrane adenyl cyclase with a subsequent elevation of intracellular cyclic AMP. The secretion of glucagon is stimulated by amino acids and other endogenous factors such as stress, starvation, hypoglycemia, and muscular exercise. Elevated blood glucose and insulin inhibit glucagon release.

Glucagon-like polypeptides, known collectively as enteroglucagon, are produced and secreted by endocrine cells of the small intestine. The role of these intestinal endocrines is unclear.

Somatostatin, usually found in the hypothalamus, is a third pancreatic hormone that inhibits both insulin and glucagon secretion. Its specific function at this site is unknown.

SPECIAL ASPECTS OF ENDOCRINE GLANDS

The separate structures of certain endocrine glands, such as the pituitary gland and the adrenal glands, originate from distinctly different embryonic tissue. For example, the neurohypophysis develops from nerve tissue, whereas the adenohypophysis represents an ectoderm outgrowth of the primitive mouth. The fusion of the neurohypophysis and adenohypophysis to form the pituitary gland results in a singular endocrine structure that secretes hormones from each separate lobe. Hormones from the neurohypophysis and adenohypophysis often act together to achieve a particular physiologic goal. In this manner, during pregnancy and after delivery, the adenohypophyseal hormone (prolactin) promotes mammary gland development and lactation and oxytocin (a hormone stored and secreted from the neurohypophysis) stimulates postpartum milk let-down. Thus, hormones from each lobe complement and support a physiologic process designed to support life for the newborn.

The adrenal medulla is derived from the same embryonic tissue as the sympathetic nervous system and shares a similar function. The adrenal cortex, however, has a different embryonic legacy and is histologically quite dissimilar from the modified nerve tissue represented in the adrenal medulla. The combination of these discrete structures to form a single gland illustrates superior biologic engineering.

Glucocorticoids, secreted from the adrenal cortex, are transported via the intra-adrenal vascular system in high concentrations to the adrenal medulla where they stimulate the synthesis of the medullary enzyme, phenethanolamine-N- methyltransferase. This enzyme stimulates the conversion of norepinephrine to epinephrine and results in medullary tissue with high epinephrine content. Therefore, glucocorticoid release, originally set in motion by a hypothalamic stimulus such as stress, ensures high epinephrine amounts immediately available for emergency functions like blood pressure elevation, respiration stimulation, slowing of digestive processes, muscle fatigue delay, blood glucose elevation, pupil dilation, and oxygen consumption increase. The close proximity and unique vascular arrangement of separate gland structures thus allow the achievement of synergistic physiologic function.

The synthesis, storage, and release mechanisms of hormones in individual endocrine glands vary considerably according to their role in maintaining life processes. For instance, the thyroid gland traps and stores iodides as organo-iodine hormones. This efficient glandular trapping mechanism for a substance (iodine) not always present in the environment is critical for maintenance of thyroid hormone levels. The thyroid gland conserves and stores an integral component of its hormone for use in the body's growth and development. Organisms are not then "required" to be continually near the sea or other environmental sources of iodine. The biosynthetic and release mechanisms for thyroid hormone involve precursor binding and incorporation into a protein (thyroglobulin) matrix. The hormone's protein storage form requires a lysis process for release. The release mechanisms of endocytosis and proteolysis are relatively inefficient and yield extremely small quantities of T_3 and T_4 for secretion into the blood for distribution to target cells.

The extensive storage of the thyroid hormone in the gland's colloid suggests the body's awareness of needing sufficient reserves because a thyroid hormone lack at any time in growth and development can adversely affect mental and physical maturation. Thus, these thyroid processes appear at first to be inefficient and extravagant, but when one considers the development price the organism pays if thyroid hormones are absent, the metabolic cost is small.

In marked contrast to the thyroid gland, the adrenal cortices synthesize and release adrenal steroids without significant storage mechanisms. In fact, synthesis of the adrenal steroids is tantamount to hormone secretion as they are immediately released to the circulation. The components and precursors of steroid hormones are ubiquitous in the diet and have no unique structural requirement, such as iodine incorporation. Adrenal steroid storage, therefore, is not as critical because the precursors acetate and cholesterol are metabolically abundant in the organism. Since the adrenal cortices are necessary for many life maintaining processes (during both development and in the mature adult), this rapid hormone turnover is not surprising.

Certain hormone spurts of activity are regulated by "biological clock" types of phenomena. A diurnal pattern represents daily (24 hour) fluctuations of hormone release related to the sleep-awake cycle. For instance, in a "normal" sleep-awake cycle, ACTH is synthesized during the night and reaches its peak concentration between 6 a.m. and 9 a.m. As the adrenal steroids are released, the negative feedback on the hypothalamus-pituitary axis that occurs with elevated blood adrenal steroids cuts off ACTH synthesis and release during the daylight-awake hours. During the midmorning until evening period, adrenal steroids are released and utilized with the ACTH levels remaining low, their lowest being at about 6 p.m. ACTH synthesis resumes during the night and another diurnal cycle begins. Certain factors such as stress and erratic sleep habits can upset these cyclic hormone release patterns.

The sudden release of large amounts of gonadotropins at the onset of puberty is another example of hormone release based upon a chronologic factor. This quiescent hypothalamus-pituitary system regulating gonadotropin release springs into activity after years of dormancy to activate the conversion of young boys and girls into men and women. The female menstrual cycle that occurs after the onset of puberty and continues for several decades, usually following a 28-day cycle with exact regularity, also illustrates a precise cyclic hormone release pattern.

In these examples of chronologic changes in hormone levels, one can visualize the differences possible in physiologic responses to drug therapy depending upon the time of administration in the cyclic pattern. Thus, the chronopharmacologic aspect of drug administration is an important factor affecting exogenous adrenocorticoid therapy (e.g., alternate-day steroid therapy).

DYSFUNCTION OF THE ENDOCRINE GLANDS

A main use of hormones or hormone analogs is replacement therapy to correct deficient hormone levels. Various glandular abnormalities in hormone synthesis, storage, or secretion account for low levels of circulating hormones. Additionally, target organ reactivity to hormones may be reduced even though the blood levels of the hormone are within the normal range.

In contrast to hypofunction, excessive hormone secretion necessitates correction by inhibiting the secretion or activity of the hormone by various means. Surgical removal (partial or total) or radioactive isotope destruction of a hyperfunctional gland are sometimes used to treat thyroid gland overactivity. Hormone analogs that block the synthesis, storage, and release of hormones are another means to counteract hyperactive states, as are drugs that inhibit or modify target organ hormone receptors.

ANTERIOR PITUITARY GLAND

HYPOFUNCTION

Pituitary dwarfism occurs when congenital deficiency of growth hormone is present. This condition is clearly apparent when the child fails to grow in physical stature at a normal rate. However, diagnosis may be delayed since the child's genetic background may reflect adult parents of small frame size. The pituitary dwarf's extremities and features are in proportion to the body trunk. Thus, this individual does not appear grotesque in any way, but is simply a small human being.

Obviously, if a "panhypopituitary" situation exists, other pituitary hormone deficiencies, such as ACTH and the gonadotropins, are also present. Human growth hormone availability has increased via genetic engineering and commercial preparations are now marketed to treat hypopituitary dwarfism. The development of radioimmunoassay techniques, which allow for a more precise differential diagnosis of hormone defiency, has greatly advanced the speedy correction of specific glandular problems.

HYPERFUNCTION

Pituitary gigantism occurs when excessive growth hormone is secreted before epiphyseal closure of the long bones. Such individuals achieve a greater than normal physical stature and are often pictured as "circus giants."

Acromegaly is the condition that occurs when excessive growth hormone is secreted in the adult after the long bones have ceased growing. The extremities and face are elongated because growth hormone still elicits an effect at those sites. A characteristic facial profile and disproportionately large extremities comprise the clinical picture of acromegaly.

POSTERIOR PITUITARY GLAND

HYPOFUNCTION

"Diabetes," from the Latin "siphon," accurately describes the clinical picture of constant thirst and profuse urine formation observed in diabetes insipidus. Insipidus, denoting flat or tasteless, contrasts to the "honeyed urine" of diabetes mellitus (sugar diabetes). A disorder of water metabolism, diabetes insipidus results from an absolute or relative deficiency in the secretion of vasopressin (ADH) from the neurohypophysis or from failure of end-organ response to the hormone.

Caused by any number of factors, neurogenic or central diabetes insipidus is characterized by deficient vasopressin release. Infection, neoplasia, or trauma destroy tissue in the hypothalamus or neurohypophysis, which leads to marked polyuria and polydipsia. Indeed, fluid loss exceeding 10 L in 1 day is sometimes noted. If an adequate thirst mechanism is operant and sufficient fluids are ingested, the physiologic balance can be maintained. If the patient becomes unconscious because of surgical procedure or trauma, severe dehydration occurs.

Nephrogenic or peripheral diabetes insipidus results from insensitivity of the kidney tubules to the action of vasopressin (ADH). Although beneficial in the treatment of neurogenic or central diabetes insipidus, vasopressin or synthetic analogs are ineffective in nephrogenic or peripheral diabetes insipidus.

THYROID GLAND

HYPOFUNCTION

Congenital hypothyroidism results in a clinical profile characterized by retarded mental and physical development, lassitude, and low energy levels. This condition is called cretinism, and such individuals are known as cretins. "Cretin" is probably derived from the Old French, meaning "little Christian," because immediately after birth and as an infant these babies are well-behaved, rarely cry, and are, in outward appearance, well-mannered new arrivals. In reality, the low amounts of thyroid hormone do not allow the "normal" energy of infants, but even more significant is the effect of the hormone deficiency upon the CNS.

Thyroid hormone is necessary for myelinization of CNS neurons, and its lack results in deficient development. Thus, cretinism undetected and uncorrected within the first few months of life has permanent effects upon intellectual capacity. The effects of hormone deficiency on growth include reduced physical stature with limbs and extremities shortened in proportion to the body trunk. This disproportionate relation contrasts markedly with hypopituitary dwarfism, in which all structures are in normal proportion to each other.

Dietary insufficiency in children is usually avoided by the use of iodized salt, high iodine content foods, or iodine-containing vitamin/mineral supplements. Hypothyroid conditions in pregnancy are corrected by use of a thyroid hormone preparation (i.e., prenatal supplement, which generally contains iodine).

In adults, hypothyroidism is manifested mainly by lassitude, bradycardia, mental dullness, and sometimes obesity. A severe hypothyroid condition in the adult is called "myxedema." Edema characterized by mucus accumulation under the skin produces a puffy appearance. These hypothyroid conditions in the adult are largely corrected by administering a thyroid hormone preparation.

HYPERFUNCTION

Graves' disease, or thyrotoxicosis, was the first disease to be recognized as related to endocrine gland hyperfunction. Excessive thyroid hormone activity may progress to "thyroid storm" and cause a clinical emergency. Hyperthyroidism is characterized by anxiety, hyperactivity, tachycardia, and exophthalmos (bulging of the eyeballs). "Popeye," the sailorman, represents a hyperthyroidism clinical picture as he exhibits high physical activity and energy levels, a lean profile, probably a fast heart beat, and the obviously protruding eyeballs.

As one might anticipate, the effects on the cardiovascular and central nervous systems are opposite to those of low thyroid hormone levels. Hyperthyroid states are treated by several means, including surgery, radioactive iodine (^{131}I) ablation, and antithyroid drugs such as methimazole.

PARATHYROID GLANDS

HYPOFUNCTION

Hypoparathyroidism results from a deficiency in parathormone (PTH) secretion or from an end-organ resistance to the hormone's activity. Symptoms of hypoparathyroidism are the consequences of lowered ionized calcium blood levels, reducing the excitability threshold of biologic membranes. Since hypocalcemia is only occasionally due to hypoparathyroidism, other etiologic factors must also be considered in hypoparathyroidism diagnosis. Common causes of hypoparathyroidism are parathyroidectomy, parathyroid disease, and trauma to the glands or to their blood supply during thyroid surgery.

Decreased concentration of plasma ionized calcium that occurs in hypoparathyroidism results in diverse neuromuscular symptoms due to the altered irritability of muscles and neurons. Paresthesias and tetany, indicating skeletal and smooth muscle involvement, are among the first noticeable clinical signs. Tetany is a condition of neuromuscular system hyperexcitability indicated by intermittent spasms of the hand and face muscles; convulsions and other evidence of CNS involvement may also occur. Chronic hypoparathyroidism is characterized by ectodermal changes, such as hair loss and grooved, brittle fingernails. Changes in dental enamel and cataract formation, as well as CNS symptoms (emotional lability, anxiety, depression, and delusions), are common in the chronic disease.

In its acute form, hypoparathyroidism is treated by raising the blood calcium through means such as an IV injection of calcium gluconate. Supplementation by intramuscular (IM) or oral administration of calcium salts is often indicated. Presently, parathormone (PTH) is rarely used in therapeutics as an adjunct drug with calcium salts. After a latent period of about 4 hours following injection, PTH raises the serum calcium; its effectiveness decreases after successive administration. In chronic hypoparathyroidism treatment, the chief therapeutic goal is to raise the serum calcium and reduce the serum phosphorus. Currently, chronic hypoparathyroidism is treated primarily with vitamin D and dietary calcium supplements.

HYPERFUNCTION

Hyperplasia or tumors of the parathyroid glands can result in primary hyperparathyroidism. In almost 90% of all primary hyperparathyroidism cases, the cause is a benign tumor of the parathyroid glands. Hyperparathyroidism may also be secondary to a negative calcium balance produced by malabsorption and renal disease. In these cases, the blood calcium is low and thus provides a stimulus for continuous PTH secretion. Hypercalciuria and hyperphosphaturia are almost always associated with primary hyperparathyroidism. A high incidence of renal calculi (kidney stones) occurs when the urinary excretion of calcium and phosphate is high. Paget's disease (osteitis deformans) and osteitis fibrosa are characterized by depletion of the bone calcium content; however, only one out of three hyperparathyroidism cases shows advanced bone changes.

Hypercalcemia causes some of the prominent symptoms of hyperparathyroidism. Thus, muscle hypotonicity with skeletal muscle weakness and smooth muscle dysfunction relates directly to elevated blood calcium. Treatment of primary hyperparathyroidism usually requires surgery to excise a portion of the hyperplastic parathyroid gland or adenoma.

ADRENAL GLANDS

HYPOFUNCTION

Hypofunction of adrenal cortical activity, usually called Addison's disease, can result from a disease process or tumor. By far, the most common form of adrenal corticol hypofunction is drug-induced, i.e., by the chronic administration of adrenal steroids or their synthetic analogs. High levels of adrenal steroids or synthetic analogs in the bloodstream suppress ACTH release from the anterior pituitary. With no trophic and stimulatory prod because of ACTH absence, the adrenal cortex becomes less functional and "lazy." After prolonged periods, adrenal cortical atrophy ensues and the person reacts inadequately to stresses such as infections or surgery. This condition develops more often when adrenal steroids are administered in a high pharmacologic dose (suprapharmacologic) as an anti-inflammatory drug, rather than as the smaller physiologic dose required for replacement therapy in adrenal cortical hypofunction.

The magnitude of life support processes affected by the adrenal cortical steroids makes survival possible only under a rigid prescribed environment if the adrenals are nonfunctional. Therefore, in extreme adrenal hypofunction, replacement therapy with adrenal corticoid preparations or ACTH is indicated. Hypofunction of the adrenal cortex may also occur when activity of the pituitary gland is deficient. Thus, in the treatment of hypopituitary dwarfism, ACTH or adrenal corticoids are part of the treatment regimen.

HYPERFUNCTION

Cushing's syndrome, a condition characterized by adrenal hyperfunction, most often results from a tumor or adrenal cortex hyperplasia. The excess of circulating adrenal corticoids profoundly affects carbohydrate, fat, and protein metabolism. A shift in fat tissue forming a "buffalo hump" on the upper back is a characteristic sign of this syndrome.

Excess amounts of circulating aldosterone and desoxycorticosterone produce salt retention and edema. A "cushingoid" syndrome is sometimes seen with adrenal corticoid or synthetic adrenal corticoid analog therapy. This iatrogenic syndrome actually proceeds while the patient's adrenal cortex becomes less functional from the negative feedback of the exogenous steroid on the hypothalamus-pituitary system.

GONADS

HYPOFUNCTION

In either sex, gonad hypofunction becomes apparent at puberty if the secondary sex characteristics fail to appear. This condition results from either a singular primary glandular deficiency or a more complex etiology involving release phenomena in the hypothalamus-pituitary system. Thus, in young girls, failure to begin a menstrual cycle at puberty could reflect a myriad of causative factors and involves extensive diagnostic tests before any therapy initiation. Replacement therapy with appropriate estrogens or androgens is usually a treatment of choice.

In males, another recognized cause of gonad hypofunction is cryptorchidism. Medical or accidental castration produces the "eunuch" appearance familiar to all late-night movie viewers of harem scenes in which a soft, plump male with a high-pitched voice is entrusted to watch over the harem entourage without danger of sexual interlude.

In females, menstruation cessation, marking the end of the ovulation cycle, often produces a post-menopausal syndrome characterized by depression, "hot flashes," and other sometimes ill-defined symptoms. Estrogens often alleviate this discomfort and therefore are effective replacement drugs for this situation.

HYPERFUNCTION

Sexual precocity in either sex occurs if an excess of the primary gonadal hormone is secreted. In contrast, an excess of androgen secretion in females or estrogen production in males produces secondary sex characteristics common to the opposite sex.

PANCREAS

HYPOFUNCTION

A common clinical manifestation of pancreas hypofunction is diabetes mellitus. In this condition, the pancreatic beta cells are incapable of synthesizing and secreting sufficient insulin for bodily needs. "Diabetes" or "siphon" accurately depicts the symptoms of polydipsia (excessive thirst) and the resulting polyuria (excessive urination) that are characteristic of diabetes mellitus. "Mellitus" refers to honey and thus "honeyed urine" was one of the first metabolic signs of diabetes mellitus noted. A predominant defect in carbohydrate metabolism that occurs in diabetes mellitus is elevation of blood glucose (hyperglycemia). This is but one reflection of other intermediary metabolism aberrations. Fat metabolism changes indicate increased lipolysis with a subsequent rise in fatty acid fragments, such as acetoacetic acid, beta-hydroxybutyric acid, and acetone. Since fats "burn in the flame of carbohydrates," the defects seen with glucose utilization tend to accentuate the elevated ketone and acid body levels. Thus, ketoacidosis commonly results from untreated diabetes mellitus. Additionally, the increased amount of glucose being synthesized from the fat catabolism products is further aggravated by conversion of amino acids into glucose. In diabetes mellitus, a breakdown or wasting of body protein occurs when the "building blocks" of protein (amino acids) undergo conversion to glucose. In essence, the body devours itself, hence the description of diabetes mellitus as a "wasting disease." This occurs even when the appetite is increased (polyphagia). Therefore, the conversion of noncarbohydrate sources of fats and proteins into glucose (gluconeogenesis) represents another significant metabolic abnormality of diabetes mellitus.

The amount of glucose in the blood passing through the islets of Langerhans determines the rate of insulin secretion. There is little evidence of nerve control of insulin secretion since complete denervation of the pancreas has little effect upon insulin secretion. When the blood sugar level is decreased sufficiently to cause hypoglycemia, the CNS stimulates the adrenal glands to produce epinephrine, which causes glucose liberation from liver glycogen. The insulin-epinephrine balance is probably the mechanism whereby the blood sugar level is promptly regulated. Other endocrine mechanisms involve somatotropin and the adrenal corticoids.

Juvenile onset diabetes (also known as Type I diabetes mellitus) is characterized by its development usually about the time of puberty and the rapid onset of a severe syndrome with a tendency toward ketoacidosis. In Type I juvenile diabetes, an absolute insulin deficiency is present. Insulin is always required to treat Type I juvenile onset diabetes and adequate titration with insulin to meet the changing everyday stresses and situations is often difficult.

Mature onset diabetes (also known as Type II diabetes mellitus) is characterized by its development after the age of 40. Usually a gradual and mild onset occurs with only a small incidence of ketoacidosis. A relative insulin deficiency exists in Type II diabetes mellitus in that plasma insulin levels are lower than normal, but there is no absolute insulin deficiency as in Type I.

Uncontrolled diabetes mellitus may be fatal due to an interference with energy liberation in the body, depletion of carbohydrate and fat stores, burning of tissue (muscle) protein resulting in emaciation of the patient which increases susceptibility to infections, and accumulation of acid products (ketoacidosis).

Several changes are common in diabetes mellitus. Microangiopathy is a disorder of the small blood vessels affecting the capillary endothelial cells and the basement membrane. The latter thickens and abnormalities occur in the polysaccharide content of the membrane and in the enzymes responsible for their synthesis. Damage to vessels is particularly evident in the eye (as diabetic retinopathy) and in the kidney glomeruli. Coronary artery disease, resulting in conditions such as myocardial infarction, is the leading cause of death in diabetes. Renal disease is another common cause of diabetes fatalities. The etiologic role of growth hormone (somatotropin) in microangiopathy production is unclear but remains suggestive since growth hormone overproduction often accompanies diabetes. The benefit of reducing the hyperglycemia of diabetes in the prognosis of microangiopathy remains undetermined.

Neuropathy, evidenced by demyelination of sensory nerves, also occurs frequently in diabetes. Hyperglycemia sensitizes the nerve fibers to unknown damaging factors. Therefore, proper blood sugar control can stop and even partially reverse these disease processes in the nerves.

Skin and genitourinary tract infections are also prevalent in diabetes. Infections of the vagina and urinary tract directly relate to excess glucose excreted in the urine; consequently, glycosuria reduction lessens the incidence of these infections.

Since diabetes mellitus has a genetic component, family history is valuable in ascertaining diabetes risk. Obesity predisposes one to the development of clinical diabetes mellitus. Insulin resistance is a common finding in obese nondiabetic patients; therefore, obesity aggravates a tendency toward diabetes mellitus by placing increased demands upon insulin reserves.

In pregnancy, decreased sensitivity to insulin

occurs, probably related to placenta lactogen and increased estrogen and progesterone levels. The increased demand for insulin during pregnancy exceeds pancreatic reserves and predisposed individuals develop diabetes symptoms.

HYPERFUNCTION

An excess of endogenous insulin occurs in pancreatic tumors or upon spontaneous hyperactivity of the islet tissue. Hyperinsulinemia also occurs in acromegaly and is most often observed clinically as hypoglycemic shock in exogenous insulin overdose. If the blood glucose level is 0.04% (a little less than ½ the normal concentration), convulsions, unconsciousness, and death may occur.

DRUGS AFFECTING THE ENDOCRINE SYSTEM

Generally, drugs affecting the endocrine system are hormones or "hormone-like" chemicals. These drugs either mimic or block hormone action on endocrine glands or target structures. Therapeutic applications of endocrine drugs are varied and they assume an important role in clinical practice.

ANTERIOR PITUITARY HORMONES

Anterior pituitary hormones (Table 6.3) have physiologic, therapeutic, and diagnostic applications in modern medicine.

Menotropins (Human Menopausal Gonadotropins; HMG). This preparation consists of gonadotropins extracted from the urine of postmenopausal women. Menotropins are standardized for follicle stimulating hormone (FSH) and luteinizing hormone (LH).

Mechanism of Action. Menotropins act as replacement therapy for gonadotropin deficiency. FSH stimulates follicle growth; LH causes ovulation and stimulates corpus luteum development although the amount of LH present in usual doses of menotropins is insufficient to elicit these responses. LH also stimulates spermatogenesis in males. Both FSH and LH stimulate cyclic AMP synthesis in the testes and ovaries by activating membrane-bound adenyl cyclase. Consequently, elevated cyclic AMP promotes sex steroid biosynthesis.

Clinical Indications. The menotropins preparation (HMG) is employed together with human chorionic gonadotropin (HCG) to promote conception in infertile women. Menotro-

Table 6.3. ANTERIOR PITUITARY PREPARATIONS.

Available products	Trade names	Daily dosage range
Clomiphene citrate	Clomid; Serophene	50 mg/day for 5 days
Corticotropin injection	Acthar; ACTH	IM or SC, 25–40 units q.i.d.; 10–25 units IV infusion in 500 ml of 5% glucose
Corticotropin injection repository	H.P. Acthar Gel; Cortropin Gel	25–40 units IM or SC q.i.d.
Corticotropin zinc hydroxide	Cortropin-Zinc	20–40 units IM q.i.d.
Cosyntropin	Cortrosyn	0.25 mg dissolved in sterile saline injected IM
Danazol	Danocrine	Individualized according to clinical situation
Menotropins	Pergonal	IM, 75 IU of FSH and 75 IU of LH daily for 9–12 days
Somatotropin*	Asellacrin; Crescormon	IM, individualized therapy
Thyrotropin	Thytropar	10 IU IM or SC daily for 1–3 days,
Protirelin	Thypinone; Relefact TRH	0.5 mg IV

* Currently not marketed in the United States

pins are effective only in ovulation failure in women who lack sufficient pituitary gonadotropins to bring about ovarian follicle development. Infertility cases that involve primary ovarian failure or organic disease of the uterus or fallopian tubes are not successfully corrected with the HMG-HCG regimen. In the sequential use of HMG and HCG, menotropins stimulate ovarian follicle development in preparation for ovulation, and the HCG subsequently administered causes ovulation.

Seventy-five percent of patients with secondary ovarian failure due to pituitary gonadotropin insufficiency ovulate after the menotropins and HCG series. Pregnancy occurs in 25% of the women who undergo this treatment and multiple births occur in about 20% of the births.

In men with primary or secondary pituitary hypofunction, menotropins have been administered concomitantly with HCG to induce spermatogenesis.

Adverse Effects/Precautions. The possibility of multiple births and adverse symptoms of ovarian overstimulation are factors that must be considered in menotropin therapy. Certain adverse effects of menotropins, including bloating and stomach or pelvic pain, are recognized as being clinically significant; these symptoms apparently result from ovarian overstimulation.

Since ovulation usually occurs 18 hours after HCG administration, intercourse should be attempted within 48 hours. During HCG therapy, the patient should have intercourse daily beginning the day HCG is administered.

Clomiphene Citrate. Clomiphene is a nonsteroidal drug that stimulates secretion of pituitary gonadotropins.

Mechanism of Action. An antiestrogenic drug, clomiphene binds to estrogen receptors in the cytoplasm of target cells. The competition for estrogen binding sites results in fewer receptors to interact with endogenous estrogen. The hypothalamus and anterior pituitary receive a signal indicating low estrogen levels and respond by increasing gonadotropin outflow. The resultant ovarian stimulation, involving ovarian follicle maturation and subsequent corpus luteum development, is responsible for this agent's designation as a "fertility drug."

Clinical Indications. In cases of infertility not due to either ovarian failure or primary pituitary dysfunction, clomiphene may be beneficial. Favorable responses in infertile females usually occur when endogenous estrogen levels are normal.

Clomiphene is being tested as an investigational drug in male infertility.

Adverse Effects/Precautions. As with the menotropins, ovarian hyperstimulation and a high incidence of multiple births occur with clomiphene use. The incidence of multiple births is less (6 to 8%) than that observed with menotropin therapy. Liver dysfunction is a contraindication in the use of clomiphene.

Danazol. A synthetic androgen, danazol suppresses pituitary gonadotropin secretion.

Mechanism of Action. Danazol inhibits the pituitary secretion of FSH and LH. The inhibition of the outflow of FSH and LH decreases estrogen production by the ovary. Danazol also binds to gonad steroid receptors and may elicit an inhibitory effect on these target organs.

Clinical Indications. Danazol renders endometrial tissue (normal and ectopic) inactive and atropic. Resolution of endometrial lesions occurs in a majority of cases.

Danazol is generally indicated in the treatment of endometriosis in patients who have not responded to other drug therapy. Danazol is also indicated in the treatment of fibrocystic breast disease and in the prophylaxis of hereditary angioedema in males and females. Additionally, this drug has been used to treat gynecomastia, infertility, menorrhagia, and precocious puberty.

Adverse Effects/Precautions. Androgenic side effects such as acne, edema, mild hirsutism, decrease in breast size, deepening of the voice, skin oiliness, and weight gain have been reported. Hypoestrogenic effects may also occur.

Adrenocorticotropic Hormone (ACTH; Corticotropin). Corticotropin, a polypeptide, is derived from the pituitaries of cattle and swine.

Mechanism of Action. Corticotropin stimulates the adrenal cortex to produce and secrete adrenocortical hormones. Adrenal function must be adequate for corticotropin to elicit this effect. Corticotropin activates membrane-bound adenyl cyclase to initiate the sequence of biochemical reactions culminating in intracellular cyclic AMP elevation. Steroidogenesis, which elevates adrenal cortical hormone levels such as hydrocortisone, is stimulated by cyclic AMP. The major metabolic step affected by the increased concentration of cyclic AMP is the oxidative cleavage of the side chain of cholesterol to form pregnenolone.

Clinical Indications. Employed in the diagnostic testing of adrenocortical function, corticotropin may also have therapeutic value in conditions that respond to corticosteroid therapy. Corticosteroids are generally used in these conditions (inflammation, collagen diseases, allergic reactions, etc.), although some clinicians feel that a corticotropin injection causes a more physiologic reaction by inducing endogenous steroid release from the adrenal cortex. Corticotropin therapy is adjunctive and the lowest effective and shortest time course dose should be employed.

Adverse Effects/Precautions. Edema, muscle weakness, gastrointestinal distress, and CNS stimulation are common side effects of corticotropin therapy (see glucocorticoids).

Cosyntropin. Cosyntropin, a synthetic peptide corresponding to the amino acid residues 1 to 24 of human corticotropin, exhibits the full corticosteroidogenic activity of natural corticotropin.

Mechanism of Action. Cosyntropin acts on the adrenal cortex to promote steroidogenesis in a manner similar to that of corticotropin. Since cosyntropin does not contain foreign animal protein, there is less likelihood of a hypersensitivity reaction occurring.

Clinical Indications. Cosyntropin is used diagnostically to determine adrenal cortical function.

Adverse Effects/Precautions. Hypersensitivity reactions are possible, although not as likely as with corticotropin.

Somatotropin* (GH; HGH). A purified polypeptide hormone, somatotropin is extracted from the human anterior pituitary gland (adenohypophysis).

Mechanism of Action. Several somatotropin actions are mediated by somatomedins, which are synthesized in the liver in response to somatotropin. Also known as the sulfation factor, somatomedins promote incorporation of sulfate into cartilaginous tissue. This sulfation factor stimulates cartilaginous growth of the long bones with resultant body weight increase. Anabolic properties of somatotropin are represented by a stimulation of intracellular amino acid transport and net nitrogen retention. Ribosomal RNA increases occur with a stimulation of protein synthesis.

Clinical Indications. The only indication for somatotropin use is growth failure due to growth hormone deficiency. Hypopituitary dwarfism is effectively treated by replacement therapy with somatotropin. Somatotropin is ineffective when dwarfism results from other factors or when epiphyseal closure has occurred.

Adverse Effects/Precautions. Since somatotropin has a diabetogenic effect, caution must be employed in patients with a personal or family history of diabetes mellitus. In susceptible patients, somatotropin therapy can lead to hyperglycemia and ketosis.

---

* In July 1985, the distribution of somatotropin was suspended and commercial somatotropin products were withdrawn from the market following disclosure that at least two young adults treated with growth hormone derived from human pituitary glands died from Creutzfeldt-Jakob disease, a rapidly fatal neurologic disease caused by a virus.

Somatrem (Genetically Engineered Human Growth Hormone). In 1986, the FDA approved the first gentically engineered human growth hormone for the long-term treatment of children who have growth failure due to lack of adequate endogenous growth hormone secretion.

Thyrotropin (TSH). A purified extract, thyrotropin is obtained from the anterior pituitary gland of cattle.

Mechanism of Action. Thyrotropin stimulates all phases of the synthesis and release of thyroxine and triiodothyronine by the thyroid gland. A primary site of thyrotropin action is thyroid cell membrane-bound adenyl cyclase. This increases the glandular concentration of cyclic AMP, which acts as a "second messenger" to stimulate thyroid hormone synthesis and secretion.

Clinical Indications. Thyrotropin is used as a diagnostic aid to differentiate between primary hypothyroidism and secondary hypothyroidism resulting from pituitary failure.

Adverse Effects/Precautions. Hypersensitivity reactions have been reported. Thyrotropin should be used with caution in patients with heart disease because of possible cardiac stimulation.

Protirelin. Protirelin, a synthetic tripeptide, is believed to be identical to thyrotropin-releasing hormone (TRH).

Mechanism of Action. Protirelin promotes thyrotropin (TSH) release from the anterior pituitary.

Clinical Indications. Protirelin is used as an adjunct in determining thyroid gland function.

Adverse Effects/Precautions. A common side effect is elevated blood pressure.

POSTERIOR PITUITARY PREPARATIONS

Posterior pituitary preparations (Table 6.4) find clinical utility in the management of diabetes insipidus and in obstetrics.

Posterior Pituitary. Posterior pituitary is a desiccated powder preparation of the posterior pituitary gland that contains the antidiuretic, vasopressor, and oxytocic principles.

Mechanism of Action. Vasopressin and oxytocin, the active hormones in posterior pituitary, act on target tissues by activating adenyl cyclase. The resultant increase in intracellular cyclic AMP causes various cellular and physiologic responses, including vascular smooth muscle stimulation and antidiuresis (vasopressin) and myometrial contraction (oxytocin).

Clinical Indications. Posterior pituitary is used as an intranasal powder for controlling the symptoms of neurogenic diabetes insipidus.

Table 6.4. POSTERIOR PITUITARY PREPARATIONS.

Available products	Trade names	Daily dosage range
Desmopressin	DDAVP; Stimate	0.5 ml-1ml daily in 2 divided doses
Lypressin	Diapid	1 or 2 sprays to one or both nostrils 4 times daily
Oxytocin, parenteral	Pitocin; Syntocinon	2-10 units IM, IV, or by IV infusion
Oxytocin, synthetic, nasal	Syntocinon	One spray into both nostrils
Posterior pituitary, intranasal	Posterior Pituitary	Individualize dosage
Posterior pituitary, injection	Pituitrin (S)	10 units SC or IM
Vasopressin	Pitressin Synthetic	5-10 units IM or SC 3 or 4 times/day
Vasopressin tannate	Pitressin Tannate in Oil	0.3-1 ml IM

Adverse Effects/Precautions. Local effects such as nasal irritation and runny nose may occur. Hypersensitivity reactions are also possible because of the animal origin (and hence antigenic nature) of posterior pituitary.

Posterior Pituitary Injection. Posterior pituitary injection is a sterile aqueous extract of the posterior pituitary gland, which contains the antidiuretic, vasopressor, and oxytocic principles.

Mechanism of Action. The mechanism of action is the same as that of posterior pituitary.

Clinical Indications. Posterior pituitary injection is used to control postoperative atony and ileus. This drug also stimulates gas expulsion and is administered before pyelography.

In surgical procedures, posterior pituitary injection promotes hemostasis. A specific use of posterior pituitary injection is in controlling the bleeding of esophogeal varices as well as functioning to combat the shock that occurs in this condition.

Posterior pituitary injection also controls symptoms of neurogenic or central diabetes insipidus.

Adverse Effects/Precautions. Increased gastrointestinal activity and uterine cramps are the most common adverse reactions. Hypersensitivity reactions are possible.

Vasopressin Injection (Antidiuretic Hormone; ADH; 8-arginine-vasopressin). Vasopressin injection, a posterior pituitary gland polypeptide, is obtained from natural sources or by chemical synthetic reaction.

Mechanism of Action. Vasopressin injection binds to membrane receptors in the kidney collecting ducts to activate adenyl cyclase. The consequent intracellular accumulation of cyclic AMP promotes the reabsorption of water, resulting in an antidiuretic effect. Vasopressin injection also has marked activity on vascular smooth muscles to produce vasoconstriction.

Clinical Indications. A major clinical use of vasopressin injection is in the control of the symptoms of diabetes insipidus in which it functions as replacement therapy for deficient endogenous vasopressin. Vasopressin injection is also used in the prevention and treatment of postoperative abdominal distention. An additional use is to remove gas shadows prior to abdominal roentgenography.

Adverse Effects/Precautions. Vasopressin injection should be used with caution in patients with vascular disease. Special care must be exercised if coronary artery disease is present because of the possible precipitation of anginal pain or myocardial infarction.

Vasopressin Tannate. Vasopressin tannate is a long-acting (24 to 96 hours) form of the antidiuretic hormone in oil.

Mechanism of Action. Its mechanism of action is the same as that of vasopressin injection.

Clinical Indications. Vasopressin tannate is used in the treatment of central or neurogenic diabetes insipidus.

Adverse Effects/Precautions. Warming the ampule in the hand facilitates equal distribution of the hormone in the solution.

Lypressin (8-lysine Vasopressin). Lypressin, a synthetic lysine vasopressin derivative, has significant antidiuretic activity but minimal effects as either a vasoconstrictor or oxytocic.

Mechanism of Action. Lypressin has a pronounced antidiuretic effect due to its effect on renal tubular cells to alter water permeability (see vasopressin injection).

Clinical Indications. Lypressin in nasal spray form is valuable in the treatment of neurogenic or central diabetes insipidus. Lypressin is less likely to cause allergic reactions or excessive fluid retention than natural preparations from an animal source.

Adverse Effects/Precautions. Local reactions (runny nose, itching nasal passages, and nasal irritation and ulceration) to the nasal spray preparation are infrequent. Systemic reactions, including headache, conjunctivitis, heartburn, abdominal cramps, and increased intestinal movements, have been reported.

Desmopressin Acetate (1-deamino-8-D-arginine Vasopressin). A synthetic arginine derivative of vasopressin (ADH), desmopressin produces prompt and prolonged antidiuretic action. Minimal vasopressor or oxytocic activity occurs at therapeutic doses.

Mechanism of Action. Desmopressin's significant antidiuretic effect is due to its activity on renal tubular cells to alter water permeability (see vasopressin injection). Desmopressin also causes a dose-dependent increase in the blood clotting factor, Factor VIII, to maintain hemostasis in patients with hemophilia A.

Clinical Indications. Desmopressin is used as replacement therapy in central or neurogenic diabetes insipidus. Parenteral desmopressin is also indicated in hemophilia A or B and in Von Willebrand's disease.

Adverse Effects/Precautions. Adverse reactions are not common with therapeutic doses. Infrequent instances of headache, nausea, mild abdominal cramps, vulval pain, mild hypertension, and facial flushing have been reported with high dosage. These side effects disappear when the dosage is lowered.

Oxytocin Injection. Prepared synthetically, oxytocin injection is chemically identical to the endogenous hormone produced in the posterior pituitary gland. Oxytocin injection is the form of oxytocin used intravenously or intramuscularly in obstetrics.

Mechanism of Action. Oxytocin injection binds to plasma membrane-bound receptors in the myometrium. Adenyl cyclase activation may be involved although the mechanism that translates receptor binding into increased frequency and contraction force is uncertain. Prostaglandin release by oxytocin may be a primary stimulus for uterine contraction.

Clinical Indications. Oxytocin injection is used intravenously for the induction or stimulation of labor. The drug also controls postpartum uterine bleeding.

Adverse Effects/Precautions. Hypertensive crises and subarachnoid hemorrhage have resulted in maternal deaths. Water intoxication after the IV infusion of oxytocin injection has precipitated convulsions and coma. Overstimulation of the uterus may present a clinical crisis to both the patient and fetus. Adverse effects on the fetus, including fetal bradycardia, are possible. Thus, the benefit-to-risk factors for each patient must be considered in the use of oxytocin injection for elective labor induction.

Synthetic Nasal Oxytocin. Synthetic nasal oxytocin is available in squeeze bottles for administration into the nostrils.

Mechanism of Action. Synthetic nasal oxytocin stimulates the smooth muscle of the mammary glands to facilitate milk ejection from lactating women. This product does not increase milk production but rather promotes milk let-down.

Clinical Indications. Synthetic nasal oxytocin is used in the initial milk let-down in postpartum females or in cases where the suckling reflex is inefficient.

Adverse Effects/Precautions. This product is administered by a single burst of the nasal spray 2 to 3 minutes before a breast feeding and presents no risk to the patient when used in this manner.

THYROID GLAND PREPARATIONS

These preparations (Table 6.5) consist of gland tissue products and the purified thyroid hormones.

Thyroid. This natural preparation is composed of cattle or swine desiccated thyroid glands. Thyroid contains liothyronine (T_3) and levothyroxine (T_4) in their natural form and ratio.

Table 6.5. THYROID GLAND PREPARATIONS.

Available products	Trade names	Daily dosage range
Levothyroxine sodium	Synthroid; Levothroid; Noroxine	0.1–0.2 mg
Liothyronine sodium	Cytomel	Initially, 5–25 mcg; individualize according to clinical condition
Liotrix	Euthroid; Thyrolar	Initiate with a 15 or 30 mg tablet; increase gradually every 1 or 2 weeks
Thyroglobulin	Proloid	Initially 32 mg; maintenance, 30–200 mg
Thyroid desiccated	Thyroid USP (various); others	65–195 mg

Mechanism of Action. Thyroid hormones exert their effects on growth and development through control of protein synthesis. The calorigenic effect is also due to an increase in protein synthesis exerted by the thyroid hormones.

Clinical Indications. The main clinical uses of thyroid are in the treatment of adult hypothyroidism, myxedema, and cretinism.

Adverse Effects/Precautions. Adverse reactions including palpitations, tachycardia, anxiety, tremors, and insomnia relate to hyperthyroidism and may be attributed to excessive thyroid dosage. Other reactions such as allergic skin reactions due to hypersensitivity are rare. Because of its cardiac stimulation effect, thyroid should be used cautiously in patients with cardiovascular disease.

Thyroglobulin. The natural storage form for thyroid hormones, thyroglobulin contains liothyronine (T_3) and levothyroxine (T_4) in a ratio of approximately 1:2.5. Thyroglobulin is obtained from cattle and swine thyroid glands.

Mechanism of Action. The mechanism of action is the same as that of thyroid, i.e., an effect on growth and development and a calorigenic effect due to protein synthesis stimulation.

Clinical Indications. Therapeutic uses include adult hypothyroidism, myxedema, and cretinism.

Adverse Effects/Precautions. The adverse effects/precautions of this product are the same as those of thyroid.

Levothyroxine Sodium (T_4; L-thyroxine). Prepared synthetically and available in both injection and oral dosage forms, levothyroxine sodium is chemically identical to the active natural thyroid hormone.

Mechanism of Action. The mechanism of action is the same as that of thyroid and thyroglobulin.

Clinical Indications. Therapeutic uses are the same as those of thyroid and thyroglobulin.

Adverse Effects/Precautions. The same precautions should be observed with this product as with thyroid and thyroglobulin.

Liothyronine Sodium (T_3; L-triiodothyronine). Liothyronine sodium is a synthetic form of l-triiodothyronine, the active natural hormone.

Mechanism of Action. This product's mechanism of action is the same as that of thyroid and thyroglobulin.

Clinical Indications. Its therapeutic uses are the same as those for thyroid and thyroglobulin. Liothyronine sodium is also used as a diagnostic aid in conjunction with ^{131}I for the T_3 suppression test.

Adverse Effects/Precautions. The adverse effects/precautions of this product are the same as those of thyroid and thyroglobulin.

Liotrix. Liotrix is a mixture of the synthetic forms of T_3 and T_4 in a 1:4 weight/ratio.

Mechanism of Action. This product's mechanism of action is the same as that of thyroid and thyroglobulin.

Clinical Uses. Its clinical uses are the same as those of thyroid and thyroglobulin.

Adverse Effects/Precautions. As with thyroid and thyroglobulin, the same adverse effects and precautions apply with this product.

ANTITHYROID DRUGS

Antithyroid drugs (Table 6.6) act on the thyroid gland to either block the release of thyroid hormones or inhibit their synthesis.

Strong Iodine Solution (Lugol's solution). Strong iodine solution consists of 5% iodine and 10% potassium iodide. The iodine undergoes reduction in the small intestine and is absorbed as iodide.

Mechanism of Action. High iodide concentrations, as provided by strong iodine solution, inhibit the release of thyroid hormones by the thyroid gland. Additionally, iodide ion, in high concentrations, inhibits its own transport into thyroid cells and thus acts to reduce the intracellular amounts available for thyroid hormone synthesis. Inhibition of the synthesis of iodotyrosine and iodothyronine also occurs with high iodide ion concentrations.

Clinical Indications. Strong iodine solution is used in conjunction with antithyroid drugs, such as methimazole, in preparation for thyroid surgery and for hyperthyroidism or thyrotoxicosis.

Adverse Effects/Precautions. Infrequent adverse reactions to oral potassium iodide may occur. Such adverse effects include skin rashes, salivary gland swelling, and "iodism" as reflected in a metallic taste, burning mouth and throat, sore teeth and gums, "headcold" symptoms, and gastrointestinal distress.

Sodium Iodide Injection. Sodium iodide injection is available in a 10 and 20% solution.

Mechanism of Action. The mechanism of action is the same as that of strong iodine solution.

Clinical Indications. The therapeutic uses for this preparation are the same as those for strong iodine solution.

Adverse Effects/Precautions. In addition to the same adverse effects/precautions as those indicated for strong iodine solution, rare hypersensitivity reactions like angioneurotic edema and laryngeal edema may occur after the IV injection of sodium iodide. Testing for idiosyncrasy to iodide is recommended before the administration of sodium iodide injection.

Sodium Iodide ^{131}I. Sodium iodide ^{131}I is available as a solution or in capsules for either oral or IV administration.

Mechanism of Action. The radioactive isotope (^{131}I) is effectively trapped, incorporated, and stored in the thyroid gland. Beta radiation is then emitted from the stored isotope in the thyroid follicle. The result is a dosage-related destruction of the thyroid parenchymal cells. Higher doses cause follicular cell pyknosis and necrosis; with properly selected doses, it is pos-

Table 6.6. ANTITHYROID DRUGS.

Available products	Trade names	Daily dosage range
Iodine products	Strong Iodine Solution; Sodium Iodide; Thyroid-Block	Oral, 2–6 drops t.i.d. for 10 days prior to thyroid surgery; 2 g IV for thyrotoxicosis
Methimazole	Tapazole	5–15 mg
Sodium iodide ^{131}I	Iodotope Therapeutic	See manufacturer's directions
Propylthiouracil (PTU)	Propylthiouracil	300 mg

sible to destroy the thyroid gland without detectable damage to surrounding tissues.

Clinical Indications. Sodium iodide ^{131}I is used in the treatment of hyperthyroidism and in selected cases of thyroid carcinoma. Thyrotropin (TSH) facilitates radioiodine uptake by the thyroid gland. Tracer amounts are used as a diagnostic aid to test for thyroid function.

Adverse Effects/Precautions. Doses of sodium iodide ^{131}I employed in the treatment of hyperthyroidism or thyrotoxicosis do not usually produce adverse reactions. In higher radiation doses, such as those used in thyroid carcinoma, depression of the hematologic system and radiation sickness may occur.

Propylthiouracil (PTU). A thioamide antithyroid drug, propylthiouracil is available in an oral dosage form.

Mechanism of Action. The thioamide derivatives (like propylthiouracil) block the synthesis of thyroid hormones. This is accomplished by blocking the incorporation of iodine into tyrosyl residues and by preventing the "coupling" of iodotyrosyl residues. These reactions are peroxidase-dependent and the ability of the thioamide derivatives to inhibit peroxidase activity relates to their antithyroid action.

Clinical Indications. The main therapeutic use of propylthiouracil is in the treatment of hyperthyroidism. The thioamide derivatives are also used to prepare the hyperthyroid patient for partial thyroidectomy or radioactive iodine therapy. They are also used in conjunction with radioiodine to hasten recovery while awaiting the effects of radiation therapy.

Adverse Effects/Precautions. Agranulocytosis is the most serious potential side effect. Other blood dyscrasias such as leukopenia and thrombocytopenia may also occur. Propylthiouracil can induce hypoprothrombinemia so care must be exercised during therapy, especially in presurgical patients.

Methimazole. Methimazole is a thioamide antithyroid drug available in an oral dosage form.

Mechanism of Action. Its mechanism of action is the same as that of propylthiouracil.

Clinical Indications. Its therapeutic uses are the same as those for propylthiouracil.

Adverse Effects/Precautions. The same care must be observed with methimazole as with propylthiouracil.

THYROID PARAFOLLICULAR C CELL HORMONE

The principal product used is a synthetic relative of naturally occurring human calcitonin.

Calcitonin-salmon. Calcitonin-salmon (Calcimar^R) is a synthetic polypeptide chemically equivalent to that obtained from the ultimobranchial glands of the salmon. It is functionally equivalent to the calcium secreted by the thyroid parafollicular C cells in mammals. An injectable form, it is employed for its effect on calcium metabolism.

Mechanism of Action. Calcitonin-salmon, with a greater potency/mg and a longer duration of action than other forms of calcitonin, acts to lower blood calcium by inhibiting the dissolution of bone (bone resorption). It also has direct renal activity and gastrointestinal effects that decrease blood calcium levels. Resistance may develop to the hypocalcemic effect that is probably due to a compensatory increase in the release of parathyroid hormone.

Clinical Indications. Paget's disease (osteitis deformans) is effectively treated with calcitonin-salmon. Another use for calcitonin-salmon is in the early treatment of hypercalcemic emergencies; however, its value is limited because of its short duration of action. Calcitonin-salmon has been FDA approved for the treatment of osteoporosis in postmenopausal women.

Adverse Effects/Precautions. Nausea occurs in about 10% of the patients in the early stages of their treatment. Local inflammatory reactions to the injection may occur. Also, hypersensitivity reactions are possible because of the protein nature of calcitonin-salmon.

PARATHYROID GLAND PREPARATIONS

Parathyroid injection is the only parathyroid gland preparation that is available commercially.

Parathyroid Injection. Parathyroid injection (Paroidin ^{R}) contains parathyroid hormone obtained from the parathyroid glands of cattle.

Mechanism of Action. Parathyroid hormone mobilizes calcium from bone. Parathyroid hormone also promotes the renal tubular reabsorption of calcium and decreases the renal tubular reabsorption of phosphate. Enhanced intestinal absorption of calcium and phosphate occurs with parathyroid hormone, probably as a result of renal conversion of calcifediol to calcitriol.

Adenyl cyclase mediates the activity of parathyroid injection on bone resorption and the renal phosphate reabsorption. The resultant elevation of intracellular cyclic AMP translates the adenyl cyclase activation into physiologic response.

Clinical Indications. There are currently no accepted therapeutic uses of parathyroid injection. For replacement therapy in hypoparathyroidism, a combination of vitamin D and calcium is the treatment of choice. Parathyroid injection is rarely employed in hypocalcemic situations because of the length of time required to reach its peak effect and its short duration of action. Calcium injections produce an immediate increase in serum calcium when a rapid response is required and vitamin D derivatives are preferred for long-term treatment because they can be given orally without any antigenic factor.

Adverse Effects/Precautions. Parathyroid injection is seldom used clinically because of its antigenic nature.

ADRENAL GLANDS PREPARATIONS

Adrenal glucocortical preparations (Table 6.7) are used as replacement drugs in cortex hypofunction or in higher doses as anti-inflammatory agents. Mineralocorticoids (Table 6.8) are used mainly to manage adrenal cortical insufficiency, as in Addison's disease.

Glucocorticoids. Cortisol (hydrocortisone) and corticosterone are the principal glucocorticoids of the adrenal cortex. Cortisol, the main glucocorticoid in the human adrenal cortex, will be discussed as the prototype glucocorticoid.

Mechanism of Action. Cortisol binds to a cytoplasmic receptor and the steroid receptor complex is translocated to the nucleus. At this site, cortisol stimulates protein synthesis by activating the transcription of messenger RNA. The translation of increased protein synthesis into physiologic response is reflected by effects on carbohydrate, protein, and fat metabolism. For example in the liver, cortisol induces synthesis of enzymes involved in gluconeogenesis, one of the prominent effects of glucocorticoids on carbohydrate and protein metabolism.

Similarly, renal effects of adrenal steroids on electrolyte metabolism may involve the synthesis of proteins that facilitate sodium ion transport.

The mechanism of anti-inflammatory action of glucocorticoids is unclear. Lysosomal stabilization, inhibition of polymorphonuclear leukocyte migration, reversal of increased capillary permeability, and suppression of fibroblast function are some proposed mechanisms for anti-inflammatory activity.

Clinical Indications. Several clinical uses of pharmacologic doses of the glucocorticoids relate to their anti-inflammatory activity. The newer synthetic glucocorticoids, which have little or no sodium-retaining activity, are usually preferred to cortisol. Initial therapy generally consists of large doses of glucocorticoids followed by gradual dosage reductions to the lowest amount that will adequately control the manifestations of the disease.

Clinical uses of glucocorticoids related to their anti-inflammatory activity include rheu-

Table 6.7. GLUCOCORTICOIDS.

Available products	Trade names	Daily dosage range
Betamethasone	Celestone	0.6–7.2 mg
Cortisone acetate	Cortone Acetate	Oral, 0.5–0.75 mg/kg; IM, 0.25–0.35 mg/kg
Dexamethasone, oral	Decadron; Hexadrol; Dexone	0.75–9 mg
Dexamethasone sodium phosphate	Decadron; Ak-Dex; others	0.5–9 mg
Fluprednisolone	Alphadrol	2.5–30 mg
Hydrocortisone	Cortef; Hydrocortone	Oral, 20–240 mg
Hydrocortisone acetate	Cortef Acetate; Hydrocortone Acetate	10–50 mg, intraarticular
Hydrocortisone cypionate	Cortef Fluid	Initially 20–240 mg
Hydrocortisone sodium phosphate	Hydrocortone Phosphate	IV, IM, or SC, 15–240 mg
Hydrocortisone sodium succinate	Solu-Cortef; A-hydroCort	IV or IM, 100–500 mg
Methylprednisolone	Medrol	Oral, 4–48 mg
Methylprednisolone sodium succinate	Solu-Medrol; A-methaPred	10–40 mg IV or IM
Paramethasone acetate	Haldrone	Oral, 2–24 mg maintenance
Prednisolone	Delta Cortef; Cortalone; others	5–60 mg
Prednisolone acetate	Meticortelone acetate; others	4–60 mg IM
Prednisolone sodium phosphate	Hydeltrasol; others	4–60 mg IM or IV
Prednisone	Deltasone; Orasone; Meticorten; Cortan; others	Initially 5–60 mg
Triamcinolone, oral	Aristocort	4–12 mg

Table 6.8. MINERALOCORTICOIDS.

Available products	Trade names	Daily dosage range
Desoxycorticosterone acetate	Doca Acetate; Percorten Acetate	10–30 mg hydrocortisone or 10–37.5 mg cortisone daily; Pellets are implanted surgically
Desoxycorticosterone pivalate	Percorten Pivalate	25–100 mg IM every 4 weeks
Fludrocortisone acetate	Florinef Acetate	0.1–0.2 mg

matoid arthritis, bronchial asthma, collagen diseases, allergic conditions, inflammatory eye disorders, and various other miscellaneous inflammatory conditions.

Dermatologic reactions, in addition to allergic skin conditions, that respond to the glucocorticoids include psoriasis, seborrheic dermatitis, and severe disorders such as erythema multiforme.

Other disease states effectively treated by glucocorticoids include the following. Blood dyscrasias, including autoimmune hemolytic anemia, are amenable to this treatment, as are certain gastrointestinal conditions such as severe exacerbation of ulcerative colitis and regional enteritis. Also, glucocorticoids, especially prednisone, are employed as a component of multiple drug therapy in neoplastic diseases.

Massive doses of glucocorticoids are sometimes employed for their antistress effect in the treatment of extensive infections, regardless of the recognized tendency of the drug to spread infection.

Another use of glucocorticoids in smaller physiologic doses is substitution therapy in primary or secondary adrenal corticol insufficiency. A natural glucocorticoid, cortisol or cortisone, is the preferred replacement drug in adrenal corticol hypofunction.

Synthetic glucocorticoids have a high anti-inflammatory potency, but they lack the significant sodium-retaining capacity common with cortisol. Prednisone and prednisolone, characterized by a separation of the anti-inflammatory component from the sodium-retaining property, were the first synthetic drugs of this type introduced into therapy.

Newer synthetic analogs of cortisol, such as dexamethasone and triamcinolone, are clinically employed in the same manner as pharmacologic doses of cortisol. These synthetic analogs may not require a salt-free diet or potassium supplementation as is always the case with extended cortisol therapy.

Of importance is the fact that glucocorticoids are not curative drugs and their benefit, in a pharmacologic dosage regimen, is most pronounced in episodic disease states. Their propensity to induce side reactions, as evidenced by endocrine toxicity as well as behavioral and ocular adverse effects, mandates that other drugs and/or procedures be attempted before instituting glucocorticoid therapy for extended periods. In every clinical situation where systemic glucocorticoid use is considered, the benefit-to-risk ratio is important. When a chronic incapacitating disease is present, the calculated risk of prolonged glucocorticoid therapy may be appropriate considering the alternative situation.

Adverse Effects/Precautions. Glucocorticoids used in the pharmacologic doses needed to achieve clinical success always produce some adverse effects. Iatrogenic Cushing's syndrome may result from high doses. Eventually, hypofunction of the adrenal cortex occurs due to suppression of ACTH release by the exogenous glucocorticoid. Peptic ulcer activation and the induction of osteoporosis (especially in postmenopausal women) are especially serious side effects that may occur with chronic glucocorticoid therapy. CNS effects, including psychoses, occur frequently. Glucocorticoids can also cause sodium and fluid retention, resulting in blood pressure elevation.

Potassium depletion is another consequence of glucocorticoid effects on electrolyte metabolism. Suppression of the hypothalamus-pituitary-adrenal axis occurs after several days of therapy; the degree of effect relates to the glucocorticoid dose and the time course of therapy. Ocular toxicity that occurs during corticosteroid therapy is manifested in increased intraocular pressure, similar to that observed in glaucoma, and a clouding of the lens (cataract).

Mineralocorticoids. Deoxycorticosterone (DOCA) and fludrocortisone (Table 6.8) are adrenal steroids with potent mineralocorticoid activity; they are only used therapeutically because of this action. Fludrocortisone has glucocorticoid activity in addition to its prominent effects on electrolytes; DOCA is devoid of glucocorticoid activity.

Mechanism of Action. DOCA and fludrocortisone act on the renal distal tubule to enhance the tubular reabsorption of sodium. The mineralocorticoids initiate RNA transcription, increasing protein synthesis. This enhanced protein synthesis that facilitates sodium transport is the probable biochemical event involved in mineralocorticoid activity in the renal tubule cell. Mineralocorticoids also promote urinary excretion of potassium and hydrogen ions.

Clinical Indications. DOCA and fludrocortisone are used as partial replacement therapy for primary and secondary adrenal cortical insufficiency in Addison's disease. These drugs are also used to treat adrenogenital syndrome in which salt loss is extensive. Sufficient supplemental glucocorticoids must always accompany mineralocorticoid therapy.

Adverse Effects/Precautions. Fludrocortisone possesses glucocorticoid activity so side effects similar to those that occur with cortisol are often encountered. Edema and increased blood volume may aggravate cardiovascular disease.

SEX HORMONE PREPARATIONS

Estrogens, progestins, and androgens find wide clinical acceptance in physiologic and pharmacologic applications.

Estrogens. Essential for development and maintenance of the female reproductive system, estrogens (Table 6.9) have prominent effects upon uterine development and the cyclic

Table 6.9. ESTROGENS.

Available products	Trade names	Daily dosage range
Chlorotrianisene	Tace	12–25 mg cyclically in menopause; 72 mg b.i.d. for 2 days to prevent postpartum breast engorgement
Diethylstilbestrol	Diethylstilbestrol	0.2–0.5 mg cyclically
Estradiol	Estrace	1 or 2 mg
Estradiol cypionate	Depo-Estradiol; others	1–5 mg IM every 3–4 weeks
Estradiol valerate	Delestrogen; others	10–20 mg IM every 4 weeks
Estrogens, conjugated	Premarin; others	Varies according to clinical situation
Estrogens, esterified	Estratab; Menest; others	0.3–1.25 mg
Estrone	Estrone Aqueous; others	IM, 0.1–0.5 mg 2 or 3 times
Estropipate	Ogen	0.625–5 mg
Ethinyl estradiol	Estinyl; Feminone	0.02–0.05 mg daily
Quinestrol	Estrovis	Initially, 100 mcg daily for 7 days, followed by 100 mcg once weekly starting 2 weeks after treatment begins

endometrial changes associated with ovulation. Primary and secondary female sex characteristics are also governed by the estrogens. Estrogens may be divided into natural estrogens (such as estradiol) that are steroid hormones and synthetic estrogens (such as diethylstilbestrol, DES) that do not contain a steroid nucleus. The following presents estradiol as the prototype estrogen.

Mechanism of Action. Estradiol binds to a macromolecular cytoplasmic receptor with the subsequent translocation of the intracellular estrogen-receptor complex to the cell nucleus. The estrogen-receptor complex increases RNA, stimulating protein synthesis. Regulation of protein synthesis by estrogens is the primary effect on target cells. High concentrations of estrogen receptors are found in the uterus, vagina, and mammary glands.

Clinical Indications. Estrogens are used extensively in the alleviation of vasomotor symptoms associated with the female climacteric syndrome. No evidence indicates that estrogens effectively treat the depression and vague nervous symptom complaints of menopausal and postmenopausal women.

Female hypogonadism and hypopituitarism respond to estrogens. In these hormone deficient states, the estrogens therapy substitutes for endogenous estrogens.

Estrogens (usually conjugated estrogens) are employed in estrogen-deficient osteoporosis. Decreased calcium deposition in bone occurs frequently in patients whose ovarian activity is absent. Estrogens are more effective in preventing osteoporosis than in reversing the process. Additionally, diet, calcium supplementation, and physiotherapy are necessary as adjunctive measures in postmenopausal osteoporosis.

Other clinical uses of estrogens include atropic vaginitis, postpartum breast engorgement, inhibition of postpartum lactation, and prostatic carcinoma.

The combination of an estrogen and a progestational steroid is used extensively as an oral contraceptive agent.

Adverse Effects/Precautions. Anorexia, nausea, and vomiting are frequent side effects of estrogen therapy. Endocrine side effects include breakthrough bleeding, "pseudo" premenstrual syndrome, and amenorrhea both during and after treatment. Breast tenderness, enlargement, and secretion may also occur.

Estrogens have increased the incidence of endometrial carcinoma. Accordingly, close surveillance of women taking estrogens is indicated to detect persistent or abnormal vaginal bleeding.

Estrogens should not be used during pregnancy.

Progestins. Progestins (Table 6.10) include progesterone and its natural and synthetic derivatives. The main endogenous progestin is progesterone, secreted largely by the corpus luteum. Progestins are responsible for transforming the proliferative endometrium into a secretory structure.

Progestin effects on the vaginal epithelium and on uterine cervical mucous secretions are opposite those of the estrogens. Progesterone withdrawal results in menstruation.

Progestins inhibit the secretion of pituitary gonadotropins, thereby preventing maturation of the graafian follicle and ovulation. Spontaneous uterine contractions are inhibited and secretory changes in the endometrium occur with progestin therapy.

Mechanism of Action. Progesterone binds to a specific cytoplasmic receptor and the progesterone-receptor complex is translocated to the nucleus. A stimulation of protein synthesis follows the resultant increase of nuclear mRNA synthesis.

Physiologic translation of these progesterone-receptor complex initiated events include development of a secretory endometrium and changing the nature of the endocervical secretion from the estrogen-stimulated watery form to a scant viscid material. Additionally, progesterone suppresses uterine contractions and prevents immunologic rejection of the fetus.

Clinical Indications. The major clinical application of these agents is in oral contraceptives. Progestins are also used in the management of secondary amenorrhea, in a sequence-regimen with estrogens in primary amenorrhea or premature ovarian failure, and in the treatment of dysmenorrhea. Functional uterine bleeding, related to anovulation at the time of the menarche, is effectively managed with progestin therapy, as is endometriosis.

The progestins are effective in maintaining pregnancy in patients with a progesterone-deficiency syndrome. Thus, in patients with endogenous progesterone deficiency, habitual abortion may be prevented with progestin therapy.

Adverse Effects/Precautions. Breakthrough bleeding, spotting, menstrual flow changes, and amenorrhea are noted side effects related to the menstrual cycle. Progestins with strong androgenic potential (such as ethisterone or norethisterone) should be avoided in pregnancy because of the danger of masculinization of the female fetus.

Potential fetal harm is a risk when progestins are used in the first trimester of pregnancy in an attempt to prevent habitual abortion. Therefore, identification of patients with progesterone-deficiency threatened abortion as candidates for progestin therapy is imperative for the rational use of these agents.

Oral Contraceptives. The most widely employed oral contraceptives contain a combination of an estrogen and a progestin, whereas single drug oral contraceptives contain low amounts of a progestin (Table 6.11). Post-coital diethystilbestrol (DES) is employed as the "morning-after pill" in selected instances.

Mechanism of Action. The estrogen contained in the combination oral contraceptives suppresses FSH and LH secretion, thereby inhibiting ovulation. This mechanism plays a

Table 6.10. PROGESTINS.

Available products	Trade names	Daily dosage range
Hydroxyprogesterone caproate	Delalutin; others	250–1000 mg
Medroxyprogesterone acetate	Amen; Provera; Curretab	5–10 mg daily for 5–10 days
Norethindrone	Norlutin	5–20 mg starting with the 5th and ending on the 25th day of the menstrual cycle
Norethindrone acetate	Norlutate; Aygestin	2.5–15 mg
Progesterone	Progelan; others	5–50 mg IM

Table 6.11. ORAL CONTRACEPTIVES.

Trade names	Progestin content	Estrogen content
Brevicon	0.5 mg Norethindrone	0.035 mg Ethinyl estradiol (EE)
Demulen	1 mg Ethynodiol diacetate	0.05 mg EE
Enovid 5 mg	5 mg Norethynodrel	0.075 mg Mestranol (ME)
Enovid-E	2.5 mg Norethynodrel	0.10 mg ME
Loestrin	1 mg and 1.5 mg Norethindrone acetate	0.02 mg and 0.03 mg EE
Lo-Ovral	0.3 mg Norgestrel	0.03 mg EE
Modicon	0.5 mg Norethindrone	0.035 mg EE
Norinyl	2 mg Norethindrone	100 mcg ME
Norlestrin	1 mg and 2.5 mg Norethindrone acetate	0.05 mg EE
Ortho-Novum 2 mg 21	2 mg Norethindrone	100 mcg ME
Ovral	0.5 mg Norgestrel	0.05 mg EE
Ovrette	0.075 mg Norgestrel	—
Ovulen	1 mg Ethynodiol diacetate	100 mcg ME

dominant role in preventing pregnancy. Another contraceptive mechanism of combination products is a change in the cervical mucus, resulting in an environment that hinders sperm migration. Combination oral contraceptives also alter the endometrium making it unsuitable for nidation.

Progestin-only contraceptives change the cervical mucus and interfere with implantation by altering the endometrium. Progestins may also suppress the secretion of gonadotropins, thereby inhibiting ovulation.

Post-coital estrogen (DES) in high doses may inhibit fertilization and nidation. Mechanisms involved include oviduct motility alteration, endometrium changes, and bleeding that results from withdrawal of high DES dosage.

Clinical Indications. Oral contraceptives are used to prevent pregnancy.

Adverse Effects/Precautions. There is a positive association between the dose of estrogens and thromboembolism. Therefore, the lowest estrogen dose that achieves a contraceptive action should be prescribed. Contraindications to oral contraceptive use include a history of thrombophlebitis and thromboembolic disorder, known or suspected breast carcinoma, liver tumors, and undiagnosed genital bleeding. Also, a higher incidence of various cardiovascular problems, including myocardial infarction, have been associated with oral contraceptive use. An increase in the risk of cardiovascular side effects from oral contraceptive use occurs with cigarette smoking; this risk increases with the number of cigarettes smoked and the patient's age. Therefore, smoking should be discouraged in women taking oral contraceptives.

Oral contraceptives with high estrogen content may cause nausea and bloating, cervical mucocorrhea and polyposis, melasma, hypertension, migraine headache, breast fullness or tenderness, and edema. Products with low estrogen content may promote early and/or mid-cycle breakthrough bleeding, increased spotting, and hypomenorrhea.

Problems associated with oral contraceptives containing high progestin amounts include increased appetite, weight gain, tiredness, hypomenorrhea, acne and oily scalp, hair loss, depression, hirsutism, monilial vaginitis, and breast regression. Products low in progestin amounts may cause late breakthrough bleeding and amenorrhea.

Androgens. Testosterone, the major androgenic hormone secreted by the male sex glands, is steroid in nature. The testicular Leydig cells are the main source of endogenous testosterone. Having masculinizing effects, testosterone is primarily responsible for the growth and development of the sex organs and secondary sex characteristics in the male. Many synthetic compounds related to testosterone (Table 6.12), including the anabolic steroids, have significant androgenic properties, especially in high doses. The metabolic effects of androgens are characterized by increases in protein anabolism and decreases in protein catabolism.

Mechanism of Action. Testosterone is biotransformed in target tissues to dihydrotestosterone, a more active form of the hormone. Dihydrotestosterone binds to a cytoplasmic receptor protein and the dihydrotestosterone-receptor complex is translocated to the nucleus. At this site, the dihydrotestosterone-receptor complex increases RNA synthesis with resultant protein synthesis stimulation.

The absence of a cytoplasmic dihydrotestosterone receptor protein is characterized by feminine development, even though a genotypic male may have normal amounts of circulating testosterone. Additionally, since skeletal muscle does not contain specific androgen receptors, the mechanism of anabolic activity of the testosterone-like agents may result from their competition with glucocorticoids for the glucocorticoid cytoplasmic receptor protein.

Pharmacologic doses of the androgenic steroids suppress endogenous testosterone release by feedback inhibition of LH. FSH release is also inhibited by large doses of exogenous androgens, decreasing spermatogenesis.

Clinical Indications. Male hypogonadism is a clear therapeutic indication for androgen replacement therapy. Other indications include selected cases of hypopituitarism, the male "climacteric," and anemia associated with hypogonadal patients. Androgens are also used for endometriosis and lactation suppression and as a palliative measure for breast carcinoma in both male and female patients.

Skeletal muscle mass increases with androgens. Another result of the increased protein anabolic activity is the growth-stimulating effect as evidenced by the promotion and stimulation of the osteoid matrix and osteoblastic activity. Thus, androgens are selectively employed to accelerate growth in children.

Androgen-anabolic steroids are used for a variety of clinical conditions including postoperative recovery to chronic debilitating diseases. The effects relate to a high protein diet with sufficient calorie intake.

Adverse Effects/Precautions. Androgens increase the rate of secretion by the sebaceous glands, resulting in an oily skin and a greater possibility of obstruction of the sebaceous glands' ducts. Androgens also stimulate body hair growth. Thus, oily skin, acne, and hirsutism are common side effects.

Masculinization of women is a common untoward effect of androgen therapy. For in-

Table 6.12. ANDROGENS.

Available products	Trade names	Daily dosage range
Ethylestrenol	Maxibolin	4 mg
Fluoxymesterone	Halotestin; Ora-Testryl; Andriol; others	2–10 mg
Methandriol	Anabol; Andriol; others	10–40 mg of the aqueous preparations
Methyltestosterone	Metandren; Android-10; Oreton Methyl; others	10–40 mg
Nandrolone decanoate	Deca-Durabolin; Analone-50	IM, 50–100 mg every 3–4 weeks
Nandrolone phenpropionate	Durabolin; others	IM, 25–50 mg weekly
Oxandrolone	Anavar	5–20 mg
Oxymetholone	Anadrol	1–5 mg/kg
Stanozolol	Winstrol	2 mg t.i.d.
Testosterone	Testosterone (various)	IM, 10–25 mg 2 or 3 times a week
Testosterone cypionate	Depo-Testosterone; others	IM, 50–200 mg every 7–14 days
Testosterone enanthate	Delatestryl; others	IM, 200 mg every 2–4 weeks
Testosterone propionate	Testex	IM, 25 mg 2 or 3 times a week

stance, when androgens are employed in female mammary carcinoma, a male pattern of voice deepening, baldness, hirsutism, and prominent musculature develops.

Edema and cholestatic jaundice are common adverse effects. Hepatic adenocarcinoma has developed in patients on androgen therapy for long periods.

Even though androgens are required for and maintain spermatogenesis, the continued exogenous androgen supply inhibits gonadotropin secretion, resulting in impotence and azoospermia.

Since long-term use of anabolic steroids involves considerable danger, the benefit-to-risk ratio must be carefully assessed.

PANCREATIC PREPARATIONS

These preparations include the naturally occurring pancreatic hormones, insulin and glucagon, as well as synthetic agents that affect the release of insulin by the pancreas.

Insulin. Endogenous insulin is secreted by the beta cells in the islets of Langerhans of the pancreas. Obtained from cattle or swine, insulin (Table 6.13) is marketed in modified preparations that vary in their onset and duration of action. The amino acid sequence in insulin extracted from swine pancreas more closely resembles human insulin, and pork insulin is generally less immunogenic than either beef or mixed forms.

All commercially available insulin products marketed in the United States are purified in that macromolecular contaminants have been largely removed by purification techniques; these products are referred to as "single peak" insulin. Human insulin is derived from synthetic processes utilizing recombinant DNA technology with strains of Escherichia coli.

Mechanism of Action. Insulin facilitates the transfer of glucose and amino acids across insulin-sensitive cell membranes into cells that would otherwise have a low permeability to these substances. Insulin-sensitive tissue includes skeletal muscle, cardiac tissue, fat cells, and leukocytes; the brain, liver, and red blood cells are considered relatively insulin-insensitive.

The cell membrane of insulin-sensitive cells contains specific receptors for this hormone. Activation of these receptors by insulin stimulates a carrier mechanism to allow transport of a non-lipid soluble substance (such as glucose) across the cell membrane into the intracellular environ. Thus, insulin promotes glucose entry into skeletal and heart muscle, fat, and leukocyctes. This site and mechanism of insulin activity is not required for glucose transport into the brain, liver, or erythrocytes.

When insulin, a key regulator of many metabolic processes, is injected into a normal or a diabetic person, several prominent biochemical events occur. Due to increased uptake of glucose by muscle and fat tissue, the blood sugar decreases. Insulin also reduces the plasma free amino acids and promotes their incorporation into muscle. In insulin deficient states such as diabetes mellitus, fatty acids are released from fat depots and are not utilized properly. Lipid fragments (like acetoacetic acid and beta-hydroxybutyric acid) accumulate in the blood; these "ketone bodies" may produce ketoacidosis in the diabetic. Insulin injection inhibits fatty acid mobilization from peripheral fat depots and increases intracellular glucose utilization. The subsequent utilization of these ketone bodies occurs as they are used as an energy source by tissues such as skeletal and cardiac muscle.

Clinical Indications. Diabetes mellitus that cannot be controlled by diet, weight reduction, and exercise or by oral hypoglycemic drugs responds favorably to insulin therapy.

Adverse Effects/Precautions. An insulin excess can result in a hypoglycemic reaction characterized by fatigue, sweating, tremors, confusion, and nervousness; respiration becomes rapid and shallow, the mouth feels numb, and the skin is moist and pale. CNS symptoms can progress to convulsions or psychoses.

Table 6.13. INSULIN*.

Available products	Trade names	Source
Insulin Injection	Actrapid	Purified pork
	Actrapid Human	Human insulin (recombinant DNA origin)
	Insulin	From pork
	Beef Regular Iletin II	Purified beef
	Humulin R	Human insulin (recombinant DNA origin)
	Pork Regular Iletin II	Purified pork
	Purified Pork Insulin	Purified pork
	Regular Iletin I	From beef and pork
	Velosulin	Purified pork
Insulin Zinc Suspension, Prompt	Semilente Iletin I	From beef and pork
	Semilente Insulin	From beef
	Semitard	Purified pork
Isophane Insulin Suspension (NPH)	Beef NPH Iletin II	Purified beef
	Humulin N	Human insulin (recombinant DNA origin)
	Insulatard NPH	Purified pork
	Isophane Insulin NPH	From beef
	Isophane Insulin NPH	Purified beef
	NPH Iletin I	From beef and pork
	Pork NPH Iletin II	Purified pork
	Protaphane NPH	Purified pork
Isophane Insulin Suspension and Insulin Injection	Mixtard	Purified pork
Insulin Zinc Suspension	Lentard	Purified pork and beef
	Lente Iletin I	From beef and pork
	Lente Iletin II	Purified beef
	Lente Iletin II	Purified pork
	Lente Insulin	From beef
	Monotard	Purified pork
	Monotard Human; Humulin L	Human insulin (recombinant DNA origin)
	Purified Beef Insulin Zinc	Purified beef
Protamine Zinc Insulin Suspension	Beef Protamine, Zinc & Iletin II	Purifed beef
	Pork Protamine, Zinc & Iletin II	Purified pork
	Protamine, Zinc and Iletin I	From beef and pork
	Protamine Zinc Insulin	From beef
Insulin Zinc Suspension, Extended	Ultralente Iletin I	From beef and pork
	Ultralente Insulin	From beef
	Ultratard	Purified beef

* Factors such as the number and size of daily doses, time of administration, and diet and exercise require continuous medical supervision depending upon the individual clinical situation.

Carbohydrate (candy or a sugar lump) readily reverses the hypoglycemic reaction in the early stages; dilute corn syrup or orange juice are also valuable should the patient become delirious or confused. Severe hypoglycemia may be counteracted by glucose (dextrose) intravenously and glucagon.

Sulfonylureas. Sulfonylureas (Table 6.14) are effective only in Type II (non-insulin-dependent) diabetic patients; these are adult-onset cases in which some endogenous insulin secretion is retained. Introduced in the 1950s, the "first generation" sulfonylureas include tolbutamide, acetohexamide, chlorpropamide, and

Table 6.14. OTHER PANCREATIC PREPARATIONS.

Available products	Trade names	Daily dosage range
Sulfonylurea:		
Acetohexamide	Dymelor	250 mg-1.5 g
Chlorpropamide	Diabinese	100–500 mg
Glipizide	Glucotrol	2.5–40 mg
Glyburide	DiaBeta; Micronase	2.5–20 mg
Tolazamide	Tolinase	100 mg
Tolbutamide	Orinase; Oramide	0.25–3 g
Glucagon:		
Glucagon	Glucagon	Varies according to individual clinical situation

tolazamide. A "second generation" of sulfonylureas, represented by glyburide and glipizide, are more potent than their predecessors because of the addition of a lipophilic side chain to the molecule.

Mechanism of Action. Sulfonylureas increase insulin secretion of the beta cells in both normal and diabetic patients. This increase may be due to enhanced beta cell sensitivity to glucose, an elevation of intracellular cyclic AMP, or a heightened calcium influx into the cell resulting in degranulation and insulin secretion.

Extrapancreatic mechanisms of sulfonylurea action that potentiate insulin action become operant after prolonged use. Plasma insulin levels return to pretreatment levels after extended treatment with the oral sulfonylurea hypoglycemic agents although glucose tolerance is retained. An increase in the number of insulin receptors on target tissues or an enhanced affinity of receptor binding sites for insulin are proposed extrapancreatic mechanisms for these drugs. An increased post-receptor tissue response to insulin could also potentiate insulin activity. Additionally, decreases in liver glucose production occur in extended sulfonylurea therapy.

Clinical Indications. The sulfonylureas are indicated as treatment for Type II (non-insulin-dependent) adult-onset diabetes mellitus that is unresponsive to diet, weight control, and exercise.

Adverse Effects/Precautions. Hypoglycemia may be considered as an adverse reaction, although it is really an extension of the pharmacologic activity of the sulfonylureas. Gastrointestinal adverse effects include nausea, vomiting, and heartburn. Hypersensitivity reactions, such as pruritus, rashes, and purpura, are also possible. Blood dyscrasias associated with the "first generation" sulfonylureas rarely occur with glyburide and glipizide.

Glucagon. A polypeptide hormone, glucagon (Table 6.14) is secreted by the alpha cells of the pancreas. The action of glucagon on carbohydrate, protein, and fat metabolism is essentially opposite that of insulin.

Mechanism of Action. Glucagon activates liver cell membrane-bound adenyl cyclase, increasing intracellular cyclic AMP levels. Increased phosphorylase activity ensues as a consequence of these elevated levels, accelerating glycogenolysis. Glycogen breakdown along with an inhibition of glycogen synthetase results in blood glucose elevation.

Additionally, increased amino acid uptake and subsequent conversion to glucose precursors promote hepatic gluconeogenesis. Because of the cyclic AMP activation of lipolysis in hepatic and adipose tissue, gluconeogenesis is further stimulated.

Clinical Indications. Glucagon is used to treat hypoglycemia in severe insulin reactions in diabetic patients. In psychiatric patients, glycogen reverses hypoglycemic reactions to insulin-shock therapy. Glucagon is also used as a diagnostic aid for the radiologic examination of the stomach, duodenum, and colon when a hypotonic state is desired.

Adverse Effects/Precautions. Occasional nausea and vomiting are glucagon's chief adverse effect. Also, a case of Stevens-Johnson syndrome (erythema multiforme) occurred after glucagon use as a diagnostic aid.

DRUG INTERACTIONS

A delicate balance usually exists when endocrine drugs are used in therapeutics. Consequently, drug interactions occupy a critical position in assessing optimal patient titration in endocrine therapy.

PITUITARY PREPARATIONS

Danazol.

Warfarin. Danazol has prolonged the prothrombin time in patients stabilized on warfarin.

Somatotropin.

Glucocorticoids. Concurrent glucocorticoid therapy may inhibit the response to somatotropin.

Oxytocin.

Sympathomimetics. Severe persistent hypertension may occur if sympathomimetic pressor amines are used concomitantly with oxytocin.

Posterior Pituitary Injection and Vasopressin.

Carbamazepine, Chlorpropamide, Clofibrate. These drugs, which potentiate ADH, may accentuate the antidiuretic activity of posterior pituitary injection or vasopressin.

THYROID GLAND PREPARATIONS

Thyroid.

Cholestyramine. Since cholestyramine binds both thyroxine and triiodothyronine in the intestine, absorption of these thyroid hormones is impaired. The current recommendation is that 4 to 5 hours should elapse between administration of cholestyramine and thyroid hormones.

Ketamine. In two patients receiving thyroid replacement, marked hypertension and tachycardia followed ketamine administration. Ketamine should probably be administered cautiously to patients on a thyroid replacement regimen.

ADRENAL GLAND PREPARATIONS

Antacids. Antacids may reduce gastrointestinal absorption of corticosteroids. Should this interaction occur, a patient stabilized on both a corticosteroid and an antacid would probably not be adversely affected due to titration to the appropriate level of the corticosteroid dose.

Barbiturates. Phenobarbital may enhance corticosteroid metabolism, possibly due to phenobarbital-induced induction of hepatic microsomal enzymes; also, hypoxemia may promote enzyme induction. Therefore, in asthma patients, barbiturates may initiate clinical problems by decreasing corticosteroid effect manifested by worsening of asthma, hypoxemia, and increased enzyme induction.

Cholestyramine. Since cholestyramine may inhibit gastrointestinal absorption of hydrocortisone, separate doses of oral hydrocortisone from cholestyramine are recommended to avoid mixing in the gastrointestinal tract.

Ephedrine. Theophylline may be preferable to ephedrine as a bronchodilator in steroid-dependent asthmatics if diminished reponses to dexamethasone occur when ephedrine is given concomitantly.

Estrogen. Estrogen-induced increases in serum cortisol-binding globulin may retard the normally rapid metabolism of hydrocortisone. Patients receiving both corticosteroids and an estrogen should be observed for evidence of excessive corticosteroid effects, necessitating a reduction of the corticosteroid dose.

Indomethacin. Increased incidence and/or severity of gastrointestinal ulceration may result from the combined effects of indomethacin and corticosteroids.

Phenylbutazone. The combined use of phenylbutazone and corticosteroids may increase the likelihood of gastrointestinal ulceration.

Salicylates. Although the frequently administered concomitant use of salicylates and corticosteroids is not contraindicated, the salicylate dosage requirement may be higher in the presence of corticosteroids. Salicylate intoxication may occur if the corticosteroid is reduced. Also, the incidence and/or severity of gastrointestinal ulceration may increase with concomitant therapy.

Vitamin A. Systemic vitamin A may inhibit the anti-inflammatory effect of systemic corticosteroids. Caution should be exercised in administering systemic vitamin A to patients receiving corticosteroids.

SEX HORMONE PREPARATIONS

Estrogen/Oral Contraceptives.

Oral Anticoagulants. Oral contraceptives may reduce the hypoprothrombinemic effect of oral anticoagulants.

Barbiturates. Concomitant administration of barbiturates and oral contraceptives may result in significant enzyme induction as indicated by spotting or breakthrough bleeding.

Benzodiazepines. Oral contraceptives apparently inhibit the metabolism of some benzodiazepines and enhance the metabolism of others. Patients taking oral contraceptives should be watched for evidence of enhanced effect of chlordiazepoxide, diazepam, and most other benzodiazepines except those which undergo glucuronide conjugation.

Smoking. Since epidemiologic evidence indicates that smoking increases the risk of cardiovascular adverse effects associated with oral contraceptive use (stroke, myocardial infarction, thromboembolism), women taking oral contraceptives should be discouraged from smoking.

Androgen/Anabolic Steroids.

Corticosteroids. Enhanced corticosteroid response may occur if methandrostenolone is administered.

Oxyphenbutazone. Since methandrostenolone may increase oxyphenbutazone plasma levels, caution should be observed in concomitant administration of these drugs.

PANCREATIC PREPARATIONS

Insulin.

Cardiotonic Glycosides. Since insulin may affect serum potassium levels, extreme caution should be exercised with concomitant administration of insulin and cardiotonic glycosides.

Thiazide Diuretics. Elevated blood glucose levels may antagonize insulin's hypoglycemic effect.

Beta-adrenergic Blocking Agents. These drugs may delay recovery from hypoglycemic episodes and may mask hypoglycemic signs and symptoms.

Other Hormones. Oral contraceptives, corticosteroids, epinephrine, and initiation of thyroid hormone replacement therapy may increase insulin requirements.

Miscellaneous Drugs. Monoamine oxidase inhibitors, phenylbutazone, sulfinpyrazone, tetracycline, alcohol, and anabolic steroids may potentiate insulin's hypoglycemic effect.

Smoking. Insulin requirements increase in diabetic patients who smoke.

Sulfonylureas.

Digitoxin. By hepatic microsomal enzyme induction, sulfonylureas may increase the metabolism of digitoxin.

Beta-adrenergic Blocking Agents. These drugs may decrease the pharmacologic effect of oral hypoglycemic agents and may mask the signs and symptoms of hypoglycemia.

Diazoxide. Concomitant administration may decrease the pharmacologic effects of both drugs due to their antagonistic activities.

Miscellaneous Drugs. Whereas some drugs (e.g., insulin, phenformin, sulfonamides, chloramphenicol, fenfluramine, oxyphenbutazone, phenylbutazone, salicylates, nonsteroidal anti-inflammatory agents, sulfinpyrazone, probenecid, monoamine oxidase inhibitors, clofibrate, and dicumarol) enhance the action of sulfonylureas and thus increase the risk of hypoglycemia, other drugs may produce hyperglcemia and may lead to loss of control. Included in this latter category are the thiazides and other diuretics, corticosteroids, phenothiazines, thyroid products, estrogens, oral contraceptives, phenytoin, nicotinic acid, sympathomimetics, calcium channel blockers, and isoniazid.

Ethanol. Hypoglycemia and hyperglycemia have both occurred with concomitant treatment. Acute alcohol intolerance, "disulfiram reaction," may also occur, especially with chlorpropamide. On the other hand, prolonged use of large amounts of alcohol may stimulate hepatic metabolism of sulfonylureas, decreasing their therapeutic effectiveness. Occasional cases of photosensitivity reactions after alcohol ingestion have occurred in patients taking tolazamide and tolbutamide.

Rifampin. By hepatic microsomal enzymes, the metabolism of chlorpropamide and tolbutamide may be stimulated, thus reducing the hypoglycemic activity of the sulfonylureas.

SUMMARY

The neuroendocrine system represents the ultimate biologic communication system involving remote control within a closed system. The endogenous hormones released by the neuroendocrine system set into motion biochemical and physiologic processes that are essential to life.

Hormones or hormone analogs are often used clinically as replacement drugs in hypofunctional glandular conditions. For example, postmenopausal women exhibiting a climacteric syndrome often respond to estrogens and diabetes mellitus patients benefit from insulin therapy.

Conversely, hormone antagonists or agents decrease glandular activity and counteract hyperfunctional glandular states. To illustrate, methimazole is effective in the treatment of hyperthyroidism, and trilostane, a synthetic steroid that blocks the adrenal cortical enzymes required for glucocorticoid synthesis, is available for treating Cushing's syndrome. Some hormone antagonists, such as the estrogen-receptor blocker clomiphene, occupy a unique place in therapy in that they activate certain related pathways due to their hormone-blocking effects.

Exogenous hormones (e.g., pituitary gonadotropins) or synthetic hormone analogs in pharmacologic or "supranormal" doses treat conditions unrelated to endocrine gland dysfunction. Adrenocorticoids, for instance, are the most effective anti-inflammatory drugs currently available for the treatment of various arthritic and collagen diseases.

Finally, normal endocrine biofeedback pathways can be intercepted to achieve a physiologic effect. Thus, by this mechanism, oral contraceptives inhibit ovulation and consequently prevent contraception. This clinical use transcends therapeutic medical practice and demands sociological, cultural, religious, and ethical considerations. Indeed, "social pharmacology" represents a new interest area that includes consideration of this issue. Additionally, the accelerated development and application of recombinant DNA techniques and the widespread use of "social drugs" are contemporary topics that fall in the realm of social pharmacology.

The importance of hormones and related drugs in modern therapeutics requires extensive integration of basic knowledge by the health care professional. A strong physiologic and biochemical substructure is the foundation for rational hormone therapy. Only with this approach can the pharmacist function as an effective supplier of information regarding endocrine therapy to both patient and physician.

SUGGESTED READINGS

Biosynthetic growth hormone. Med Lett Drugs Ther, 27:101, 1985.
Corticosteroid aerosols for asthma. Med Lett Drugs Ther, 27:5, 1985.
Crouch, J.E.: Essential Human Anatomy. Philadelphia, Lea & Febiger, 1982.
Czech, M.P.: The nature and regulation of the insulin receptor. Structure and function. Annu Rev Physiol, 47: 357, 1985.
Fink, G.: Feedback actions of target hormones on hypothalamus and pituitary, with special reference to gonadal steroids. Annu Rev Physiol, 41:571, 1979.
Fletcher, A., and Atkins, J.D.: A review of glipizide and glyburide second generation sulfonylureas. Am Col Apoth Profess Pract Newsletter, 5, November 1984.
Gilman, A.G., et al. (eds.): The Pharmacological Basis of Therapeutics. 7th ed. New York, Macmillan Publishing Co., Inc., 1985.
Habener, J.F.: Regulation of parathyroid hormone secretion and biosynthesis. Annu Rev Physiol, 43:211, 1981.
Hansten, P.D.: Drug Interactions. 5th Ed. Philadelphia, Lea & Febiger, 1985.
Huff, P.S.: Second generation oral hypoglycemic agents. US Pharmacist, 10:51, 1985.
Jackson, O.G.P., Eden, S., and Jansson, J.-O.: Mode of action of pituitary growth hormone on target cells. Annu Rev Physiol, 47:483, 1985.
Kastrup, E.K., and Boyd, J.R. (eds.): Drug Facts and Comparisons. Philadelphia, J.B. Lippincott Co., 1985.
Katzenellenbogen, B.S.: Dynamics of steroid hormone receptor action. Annu Rev Physiol, 42:17, 1980.
Labrie, F., et al.: Mechanism of action of hypothalamic hormones in the adenohypophysis. Annu Rev Physiol, 41:555, 1979.
Leichter, S.: The team approach to diabetes care. A growing role for pharmacists. NARD J, 106:57, 1984.
Leung, P.C.K., and Armstrong, D.T.: Interactions of steroids and gonadotropins in the control of steroidogenesis in the ovarian follicle. Annu Rev Physiol, 42:71, 1980.
McCann, S.M.: Physiology and pharmacology of LHRH and somatostatin. Annu Rev Pharmacol Toxicol, 22:491, 1982.
McEwen, B.S.: Binding and metabolism of sex steroids by the hypothalamic-pituitary unit. Physiological implications. Annu Rev Physiol, 42:97, 1980.
Meites, J., and Sonntag, W.E.: Hypothalamic hypophysiotropic hormones and neurotransmitter regulation. Current views. Annu Rev Pharmacol Toxicol, 21:295, 1981.
Melby, J.C.: Clinical pharmacology of systemic corticosteroids. Annu Rev Pharmacol, 17:511, 1977.
Problems with growth hormone. Med Lett Drugs Ther, 27:57, 1985.
Rahwan, R.G.: Antiabortifacient and fertility-inducing drugs. AJPE, 49:86, 1985.
Reiter, E.O., and Grumbach, M.M.: Neuroendocrine control mechanisms and the onset of puberty. Annu Rev Physiol, 44:595, 1982.
Sterling, K., and Lazarus, J.H.: The thyroid and its control. Annu Rev Physiol, 39:349, 1977.
Trilostane for Cushing's syndrome. Med Lett Drugs Ther, 27: 85, 1985.
Unger, R.H., Dobbs, R.E., and Orci, L.: Insulin, glucagon, and somatostatin secretion in the regulation of metabolism. Annu Rev Physiol, 40:307, 1978.

CHAPTER EXAMINATION

A 50-year-old female patient has recently undergone surgery for Hashimoto's thyroiditis. This resulted in partial thyroidectomy, necessitating replacement therapy with a thyroid preparation. The patient complains of anxiety and her husband confirms that she "overreacts" to almost any situation. They request that you call her physician for a possible medication change.

1. Early signs of excess thyroid hormone activity are
   a. tachycardia and anxiety
   b. lassitude and loss of appetite
   c. myxedema and bradycardia
   d. depression and melancholia
2. Liotrix, a physiologic mixture of synthetic thyroid hormones, is
   a. a 4 to 1 mixture of triiodothyronine and thyroxine
   b. a 100 to 1 mixture of triiodothyronine and thyroxine

c. a 1 to 4 mixture of triiodothyronine and thyroxine
d. available as thyrotropin
3. Thyroxine
   a. is extensively bound by blood albumen
   b. stimulates protein synthesis by decreasing RNA levels
   c. synthesis is increased by TSH
   d. all of the above
4. Levothyroxine is
   a. a potent antithyroid drug
   b. largely converted to liothyronine peripherally
   c. used extensively as a diagnostic aid to test thyroid reserve
   d. the drug of choice for Graves' disease

A 41-year-old male patient is being treated for debilitating rheumatoid arthritis with alternate-day doses of prednisolone.

---

5. Which of the following situations would warrant special attention in this patient's therapeutic regimen?
   a. The patient starts buying large quantities of an OTC antacid.
   b. The patient's wife says he is "acting strangely" lately.
   c. The patient informs you that the fortified formula vitamin you recommended is "great" and that he feels high all the time.
   d. all of the above
6. The patient has been taking prednisolone for several months. Prolonged use of prednisolone could result in
   a. adrenal cortical hyperplasia
   b. stimulation of endogenous ACTH secretion
   c. the need for special precautions if surgical procedure is being considered for this patient
   d. an exaggerated response to an ACTH diagnostic test
7. Adrenal glucocorticoids and their synthetic analogs
   a. stimulate glucose formation and decrease the rate at which the body's tissues burn the sugar
   b. promote gluconeogenesis
   c. have a protein anabolic effect
   d. a and b
8. The biosynthesis and secretion of glucocorticoid hormones follow a diurnal rhythm. The adrenal cortex secretes large amounts of glucocorticoids during an ordinary cycle of sleep and wakefulness
   a. between 6:00 and 9:00 a.m.
   b. around noon
   c. between 6:00 and 9:00 p.m.
   d. about midnight
9. Adrenal insufficiency occurs in
   a. Cushing's syndrome
   b. Addison's disease
   c. pheochromocytoma
   d. acromegaly
10. The anti-inflammatory activity of synthetic corticosteroids relates to
    a. membrane stabilization
    b. an interference with the movement of polymorphonuclear leukocytes from the blood to the site of injury or irritation
    c. prevention of the release of prostaglandin and bradykinin
    d. all of the above

A 19-year-old male college varsity athlete requests your opinion on the advisability of taking anabolic steroids to better his chances at the Olympic tryouts. In your discussion with him, the following questions are important to your view of the inadvisability of using these drugs in his situation.

---

11. Oxandrolone and ethylestrenol are androgen-anabolic agents used to promote weight gain and as adjunctive therapy in osteoporosis. These agents
    a. are protein anabolic agents that reverse catabolic or tissue depleting processes
    b. suppress the gonadotropic functions of the pituitary
    c. may exert a direct effect upon the testes
    d. all of the above
12. Endogenous androgens are
    a. responsible for the growth spurt of adoles-

cence and for the termination of linear growth by fusion of the epiphyseal growth centers
b. synthesized to some extent in the adrenal medulla
c. responsible for the normal growth and development of the female sex organs and for maintenance of secondary sex characteristics
d. secreted mainly from the anterior pituitary gland

13. Large doses of exogenous androgens
    a. suppress spermatogenesis
    b. stimulate gonadotropin release
    c. are employed in prostatic carcinoma
    d. induce lactation in females

14. The most serious adverse reaction reported with prolonged androgen anabolic steroid therapy is
    a. dehydration due to sodium loss from the body
    b. hepatoxicity, including cholestatic jaundice
    c. a feminization in male patients
    d. CNS depression that may result in coma

A 46-year-old female suffering from the climacteric syndrome has been receiving conjugated estrogens for several months. In addition to their use in postmenopausal syndrome, estrogens have other therapeutic indications.

---

15. Which of the following concurrent clinical conditions would most likely benefit from estrogen therapy?
    a. migraine
    b. osteoporosis
    c. glaucoma
    d. Graves' disease

16. Estrogens are secreted by the ovaries in response to the pituitary release of
    a. LH
    b. somatotropin
    c. FSH
    d. ICSH

17. Which of the following concurrent disease states might be aggravated by estrogen therapy?

    a. congestive heart failure (CHF)
    b. bronchial asthma
    c. migraine
    d. all of the above

A 32-year-old female has been taking a combination estrogen-progestin oral contraceptive for several years. After recently moving to your city, she sees a new physician who prescribes a different combination oral contraceptive. She calls your pharmacy and complains that she is gaining weight and has developed acne and an oily skin.

---

18. These noxious symptoms probably indicate which of the following?
    a. an excess of estrogen
    b. an excess of progestin
    c. insufficient estrogen
    d. insufficient progestin

19. Contraindications in patients taking oral contraceptive agents include
    a. acne, obesity, and halitosis
    b. irregular menstrual cycles, urinary tract infections, and hirsutism
    c. a history of thrombophlebitis, bronchial asthma, and carcinoma of the endometrium
    d. a history of renal calculi and hypertension

20. Which of the following is the most prominent effect of combination oral contraceptives in pregnancy prevention?
    a. The estrogens suppress the release of FSH and LH thereby inhibiting ovulation.
    b. The estrogens and progestins increase FSH release by the pituitary.
    c. The estrogens and progestins increase LH release by the pituitary.
    d. The resultant decrease in FSH and LH causes the graafian follicle to rupture prematurely.

A 60-year-old diabetic male patient has confided to you that his life situation is stressful and he has started relaxing with a "few drinks a day."

21. The patient drinks excessively one evening and wakes up with symptoms of clammy skin and incoherent speech.
    This is probably due to
    a. hypoglycemia
    b. hyperglycemia
    c. bad liquor
    d. dehydration
22. Patients taking sulfonylureas, especially chlorpropamide, and wanting to consume alcohol should be cautioned about
    a. an excessive depressant effect on the CNS
    b. a "disulfiram-like" reaction
    c. increased intraocular pressure
    d. b and c
23. Sulfonylureas are useful in the management of
    a. Type I diabetes mellitus
    b. insulin-dependent diabetes mellitis
    c. Type II diabetes mellitus
    d. diabetes insipidus
24. The most important long-term benefit from treatment with sulfonylureas is
    a. potentiation of insulin action
    b. increased insulin production
    c. decreased insulin production
    d. increased numbers of beta cells
25. Propranolol is additionally prescribed on a regular basis for this patient. After a period of alcohol abstinence following his "bad experience," he again has a night on the town and consumes excess alcohol. The following morning he jumps out of bed and heads to the country club feeling great and ready for a round of golf. Shortly, he becomes incoherent and has cold, clammy skin. The propranolol may have been responsible for initially masking an adverse reaction because
    a. beta-adrenergic blockers, such as propranolol, greatly speed the metabolism of alcohol
    b. propranolol produces excess hyperglycemia, thereby blocking the adverse reaction
    c. propranolol blocks the symptoms of hypoglycemia
    d. of a blocking of the intestinal absorption of alcohol

ANSWER KEY

1. a	14. b
2. c	15. b
3. c	16. c
4. b	17. d
5. d	18. b
6. c	19. c
7. d	20. a
8. a	21. a
9. b	22. b
10. d	23. c
11. d	24. a
12. a	25. c
13. a	

chapter 7

RESPIRATORY SYSTEM

CHAPTER OBJECTIVES

After studying this chapter, you should be able to:
1. Describe the functions of the essential organs of the respiratory system.
2. Discuss the characteristics of the respiratory unit (alveolus) of the lung.
3. Define bronchial asthma.
4. Name several drugs that relax bronchiolar smooth muscle.
5. Explain the role of adenosine 3′, 5′- monophosphate (cyclic AMP) in the action of beta-adrenergic agonists on bronchiolar smooth muscle.
6. List several expectorants and mucolytic drugs used in medical practice.
7. Elaborate on the mechanism of bronchodilator action of theophylline and aminophylline (theophylline ethylenediamine).
8. Discuss the value of histamine (H_1) blockers in the treatment of allergic rhinitis.
9. Describe the major adverse reactions that occur with the histamine (H_1) blockers.
10. Discuss the role of antibiotics in treating respiratory infections.

INTRODUCTION

Respiratory system disease is managed by reducing airway obstruction; two primary methods employed are improvement of respiratory tree passage diameter and removal of retained secretions. Bronchial asthma and chronic obstructive pulmonary disease (COPD) are examples of respiratory diseases amenable to drug therapy.

Upper respiratory tract dysfunction can result from allergy, infection, anatomic factors, trauma, or tumor development. Allergic reactions are commonly associated with histamine release and symptoms such as swollen mucous membranes and profuse secretions.

Pathogenic microorganisms may breech the respiratory tract and have cytotoxic effects. The symptoms of respiratory infection include hypertrophy, vacuolization, and necrosis. An acute inflammatory response, including fever, redness, swelling, and pain, follows infection. The majority of acute infections of the upper respiratory tract (i.e., the common cold) are viral in nature and do not respond to antibacterial therapy. However, antibacterial therapy may be indicated in individual cases to prevent or treat secondary infection and complications.

Drugs often contribute to the effective management of respiratory diseases. For example, antihistamines relieve nasal fluid accumulation; bronchodilators open partially blocked air passages; mucolytics change the characteristics of respiratory fluid; and antitussives relieve nonproductive coughs. Additionally, antibiotics are beneficial in certain infections, and corticosteroids reduce respiratory tract inflammation.

ANATOMY AND PHYSIOLOGY OF THE RESPIRATORY SYSTEM

The respiratory system is an air-supply system of passages that begin at the nose and mouth and eventually end in sac-like structures called alveoli (Figure 7.1). The mouth and nasal passages lead into the pharynx; the latter divides into the esophagus (see Chapter 8) and the trachea. By branching into two bronchi, the trachea delivers air (oxygen) to the lungs. Each bronchus progressively divides into bronchioles. These structures receive autonomic innervation to their smooth muscle that governs bronchiole diameter and hence, the airway resistance.

Bronchial smooth muscle is under neural and neuroendocrine control. Activation of beta-adrenergic receptors in the musculature causes bronchodilation. Conversely, parasympathetic stimulation (via the vagus nerve) produces vasoconstriction. In a normal physiologic state, these autonomic mechanisms are balanced.

The bronchioles lead to the alveolar ducts to the alveoli (Figure 7.2). The alveolar membrane consists of a thin layer of cells surrounded by pulmonary capillaries, the site of respiration (oxygen-carbon dioxide exchange). Thus, the membrane for gas exchange between blood and air lies deep within the thorax and is characterized by its division into millions of subsections at the ends of minute branches of a hollow tracheobronchial tree. The pulmonary membrane is protected (by virtue of its location) against trauma, dehydration, and freezing. The delicate pulmonary membrane represents an extremely fragile barrier between the external environment and body fluids.

RESPIRATORY SYSTEM

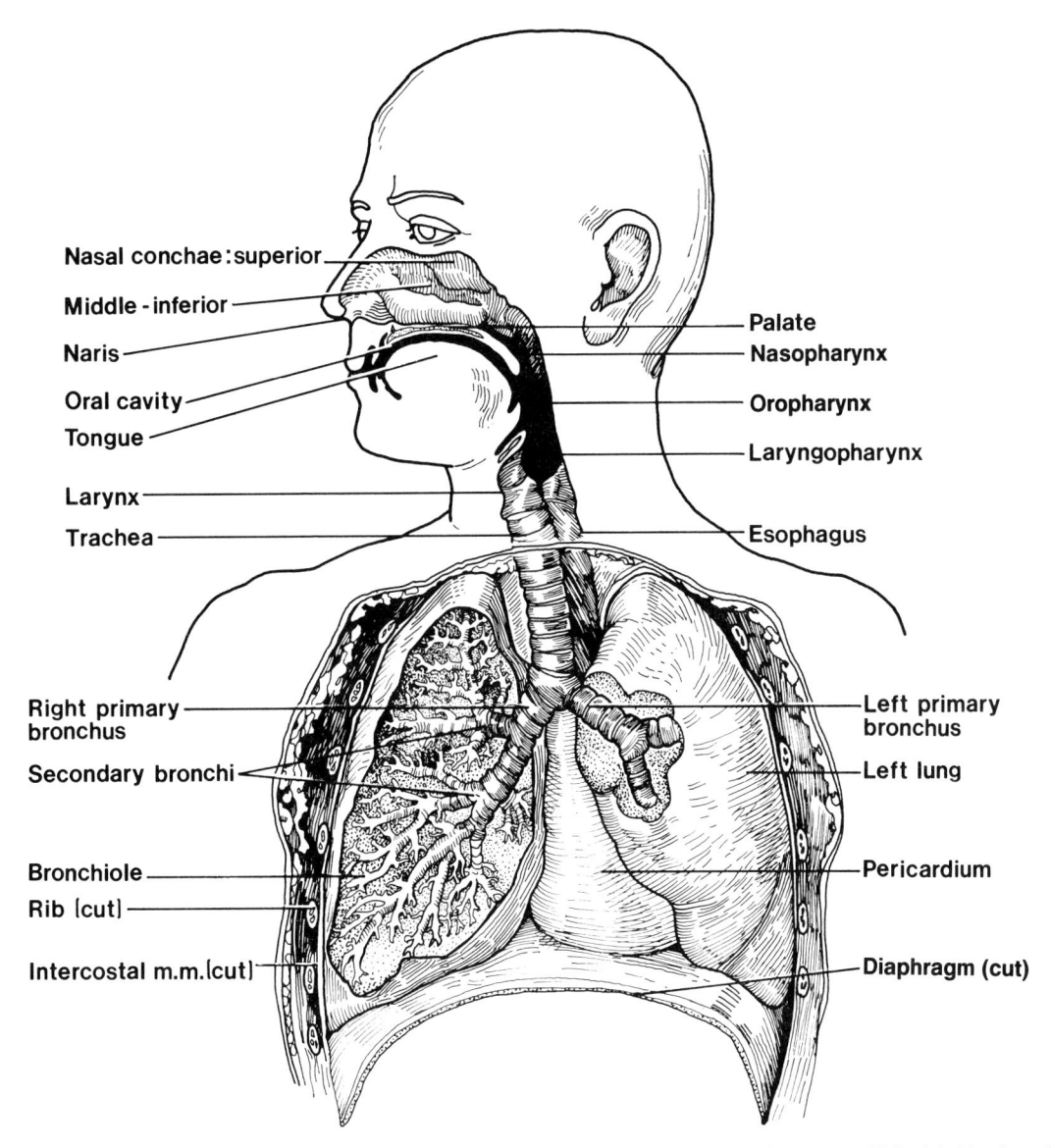

Fig. 7.1 *Human respiratory system.* (From Crouch, J.E.: Essential Human Anatomy. Philadelphia, Lea & Febiger, 1982.)

Respiratory movements deliver oxygen and remove carbon dioxide. The two lungs, essentially elastic air-sacs, are suspended on either side of an airtight thoracic cavity (Figure 7.1). The sternum, ribs, and diaphragm form the movable walls of the thoracic cavity. Expansion of this cavity reduces pressure within the cavity. The intracavity pressure is less than the atmospheric pressure so that when air enters the thoracic cavity, the lungs expand.

Two concurrent mechanisms accomplish this respiratory process. The relaxed diaphragm (Figure 7.1), a dome-shaped muscle, extends upward into the thoracic cavity. As the diaphragm contracts, it flattens and moves downward into the abdomen, which increases the longitudinal size of the thoracic cavity. The simultaneous contraction of the external intercostal muscles raises the ribs—bony structures attached to the spinal vertebrae and joined to-

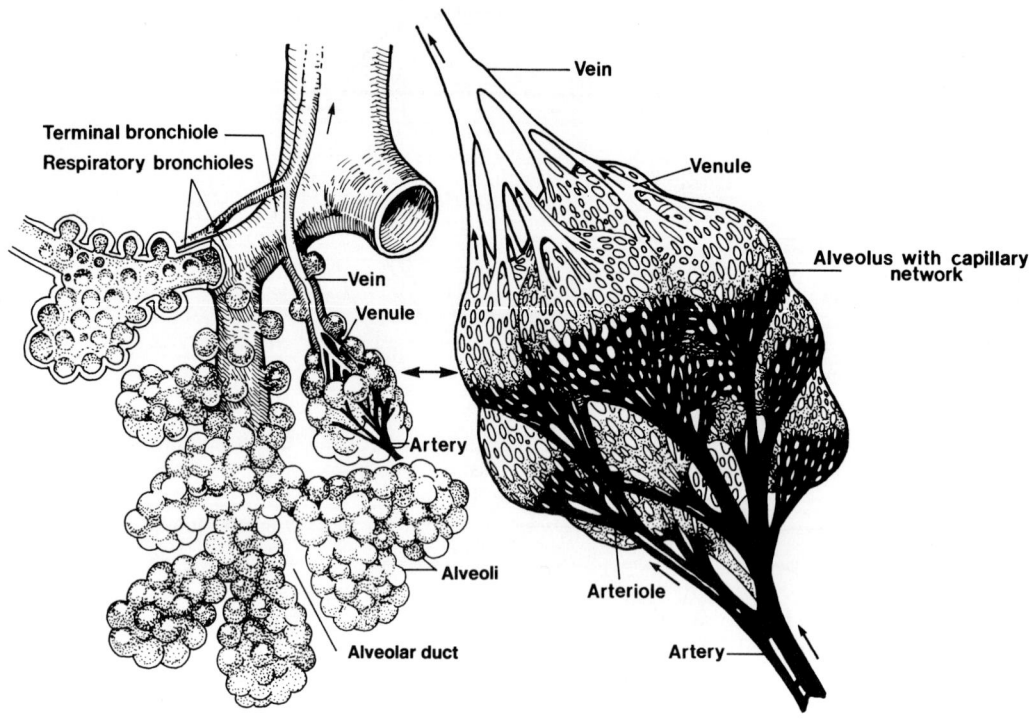

Fig. 7.2 Respiratory unit of lung - alveolus. (From Crouch, J.E.: Essential Human Anatomy. Philadelphia, Lea & Febiger, 1982.)

gether at the sternum. Thus, the elevated and forward movement of the sternum increases the diameter of the chest cavity. Inspiration of air is achieved by simultaneous movements of the diaphragm and ribs that expand the thoracic cavity and fill the lungs with air. Expiration then follows passively (unless, of course, the breath is held).

An increase in the carbon dioxide pressure (pCO_2) is a potent respiratory stimulant in nonexercising individuals, as well as a probable dominant factor in the chemical regulation of respiration. Specialized, structurally discrete inspiratory and expiratory centers in the medulla oblongata are activated by carbon dioxide.

Chemoreceptor reflex activity, involving receptors in the carotid and aortic bodies, are stimulated by carbon dioxide. The pronounced respiratory response to carbon dioxide is mediated almost entirely by direct stimulation of central nervous system (CNS) centers or by activation of peripheral chemoreflex (pCO_2 sensitive) influence on these centers.

The respiratory movements do not clear the lungs of inspired air with each breath. A semirigid bellows-like system intermittently replaces only a small part of the alveolar gas with fresh new air from the atmosphere. Some "dead space" air enters and is expelled without ever participating in gas exchange. A large residual gas volume minimizes the degree to which each new breath affects the composition of gas in diffusion exchange with the blood.

The inefficient respiratory design favors retention of metabolically produced carbon dioxide, thereby maintaining a stable blood and tissue carbon dioxide pressure (much higher than in the ambient atmosphere). Actually, maintenance of carbon dioxide homeostasis is more important than precise control of oxygen because so many metabolic functions depend upon the H^+ concentration of the biologic fluids in which they occur. Thus, respiration functions not only as an oxygen uptake-carbon dioxide removal vehicle, but also as an active participant in regulating the internal cellular environment.

Inhaled air is cleaned and humidified before its delivery to the alveoli. The nasal cavities are lined with highly vascular mucous membranes and ciliated epithelial cells; following this passage, inspired air is warmed, humidified, and filtered. Trapped dust particles, bacteria, and other foreign matter are carried by mucus toward the pharynx via nasal ciliary movement. As air passes through the trachea, bronchia, and bronchioles, further humidification and filtration occur. Cilia propel the foreign particles reaching these sites upward toward the oral cavity where they are either expelled or swallowed.

The cough, an important physiologic mechanism, clears the respiratory passages of foreign material and excess secretions. As coughing serves a useful purpose in some situations, indiscriminate suppression of the cough reflex is not always advisable. The cough reflex is complex and involves both the central and peripheral nervous systems, as well as the bronchial tree smooth muscle.

Irritation of the bronchial mucosa causes bronchoconstriction, which in turn activates special stretch receptors (cough receptors) located in the tracheobronchial passages. Afferent vagal neuron conduction to the CNS follows stimulation of these cough receptors. Several central centers, distinct from those involved in respiration, participate in the cough reflex.

Connected to the respiratory system by the eustachian tube, the ear is protected by the location of its most delicate parts within hard bony areas of the head (Figure 7.3). Largely ornamental, the external ear directs sounds into the ear canal. Penetrating about 2.54 cm into the head, this minute canal ends at the tympanic membrane (eardrum). The pale-pink, concave eardrum seals the middle ear, an air-filled cavity surrounded by thin, bony walls. Other components of the ear are an opening that leads to the mastoid bone and the eustachian tube, a tubular passage about 3.8 cm long that opens into the throat.

Sound waves enter the external ear canal and cause the eardrum to vibrate. Air on either side of the eardrum must be at equal pressures for the eardrum to vibrate freely; pressures are ordinarily equalized by air that can move both ways through the eustachian tube. In the middle ear,

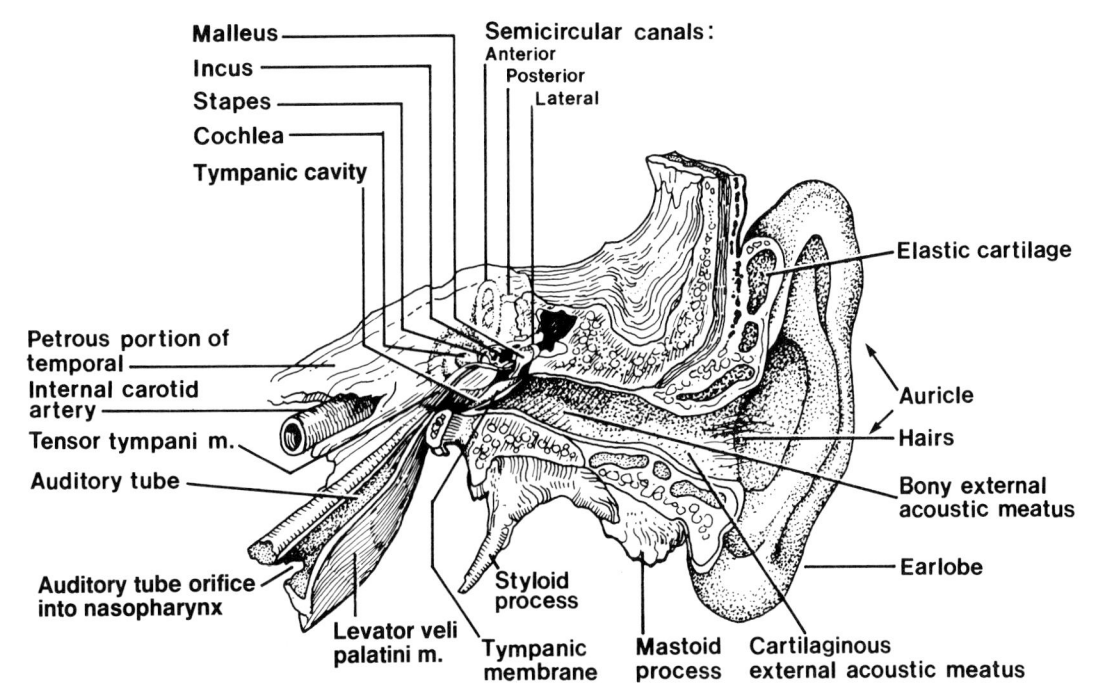

Fig. 7.3 Ear. (From Crouch, J.E.: Essential Human Anatomy. Philadelphia, Lea & Febiger, 1982.)

a chain of ossicles (i.e., tiny bones comprising the eardrum-attached malleus or hammer; incus or anvil; and stapes or stirrup) amplify these vibrations from the eardrum.

In the inner ear, the footplate of the stapes, in contact with the oval window of the snail-shaped cochlea, then transmits the vibrations to fluid in the labyrinth. A tubular, bony structure, the cochlea is lined with a membrane that contains thousands of feathery hair cells tuned to vibrate to different sounds. Nerve endings are contained in the organ of Corti, the center of the sense of hearing, which is slightly elevated over the floor of the tube forming the cochlea. Hair cells stimulate individual nerve cells whose fibers merge into the acoustic nerve; this nerve of hearing then carries impulses to auditory centers of the brain where sound is "heard."

Located near the cochlea are three semicircular canals which lie in planes at right angles to one another. The fluid found in these canals (semicircular duct) responds to movements and transmits information to the brain (via the vestibular nerve) about positions of the body. Thus, in addition to its essential function in hearing processes, the ear is also important as an organ of equilibrium.

Dizziness, vomiting, and balance disturbances may result from inflammation of the labyrinth (cochlea, semi-circular canals, and several small structures). Although these problems usually disappear within a few days, they sometimes advance to severe pain, fever, and deafness in the affected ear.

DISORDERS OF THE RESPIRATORY SYSTEM

Disorders of the respiratory system may be either acute or chronic and often involve allergic responses. Inhaled air may contain allergens, irritants, and/or infectious organisms, any of which could initiate a disease process.

ALLERGY

Two types of clinical allergic reactions include the nasal allergy often manifested as seasonal allergic rhinitis (hay fever) and bronchial asthma. These allergies, which involve the respiratory tract, are termed Type I hypersensitivity reactions. A Type I reaction is an immediate or anaphylactic response involving the formation of a specific class of antibodies called reagins. These antibodies belong to the immunoglobulin E (IgE) group and form in response to antigenic stimulus (perhaps an allergen such as hay pollen). The IgE protein is usually present in minute quantities in the blood, but after allergen exposure, especially large amounts are found.

The circulating IgE antibodies attach to blood basophils and to mast cells found in blood vessels of the nasal mucosa and lungs, thereby sensitizing these cells. At a later time when re-exposure to the allergen occurs, the foreign protein (allergen) combines with the IgE antibodies attached to the cell surfaces. The IgE-allergen reaction results in the release of autacoids, such as histamines, bradykinin, and slow reacting substance of anaphylaxis (SRS-A), from the sensitized mast cells and basophils. The release of histamine and other autacoids from their bound form in the cell results in their reaction with specialized receptors in the mucous membranes of the respiratory tract and bronchial smooth muscle (as well as the skin).

The pharmacologic interaction between histamine and target receptors produces the clinical picture of rhinitis, such as edema in the nasal mucous membranes. Histamine, bradykinin, and SRS-A all produce constriction of the bronchioles and the consequent wheezing and respiratory distress characteristic of bronchial asthma.

Histamine is found in a bound form in high concentrations in the lungs, skin, and gastrointestinal tract. Its release in free form participates in the body's inflammatory defense mechanisms against tissue injury, gastric acid secretion, and in the pathophysiology of allergy.

The freed histamine reacts with at least two types of histamine receptors designated as H_1 and H_2. Bronchial smooth muscle contraction and vascular effects that result in edema of nasal mucous membranes are the product of H_1 receptor activation. Gastric hydrochloric acid secretion is stimulated by histamine-H_2 receptor interaction. Both H_1 and H_2 receptors participate in the complex cardiovascular responses to released histamine.

Histamine is synthesized from the amino acid histidine by the action of histidine decarboxylase (Figure 7.4). Histamine is formed and concentrated in secretory granules of mast cells and basophils where it is bound by ionic forces to a heparin-protein complex. The allergen-IgE globulin interaction produces an increase in the cell membrane to calcium (Ca^{++}). The influx of Ca^{++} and metabolic energy are required for the extrusion of the granule contents (histamine) by the process of exocytosis.

This histamine release process occurs in two stages; the first is an extrusion of the granules into extracellular fluid. The second step involves the exposure of the granules to the cations in the extracellular fluid. Histamine is then released into the external environment by ion exchange. The free histamine becomes available to react with histamine receptors, an apparent component of the cell surface.

H_1 receptors are preferentially activated by 2-methylhistamine, whereas 4-methylhistamine has a special affinity for H_2 receptors. Preferential agonists are utilized in the search for specific histamine blocking drugs that inhibit only one type of receptor (H_1 or H_2).

Histamine interacts with receptors on target tissues to induce changes in the plasma membrane; it also causes an altered permeability of the plasma membrane to sodium (Na^+) and calcium (Ca^{++}). An opening of Ca^{++} channels results in an increase in the intracellular Ca^{++}, as does a release of Ca^{++} from intracellular stores. The release mechanism involves the breakdown of phosphatidyl inositides to form inosityl triphosphate. Histamine effects on cyclic AMP and guanosine 3', 5'-monophosphate (cyclic GMP) levels relate to pharmacologic response because of their function in modulation or modification of ionic permeability.

DISEASES/DISORDERS OF THE NOSE, THROAT, AND EAR

The nasal passages and throat allow growth of airborne organisms that are generally not disease-causing. The nose and pharynx contain

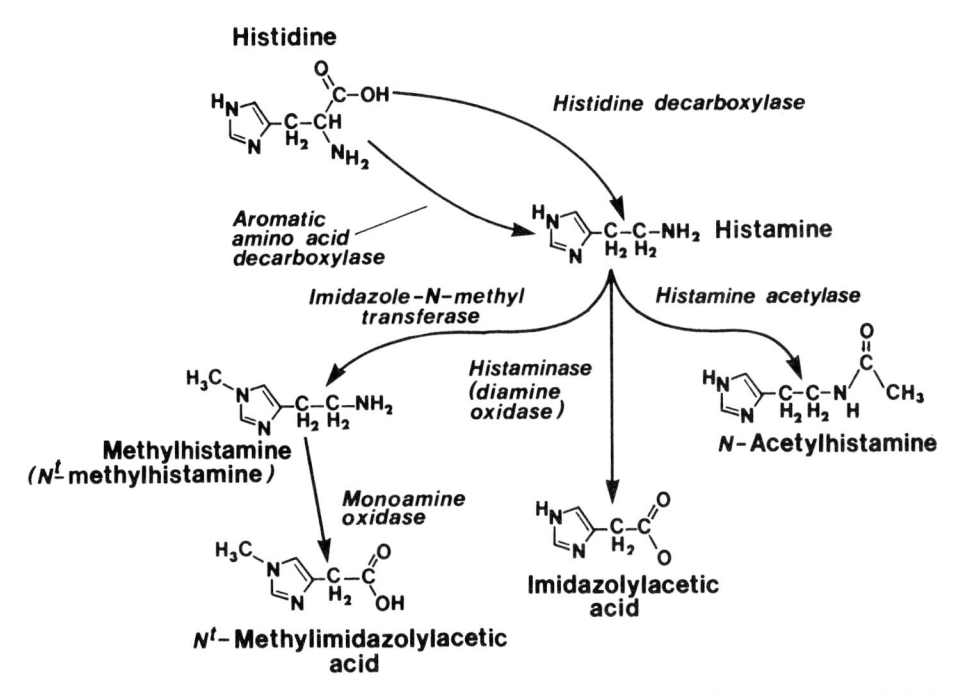

Fig. 7.4 Histamine biosynthesis and metabolism. (Modified from Bowman, W.C., and Rand, M.J.: Textbook of Pharmacology. 2nd Ed. Oxford, Blackwell Scientific Publications, 1980.)

many potentially pathogenic organisms should they become either invasive or dominant microorganisms. Healthy individuals ordinarily have adequate immunologic and mechanical protection to prevent such problems.

ACUTE RHINOSINUSITIS

Most nasal inflammatory disorders involve, at least to some degree, the paranasal sinuses. A mucous or purulent discharge characterizes acute rhinosinusitis. A thin, watery discharge is typical of an allergic reaction or a viral infection, whereas a purulent discharge usually indicates bacterial infection.

Persistent congestion for over a week and the presence of a purulent discharge are signs of progression to bacterial infection. Recurrent, incompletely resolved bacterial infections can cause mucosal ulcerations.

ALLERGIC RHINITIS

Allergic rhinitis occurs either seasonally or perennially. Common symptoms of this disorder are nasal stuffiness and discharge, sneezing, eye irritation, and itching of the eyes, nose, and throat. Early treatment consists of either removing the causative allergen or limiting exposure to the responsible irritant.

ACUTE LARYNGOTRACHEOBRONCHITIS

Viral or bacterial infections can cause acute inflammation of the larynx and tracheobronchial tree. Additional etiologic factors are inhalation of irritating substances or allergens. The bacteria most commonly implicated in laryngotracheobronchitis are Staphylococcus aureus, streptococci, Hemophilus influenzae, and Streptococcus pneumonia. Additional causative agents are the adenoviruses, ECHO virus, and influenza virus.

Characterized by a low-grade fever, malaise, hoarseness, and productive cough, this condition often follows a common cold and is usually mild in adults. Because of the small size of the infant larynx, the obstruction by edema and inflammation is sometimes life-threatening and constitutes a pediatric emergency.

MUCOMYCOSIS

Fungal infections of the nasal and paranasal tissues most often affect poorly controlled diabetics or renal transplant patients. A commonly seen fungal external ear infection, aspergillosis, also occurs in the nose and paranasal sinuses.

NASAL FURUNCLES (NASAL BOILS)

Boils are painful nodules formed by circumscribed inflammation of the corium and subcutaneous tissue, enclosing a central slough or "core." These result mainly from staphylococci that enter the skin through hair follicles. Furuncles may occur chronically as recurring infections.

PHARYNGITIS (COMMON SORE THROAT)

Pharyngitis, a common illness, has numerous causes; among these are infectious organisms, nonspecific irritants, and chemical pollutants. Many sore throats are viral, and the potentially serious streptococcal sore throat is relatively uncommon. Generally, except in situations like a rheumatic fever epidemic, throat culture results dictate the specific chemotherapy.

Infectious mononucleosis, a viral infectious disease, often presents as pharyngitis. Diphtheria and pertussis are infectious diseases that are characterized by pharyngitis.

The value of adenoidectomy and tonsillectomy in patients with recurrent infections of the adenoids or tonsils remains a controversial clinical question. Repeated regimens of antibacterial drugs with symptomatic management is the present favored medical treatment of resistant infections at these sites (adenoids and/or tonsils).

OTITIS MEDIA

Generalized nose and throat infections often include middle ear involvement. Inflammation of the middle ear (otitis media) is commonly associated with earache. The treatment of otitis media includes restoration of eustachian tube function, ventilation of the middle ear, and treatment of the infection. Purulent or chronic suppurative otitis media usually indicates a middle ear infection that has persisted for several weeks.

Secretory (serous) otitis media is the most common form of deafness in children. An accumulation of thin serous fluid or more commonly, thick tenacious mucus ("glue ear") characterizes this condition. Earache is either minimal or absent with this disorder that rarely affects adults. Persistent fluid behind the eardrum may result in damage followed by otic discharge and accompanied by prolonged (months) hearing loss. Permanent deafness rarely results.

MASTOIDITIS

Acute mastoiditis represents a definite progression from upper respiratory infection to acute otitis media to acute mastoiditis. Surgical procedures are usually employed, although certain cases of acute mastoiditis respond to chemotherapy if adequate middle ear drainage is accomplished.

CHRONIC OBSTRUCTIVE PULMONARY DISEASE (COPD)

Chronic obstructive pulmonary disease (COPD) identifies a group of lung disorders that are characterized by airflow obstruction, ventilation-perfusion abnormality, and hypoxic respiratory failure. Emphysema, chronic bronchitis, and bronchial asthma are examples of COPD.

EMPHYSEMA

Enlargement of the alveoli with loss of elasticity and wall rupture characterize pulmonary emphysema. Morphologic changes are an enlargement of air spaces distal to the terminal bronchiole with destruction of the alveolar walls. Severe emphysema often coexists with chronic bronchitis and represents a principal cause of chronic respiratory failure.

Two major forms of emphysema are centrilobular and panacinar; of these, the former is the most common. In centrilobular emphysema, lesions are located at the center of the pulmonary lobules. The enlarged spaces represent primarily damaged respiratory bronchioles rather than alveoli. Centrilobular emphysema occurs almost exclusively in cigarette smokers.

Panacinar emphysema usually involves all portions of the lobules and all lobes of the lungs. A lesser association with smoking is seen with panacinar emphysema than with centrilobular emphysema. A relation is noted of panacinar emphysema to an impaired ability to counteract proteolytic enzymes released by alveolar macrophages and other leukocytes.

CHRONIC BRONCHITIS

Functionally, chronic bronchitis is defined as a condition characterized by a persistent productive cough for 3 months of the year for at least 2 consecutive years. Cigarette smoking clearly relates to this pulmonary disease. Infections of the respiratory tract often cause a pronounced worsening of chronic bronchitis.

In this disease, connective tissue thickens the bronchial walls that are also infiltrated by inflammatory cells. Mucous gland secretions increase, and airflow obstruction results from mucous plugs and collapse of peripheral airway passages.

Chronic bronchitis and emphysema frequently coexist in many patients. If emphysema is the overriding component, dyspnea and hyperventilation are dominant features, with minimal disturbance of blood gases and little production of sputum. When chronic bronchitis predominates, the patient is hypoxic, cyanotic, and polycythemic with the production of copious amounts of sputum. Cor pulmonale and right ventricular cardiac failure are frequent sequelae in severe chronic bronchitis patients.

ASTHMA

Bronchial asthma attacks are indicated by wheezing and marked respiratory difficulty. Paroxysmal narrowing of airway passages (bronchiolar constriction) characterizes asthma (see Chapter 2).

The bronchi and bronchioles are usually

plugged with mucus and thickening of the basement membrane, smooth muscle hyperplasia, and enlargement of the mucous glands with subsequent increased secretion of mucus, edema, and leukocyte infiltration. Type I hypersensitivity (allergic) reactions are involved in most bronchial asthma patients.

BACTERIAL/VIRAL INFECTIOUS DISEASES OF THE LOWER RESPIRATORY TRACT

The lower respiratory passages, which are located below the pharynx, are usually sterile. The trachea and lungs have no normal flora and hence, organisms that reach this region ordinarily cause infection. Immunologic and predisposing factors also contribute to the development of clinical disease.

PNEUMONOCOCCAL PNEUMONIA

The pathogenicity of Streptococcus pneumoniae resides in its ability to reproduce rapidly and to resist phagocytosis by virtue of its thick surrounding polysaccharide capsule. Hyaluronidase (an enzyme that enables the micro-organism to enter cells and tissues) and hemolysin are also produced by Streptococcus pneumoniae.

Lobar pneumonia involves either an entire lobe or a large portion of it. About 90% of all lobar pneumonia cases are caused by pneumonococci; the remaining cases often result from Klebsiella pneumoniae (Friedlander's bacillus) or Staphylococcus aureus.

Pneumonococcal pneumonia is characterized by a rapid onset with chills and high fever, "rusty" sputum, cyanosis, and pleural inflammation. The infection spreads rapidly through one or more lung lobes with dilation and congestion of alveolar capillaries. Extensive alveolar edema containing pneumonococci is also present. Large numbers of polymorphonuclear leukocytes migrate into the alveoli to accomplish limited phagocytosis.

A key feature of the pathogenesis of lobar pneumonia is consolidation or the formation of a semisolid mass of exudate containing fibrin. This affected region of the lung is virtually nonfunctional. Inspiratory rales cease when consolidation occurs (much like the silence of the "eye" of a hurricane) and then reappear as consolidation begins to clear. A crisis occurs between the fifth and tenth days after infection onset. In the recovering patient, a rapid diminution of symptoms results from the production of anticapsular opsonins and subsequent massive leukocyte phagocytosis and destruction of the pneumonococci.

Resolution, evidenced by the enzymatic digestion and liquefication of the alveolar exudate, is a progression in the healing process. Following expulsion or absorption of the resolution fluids, regeneration of the alveolar lining to a normal state occurs.

BRONCHOPNEUMONIA

Bronchopneumonia is a patchy invasion and consolidation of the lung, usually involving several lobes. Organisms associated with this disease include Pseudomonas aeruginosa, staphylococci, streptococci, pneumonococci, Hemophilus pertussis, and enteric organisms. Mycotic infections of the lung often have a bronchopneumonic distribution. Ulceration of the bronchial mucosa is common, along with alveolar necrosis and abscess formation.

LEGIONNAIRE'S DISEASE

The causative organism, Legionella pneumophilia, does not grow on routine bacteriologic media and requires special techniques for detection. The 1976 outbreak of the disease (so named for the American Legion conventioners who apparently contacted the disease from contaminated dust in the air-conditioning system of a Philadelphia hotel) in the United States was the first time this respiratory infection was recognized. Bronchopneumonia and marked intra-alveolar exudation characterize Legionnaire's disease.

VIRAL PNEUMONIA (PRIMARY ATYPICAL PNEUMONIA)

Influenza viruses, rhinoviruses, Coxsackie, and ECHO viruses are among the causative agents in viral pneumonia. This type of pneumonia is usually patchy and predominantly interstitial. The alveolar septa are thickened, edematous, and infiltrated by macrophages. A pneumonia caused by Mycoplasma pneumoniae is clinically indistinguishable from viral pneumonia.

TUBERCULOSIS (TB)

Tuberculosis is an acute or chronic communicable disease caused by Mycobacterium tuberculosis. Although the lung is usually involved, the organism may invade any other organ or tissue. "Tuberculosis" is derived from the word "tubercle" (small potato), an apt description of the infectious lesion.

Mycobacterium tuberculosis produces no significant toxins in tuberculosis infection. Its pathogenicity lies in the capacity to survive and grow slowly within host cells, as well as its ability to induce cell-mediated immunity or delayed hypersensitivity to its proteins.

Tuberculosis was once a major cause of death in the United States and remains as such in many areas of the world. Malnutrition, chronic disease, and alcoholism are all predisposing factors in tuberculosis development. As there is a great deal of natural resistance to tuberculosis, probably no more than 5% of the people in the United States now infected with Myobacterium tuberculosis will develop clinical disease.

Tuberculosis is usually spread by respiratory droplet infection. The inhaled tubercle bacilli become implanted upon the alveolar surfaces of the lung. Tubercle bacilli are phagocytized by macrophages, although the bacilli continue to grow within the phagocytes in a symbiotic relationship.

A minimal inflammatory response occurs initially, but after 1 or 2 weeks, a cell-mediated hypersensitivity to the tubercle bacillus develops. Mycobacterium tuberculosis migrate to the nearby hilar lymph nodes where they are trapped. During the second week of infection, sensitivity to the organism develops and results in the formation of soft tubercles, both at the point of initial infection and within the regional lymph nodes. Also, the phagocytes acquire the capacity to inhibit the growth of ingested bacilli.

Granulation occurs and necrosis follows in the infected tissue with the formation of a lesion with a caseous or "cheesy" center. Progressive fibrosis walls off the focus and often the necrotic center becomes calcified or ossified (the condition often called "closed" tuberculosis). The primary lesion is termed Ghon focus, and the combination of this state with lymph node involvement is called a Ghon complex; the latter is usually visible by x-ray examination.

Secondary tuberculosis results from either repeated exposure to or reactivation of a primary focus ("open" tuberculosis) where organisms previously trapped within calcified lesions are released. The immunity developed from the primary infection is overcome and hypersensitivity leads to significant lung damage. The secondary lesion is ordinarily located at the top of the lung, the site of the greatest oxygen supply. The risk of developing secondary tuberculosis is appreciably lower than primary tuberculosis. Cavitation, resulting in bronchogenic dissemination, occurs readily and is the anatomic hallmark of secondary tuberculosis.

The clinical symptoms of tuberculosis include cough, chest pain, and weight loss (the term "consumption" was applied to TB since it seemed as though the body consumed itself). Fever, often mild during the day, worsens in the afternoon and breaks at night producing the "night sweats," a characteristic of clinical tuberculosis. With advancing disease, the cough becomes more distressing and yields increasing amounts of sputum, often of a purulent nature. Hemoptysis (spitting of blood) occurs in about 50% of the cases of pulmonary tuberculosis.

INFECTIOUS FUNGAL DISEASE

The lungs represent the most common deep structures invaded by pathogenic fungi. Clinically, fungal diseases range from an acute pneumonitis to a chronic process resembling tuberculosis. Fungi cause tissue damage primarily by virtue of a host hypersensitivity reaction induced by the fungal protein.

CANDIDIASIS (MONILIASIS)

The bronchial mucosa is the respiratory focus of Candida albicans infection. Pulmonary candidiasis usually occurs as an acute or subacute disease similar to bacterial pneumonia. A mucoid or gelatinous sputum, rather than purulent as in bacterial pneumonia, is characteristic of candidiasis.

NOCARDIOSIS

Caused by Actinomyces (Nocardia) asteroides, pulmonary nocardiosis occurs as an acute bronchopneumonia with abscess formation. Nocardiosis occasionally resembles tuberculosis; an associated emphysema is also possible.

ACTINOMYCOSIS

Actinomycosis ("lumpy jaw"), caused by Actinomyces bovis, usually affects cattle and hogs. The formation of slowly developing granulomas progressing to purulent abscesses characterizes this disease. Although the infection ordinarily affects the jaws and mouth, it may also spread to the lungs.

ASPERGILLOSIS

Aspergillosis fumigatus invades a pre-existing cavity to form an aspergilloma ("fungus ball") or causes multiple lung foci of tissue necrosis. Pneumonitis, a tuberculosis-like chronic granulomatous process, or a pseudomembranous tracheobronchitis are other less frequent manifestations of this disease.

HISTOPLASMOSIS

Histoplasma capsulatum infection is endemic in the east-central part of the United States. In this region, the infection is asymptomatic or mild. Lymphatic involvement and peripheral calcifications identical to those of the Ghon complex are present in histoplasmosis.

Clinical symptoms of histoplasmosis include diffuse pneumonitis, disseminated nodule miliary (resembling the size of millet seed) involvement, and a chronic cavitary process similar to that of secondary tuberculosis.

COCCIDIOIDOMYCOSIS (SAN JOAQUIN FEVER)

The causative agent of coccidioidomycosis is Coccidioides immitis. The condition is endemic in the southeastern United States and in the San Joaquin Valley of California (90% of the long-term Valley residents show a positive skin test denoting exposure to the organism). This infection is asymptomatic or presents itself as a pneumonitis or a chronic tuberculosis-like disease. Fatalities may result if the fungus becomes disseminated throughout the body.

NORTH AMERICAN BLASTOMYCOSIS

Pulmonary blastomycosis, caused by Blastomyces dermatidis, occurs most frequently in the southeastern United States. This disease resembles histoplasmosis and coccidioidomycosis in that it is sometimes asymptomatic. Also, like these other fungal infections, pulmonary blastomycosis either presents as an acute, self-limited pneumonitis or progresses to a life-threatening disseminated process.

CRYPTOCOCCOSIS

Cryptococcus neoformans, the causative organism, invokes pulmonary involvement that results in a low-grade fever and cough. The condition may also be entirely asymptomatic.

PULMONARY TUMORS

Carcinomas of the lungs and accessory structures are the leading cause of cancer death (30 to 35%) in American men. The most common type of lung cancer (90% of all cases) is bronchogenic carcinoma.

BRONCHOGENIC CARCINOMA

Bronchogenic carcinoma originates in the bronchial mucosa. This cancer usually affects middle-aged males (primarily between 50 to 60 years of age) who are heavy smokers. The disease is most often a squamous cell carcinoma, but it may also be a bronchial carcinoid or undifferentiated tumor (either "oat cell" pattern or large cell pattern). Oat cell carcinoma, a small cell tumor, is an extremely rapidly growing lesion that is often inoperable at the time of diagnosis.

The incidence of bronchogenic carcinoma has increased at alarming rates since the late 1940s. The relationship of smoking and the development of bronchogenic carcinoma is well established; however, investigation continues on the role of smoking as a nonspecific irritant or a promoting influence. Exposure to certain dusts and ores also increases the risk of developing bronchogenic carcinoma. For example, lung cancer is a frequent sequela in asbestosis patients. As the preceding indicates, bronchogenic carcinoma is largely a preventable disease.

Cough, wheezing, and hemoptysis are the primary symptoms of bronchogenic carcinoma. Lung cancer frequently metastasizes to other areas, including the chest wall, ribs, or spine. Neurologic symptoms (headache, seizures, or paralysis) are sometimes caused by a secondary brain tumor as a result of metastasis from the lung carcinoma.

CARCINOMA OF THE LARYNX

In comparison to lung carcinoma, larynx cancer occurs rarely. It usually develops after the age of 40 and affects men seven times more often than women. Environmental irritants that produce chronic inflammation are often implicated as etiologic factors in the development of larynx cancer.

About 95% of all laryngeal carcinomas are squamous cell lesions with the tumor located directly on the vocal cords. Larynx carcinoma is clinically manifested as a persistent hoarseness. Progression leads to pain, difficulty in swallowing, and hemoptysis.

BENIGN LESIONS OF THE LARYNX

Polyps ("singer's nodes") and papillomas are benign lesions usually found on or near the vocal cords. Since hoarseness is a primary symptom, these conditions require differentiation from carcinoma. Multiple laryngeal papillomas, probably of viral origin, which sometimes occur in children tend to regress at puberty.

DRUGS USED IN RESPIRATORY DISORDERS AND INFECTIONS

These drugs include antihistamines and bronchodilators for symptomatic management of respiratory disease. In addition, anti-infectives combat invading pathogenic microorganisms.

ANTIHISTAMINES, H_1 RECEPTOR BLOCKERS

Antihistamines (Table 7.1) are classically designated as H_1 histamine receptor blockers. These drugs competitively antagonize histamine at the H_1 receptor sites, but they neither inhibit histamine release nor bind with histamine to inactivate it. Antibody production or the antigen-antibody reaction are not inhibited by antihistamines.

In addition to blocking H_1 receptors, antihistamines often possess anticholinergic activity, and some have antiserotonin action. Individual antihistamines are characterized by possessing clinically significant antipruritic activity (trimeprazine), antiemetic effect (promethazine), and local anesthetic action (tripelennamine).

Often present in combination cough-cold medications, antihistamines modify the symptoms of the common cold, but they do not alter the course of the viral disease. Antihistamines with predominant sedative properties are used as sleep-aids in the treatment of insomnia. Should a patient become refractory to the effects of a particular antihistamine, switching from one chemical class of antihistamine to another may restore responsiveness.

Generally, antihistamines are remarkably nontoxic drugs when used properly. However, in cases of improper use, central nervous stimulation and convulsions have occurred, especially in infants and children who ingested large doses. This reaction is interesting considering that excessive drowsiness and sedation ordinarily result from therapeutic dosage or moderate overdosage with antihistamines.

Table 7.1. ANTIHISTAMINES.

Available products	Trade names	Daily dosage range
Azatadine maleate	Optimine	1 or 2 mg b.i.d.
Brompheniramine maleate	Dimetane; Bromphine; others	4 mg q. 4–6 hrs
Buclizine	Bucladin	50 mg
Carbinoxamine maleate	Clistin	4–8 mg t.i.d. or q.i.d.
Chlorpheniramine maleate	Chlor-Trimeton; others	4 mg q. 4–6 hrs
Clemastine fumarate	Tavist	2.68–8.04 mg
Cyclizine	Marezine	50–200 mg
Cyproheptadine HCl	Periactin	4–20 mg/kg
Dexchlorpheniramine maleate	Polaramine; Dexchlor; Poladex T.D.	2 mg q. 4–6 hrs
Dimenhydrinate	Dramamine; others	50–400 mg
Diphenhydramine HCl	Benadryl; others	25–50 mg t.i.d or q.i.d.
Diphenylpyraline HCl	Hispril	5 mg q. 12 hrs
Meclizine	Meclizine HCl; Antivert; others	25–50 mg
Methdilazine HCl	Tacaryl	8 mg b.i.d.-q.i.d.
Phenindamine tartrate	Nolahist	25 mg q. 4–6 hrs
Promethazine HCl	Phenergan; others	25 mg
Pyrilamine maleate	Pyrilamine Maleate	25–50 mg t.i.d.
Terfenadine	Seldane	60 mg b.i.d.
Trimeprazine	Temaril	2.5 mg q.i.d.
Tripelennamine HCl	Pelamine; PBZ	25–50 mg q. 4–6 hrs
Triprolidine HCl	Actidil; Bayidyl	2.5 mg q. 4–6 hrs

The antihistamines are divided into groups or types based upon their chemical structures. All the antihistamines bear a chemical relationship to histamine, but the individual groups have pharmacologic and toxicity profiles characteristic of that particular group. The chemical types of antihistamines are ethanolamines, ethylenediamines, alkylamines, phenothiazines, piperazines, and piperidines. A discussion of a representative prototype of each antihistamine class follows.

Ethanolamine Antihistamines. Diphenhydramine, dimenhydrinate, and carbinoxamine are examples of the ethanolamine class of antihistamines. Diphenhydramine has pronounced sedative action.

Mechanism of Action. Diphenhydramine competitively antagonizes histamine at the H_1 receptor site. This drug has significant sedative and muscarinic blocking (atropine-like) effects.

Clinical Indications. Diphenhydramine is indicated for the symptomatic treatment of perennial and seasonal allergic rhinitis; allergic conjunctivitis; mild, uncomplicated urticaria and angioedema; amelioration of allergic reactions to blood or plasma; dermagraphia; and as adjunctive therapy in anaphylaxis. Other of its uses are in the treatment of motion sickness, as a sleep-aid, and for selected cases of parkinsonism. A parenteral form of diphenhydramine is available when use of the oral form is impractical. Indications for the parenteral form include allergic reactions to blood or plasma and as an adjunct in anaphylaxis, motion sickness, and parkinsonism.

Adverse Effects/Precautions. The most frequent adverse reactions to diphenhydramine are drowsiness and sedation. These reactions somewhat limit the drug's use in the daytime, especially for patients who must drive or perform tasks requiring alertness. Gastrointestinal distress is also possible with this drug.

Patients with a history of urinary retention, bronchial asthma, increased intraocular pressure, hyperthyroidism, cardiovascular disease, or hypertension should use diphenhydramine with caution because of the drug's atropine-like effects.

Ethylenediamine Antihistamines. Examples of this class of antihistamines are tripelennamine and pyrilamine. Tripelennamine is a relatively specific histamine antagonist at H_1 receptor sites.

Mechanism of Action. Tripelennamine blocks the action of histamine at H_1 receptor sites. Sedative activity is not pronounced with this drug, although somnolence occurs in many patients receiving tripelennamine.

Clinical Indications. Tripelennamine is used to relieve symptoms associated with perennial and seasonal allergic rhinitis. Other indications include vasomotor rhinitis, allergic conjunctivitis due to allergens and foods, uncomplicated urticaria and angioedema, amelioration of allergic reactions to blood or plasma, dermagraphia, and as an adjunct to epinephrine and other usual measures in anaphylaxis.

A tripelennamine cream is available for the temporary relief of itching due to minor skin disorders, poison ivy and poison oak dermatitis, hives, sunburn, and non-poisonous insect bites and stings.

Adverse Effects/Precautions. Gastrointestinal side effects are common with tripelennamine. Drowsiness may also occur, necessitating cautious use if patient alertness is required.

A drug abuse warning involves the intravenous injection of oral preparations of tripelennamine and pentazocine ("T's and Blues") to serve as a substitute for heroin. Although neurologic complications occur, pulmonary disease is the most frequent and severe complication of the IV injection of "T's and Blues."

Alkylamine Antihistamines. Chlorpheniramine, brompheniramine, and triprolidine are representatives of the alkylamine class of antihistamines. Chlorpheniramine and its chemical relatives are among the most potent H_1 blocking drugs.

Mechanism of Action. Chlorpheniramine blocks the action of histamine at H_1 receptor sites. Drowsiness is less common with chlorpheniramine than with antihistamines in the other chemical classes. Chlorpheniramine possesses anticholinergic (drying) activity.

Clinical Indications. This antihistamine is indicated for perennial and seasonal allergic rhinitis; vasomotor rhinitis; allergic conjunctivitis; mild, uncomplicated urticaria and angioedema; amelioration of allergic reaction to blood and plasma; and as an adjunct to epinephrine and other standard procedures in anaphylaxis. An injection is available for uncomplicated allergic reactions of the immediate type and for use as an adjunct to anaphylaxis when use of the oral form of the drug is impractical.

Chlorpheniramine is highly suitable for daytime use because of the low incidence of drowsiness with this drug.

Adverse Effects/Precautions. The side effects of chlorpheniramine are the same as those reported for the other antihistamines.

Phenothiazine Antihistamines. Promethazine, a phenothiazine antihistamine, is a potent sedative that also has antiemetic activity. This drug was introduced several decades ago for the treatment of allergic conditions. Early clinical observations confirmed the drug's sedative and anti-motion sickness properties.

Mechanism of Action. Promethazine antagonizes the action of histamine at H_1 receptors. High anticholinergic activity occurs with promethazine, along with prominent CNS actions, including sedative and antiemetic effects.

Clinical Indications. In addition to the usual indications (such as allergic conditions) for H_1 receptor blocking drugs, promethazine is also used for the active and prophylactic treatment of motion sickness; preoperative, postoperative, or obstetrical sedation; and as an antiemetic in the control of nausea and vomiting associated with surgical procedures, anesthesia, and postoperative recovery. Another of the drug's uses is as a sedative to allay apprehension and support sleep.

Adverse Effects/Precautions. Adverse reactions include drowsiness, sedation, epigastric distress, and atropine-like effects that include urinary retention, blurred vision, xerostomia, and constipation. Of all the antihistamines, the phenothiazines are the most likely to cause blood dyscrasias.

Piperazine Derivatives. Piperazine derivatives include cyclizine, chlorcyclizine, and meclizine. Cyclizine and meclizine are valuable in the treatment and prophylaxis of motion sickness; chlorcyclizine is used mainly for the usual antihistamine indications. Hydroxyzine, useful in treating skin allergies, has considerable CNS depressant action (see Chapter 1).

Cyclizine. Cyclizine is frequently employed in both the prevention and control of motion sickness.

Mechanism of Action. In addition to antagonizing histamine at H_1 receptors, cyclizine has pronounced antiemetic and anticholinergic properties. A prominent ancillary activity is its reduction in the sensitivity of the labyrinthine apparatus of the ear. An effect on nerve pathways from the chemoreceptive trigger zone (CTZ) to the vomiting center, other CNS centers, or peripheral nerve pathways may mediate the drug's antiemetic activity.

Clinical Indications. Cyclizine is used mainly to treat motion sickness-induced nausea and vomiting.

Adverse Effects/Precautions. Reports of numerous adverse reactions including urticaria, drug rash, drowsiness, restlessness, excitement, and euphoria have followed cyclizine administration. Anticholinergic (atropine-like) side effects (such as xerostomia, blurred vision, constipation, and urinary retention) are also possible. Cholestatic jaundice is still another possible side effect.

Piperidines. Terfenadine, a piperidinebutanol derivative, was recently introduced as a nonsedating antihistamine.

Mechanism of Action. Terfenadine, a histamine H_1 receptor blocking drug, binds mainly to peripheral H_1 receptors.

Clinical Indications. Terfenadine is indicated in the treatment of seasonal allergic rhinitis. The drug is also apparently effective in treating perennial allergic rhinitis and histamine-related skin disorders (such as chronic idiopathic urticaria), but it has not yet received FDA approval for these indications.

Adverse Effects/Precautions. Terfenadine has minimal sedative and anticholinergic properties. Side effects reported for this drug include headache, drowsiness, fatigue, dry mouth, sore throat, nausea, nasal stuffiness, cough, weakness, dizziness, and abdominal distress.

ANTIBACTERIAL DRUGS

Bacteria and related organisms such as the myoplasmas, rickettsiae, and chlamydiae are designated as prokaryotic cells. Cytoplasm in prokaryotic cells includes a diffuse nuclear area containing deoxyribonucleic acid (DNA) but not surrounded by a nuclear membrane. These cells contrast with eukaryotic cells that contain at least one clearly defined nucleus enclosed by a discrete nuclear membrane (such as typical animal cells). Distinct mitochondrial organelles are located in the plasma membrane and in a system of internal membranes. Ribosomes and ribonucleic acid (RNA) are present in the nuclear environ, and protein synthesis proceeds by mechanisms common to eukaroytic cells.

Bacteria (such as Actinomyces and Streptomyces) are branching filamentous organisms which resemble fungi in morphology. Actinomyces may be pathogenic in man, but Streptomyces contains no pathogenic species. In fact, Streptomyces is interesting because many species produce therapeutically valuable antibiotics.

A lower group of bacteria produces clinical disease under specific situations. Simpler in shape, this bacteria group has a diameter of about 1 μm and are either spherical (cocci), short chain straight cylinders (bacilli), slightly curved cylinders (vibrios), or rigid spiral rods. The cocci group formations represent various patterns: diplococci (pairs), staphylococci (variably sized clusters), and streptococci (chains).

Pathogens of these bacteria types damage the host cells, whereas commensals represent parasitic organisms that coexist with host cells without causing damage. Commensals include oral bacteria that play an important role in digestion by initiating the breakdown of food. The distinction between commensals and pathogens is not complete; for example, bacteria that is present as normal flora in the gastrointestinal tract may become pathogenic if they gain access to the genitourinary tract. Components of the basic structure of bacteria and processes that occur within the organism are sites of action of antibacterial drugs (Figure 7.5).

The rigid bacterial cell wall is composed of a mucopeptide in which the amino sugars N-acetyl-D-glucosamine and N-acetylmuramic acid are joined alternately into linear chains that are cross-linked by peptides. Cell wall synthesis takes place in the cytoplasm, within the plasma membrane, and on the outer surface of the plasma membrane. An extracellular colloid layer (consisting of polysaccharides, polypeptides, and proteins) is secreted by the bacterium. This outside, outermost layer gives the bacteria highly specific immunologic properties.

Composed mainly of lipoprotein, the plasma membrane offers little rigidity and depends upon the cell wall for protection and support. Phospholipids, with smaller amounts of glycolipids, are the major bacterial lipids. Sterols are not found in the bacterial plasma membrane. Transport of nutrients and other substances occurs at the plasma membrane. The enzymes and carrier proteins concerned with membrane transport, metabolic enzymes, and enzymes involved with cell wall synthesis are found in the plasma membrane. The cytochrome system of the bacterial cell is also located in the plasma membrane, in contrast with eukaryotic cells where the mitochondria fulfill this role. One or more intracellular condensations of DNA are present in all bacteria, as are large numbers of ribosomes and RNA.

Bacteria are divided empirically into two classes depending upon their reaction to certain dyes (gram stain). Those bacteria that retain a methyl violet stain after exposure are designated as gram-positive; others that lose the methyl violet and take up a counterstain are termed gram-negative. The amino acid and lipid profile of the bacterial cell wall determine whether an organism is gram-positive (gram +) or gram-negative (gram −).

Bacterial pathogenicity is determined by the invasiveness and toxigenicity characteristics of the organism. Invasiveness denotes the capacity of the pathogenic organism to multiply rap-

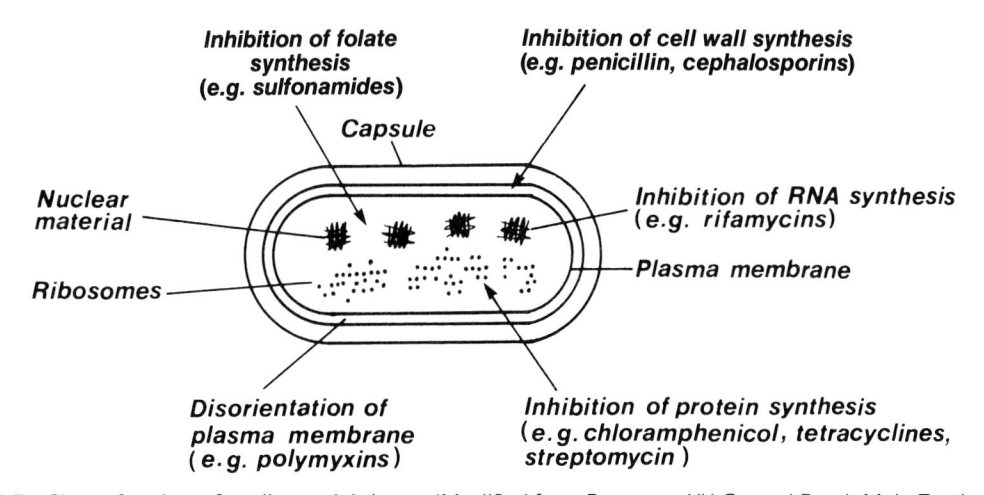

Fig. 7.5 Sites of action of antibacterial drugs. (Modified from Bowman, W.C., and Rand, M.J.: Textbook of Pharmacology. 2nd Ed. Oxford, Blackwell Scientific Publications, 1980.)

Table 7.2. ANTIBACTERIAL DRUGS USED IN PULMONARY INFECTIONS.

Available products	Trade names	Daily dosage range
Amikacin sulfate	Amikin	15 mg/kg
Amoxicillin	Amoxil; Polymox; others	500 mg q. 8 hrs
Ampicillin	Omnipen; Polycillin; others	Individualize according to clinical situation
Azlocillin sodium	Azlin	200–300 mg/kg in 4–6 divided doses
Bacampicillin HCl	Spectrobid	400 mg q. 12 hrs
Carbenicillin disodium	Geopen; Pyopen	IV, 400–500 mg/kg
Cefaclor	Ceclor	250 mg q. 8 hrs
Cefadroxil	Duricef; Ultracef	1 g in 2 divided doses
Cefamandole nafate	Mandol	500 mg–1 g q. 4–8 hrs
Cefonicid sodium	Monocid	1 g
Cefoperazone sodium	Cefobid	2–4 g in divided doses q. 12 hrs
Ceforanide	Precef	IM or IV, 0.5–1 g q. 12 hrs
Cefotaxime sodium	Claforan	1 g q. 6–8 hrs
Cefoxitin sodium	Mefoxin	1–2 g q. 6–8 hrs
Ceftizoxime sodium	Cefizox	1 or 2 g q. 8–12 hrs
Cefuroxime sodium	Zinacef	750 mg–1.5 g q. 8 hrs
Cephalexin	Keflex	1–4 g
Cephalothin sodium	Keflin; Seffin	500 mg–1 g 4–6 hrs
Cephapirin sodium	Cefadyl	500 mg–1 g q. 4–6 hrs
Cephradine	Anspor; Velosef	500 mg q. 12 hrs
Clindamycin	Cleocin HCl; Cleocin Phosphate	150–300 mg q. 8 hrs
Cloxacillin sodium	Cloxapen; Tegopen	250 mg q. 6 hrs
Colistimethate sodium	Coly-Mycin M	2.5–5 mg/kg
Cyclacillin	Cyclapen-W	250 mg q. 6 hrs
Demeclocycline HCl	Declomycin	4 divided doses of 150 mg each
Dicloxacillin sodium	Dynapen; Dycill; others	125 mg q. 6 hrs
Doxycycline	Vibramycin IV; Doxy 100; Doxy 200	200 mg IV followed by 100–200 mg daily
Erythromycin	E.E.S.; Ilosone; others	250 mg q. 6 hrs
Gentamicin	Garamycin; Apogen; others	3 mg/kg
Hetacillin	Versapen; Versapen-K	225–450 mg q.i.d.
Kanamycin sulfate	Kantrex; Kanamycin Sulfate; Klebcil	15 mg/kg
Lincomycin	Lincocin	Oral, 500 mg q. 8 hrs
Methacycline HCl	Rondomycin	600 mg in 4 divided doses
Methicillin sodium	Celbenin; Stapcillin	IM, 1 g q. 4–6 hrs
Mezlocillin sodium	Mezlin	200–300 mg/kg in 4–6 divided doses
Minocycline HCl	Minocin IV	200 mg followed by 100 mg q. 12 hrs
Moxalactam disodium	Moxam	2–6 g in divided doses q. 8 hrs
Nafcillin sodium	Nafcil; Unipen; Nallpen	IM, 500 mg q. 6 hrs
Netilmicin sulfate	Netromycin	1.5–2 mg/kg
Oxacillin sodium	Bactocill; Prostaphlin	Oral, 500 mg q. 4–6 hrs
Oxytetracycline	Oxymycin; Terramycin IM	250 mg
Penicillin G	Penicillin G Potassium; Pfizerpen; Pentids	Individualize according to clinical situation
Penicillin G Benzathine	Bicillin L-A; Permapen; Bicillin	Individualize according to clinical situation
Penicillin V	Penicillin V	250–500 mg
Penicillin V Potassium	Pen-Vee K; V-Cillin K; others	Individualize according to clinical situation
Piperacillin sodium	Pipracil	IM, 6–8 g in divided doses
Polymyxin B sulfate	Polymyxin B Sulfate; Aerosporin	15,000–25,000 units/kg
Spectinomycin	Trobicin	Inject 5 ml IM for a 2 g dose
Streptomycin sulfate	Streptomycin Sulfate	Individualize according to clinical situation
Sulfamethoxazole	Ganatol; Urobak	2 g
Tetracycline HCl	Achromycin; Sumycin; others	Oral, 1–2g in 2 or 4 equal doses
Ticarcillin disodium	Ticar	200–300 mg/kg by IV infusion in divided doses
Tobramycin sulfate	Nebcin	3 mg/kg
Trimethoprim	Proloprim Trimpex	100 mg q. 12 hrs
Troleandomycin	Tao	250–500 mg q.i.d.
Vancomycin	Vancocin	500 mg q. 6 hrs

idly at the site of infection and overwhelm the defense mechanisms of the host. If organisms spill over into the blood, bacteremia occurs and spreads to other tissues. Septicemia results if the defense mechanisms of the blood are overwhelmed. Bacterial toxigenicity, due to either bacterial exotoxins and/or endotoxins, results in specific damage to host tissues.

Exotoxins are polypeptide or protein toxins formed by some gram-positive bacteria including Streptococcus pyogenes, Clostridia, and Corynebacterium diphtheriae. Endotoxins are derived from cell wall components of many gram-negative and some gram-positive bacteria. The endotoxins are released upon disintegration of the pathogenic bacteria following destruction by the host's defense mechanisms. Endotoxins are less specific in their action than are exotoxins. Organisms that produce endotoxins include Salmonella typhi (typhoid fever), Shigella dysenteriae (dysentery), and Pasteurella pestis (bubonic plague).

The chemotherapy of bacterial infections depends upon a selective toxicity. Specifically, there is a much greater cytotoxic effect on the infecting organism than on the host.

GENERAL MECHANISMS OF ANTIBACTERIAL ACTION

Antibacterial drugs (Tables 7.2–7.5) inhibit or kill invading organisms by several methods. One mechanism involves an interference with bacterial cell wall synthesis, resulting in the cell bursting in a hypotonic environment. A selective toxicity is noted because cell walls are not a component of the cells of the host. The penicillins and cephalosporins are antibiotics that act by this mechanism.

Another antibacterial mechanism depends upon an impairment of protein synthesis, either by interfering with the synthesis of RNA (e.g., rifamycin) or more frequently, by an action on ribosomes. Aminoglycosides, tetracyclines, and chloramphenicol are antibiotics that act in this manner. The selective toxicity of these drugs is attributed to diffusion barriers in resistant cells (host cells) or differences in the binding sites and target enzymes in sensitive cells (certain pathogenic bacteria), as compared to insensitive cells (host cells).

Antibacterial drugs can also act as antimetabolites in that they inhibit essential metabolic reactions within the cytoplasm of the organism.

Table 7.3. **ANTIBACTERIAL DRUGS USED FOR INITIAL TREATMENT OF EAR, NOSE, AND THROAT DISORDERS.**

Available products	Trade names	Daily dosage range
Amoxicillin	Various	250 mg
Ampicillin	Various	500 mg
Cloxacillin	Various	500 mg
Dicloxacillin	Various	125 mg
Penicillin V	Various	250 mg

Table 7.4. **ANTITUBERCULOSIS DRUGS.**

Available products	Trade names	Daily dosage range
First-Line:		
Isoniazid	Isoniazid; Laniazid; Nydrazid	Oral, 5 mg/kg
Rifampin	Rifadin; Rimactane	Oral, 600 mg
Second-Line:		
Ethambutol HCl	Myambutol	Oral, 15 mg/kg
Pyrazinamide	Pyrazinamide	Oral, 20–35 mg/kg
Streptomycin sulfate	Streptomycin Sulfate	IM, 1 g
Tertiary:		
Aminosalicylate sodium	Teebacin; P.A.S. Sodium	Oral, 14–16 g in 2–3 divided doses
Capreomycin	Capastat Sulfate	IM, 1 g
Cycloserine	Seromycin	Oral, 500 mg–1 g in divided doses
Ethionamide	Trecator-SC	Oral, 0.5–1.0 g in divided doses
Kanamycin	Kanamycin Sulfate; Kantrex; Klebcil	IM, 0.5–1 g

In order for drugs, such as the sulfonamides, to be clinically useful, the inhibited reaction must be essential to the infecting organism but not to the host.

Permeability changes in the plasma membrane as a result of structural disorientation by the antibacterial is a fourth antimicrobial mechanism. Drugs such as polymyxin B and colistin cause permeability changes in the plasma membrane of sensitive cells (certain pathogens) but do not bind to insensitive cells (host cells). The reasons for this selective toxicity remain obscure.

Antibacterial drugs are either bacteriostatic or bacteriocidal. The former inhibit the growth and reproduction of susceptible organisms, allowing the host defense mechanisms to better repel the infection. Sulfonamides and trimethoprim are examples of bacteriostatic antibacterial drugs. Whereas bacteriostatic drugs act mainly by inhibiting protein synthesis, bacteriocidal drugs kill susceptible invading organisms and usually act by interference with cell wall synthesis.

Antibacterial drugs usually have a selective toxicity toward different species of organisms; penicillin G, for example, acts mainly against gram-positive bacteria. An antibiotic (e.g., tetracycline) is designated as a broad spectrum antibiotic because it demonstrates toxicity against a wide range of gram-positive and gram-negative organisms. If organisms of the body's natural flora are killed, an imbalance that favors resident pathogens formerly held in check by these "friendly" organisms may cause a superinfection. Candidiasis is one example of a superinfection that sometimes occurs after inadequate tetracycline therapy.

The major current therapeutic problem associated with antibacterial therapy is the emergence of drug resistant strains of organisms that were previously sensitive to a particular antibacterial. Using adequate doses of antibacterials for a sufficient period of time to assure that the host has overcome the infecting organism may minimize the problem of drug-resistance.

Table 7.5. ANTIFUNGAL DRUGS.

Available products	Trade names	Daily dosage range
Miconazole	Monistat i.v.	Variable
Ketoconazole	Nizoral	200 mg
Amphotericin B	Fungizone	1 mg/kg

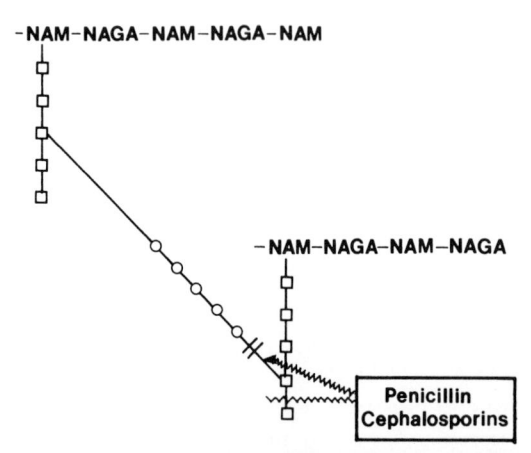

Fig. 7.6 *Cross-linking of peptidoglycan strands and site of action of penicillin and cephalosporins.* (From Goth, A.: Medical Pharmacology. 11th Ed. St. Louis, C.V. Mosby, 1984.)

ANTIBACTERIAL DRUGS THAT AFFECT CELL WALL SYNTHESIS

The multiple step formation of N-acetylmuramic acid (NAM) pentapeptide, an important starting material in cell wall synthesis, begins with UTP-activated N-acetylglucosamine (NAGA). The reaction proceeds within the cell, and finally terminates by the addition of the dipeptide D-alanyl-D-alanine to the three amino acids residues (alanine, D-glutamic acid, and lysine) that are attached by previously formed peptide bonds (Figure 7.6). Prior conversion of L-alanine to D-alanine is required, followed by dipeptide formation, to form the D-alanyl-D-alanine dipeptide.

Peptidoglycan formation occurs when the precursor molecules (after being anchored to the phospholipid in the plasma membrane) are transported through the membrane where they are covalently bound to pre-existing portions of the bacterial cell wall. The linear polymer of the repeating units of the cell wall is thus formed.

Cross-linkage of the peptidoglycans is the

final phase of the bacterial cell wall synthesis. Transpeptidation occurs when the D-alanine (fourth residue) of the peptide side chain of one muropeptide chain is attached to an adjacent muropeptide-glycopeptide polymer through a short polypeptide bridge (consisting of five glycine units) to the epsilon-amino group of lysine (Figure 7.7). The fifth residue (also D-alanine) is released in the transpeptidase reaction. The result is a lattice-like structure forming an envelope around the cell. This net-like envelope is closed on all sides and is a completely covalently bound structure. Depending upon the nature of the cross-linking, the meshwork is either tightly woven, as in the case of Staphyloccocus aureus, or is loosely woven, as represented by Escherichia coli.

In gram-positive bacteria, the cross-linked peptidoglycans form the most important rigid support of the cell. The cell wall protects the underlying membrane from damage by the high internal osmotic pressure concentration of solutes within cells present when bacteria are growing in media of normal osmolarity. Unless the bacterial cell is maintained in a medium of high osmolarity, damage to the underlying cell membrane occurs with the resultant loss in the ability to concentrate amino acids and other solutes within the cell. Damage to the cell leads to death of the cell and perhaps lysis.

PENICILLINS

In 1928, Sir Alexander Fleming began the modern era of antibiotic therapy when he astutely observed an air-contaminated culture plate upon which staphylococci were growing. Fleming's attention was drawn to a bacteria-free zone surrounding a mold colony growing on the culture plate. An extract of the Penicillium mold grown in culture selectively killed certain bacterial species without harming leukocytes. Fleming named the antibacterial substance "penicillin." In 1940, Flory isolated penicillin from Penicillin notatum, and Abraham, Flory's colleague at Oxford, described its first clinical use against several gram-positive bacterial infections.

In 1941, concentrated cultures were sent to the United States from Britain to enable contin-

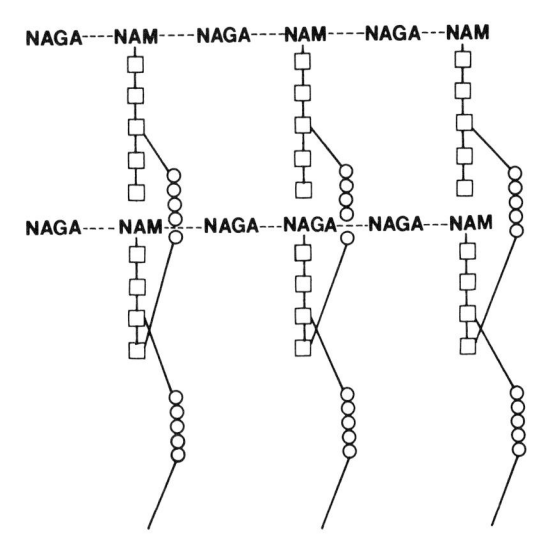

Fig. 7.7 Cross-linking of peptidoglycans by a pentaglycine bridge. (From Goth, A.: Medical Pharmacology. 11th Ed. St. Louis, C.V. Mosby, 1984.)

ued work on the isolation with less distraction from the active war conditions then present in England. Several reasons account for the acceleration of penicillin production; among these were the discovery of cornsteep liquor as a prime growth medium for Penicillium, the isolation of higher yield strains of Penicillium, the use of submerged cultures, and the interest of pharmaceutical manufacturers with expertise in vat fermentation.

The more recently introduced penicillins are designated as semisynthetic, so named as they are a product of structural modification of the basic penicillin obtained by fermentation. Penicillinase-resistant penicillins, among the semisynthetic group, are valuable because many bacterial species, once sensitive to the early agents (penicillin G), have developed resistance. Penicillin is susceptible to hydrolytic action by penicillinase (beta-lactamase); the elaboration of this enzyme by resistant organisms greatly reduced the antibiotic's effectiveness against the pathogen.

The penicillin molecule is basically a system of two fused rings, one of which is a saturated thiazolidine ring and the other is a beta-lactam ring. The fused ring, with the substituent groups (one amino, one carboxyl, and two methyl) is designated as 6-aminopenicillanic acid (6-APA). The sidechains are acyl groups in amide linkage with 6-APA and determine absorption, stability to degradation, and antibacterial activity. 6-APA, without an akyl group sidechain, is devoid of antibacterial activity. This highly strained and unstable system is especially labile to acid (gastric hydrochloric), bases (enterodigestive juices), and hydrolytic enzymes (penicillinase).

In the 1940s, benzylpenicillin (Penicillin G) was the first natural penicillin to achieve clinical prominence. A decade later, phenoxymethyl penicillin (Penicillin V), an acid-resistant penicillin, was synthesized in Penicillin chrysogenum culture broths. Phenoxymethylpenicillin, being acid-resistant, was deemed more suitable for oral administration. The 1950s was a time in which penicillinase-producing staphylococci became a critical public health problem; penicillinase-resistant penicillins were developed to combat these resistant bacterial strains.

Research on penicillin synthesis in the past three decades has yielded many semisynthetic forms which have special clinical advantages. The penicillin family currently includes natural, acid stable, penicillinase-resistant, ampicillins, and extended antibacterial spectrum members (Table 7.6).

Natural Penicillins. Penicillin G, benzylpenicillin, is a naturally occurring antibiotic.

Mechanism of Action. Penicillin G inhibits the synthesis of the bacterial cell wall mucopeptide. Cross-linking of the peptidoglycans that compose the mucopeptide is accomplished by a transpeptidation reaction. Penicillin G binds the transpeptidase and competitively inhibits the transpeptidation reaction. The lack of the peptide cross-linking inhibits the synthesis of the developing bacterial cell wall. The penicillin G molecule may actually bind covalently to the site on the enzyme (transpeptidase) that is ordinarily accepted by D-alanyl-D-alanine.

Table 7.6. SIGNIFICANT DIFFERENCES OF THE PENICILLINS.

Agent	Routes	Penicillinase-resistant	Acid stable
Penicillin G	IM, IV, Oral	No	No
Acid stable			
Penicillin V	Oral	No	Yes
Penicillinase-resistant			
Methicillin	IM, IV	Yes	No
Nafcillin	IM, IV, Oral	Yes	Yes
Oxacillin	IM, IV, Oral	Yes	Yes
Cloxacillin	Oral	Yes	Yes
Dicloxacillin	Oral	Yes	Yes
Ampicillins			
Ampicillin	IM, IV, Oral	No	Yes
Hetacillin	Oral	No	Yes
Bacampicillin	Oral	No	Yes
Amoxicillin	Oral	No	Yes
Cyclacillin	Oral	No	Yes
Extended spectrum			
Carbenicillin	IM, IV, Oral*	No	Yes*
Ticarcillin	IM, IV	No	**
Mezlocillin	IM, IV	No	**
Piperacillin	IM, IV	No	**
Azlocillin	IV	No	**

* Indanyl derivative
** Available only for IM and/or IV use

The bacterial cell with the defective cell wall, designated as an "L-form" or protoplast, would then swell and burst open from its own high internal pressure, which is very high in contrast to all body fluids.

Penicillin G is bacteriocidal against organisms when adequate concentrations are present, and the antibiotic is more effective during active multiplication of the bacteria. Bacteriostatic effects are noted when inadequate concentrations of penicillin G are used.

Mammalian cells possess an outer plasma membrane rather than a rigid cell wall. A selective toxicity is then evident due to the interaction of penicillin with a biochemical process common to bacteria but not operant in human host cells. Compared to the other antibiotics, penicillin comes close to being the ideal chemotherapeutic agent.

Clinical Indications. Penicillin G is used in streptococcal infections, such as acute bacterial pharyngitis ("strep throat"). Infections of the respiratory tract caused by pneumonococci, including pneumococcal pneumonia and otitis media, are also effectively treated with parenteral (IM) penicillin G procaine. Other respiratory ailments responsive to penicillin G include actinomycosis, fusospirochetal infections of the oropharynx and lower respiratory tract, and diphtheria (as an adjunct to diphtheria antitoxin).

Oral preparations of penicillin G should be taken on an empty stomach for optimal absorption. Administration of penicillin G preparations by the parenteral route is necessary for treating severe infections.

Adverse Effects/Precautions. Hypersensitivity reactions, at an incidence rate from 1 to 10%, are the most common adverse effect of penicillin G. Frequently occurring reactions include skin eruptions, such as urticaria (hives), and exanthemous rashes of various types. Patients with previously demonstrated hypersensitivity and those with a medical history of allergy, asthma, allergic rhinitis, or urticaria are more likely to experience hypersensitivity reactions.

Anaphylaxis, the most severe reaction (at an estimated incidence of 0.01 to 0.05%), usually occurs following parenteral injection of this drug. Direct tissue damage, evidenced by CNS neurotoxicity, is possible with excessively high serum levels. Lethargy, neuromuscular irritability, hallucinations, and seizures are additional potential problems.

Intravenous aqueous penicillin G should be administered slowly to avoid the possibility of adverse effects related to electrolyte imbalance that may result from the sodium or potassium content of the penicillin preparation.

Acid-Stable Penicillin. Penicillin V (phenoxymethyl penicillin) has a phenoxy sidechain, rather than a benzyl, from the 6-AMA basic nucleus.

Mechanism of Action. Penicillin V is more resistant to stomach acid and thus gives higher plasma levels than equal oral doses of penicillin G. Penicillin V inhibits bacterial cell wall synthesis by blocking cross-linking of the peptidoglycans that form the latticework of the structure.

Clinical Indications. The indications for penicillin V are the same as those of penicillin G; among these are streptococcal and pneumonococcal infections and fusospirochetosis (Vincent's infection).

Adverse Effects/Precautions. As with penicillin G, hypersensitivity reactions are the most serious potential adverse effect. Only oral preparations of penicillin V are marketed, rendering the possibility of anaphylaxis (usually seen with parenteral administration) less likely.

Penicillinase-resistant Penicillins. The penicillinase-resistant penicillins include methicillin, nafcillin, oxacillin, cloxacillin, and dicloxicillin.

Mechanism of Action. The semisynthetic penicillinase-resistant penicillins inhibit the synthesis of the bacterial cell wall mucopeptides in a manner similar to that of penicillin G. These penicillins are especially resistant to staphylococcal penicillinase. Currently, many staphylococcal infections, whether hospital or community acquired, are resistant to treatment by either penicillin G or V.

Clinical Indications. The principal indication for penicillinase-resistant penicillins is in the treatment of infections due to penicillinase-producing staphylococci. These antibiotics are recommended as initial therapy in staphylococcal infections until culture and sensitivity results are known. Using an oral penicillinase-resistant penicillin is presently advocated for the initial treatment of all gram-positive infections of mild to moderate severity.

Adverse Effects/Precautions. Hypersensitivity reactions are the most serious potential adverse effect of these antibiotics. Methicillin, administered only parenterally, is possibly nephrotoxic. Recently detected staphylococcal strains are now appearing that are "methicillin-resistant," in which drug inactivation is not dependent upon penicillinase.

Ampicillins. The ampicillins include ampicillin; amoxicillin and cyclacillin (close chemical relatives of ampicillin); and hetacillin and bacampicillin (antibiotics that are hydrolyzed to ampicillin).

Mechanism of Action. The ampicillin penicillins inhibit the biosynthesis of bacterial cell wall mucopeptides. Specific aspects of antibacterial activity resemble those of penicillin G.

Clinical Indications. The broader spectrum of antibacterial activity and acid-resistant properties of the ampicillins render them valuable chemotherapeutic agents. Tonsillitis, pharyngitis, and otitis media caused by Group A beta-hemolytic streptococci are clinical indications for heptacillin. Since ampicillin is extremely active against the pathogens responsible for many pediatric bacterial infections, it is especially effective in treating serious infections in young children. Hemophilus influenzae, a common causative agent in childhood otitis media, is particularly sensitive to ampicillin.

Adverse Effects/Precautions. Ampicillin occasionally causes a skin rash apparently unrelated to the penicillin-type allergic dermatitis. The ampicillin-induced rash occurs almost always if the patient has infectious mononucleosis. Diarrhea, a common adverse reaction with ampicillin, occurs less frequently with amoxicillin. Typical hypersensitivity reactions are possible with the ampicillins.

Extended Spectrum Penicillin. Carbenicillin has a greater activity than ampicillin against Pseudomonas aeruginosa and enterobacter and Serratia organisms. Ampicillin-resistant strains of Proteus may also respond to carbenicillin therapy. The carbenicillin-like antibiotics (available for parenteral administration) have a similar extended spectrum; these antibiotics include ticarcillin, piperacillin, mezlocillin, and azlocillin.

Mechanism of Action. The extended spectrum penicillins inhibit biosynthesis of the bacterial cell wall in a manner similar to that of the other penicillins.

Clinical Indications. Carbenicillin and the carbenicillin-like extended antibiotics are indicated primarily for infections resultant from Pseudomonas aeruginosa, Proteus, and certain strains of Escherichia coli. Severe systemic infections due to Hemophilus influenzae and Streptococcus pneumoniae also respond to these antibiotics.

Lower respiratory tract infections caused by Klebsiella pneumoniae, Proteus mirabilis, Serratia species, and Bacteroides species are often responsive to the parenteral administration of piperacillin, mezlocillin, or azlocillin. Ticarcillin has greater potency than carbenicillin against the highly pathogenic and difficult gram-negative bacilli, such as Pseudomonas species. Piperacillin, mezlocillin, and azlocillin, extended spectrum relatives of carbenicillin, are often used in combination with the aminoglycosides.

Adverse Effects/Precautions. Hypersensitivity reactions may occur with the extended spectrum carbenicillin-like penicillins. Due to their high sodium content (1 g of carbenicillin contains 6 meq of Na$^+$), these antibiotics in high doses may cause sodium overload in renal and cardiac patients.

Cephalosporins. The cephalosporins are beta-lactam antibiotics that act to inhibit the biosynthesis of the bacterial cell wall. These antibiotics are derivatives of 7-aminocephalosporinic acid compared to the parent nucleus of penicillin, 6-aminopenicillanic acid. The antibacterial spectrum of the "first generation" cephalosporins (cephalothin, cephapirin, cephalexin, and cefazolin) resembles the penicillinase-resistant penicillins. Hemophilus influenzae is especially sensitive to cefaclor and cefamandole, "second generation" cephalosporins.

The "third generation" or most recently developed cephalosporins include moxalactam, cefadroxil, and cefotaxime. These antibiotics are more active than the earlier cephalosporins against a wide spectum of gram-negative organisms and thus resemble the extended spectrum penicillins.

Mechanism of Action. Cephalosporins bind to the transpeptidase responsible for the crosslinking of peptidoglycans in the bacterial cell wall in the same manner as the penicillins. Generally speaking, a loss of gram-positive efficacy with increased effectiveness against gram-negative and resistant organisms characterizes the progression from first to third generation. Cefoxitin (a cephamycin) and moxalactam (a beta-lactam) are included with the cephalosporins because of their structural pharmacologic similarity.

Clinical Indications. Most cephalosporins are effective in the treatment of respiratory infections (such as tonsillitis, pharyngitis, and lobar pneumonia) caused by Streptococcus pneumoniae and Group A beta-hemolytic streptococci.

Adverse Effects/Precautions. The cephalosporins share the toxicity profile of the penicillins. Common adverse effects are hypersensitivity reactions; gastrointestinal disturbances occur most frequently with oral administration of these drugs. Rash, fever, eosinophilia, SGOT elevation, neutropenia, and anaphylactoid reactions are also possible. Pseudomembraneous colitis, attributed to Clostridia overgrowth, may occur due to alteration of the normal colon flora.

Cycloserine. Structurally similar to D-alanine, cycloserine is an amino acid critical to bacterial cell wall synthesis.

Mechanism of Action. In bacterial cell wall synthesis, a conversion of L-alanine to D-alanine is the important initial reaction in the formation of the dipeptide D-alanyl-D-alanine. This conversion or racemization step is followed by dipeptide formation through the action of D-alanyl-D-alanine synthetase. Cycloserine inhibits both the racemase and synthetase reactions.

The similarity in structure of cycloserine to D-alanine explains the drug-enzyme binding to the D-alanine enzyme site. A preferential binding factor of 100 in favor of the cycloserine-enzyme binding makes the drug an effective blocker of the synthesis of the pentapeptide precursor of bacterial cell wall synthesis.

Clinical Indications. Cycloserine is used only in the treatment of tuberculosis, especially in resistant cases.

Adverse Effects/Precautions. Adverse reactions to cycloserine include headache, psychosis, and seizures. Allergic skin rash is also possible.

Vancomycin. Vancomycin, a glycopeptide antibiotic, is obtained from Streptomyces orientalis isolated from Indonesian and Indian soil samples.

Mechanism of Action. Vancomycin binds to the D-alanyl-D-alanine precursor sites to hinder polymerization of peptidoglycans.

Clinical Indications. Parenteral vancomycin is used to treat severe staphylococcal pneumonia (including methicillin-resistant strains). Serious systemic infections in patients allergic to both the penicillins and cephalosporins respond well to vancomycin.

Adverse Effects/Precautions. "Red neck syndrome," characterized by chills, fever, paresthesias, and erythema of the neck and back, is a specific adverse reaction sometimes encountered with vancomycin. This drug is administered intravenously because of its irritation to tissues; also, IM injections of vancomycin cause pain and necrosis. Ototoxicity and nephrotoxicity may occur with this drug.

Bacitracin. Obtained from a special strain of Bacillus subtilus, bacitracin is a polypeptide antibiotic. In 1943, the Tracy-I strain of Bacillus subtilus was isolated from the damaged tissue and street dirt present in a compound fracture in a girl named Tracy.

Mechanism of Action. Bacitracin inhibits the polymerization of peptidoglycans by blocking regeneration of carrier phospholipid that is necessary for the formation of the bacterial cell wall.

Clinical Indications. Bacitracin is ordinarily used only for topical (skin) infections. The use of IM bacitracin is limited to the treatment of infants with pneumonia and empyema caused by staphylococci with known sensitivity to the drug.

Adverse Effects/Precautions. Bacitracin, given intramuscularly, may cause renal failure due to tubular and glomerular necrosis. Careful monitoring of renal function is necessary during parenteral bacitracin therapy.

Isoniazid. Isoniazid (isonicotinic acid hydrazide, INH) is considered as a primary agent in the treatment of tuberculosis.

Mechanism of Action. Isoniazid inhibits the biosynthesis of mycolic acids, important constituents of the mycobacterial cell wall. Mycolic acids are unique to mycobacteria, a fact that may explain the high degree of cytoxic specificity for isoniazid. This drug also elicits its bactericidal action by inhibiting lipid and nucleic acid synthesis in the reproducing organism.

Clinical Indications. Isoniazid is used to treat pulmonary tuberculosis; both isoniazid and rifampin are considered as primary first-line drugs in the treatment of this disease.

Adverse Effects/Precautions. Among the reported adverse reactions are rash, fever, jaundice, and peripheral neuritis. The most frequent toxic effects occur on the CNS and liver.

Pyridoxine (vitamin B_6) deficiency is occasionally noted in patients taking high doses of isoniazid; also, peripheral neuritis may occur in 10 to 20% of isonoazid recipients if prophylactic pyridoxine is not given. Severe and sometimes fatal hepatitis has been associated with isoniazid therapy; the risk of hepatitis apparently increases with the daily consumption of alcohol.

ANTIBACTERIAL DRUGS THAT AFFECT PROTEIN SYNTHESIS

Protein biosynthesis begins at the amino end and proceeds in sequence to the carboxy terminal of the finished protein. Initiation starts with the formation of a complex that consists of the 30S (mRNA, messenger RNA) ribosomal subunit and three initiator proteins designated as F1, F2, and F3 (Figure 7.8). The mRNA-30S subunit complex, along with initiation factors F1 and F2, guanosine triphosphate (GTP), and Mg^{++}, binds to N-formylmethionyl tRNA (a special initiation transfer RNA) at the initiation codon (AUG) on mRNA. The anticodon triplet is put into the proper position relative to the starting signal (AUG) with the aid of the third initiation factor, F3. The 50S subunit then associates to form the complete 70S ribosomal complex.

Elongation of the peptide chain begins with the codon-directed binding of the first aminoacyl tRNA to the acceptor site after attachment of the initiation unit, formylmethionyl tRNA. A new peptide bond forms when the alpha-amino group of aminoacyl tRNA reacts with the activated carboxy terminal residue of the peptidyl tRNA. Translocation of the newly synthesized peptidyl tRNA and mRNA from acceptor to donor site must occur so that the acceptor site can again accept the next incoming aminoacyl tRNA that contains the appropriate triplet codon.

Termination of the peptide chain begins with recognition of a signal in the mRNA and ends when the full 70S ribosome separates from the mRNA and dissociates into its component 30S and 50S subunits. The 30S and 50S components are then available for re-entry into the cycle; Figure 7.9 summarizes this process of bacterial protein synthesis.

AMINOGLYCOSIDES

Neomycin, streptomycin, kanamycin, gentamicin, tobramycin, amikacin, and netilmicin are members of the aminoglycoside group of antibiotics that inhibit bacterial protein synthesis. Each of the aminoglycosides consists of two or more amino sugars that are joined by glycosidic linkage to a central hexose nucleus. These drugs are bactericidal agents routinely used to treat serious infections caused by numerous gram-negative bacilli and some gram-positive organisms. Streptococci, pneumonococci, clostridia, anaerobes, and fungi are resistant to the aminoglycosides. The principal clinical use of the aminoglycosides is in the treatment of infections caused by Pseudomonas, Escherichia coli, Proteus, Klebsiella, and Enterobacter.

The aminoglycosides have similar pharmacologic and bactericidal profiles. As these antibiotics are poorly absorbed by the oral route, they are usually administered intravenously or intramuscularly (except neomycin).

Streptomycin. Streptomycin was isolated as the result of a structured, well-planned search for antibiotics. In 1943, Waksman discovered a strain of Streptomyces griseus that synthesized a potent antibacterial substance, appropriately designated as streptomycin. Thus, streptomycin's availability for the past four decades accounts for the extensive therapeutic and toxicologic data accumulated on aminoglycosides in general and on this antibiotic in particular.

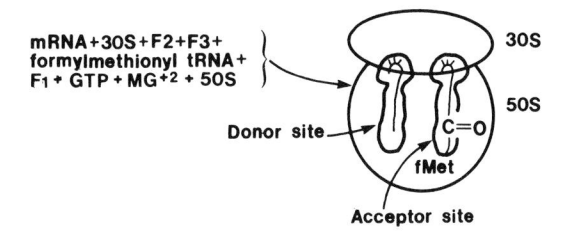

Fig. 7.8 Initiation step of bacterial protein synthesis. (From Gringuaz, A.: Drugs. How They Act and Why. St. Louis, C.V. Mosby, 1978.)

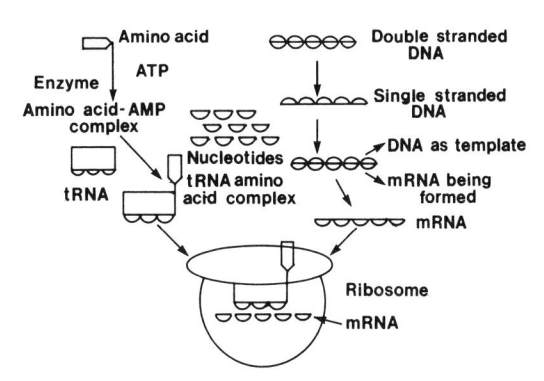

Fig. 7.9 Protein synthesis. (From Gringuaz, A.: Drugs. How They Act and Why. St. Louis, C.V. Mosby, 1978.)

Mechanism of Action. Streptomycin inhibits bacterial protein synthesis by interfering with the binding of bacterial aminoacyl tRNA to the 30S ribosomal subunit.

Clinical Indications. The main clinical value of streptomycin is in the treatment of tuberculosis. Resistance to streptomycin may occur rapidly due to induction by R factors.

Adverse Effects/Precautions. Ototoxicity and nephrotoxicity are direct toxic effects induced by streptomycin. Neuromuscular blockade, resulting in aggravation of myasthenia gravis, is another adverse effect of this antibiotic. An exacerbation of the muscle relaxant property occurs with certain general anesthetics and neuromuscular blocking agents employed in surgical procedures.

One form of resistance to streptomycin's antibacterial action relates to enzyme induction. Specifically, streptomycin is rendered inactive as an antibacterial when R factors induce enzymes that acetylate or phosphorylate the drug. Resistance occurs more rapidly with streptomycin than with the other aminoglycosides. Resistance to streptomycin is also acquired by a single mutational step.

Gentamicin. Gentamicin is currently the aminoglycoside antibiotic used most frequently. The -micin suffix (rather than -mycin) denotes the source as Micromonospora purpura (instead of a Streptomyces species).

Mechanism of Action. By binding to the 30S ribosomal subunit, gentamicin inhibits bacterial protein synthesis.

Clinical Indications. Gentamicin is an important antibiotic in the treatment of serious gram-negative bacillary infections (including pneumonia and otitis). The drug is effective in infections caused by sensitive strains of Pseudomonas aeruginosa, Proteus species, Escherichia coli, Klebsiella-Enterobacter-Serratia species, Citrobacter, and Staphylococcus species. On the other hand, gentamicin is totally ineffective in treating pneumonia caused by Streptococcus pneumoniae, the most common community-acquired pneumonia.

Adverse Effects/Precautions. A serious adverse reaction to gentamicin is ototoxicity; the direct toxic effects are manifested by both vestibular and auditory dysfunction. Nephrotoxicity is another important adverse effect of gentamicin therapy.

Other side effects that resemble those of streptomycin include nausea, vomiting, headache, an increase in serum transaminases (SGOT), and transient macular rashes.

Tobramycin. Tobramycin and gentamicin have similar structural and pharmacologic properties and toxicity profiles. The main difference between these drugs is the greater potency of tobramycin in Pseudomonas aeruginosa infections.

Kanamycin. Kanamycin, an aminoglycoside antibiotic with a limited spectrum of action and a toxicity profile similar to that of streptomycin, is primarily used parenterally against serious gram-negative bacilli infections.

Amikacin. Effective in gram-negative bacterial infections, amikacin is a semisynthetic aminoglycoside derived from kanamycin.

Netilmicin. Netilmicin is a semisynthetic aminoglycoside antibiotic derived from sisomicin. Available in a parenteral form, this drug is used in the short-term treatment of patients with serious or life-threatening gram-negative bacterial infections. The same warnings and precautions for other injectable aminoglycosides also apply to netilmicin.

TETRACYCLINES

The tetracyclines, commonly referred to as broad-spectrum antibiotics, are derivatives of the polycyclic (4 rings) structure, naphthacenecarboxamide. The initial tetracyclines, introduced in 1947, were developed as a result of extensive screening of antibiotics from soil organisms. Chlortetracycline (derived from Streptomyces aureofaciens), oxytetracycline (obtained from Streptomyces rimosus), and tetracycline (a semisynthetic antibiotic derived from chlortetracycline) were the first clinically available tetracyclines. Demeclocycline is obtained from a mutant strain of Streptomyces aureofaciens; methacycline, doxycycline, and minocycline are all semisynthetic tetracyclines.

Mechanism of Action. Tetracyclines are more specific for passage through bacterial plasma membranes, compared to mammalian plasma membranes, because of their ability to chelate Mg^{++} in the bacterial membrane. Inhibition of bacterial protein synthesis results from the interaction with the 30S ribosomal subunit. The drug-30S subunit combination prevents the binding of aminoacyl tRNA to the acceptor site on the ribosome; this drug-30S subunit binding is reversible. At usual therapeutic doses, the tetracyclines are bacteriostatic. They also have similar antimicrobial spectra and cross-resistance among them is common.

Clinical Indications. Tetracyclines are widely used in the treatment of infections caused by Mycoplasma pneumoniae (PPLO), Hemophilus influenzae, and respiratory disease resultant from rickettsiae and the agents of psittacosis and ornithosis. Extremely lipid-soluble, doxycycline and minocycline readily penetrate into the cerebral spinal fluid, the eye, and the prostate. Oxytetracycline is the least lipid soluble tetracycline. Minocycline readily enters the saliva and is effective in the treatment of asymptomatic carriers of Neisseria meningitidis to eliminate meningococci from the nasopharynx. Since doxycycline is not significantly dependent upon the kidney for excretion, this tetracycline is useful in patients with impaired renal function. Also, doxycycline's slower elimination allows for its administration at less frequent intervals.

Tetracyclines should generally be taken with a full glass of water on an empty stomach; however, doxycycline and minocycline may be taken with milk or food.

Adverse Effects/Precautions. Superinfection by bacterial or fungal organisms may result in secondary infection. The development of serious staphylococcal gastroenteritis is sometimes life-threatening.

Side effects include gastrointestinal distress (oral administration may precipitate esophageal ulcers), skin rash, and abnormal development of enamel deposition in teeth ("mottled"teeth). Tetracyclines are also taken up by chelation in bone. Other adverse effects include a negative nitrogen balance and hepatatoxicity. Antianabolic action has also occurred with high doses of tetracyclines.

All tetracyclines may induce photosensitivity; demeclocycline is the one most likely to cause severe phototoxic reactions. Thus, avoidance of exposure to sunlight or sunlamps is recommended. Minocycline sometimes produces severe vertigo and nausea.

MACROLIDES

The macrolide antibiotics are large molecular weight compounds with long chain aliphatic acid lactone rings that are attached to one or more drug sugars by glycosidic linkage. The macrolides, which are bactericidal or bacteriostatic at therapeutic concentrations, include erythromycin and troleanomycin (triacetylloleanomycin).

Erythromycin. Erythromycin was discovered in 1952 as a metabolic product in a strain of Streptomyces erythreus. The soil sample examined was collected in the Phillipine Archipelago.

Mechanism of Action. Erythromycin binds to the 50S ribosomal subunit and thereby inhibits bacterial protein synthesis in susceptible organisms. The interaction between erythromycin and the ribosome is reversible and occurs only when the 50S subunit is free from tRNA molecules from the early-formed peptide chains. Thus, erythromycin does not affect the production of small peptides, but it inhibits the synthesis of highly polymerized homopeptides.

Clinical Indications. Erythromycin is effective in pneumonococci and Mycoplasma pneumoniae infections; infections of the lower respiratory tract; and in the treatment of acute bacterial pharyngitis, tonsillitis, and otitis media, including those caused by Hemophilus influenzae.

The estolate ester of erythromycin rapidly penetrates the bacterial cell and is hydrolyzed to the active moiety. The estolate ester is also more acid resistant and is orally absorbed more efficiently than other erythromycin forms. Erythromycin ethylsuccinate is another ester that is adequately absorbed following oral administration.

Erythromycin is recommended for the treatment of pneumonia caused by Legionella pneumophila or L. micdadei (Legionnaire's disease). Another of its uses is to eliminate the carrier state in pertussis (whooping cough) and diphtheria.

Adverse Effects/Precautions. Reported allergic reactions include fever, eosinophilia, and skin eruptions. Cholestatic jaundice occurs primarily with erythromycin estolate. Large doses of oral erythromycin may produce epigastric distress. Transient hearing impairment sometimes results from large IV doses of the gluceptate or lactobionate or from extremely high oral doses of the estolate.

Troleandomycin. Troleandomycin, a macrolide antibiotic, acts against Streptococcus pyogenes and Streptococcus pneumoniae.

Mechanism of Action. Troleandomycin inhibits bacterial protein biosynthesis by binding with the 50S ribosomal subunit.

Clinical Indications. Troleandomycin is indicated in pneumonococcal pneumonia caused by susceptible strains of Streptococcus pneumoniae and for Group A beta-hemolytic streptococcal infections of the upper respiratory tract.

Adverse Effects/Precautions. Frequent adverse reactions to this drug are abdominal cramping and discomfort. Allergic cholestatic hepatitis may also occur with troleandomycin use.

LINCOMYCIN AND STRUCTURALLY RELATED ANTIBIOTICS

Lincomycin, the first commercially available lincosamide antibiotic, was isolated from Streptomyces lincolnensis contained in a soil sample collected near Lincoln, Nebraska. Clindamycin, closely related to lincomycin, has replaced lincomycin because of the former's greater activity and fewer adverse reactions.

Clindamycin. A congener of lincomycin, clindamycin differs only in a chlorine substitution of the 7-methyl group.

Mechanism of Action. Clindamycin, which is bactericidal or bacteriostatic, binds exclusively to the 50S ribosomal subunit and thereby inhibits bacterial protein synthesis.

Clinical Indications. Clindamycin is indicated in severe anaerobic respiratory infections, such as empyema, anaerobic pneumonia, and lung abscess. Serious streptococcal, staphylococcal, and pneumonococcal respiratory infections are additional indications for clindamycin therapy. This drug should be reserved for serious infections in which less toxic antimicrobial agents are inappropriate.

Adverse Effects/Precautions. Severe pseudomembranous colitis (sometimes fatal) has developed in some patients receiving clindamycin. Persistent, severe diarrhea and abdominal cramps, as well as possible fecal passage of blood and mucus, clinically characterize this disease.

Adverse effects include gastrointestinal irritation, neutropenia, eosinophilia, rashes, and elevated serum glutamic-oxaloacetic transaminase (SGOT).

Rifampin. The rifamycins are a group of macrocyclic antibiotics that are isolated from Streptomyces mediterranei. Rifampin is a semisynthetic derivative of rifamycin B.

Mechanism of Action. Rifampin, which inhibits nucleic acid synthesis in mycobacteria and other micro-organisms, interacts with DNA-dependent RNA polymerase to block chain formation in RNA synthesis. Protein synthesis is thus reduced in susceptible organisms.

Clinical Indications. Rifampin is used concurrently with at least one additional antituberculosis drug to treat pulmonary tuberculosis. Another of rifampin's clinical indications is in the treatment of asymptomatic carriers of Neisseria meningitidis.

Adverse Effects/Precautions. Nausea, vomiting, rash, and fever are common adverse reactions to rifampin. Jaundice has been reported in elderly patients and those with concurrent hepatic disease. A potent inducer of hepatic microsomal enzymes, rifampin decreases the activity of many drugs by speeding their metabolism.

ANTIBACTERIAL DRUGS THAT ACT PRIMARILY AS ANTIMETABOLITES

Drugs may block the action of vital bacterial metabolites to elicit a cytotoxic effect on the microorganism.

SULFONAMIDES

Sulfonamides were the first effective systemic chemotherapeutic agents used in the prophylaxis and treatment of bacterial infections. These drugs have a broad antibacterial spectrum that includes both gram-positive and gram-negative organisms.

Sulfonamides, structural analogs and competitive antagonists of para-aminobenzoic acid (PABA), prevent the bacterial utilization of PABA for the synthesis of folic acid. Organisms that require exogenous folic acid and do not synthesize it are not sensitive to PABA inhibition.

Certain sulfonamides are combined with a penicillin or erythromycin to treat otitis media caused by Hemophilus influenzae. However, the major clinical utility of sulfonamides is in the treatment of urinary tract infections; Chapter 9 contains a discussion of the therapeutic characteristics of these drugs.

Ethambutol. Ethambutol is an orally effective chemotherapeutic agent that is used in the treatment of tuberculosis.

Mechanism of Action. Ethambutol apparently inhibits the synthesis of one or more essential metabolites in Myobacterium species, including Myobacterium tuberculosis.

Clinical Indications. Ethambutol is used concurrently with at least one other antituberculosis drug in the treatment of pulmonary tuberculosis.

Adverse Reactions/Precautions. Ethambutol, which has essentially replaced aminosalicylic acid in tuberculosis chemotherapy, may cause decreases in visual acuity due to optic neuritis; patients receiving this drug may also lose their ability to differentiate red from green. These ocular side effects are generally reversible, but recovery may take as long as 1 year. Other adverse reactions include pruritus, joint pain, gastrointestinal distress, abdominal pain, and confusion.

AMINOSALICYCLIC ACID (PARA-AMINOSALICYCLIC ACID; PAS)

Due to its structural similarity to para-aminobenzoic acid (PABA), aminosalicyclic acid acts as an antimetabolite in bacterial metabolism. More active and less toxic drugs are preferred over aminosalicyclic acid in antituberculosis therapy.

ANTIMICROBIAL DRUGS THAT ALTER PLASMA MEMBRANE PERMEABILITY

Certain antibiotics change the permeability characteristics of the bacterial plasma membrane to allow essential metabolites to leak out.

Polymyxin B. Polymyxin B is a cationic, basic peptide antibiotic that is isolated from various strains of Bacillus polymyxa.

Mechanism of Action. Polymyxin B, a surface-active agent, has an intramolecular separation of lipophilic and lipophobic groups. After interacting with the bacterial plasma membrane phospholipids, this drug then penetrates into the structure. A disruption of the structural integrity of the plasma membrane occurs with the subsequent leakage of essential substances out of the organism.

Clinical Indications. Polymyxin B is indicated for treatment of respiratory infections that are caused by susceptible strains of Pseudomonas aeruginosa. Carbenicillin and gentamicin have largely replaced the use of Polymyxin B, except in resistant infections.

Adverse Effects/Precautions. The most significant adverse reaction to polymyxin B is nephrotoxicity; pain is also common after IM injection. Facial flushing, dizziness, paresthesias, and generalized weakness may occur.

Miconazole. Miconazole, a synthetic imidazole derivative, has broad-spectrum antifungal activity.

Mechanism of Action. By altering the permeability of the fungal plasma membrane, miconazole exerts its fungicidal effect.

Clinical Indications. Miconazole is used in the treatment of systemic coccidioidomycosis, candidiasis, petriellidosis, paracoccidioidomycosis, and cryptococcosis. Miconazole should be given by IV infusion.

Adverse Effects/Precautions. Adverse effects include nausea, vomiting, thrombocytopenia, and fever. Integumentary reactions, such as phlebitis, pruritus, and rash, may necessitate discontinuation of treatment with miconazole.

Ketoconazole. Ketoconazole is a broad-spectrum imidazole antifungal drug.

Mechanism of Action. Ketoconazole inhibits the synthesis of ergosterol, a prime fungal plasma membrane constituent, thereby increasing permeability and leakage of essential cellular components.

Clinical Indications. Ketoconazole is used in systemic fungal infections including oral thrush, blastomycosis, coccidioidomycosis, histoplasmosis, and paracoccidioidomycosis.

Adverse Effects/Precautions. Ketoconazole has been associated with hepatotoxicity, including some fatalities. Frequent adverse reactions are gastrointestinal complaints, including nausea, vomiting, and abdominal pain.

Amphotericin B. Obtained from Streptomyces nodusus, amphotericin B is a polyene antibiotic that has broad-spectrum antifungal activity.

Mechanism of Action. Amphotericin B binds to sterols in the fungus plasma membrane to alter its permeability. Essential metabolites then leak out, resulting in a fungistatic or fungicidal effect. A possible explanation for the joint host-fungus toxicity is that mammalian cells also contain sterols.

Clinical Indications. Amphotericin B is frequently the sole effective treatment of potentially fatal fungal infections. This drug is used to treat systemic fungal infections, including cryptococcosis, North American blastomycosis, disseminated candidiasis, coccidiodomycosis, and histoplasmosis.

Adverse Effects/Precautions. Practically all patients receiving amphotericin B show some toxic effects: fever, chills, headache, anorexia, and generalized pain of the muscles and joints. Renal function is impaired in more than 80% of the patients on this drug therapy that also frequently produces normochronic, normocytic anemia. Hospitalization is necessary for all patients receiving amphotericin B.

DRUGS USED IN RESPIRATORY TRACT OBSTRUCTION

Certain drugs (Table 7.7) act to improve breathing and ventilation by dilating bronchioles, altering viscosity of respiratory secretions, and reducing nonproductive coughing.

BRONCHODILATORS

Chapter 2 contains a complete discussion of the beta-adrenergic agonists, including epinephrine, ephedrine, isoproterenol, albuterol, and terbutaline, whose mechanism of action involves increasing the levels of intracellular cyclic AMP in the bronchiole smooth muscle to induce bronchodilation. Increased cyclic AMP enhances binding of Ca^{++} to the cell membrane and endoplasmic reticulum, thereby reducing myoplasmic Ca^{++}. The smooth muscles of the bronchioles are consequently relaxed due to the reduction of free Ca^{++} for the contractile elements. Beta-adrenergic agonists also increase cilial beat frequency and reduce mucous gland secretion and mast cell degranulation.

The methylxanthines, such as theophylline and aminophylline, increase intracellular cyclic AMP by inhibiting phosphodiesterase. Thus, the effectiveness of both groups of drugs is

Table 7.7. DRUGS USED IN RESPIRATORY TRACT OBSTRUCTION.

Available products	Trade names	Daily dosage range
Bronchodilator drugs		
Adrenergic Type (also see Table 2.7):		
Albuterol	Proventil; Ventolin	Oral, 2 or 4 mg t.i.d. or q.i.d.
Ephedrine sulfate	Ephedrine Sulfate	25–50 mg, oral
Epinephrine	Adrenalin Chloride; Vaponefrin; others	0.2–0.5 mg SC or IM
Ethylnorepinephrine HCl	Bronkephrine	SC or IM, 0.5–1.0 ml
Isoetharine HCl	Arm-a-Med; Dispos-a-Med; others	Variable
Isoproterenol HCl	Isuprel; Aerolone	Inhal. of 1 : 100 or 1 : 200 solution; 10–15 mg, subling.
Metaproterenol sulfate	Alupent; Metaprel	2 or 3 inhal. every 3 or 4 hrs; 20 mg orally t.i.d. or q.i.d.
Terbutaline sulfate	Brethine; Bricanyl	5 mg orally t.i.d. at 6 hr intervals; SC, 0.25 mg
Theophylline or Methylxanthine Type:		
Aminophylline	Aminophylline; Amoline; others	Variable
Dyphylline	Dilor; Lufyllin; Neothylline	Up to 15 mg/kg; 250–500 mg IM
Oxtriphylline	Choledyl	200 mg q.i.d.
Theophylline	Elixophyllin; Slo-Phyllin; Theo-Dur; others	Variable
Theophylline sodium glycinate	Synophylate	330–660 mg q. 6–8 hrs
Expectorants		
Ammonium chloride	—	300 mg orally
Guaifenesin	Glycotuss; Hytuss; Robitussin; others	100–400 mg q. 4–6 hrs
Iodinated glycerol	Organidan	30–60 mg
Ipecac	—	0.5–2 ml orally
Potassium iodide	—	300 mg orally
Sodium iodide	—	300 mg orally
Terpin hydrate	—	85 mg q. 2–4 hrs
Mucolytic agents		
Acetylcysteine	Mucomyst	1–10 ml of 20% solution by nebulizer; 1–2 ml by instillation
Corticosteroids		
Beclomethasone diproprionate	Vanceril; Beclovent	2 inhalations: 0.8 mg t.i.d. or q.i.d.
Dexamethasone sodium phosphate	Decadron Phosphate; Respihaler	3 inhalations t.i.d. or q.i.d.
Hydrocortisone sodium phosphate	Hydrocortisone Phosphate	Variable
Hydrocortisone sodium succinate	Solu-Cortef; A-hydroCort	100–500 mg IV or IM
Methylprednisolone sodium succinate	Solu-Medrol; A-methaPred	10–40 mg IV
Prednisolone sodium phosphate	Hydeltrasol; others	4–60 mg IV or IM
Triamcinolone Acetonide	Azmacort	2 inhalations t.i.d. or q.i.d.

based upon the common property of increasing intracellular cyclic AMP levels.

XANTHINE DERIVATIVES

Xanthine derivatives include theophylline preparations that relax the smooth muscle of the bronchi and pulmonary blood vessels. Additionally, theophylline preparations may stimulate the CNS (including the respiratory center), induce diuresis, and produce weak positive cardiac chronotropic and inotropic effects.

Mechanism of Action. Theophylline inhibits phosphodiesterase in a competitive manner, resulting in an increase of cyclic AMP. Endogenous epinephrine is released in response to this cyclic AMP elevation. Theophylline (by its effect on cyclic AMP) may inhibit the release of slow reacting substance of anaphylaxis (SRS-A) and histamine.

Clinical Indications. The theophylline salts and its derivative, dyphylline, are used for the symptomatic relief or prevention of bronchial asthma. These preparations are also used to treat reversible bronchospasm associated with chronic bronchitis and emphysema.

Theophylline is adequately absorbed from the gastrointestinal tract and the clearance rate determines the drug's dosage. Aminophylline (theophylline ethylenediamine) is administered either by slow IV injection, orally, or rectally. Oxitriphylline (more soluble than theophylline) is readily absorbed after oral administration.

Adverse Effects/Precautions. Blood levels of theophylline slightly over the therapeutic serum range may produce nausea, vomiting, diarrhea, headache, insomnia, and irritability. Higher blood concentrations may lead to hyperglycemia, hypotension, cardiac arrhythmias, and tachycardia. Convulsions, shock, and death have resulted from excessive blood levels of aminophylline, as may occur with IV administration.

ANTICHOLINERGIC, ANTIMUSCARINIC BRONCHODILATOR DRUGS

Ipratropium Bromide. Ipratropium bromide (Atrovent[R]) is a poorly absorbed bronchodilator that is administered by inhalation aerosol.

Mechanism of Action. Ipratropium antagonizes the action of acetylcholine at parasympathetic, postganglionic effector cells by competing with acetylcholine for receptor sites. This antimuscarinic action results in bronchodilation.

Clinical Indications. Ipratropium is used primarily as a bronchodilator in chronic bronchitis and emphysema. It is also indicated for asthma patients who find adrenergic agonists unsuitable (i.e., poor control, adverse effects).

Adverse Effects/Precautions. Because of its poor systemic absorption, ipratropium is relatively free of side effects. However, adverse effects reported include cough, nausea, palpitations, and dry mouth.

MUCOLYTIC DRUGS

Mucolytic drugs (expectorants) alter sputum viscosity and/or increase the volume of respiratory fluids to facilitate expectoration.

Acetylcysteine (N-acetylcysteine). Acetylcysteine, a nebulized mucolytic agent, loosens viscid sputum and improves expectoration.

Mechanism of Action. The viscosity of pulmonary mucous secretions relates to the concentration of mucoprotein in the secretory fluid, the presence of disulfide bonding between the mucoproteins, and, to some extent, DNA. The mucolytic action of acetylcysteine depends upon the sulfhydry group in its structure that acts to cleave disulfide linkages. This results in depolymerization of the mucoprotein complexes and a decrease in mucus viscosity. Liquefaction occurs shortly (1 minute) after inhalation with a maximal effect happening after 5 to 10 minutes.

Clinical Indications. Acetylcysteine is used as an adjunct in the treatment of chronic respiratory disorders such as emphysema, emphysema with bronchitis, and asthmatic bronchitis. Acute respiratory conditions, including pneumonia and tracheobronchitis, are also amenable to acetylcysteine, as are the respiratory complications of cystic fibrosis.

Adverse Effects/Precautions. Although adverse effects are infrequent with acetylcysteine, bronchospasm, stomatitis, severe bronchorrhea and rhinorrhea, nausea, and vomiting may occur.

Guaifenesin (Glyceryl Guiacolate). Guaifenesin is an expectorant commonly found in proprietary cough/cold mixtures.

Mechanism of Action. Guaifenesin enhances the output of respiratory tract fluid by reducing its adhesiveness and surface tension. A reflex initiated by irritation of the stomach apparently mediates this action.

Clinical Indications. Guaifenesin may assist in the symptomatic relief of dry, unproductive coughs and the presence of mucus in the respiratory tract.

Adverse Effects/Precautions. Nausea, vomiting, and gastric disturbances may occur with this drug.

Terpin Hydrate. Terpin hydrate is a bitter, colorless, crystalline compound sometimes used in chronic cough. The favored clinical preparation is terpin hydrate elixir.

Mechanism of Action. Terpin hydrate acts by direct stimulation of respiratory tract secretory glands to increase the fluid output.

Clinical Indications. Terpin hydrate is used for the symptomatic relief of coughs due to colds and minor bronchial irritations.

Adverse Effects/Precautions. Terpin hydrate elixir, due to its high alcohol content, may cause drowsiness. Epigastric pain sometimes occurs, especially on an empty stomach.

Iodine Products. Potassium iodide, iodinated glycerol, and hydriotic acid are active expectorants.

Mechanism of Action. Iodides enhance the secretion of respiratory fluid, thereby decreasing the viscosity. The iodides may promote the breakdown of fibrinoid material in inflammatory exudates.

Clinical Indications. Iodide products are potentially useful in the symptomatic treatment of chronic pulmonary diseases that are complicated by tenacious mucus. These conditions include bronchial asthma, chronic bronchitis, and pulmonary emphysema.

Adverse Effects/Precautions. Thyroid adenoma, goiter, and myxedema are possible with use of the iodine products, as are hypersensitivity reactions. Metallic taste, stomatitis, increased salivation, ulceration of mucous membranes, and gastric disturbances indicate chronic iodide poisoning that occurs with prolonged therapy. More advanced chronic iodide poisoning is manifested by headache, pulmonary edema, swelling and tenderness of the salivary glands, and severe skin eruptions.

CORTICOSTEROIDS

Corticosteroids (see Chapter 6) are sometimes used in allergic rhinitis. At the height of the pollen season, an aerosol of dexamethasone, or a similar agent, suppresses inflammation of the nasal mucosa in patients with seasonal allergic rhinitis.

Oral administration of prednisone or methylprednisone on a count-down regimen is generally considered safe for treating seasonal allergic rhinitis. A high loading dose, with subsequent reductions in doses over a period of about 5 days, appears safe and rarely produces the adverse effects seen when corticosteroids (Table 7.7) are taken for prolonged periods.

NASAL DECONGESTANTS

Sympathomimetics (see Chapter 2), such as phenylpropanolamine and pseudoephedrine, are often used alone or in combination with an antihistamine to treat nasal congestion and associated symptoms of allergic rhinitis. The effectiveness of oral antihistamine-decongestant mixtures in the treatment of otitis media in children remains controversial.

ANTITUSSIVES

Although antitussives (Table 7.8) are defined as drugs that are effective against coughs or that suppress coughs, they are often used in conjunction with expectorants, i.e., drugs that promote removal of respiratory material (sputum). Antitussives (such as codeine and dextromethorphan) usually act by depressing the medullary cough center in the CNS.

Table 7.8. ANTITUSSIVES.

Available products	Trade names	Daily dosage range
Centrally acting antitussives		
Narcotic Antitussive-Analgesics:		
Codeine	Codeine Sulfate; Codeine Phosphate	10–20 mg q. 4–6 hrs
Hydrocodone bitartrate	Dicodid	5 mg q. 4–6 hrs
Non-narcotic Antitussives:		
Chlophedianol HCl	Ulo	25 mg t.i.d. or q.i.d.
Dextromethorphan HBr	Chloraseptic; Cough Control; Sucrets Cough Control; others	10–30 mg q. 4–8 hrs
Diphenhydramine HCl	Diphen Cough; Noradryl Cough; others	25 mg q. 4 hrs
Noscapine	Tusscapine	15–30 mg at 4–6 hr intervals
Peripherally acting antitussives		
Expectorants, Demulcents, and Vehicles:		
Acacia Syrup	—	—
Ammonium chloride	—	300 mg
Benzonatate	Tessalon Perles	100–600 mg
Glycyrrhiza Syrup	Licorice Syrup	—
Guaifenesin	Glycotuss; Hytuss; Robitussin; others	100 mg
Ipecac Syrup	In Ipsatol	5 ml
Honey	—	—
Hydriodic Acid Syrup	—	5 ml
Potasssium iodide	—	300 mg
Sodium iodide	—	100 mg
Terpin hydrate	—	85 mg q. 2–4 hrs
Tolu Balsam Syrup	—	—
White Pine Syrup	—	—
Wild Cherry Syrup	—	—

The pharmacologic properties of codeine, a narcotic opioid, are discussed in Chapter 1. Dextromethorphan is a non-narcotic antitussive; however, it is a potential drug of abuse, as is codeine. Physical dependence is not a problem with antitussive use of these drugs, but massive doses of either can cause respiratory depression.

DRUGS USED IN LUNG CARCINOMA

Chemotherapy for lung carcinoma includes combinations of the following drugs: cyclophosphamide, doxorubicin, vincristine, etoposide, cisplatin, methotrexate, and lomustine. Chapter 4 contains a detailed discussion of these agents. Ordinarily, chemotherapy is used in combination with surgery and/or radiotherapy in the treatment of lung carcinoma.

DRUG INTERACTIONS

Concurrent use of two or more anti-infectives often compounds an adverse reaction common to the individual drugs. Also, potential antagonism of the penicillins' bacteriocidal action may occur with concomitant use of antibiotics (e.g., tetracyclines) that block protein synthesis.

AMINOGLYCOSIDES

Amphotericin B. Combined use of amphotericin B and gentamicin may produce renal function deterioration.

Cephalosporins. Gentamicin and cephalothin evidently have additive nephrotoxic effects in some predisposed patients.

Ethacrynic Acid. The ototoxicity produced by ethacrynic acid possibly adds to or potentiates the ototoxicity of aminoglycoside antibiotics.

Neuromuscular Blocking Agents. Kanamycin, tobramycin, gentamicin, neomycin, and streptomycin all produce neuromuscular blockade. Thus, enhanced blockade of skeletal muscle relaxants is possible with concomitant use of neuromuscular blocking agents and aminoglycoside antibiotics.

ANTIHISTAMINES

Ethanol; CNS Depressants. Additive depressant effects occur with concomitant use of antihistamines and alcohol and other CNS depressants (antianxiety agents, depressant analgesics, hypnotics, sedatives, and tranquilizers).

Epinephrine. Diphenhydramine, tripelennamine, and chlorpheniramine enhance the effects of epinephrine.

MAO Inhibitors. MAO inhibitors both prolong and intensify the drying (anticholinergic) effects of antihistamines.

OTHER ANTIBIOTICS/ANTIBACTERIALS

Amphotericin B.

Digitalis Glycosides. Potassium depletion frequently results when amphotericin B and digitalis are used concomitantly.

Chloramphenicol.

Penicillins. Chloramphenicol, a bacteriostatic drug, evidently interferes with the action of bacteriocidal agents, such as the penicillins. Chloramphenicol (and other agents that block protein synthesis) may alter the bacteriocidal effect of penicillin and other drugs that block cell wall synthesis.

Erythromycin.

Theophylline. Close monitoring of patients receiving both drugs is necessary because erythromycin apparently inhibits the metabolism of theophylline.

Lincomycin.

Kaolin-Pectin. Another form of diarrheal control is recommended since kaolin-pectin mixtures inhibit the absorption of orally administered lincomycin.

Penicillin.

Tetracyclines. As bacteriostatic agents, tetracyclines apparently interfere with other bactericidal agents such as the penicillins. Although antibiotic antagonism is not a major component of clinical medicine, health professionals should recognize the reported occurrences of tetracycline antagonism of penicillin. Also, since certain manufacturers' product information may contain warnings against concomitant use of tetracyclines and penicillins, potential medico-legal problems are possible should patients have difficulty while using such a combination.

Rifampin.

Digitalis. Apparently through induction of hepatic microsomal enzymes, rifampin may enhance the hepatic metabolism of digitoxin. Since enzyme induction is less of a problem with digoxin than with digitoxin, digoxin is probably a better choice for patients receiving rifampin.

Sulfonamide.

Para-aminobenzoic Acid (PABA). Sufficient doses of PABA antagonize the antibacterial effect of the sulfonamides. Therefore, administration of PABA to patients also receiving antibacterial sulfonamides is discouraged.

Tetracycline.

Antacids that Contain Divalent or Trivalent Cations. Antacids such as aluminum, calcium, or magnesium impair the absorption of orally administered tetracyclines. Patients should not receive tetracyclines within 1 to 2 hours of administration of antacids that contain divalent or trivalent cations.

Oral Contraceptives. Since tetracycline may decrease the pharmacologic effects of oral contraceptives, alternative methods of birth control are advisable for women receiving tetracycline therapy.

Milk and Dairy Products. Milk and dairy products reduce the absorption of tetracyclines. This interaction necessitates a lengthy time lapse between ingestion of milk and dairy products and administration of tetracyclines for optimal drug absorption.

Methoxyflurane. Since a severe, combined nephrotoxic action may occur, caution is advised in administering tetracycline to patients who soon will or recently have undergone methoxyflurane anesthesia.

SUMMARY

The goals in management of respiratory tract disease include reduction of airway obstruction by improvement of respiratory tree caliber and removal of retained secretions. If infectious disease is present, appropriate antimicrobial therapy is usually indicated.

Complex diseases (e.g., bronchial asthma) require extensive diagnostic and therapeutic measures. Among these are repeated assessment of ventilatory function, avoidance of known precipitating factors, and a logical approach to the use of a myriad of drugs, including bronchodilators and corticosteroids.

In respiratory diseases, a clinical distinction between acute and chronic disorders is necessary. Oftentimes, prompt therapy with an aerosol or parenteral adrenergic drug is life-saving in an acute bronchial asthma attack. Likewise, an acute onset or exacerbation of bronchitis or pneumonia may respond to immediate therapy with antibacterial drugs. Chronic respiratory disease, however, is managed in a more holistic manner that emphasizes life style alterations; diet, place of residence, and physical activity are usual considerations in this treatment protocol.

From the pharmacologic viewpoint, more specific acting agents, such as the beta$_2$-adrenergic agonists, offer immediate benefit without many of the adverse reactions of the earlier drugs. Additionally, current research promises to broaden and improve methods for respiratory disease prevention and treatment.

SUGGESTED READINGS

Appelt, G.D.: The safety of phenylpropanolamine. J Clin Psychopharmacol, 3:332, 1983.

Choice of antimicrobial drugs. Med Lett Drugs Ther, 28:33, 1986.

Diamond, L., et al.: An evaluation of triprolidine and pseudoephedrine in the treatment of allergic rhinitis. Ann Allergy, 47:87, 1981.

Gilman, A.G., et al. (eds.): The Pharmacological Basis of Therapeutics. 7th Ed. New York, Macmillan Publishing Co., Inc., 1985.

Gossel, T.A.: How to help your patients self-treat their asthma. US Pharmacist, 11:22, 1986.

Hansten, P.D.: Drug Interactions. 5th Ed. Philadelphia, Lea & Febiger, 1985.

Hodge, N.A.: Seasonal allergic rhinitis. Its etiology and management. Am Druggist, 179:39, 1979.

Jacknowitz, A.I.: Seasonal allergic rhinitis. US Pharmacist, 11:10, 1986.

Jawetz, E.: The use of combinations of antimicrobial drugs. Annu Rev Pharmacol, 8:151, 1968.

Job, M.L., Matthews, H.W., and Shulman, E.M.: Your guide to therapy of systemic fungal infections. US Pharmacist, 11:41, 1986.

Kastrup, E.K., and Boyd, J.R. (eds.): Drug Facts and Comparisons. Philadelphia, J.B. Lippincott Co., 1985.

La Piana, L.J.: Why & how pharmacists help people with allergies. Pharmacy Times, 52:28, 1986.

Pentamidine for Pneumocystis carinii pneumonia. Med Lett Drugs Ther, 27:6, 1985.

Safety of antimicrobial drugs in pregnancy. Med Lett Drugs Ther, 27:93, 1985.

Schnore, S.K., et al.: Are antihistamine-decongestants of value in the treatment of acute otitis media in children? J Family Pract, 22:39, 1986.

Stewart, G.T.: Allergy to penicillin and related antibiotics. Antigenic and immunochemical mechanism. Annu Rev Pharmacol, 13:309, 1973.

Tashkin, D.P., et al.: Comparison of anticholinergic bronchodilator ipratropium bromide with metaproterenol in chronic obstructive pulmonary disease. Am J Med, 81: 59, 1986.

Terfenadine. A non-sedating antihistamine. Med Lett Drugs Ther, 27:65, 1985.

CHAPTER EXAMINATION

A middle-aged female with a cold has taken diphenhydramine capsules for 4 days. Feeling tired and woozy, she asks her pharmacist about alternate medications.

1. The pharmacist recommends terfenadine because
   a. the patient really needs an H_2 blocker
   b. it is a new H_1 blocker with less incidence of drowsiness
   c. of its antiviral action
   d. it is most effective against gram-positive organisms

2. Diphenhydramine
   a. rarely produces sedation
   b. is used only to treat motion sickness
   c. is a type of H_1 blocker that commonly produces drowsiness
   d. acts as an antiviral agent

3. The class of H_1 blocking drugs that is most likely to produce gastrointestinal upset is the
   a. alkylamine series
   b. phenothiazine series
   c. ethanolamine series
   d. ethylenediamine series

4. Types of drugs commonly found in cough/cold/allergy combinations are
   a. antihistamines, adrenergic agonists, and antitussives
   b. antiviral agents, antibacterial drugs, and bronchodilators
   c. antihistamines, cholinergic agonists, and antiviral drugs
   d. antibiotics, adrenergic blocking drugs, and antitussives

5. Terfenadine, tripelennamine, and diphenhydramine
   a. inhibit the synthesis of histamine
   b. activate histaminase
   c. bind reversibly to histamine
   d. competitively antagonize histamine by attaching to H_1 receptors

An elderly male with chronic bronchitis and a history of cigarette smoking is taking a theophylline elixir in addition to medication for congestive heart failure. His physician adds terbutaline to the treatment regimen.

6. A respiratory disease frequently associated with chronic bronchitis is
   a. emphysema
   b. ulcerative lung abscess with emphysema
   c. tuberculosis
   d. oat cell lung carcinoma

7. Theophylline
   a. lowers intracellular cyclic AMP in bronchiolar smooth muscle
   b. inhibits phosphodiesterase to induce bronchodilation
   c. is a specific beta$_2$-adrenergic agonist
   d. markedly depresses the CNS

8. Terbutaline
   a. is contraindicated in bronchial asthma
   b. inhibits phosphodiesterase
   c. is a beta$_2$-adrenergic agonist
   d. has a stimulatory effect on the myocardium

9. The patient develops an acute respiratory infection. Antibiotics are indicated and a culture demonstrates that a streptococcal infection is responsible. Drugs effective against these organisms are
   a. cyclacillin, penicillin G, and ampicillin
   b. amphotericin B, miconazole, and ketoconazole
   c. kanomycin, gentamicin, and polymyxin B
   d. chloramphenicol, bacitracin, and isoniazid

10. Important mechanisms operant in antibiotic activity include
    a. binding to bacterial cell mitochondria and activation of adenyl cyclase
    b. cleaving of the 30S and 50S ribosomal subunits and inhibition of bacterial phospholipid synthesis
    c. inhibiting bacterial cell wall biosynthesis and binding to the 50S subunit of bacterial ribosomes
    d. bacterial cell lysis due to Mg^{++} chelation and inhibition of the synthesis of ATPase

A female child receives amoxicillin for a respiratory Hemophilus influenzae infection. The therapy does not produce improvement, and the child's concerned parents consult her physician.

11. Certain strains of Hemophilus influenzae are
    a. resistant to amoxicillin therapy
    b. responsible for bacterial meningitis
    c. especially susceptible to amoxicillin
    d. all of the above
12. Amoxicillin is
    a. an orally effective semisynthetic penicillin that is penicillinase-susceptible
    b. not active against most strains of Hemophilus influenzae
    c. used exclusively for infections caused by penicillinase-producing staphylococci
    d. not effective orally
13. Two common adverse reactions to amoxicillin are
    a. maculopapular rash and diarrhea
    b. ototoxicity and nephrotoxicity
    c. agranulocytosis and thrombocytopenia
    d. blurred vision and constipation
14. Their call to the physician results in hospitalization of the child. Parenteral administration of carbenicillin produces rapid improvement and the child is discharged. Carbenicillin is
    a. effective in many severe infections due to ampicillin-resistant Hemophilus influenzae
    b. a penicillinase-resistant antibiotic
    c. effective against the secondary viral infection seen in this patient
    d. all of the above
15. Amoxicillin and carbenicillin
    a. bind with the 30S bacterial ribosomal subunit to inhibit protein synthesis
    b. block PABA reactions in bacterial metabolism
    c. cause leakage of nutrients from the bacterial plasma membrane
    d. inhibit cross-linking of the peptidoglycan strands in the cell wall

A middle-aged chronic alcoholic comes into the free clinic and complains of chest pains with hemoptysis of about a year's duration.

16. A communicable disease that should be considered is
    a. otitis media
    b. emphysema
    c. bronchial asthma
    d. tuberculosis
17. Isoniazid and rifampin are prescribed for the patient. Isoniazid is
    a. a specific drug for chronic emphysema
    b. an antibiotic produced by several Streptomyces species
    c. generally used alone in the treatment of respiratory disease
    d. none of the above
18. Isoniazid therapy
    a. may produce pyridoxine (vitamin B_6) deficiency
    b. is based upon beta$_2$-adrenergic receptor activation
    c. often cures the hepatitis associated with alcoholism
    d. none of the above
19. The patient's friend, complaining of a cough and sore throat, visits the clinic. The physician prescribes a cough preparation that contains dextromethorphan. An antibiotic choice to enhance this regimen is
    a. chloramphenicol
    b. polymyxin B
    c. penicillin G
    d. miconazole
20. Dextromethorphan
    a. activates stretch receptors in the oropharyngeal area
    b. depresses the cough center in the medulla oblongata
    c. has extensive addiction potential
    d. is a naturally occurring opium alkaloid

ANSWER KEY

1. b	11. d
2. c	12. a
3. d	13. a
4. a	14. a
5. d	15. d
6. a	16. d
7. b	17. d
8. c	18. a
9. a	19. c
10. c	20. b

chapter 8

DIGESTIVE/ GASTROINTESTINAL SYSTEM

CHAPTER OBJECTIVES

After studying this chapter, you should be able to:

1. Discuss the rational therapy for peptic ulcer and the problems involved in treating it.
2. Describe the difference between systemic and nonsystemic antacids and list examples of both types.
3. Discuss "acid-rebound" and name three drugs that may produce this effect.
4. Outline in detail (including the mechanism) four drug interactions that may occur with antacids.
5. Name two antacids with high sodium content and discuss their use in patients with cardiovascular disease. Name two antacids that have relatively low sodium content.
6. Explain why aluminum and magnesium compounds are combined in antacid preparations.
7. Name two bile salt preparations and discuss their therapeutic usefulness.
8. Discuss proposed mechanisms of sucralfate activity in the treatment of duodenal ulcer.
9. List the most common drug interactions that occur with anticholinergics/antispasmodics.
10. Differentiate between histamine activity attributed to H_1 and H_2 histamine receptors.
11. Describe the pharmacologic effects produced by H_2 receptor blockade.
12. Discuss the mechanism of action of cimetidine and ranitidine.
13. Discuss the anthracene-type cathartics, i.e., their active ingredients, mechanism of cathartic action, and unusual reactions/adverse effects sometimes noted.
14. Name several OTC bulk laxatives and describe the mechanism(s) involved in their laxative action.
15. Name a cascara-type ingredient that is combined with docusate for use as a combination laxative product.
16. Name two widely employed gastrointestinal absorbents.
17. Discuss the pharmacologic properties of diphenoxylate.
18. Describe the mechanism of action of phenothiazines in controlling emesis.
19. Discuss antibiotic therapy for infectious diseases of the gastrointestinal tract.
20. Describe the incidence of helminthiasis and name several anthelminthic agents.

INTRODUCTION

The digestive/gastrointestinal system is susceptible to both functional and infectious disorders. The functional disorders may involve either deficiency or excessive amounts of enzymes and/or factors necessary for digestive and absorptive processes. The cause of certain disorders, such as peptic ulcer, remains obscure, although symptomatic treatment allows some management of the pathophysiologic processes. Patients' gastrointestinal disorders, which are sometimes related to their emotional state, may worsen due to stress or anxiety.

Infectious gastrointestinal diseases usually involve microorganism invasion of the intestinal mucosal lining and sometimes in the blood stream. The resultant systemic infection may spread to other body organs, including the liver. Helminth infestation usually occurs "outside the body" in the intestinal lumen (as with tapeworm infestation) or in the anal or perianal region (as with pinworm infestation). Anemia and other consequences of helminth infestations are often debilitating. The expansive list of both OTC and Rx drugs is indicative of the widespread occurrence and pervasiveness of the gastrointestinal disorders.

ANATOMY AND PHYSIOLOGY OF THE DIGESTIVE/ GASTROINTESTINAL SYSTEM

An open-ended tube, the digestive system passes through the body from the mouth to the anus (Figure 8.1). Digestion of ingested foodstuffs occurs at various sites along the gastrointestinal tract and wastes are excreted without ever actually being inside the body since they are actually surrounded by it. Absorption of materials takes place only at specialized locations where anatomic and physiologic factors favor the mucosal cell-blood stream interchange of nutrients. The upper part of the small intestine portion of the gastrointestinal tract is an ideal absorption site because the nature of the intestinal wall cells, digestive enzymes, and the blood supply are optimal for the absorption of materials into the body.

Over 9 m long, the digestive tract is continuous with its bulges, turns, and regions that have special functions. Valves at various sites along the tract regulate passage of the ingested, partially digested mass along the gastrointestinal system. Layers of muscle along the digestive tube propel foodstuffs and eventually expel wastes. Thus, the muscular tube system acts as a "conveyer belt" with the eventual product being the remains of materials not taken into the body.

MOUTH AND ESOPHAGUS

Digestion starts in the mouth where salivary enzymes initiate breakdown of foods. The salivary glands secrete a watery juice containing an amylase-type enzyme (ptyalin) that starts the starch breakdown to simple sugars. Three salivary glands are located on each side of the face (Figure 8.2): the parotid gland is front of and below the ear, the sublingual is below the tongue, and the submaxillilary is below and behind the tongue.

The bolus of chewed and mixed masticated food is forced into the back of the oral cavity where it enters the esophagus. The process of peristalsis begins at this site and the "milking" contraction and relaxation of the muscles propel the food mass. Thus, the encircling muscles constrict behind the bolus in concert with muscular relaxation in front of the mass, resulting in passage of the food along the digestive tract.

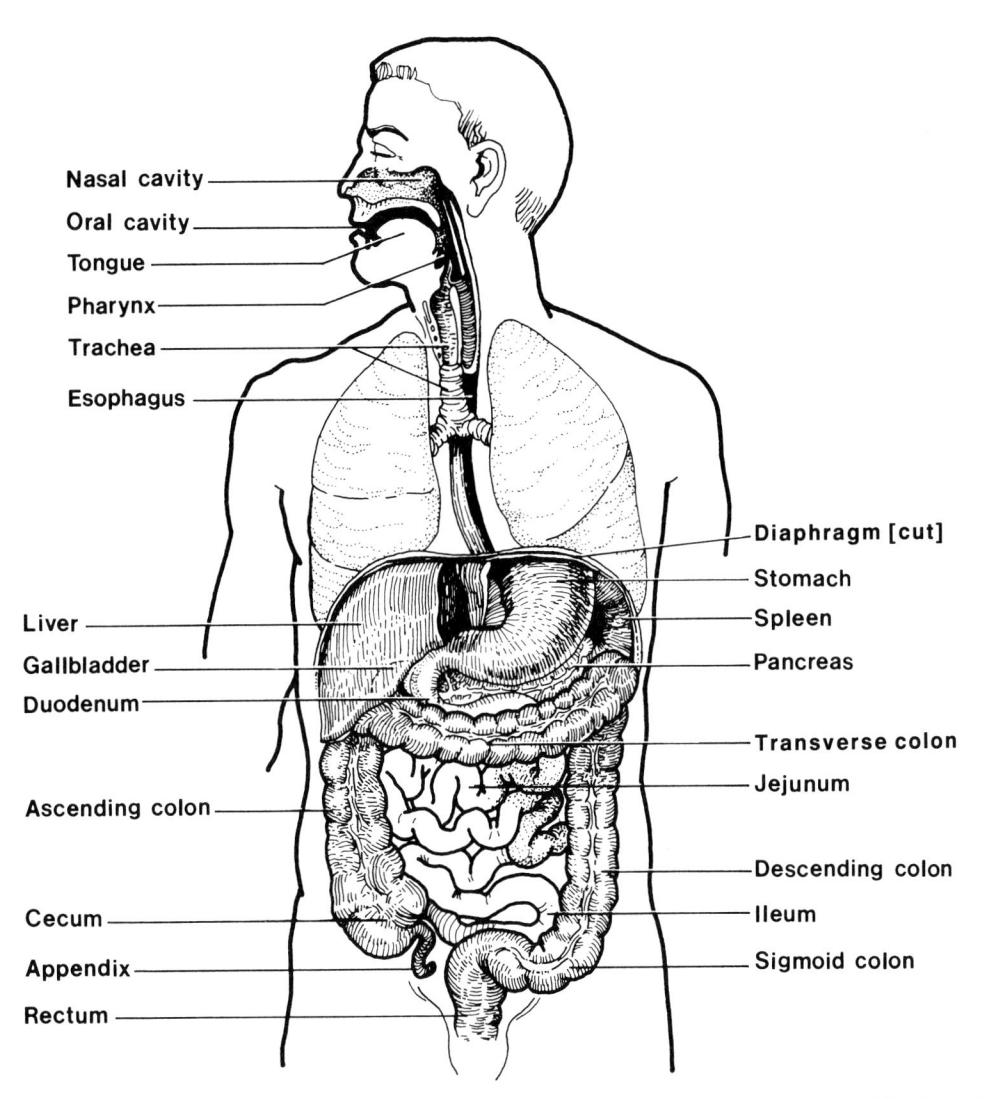

Fig. 8.1 Digestive system. (From Crouch, J.E.: Essential Human Anatomy. Philadelphia, Lea & Febiger, 1982.)

A valve, the cardia, is located at the junction of the esophagus and the stomach. A ringlike muscle, the cardia prevents backflow of materials (from the stomach) and regulates the release of the food mass into the stomach from the esophagus.

Peristalsis, along with gravity, delivers the food mass to the esophageal-stomach junction. The lower espohageal sphincter (LES) is a physical barrier whose tone determines the passage of food into the stomach. This sphincter also prevents the reflux of gastric contents into the lower esophagus. The LES relaxes in the basal state and contracts with swallowing. The autonomic influence is characterized by relaxation with beta-adrenergic activation or cholinergic inhibition. Thus, gastroesophageal reflux is likely with anticholinergic or beta-adrenergic agents. Additionally, alcohol, smoking, and fatty foods lower LES tension and predispose the individual to reflux.

STOMACH

The stomach consists of the cardia, fundus, body, and pylorus (Figure 8.3). A different type of mucosa characterizes each anatomic region.

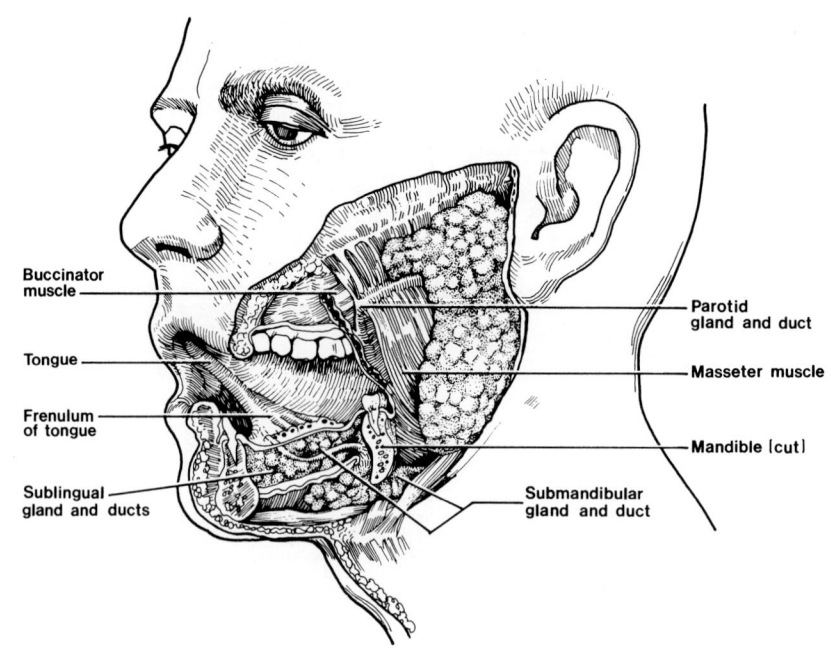

Fig. 8.2 Salivary glands. (From Crouch, J.E.: Essential Human Anatomy. Philadelphia, Lea & Febiger, 1982.)

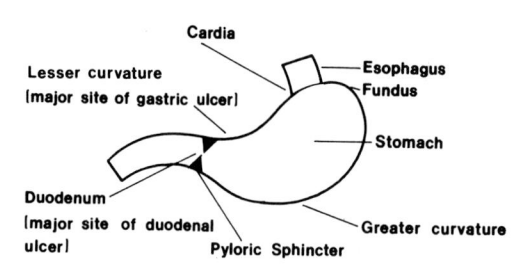

Fig. 8.3 Stomach-duodenum region. (Modified from Pastewski, B.M.: Peptic ulcer disease and its medical management. American Druggist, 182:36, 1980.)

The gastric mucosa, which lines the fundus and the body, contains surface mucous cells, mucous neck cells, argentaffin cells, parietal cells, and chief cells. Parietal cells secrete hydrochloric acid and intrinsic factor; secretion of the latter is the stomach's only essential function. Intrinsic factor is necessary for the absorption of vitamin B_{12}; when intrinsic factor is absent, vitamin B_{12} stores are exhausted, resulting in death (as in untreated pernicious anemia).

Pepsinogen is released from the chief cells and is converted to pepsin by the action of hydrochloric acid. An alkaline mucous secretion from the epithelial mucosal cells protects the stomach lining from the HCl-pepsin complex. The mucosal cells, which line both the antrum and prepyloric canal, secrete gastrin and a protective mucus.

Autonomic innervation to the stomach is by the parasympathetic division via the vagus nerve. The preganglionic vagal fibers synapse with the intrinsic plexus and postganglionic fibers, which lead to the gastric muscles and secretory glands. Vagotomy decreases without completely eliminating local reflexes, such as those involved with gastric secretion.

GASTRIC SECRETION

Gastric secretion occurs at different rates termed cephalic, gastric, and intestinal. These food-initiated phases continue for several hours. The cephalic and gastric phases stimulate gastric secretions, whereas the intestinal phase, although mildly stimulatory, promotes negative feedback to inhibit gastric secretions.

The thought, smell, taste, chewing, and swallowing of food initiates a parasympathetic response through the vagus nerve. Pepsinogen, hydrochloric acid, and gastric secretion are stimulated by the acetylcholine that the postganglionic vagal fibers release.

Food in the stomach increases gastric secretion by both direct and indirect mechanisms. The distention of the gastric mucosa by the physical presence of food results in a release of gastric secretions. Amino acids and peptides (formed by protein breakdown) indirectly cause the secretion of gastrin. Gastrin is an important mediator in the release of hydrochloric acid and pepsinogen secretion by the parietal and chief cells, respectively. The parasympathetic division of the autonomic nervous system (ANS) has an important activating influence on the gastric phase of secretion.

Food also stimulates the release of gastrin by several mechanisms, including mechanical distention of the antrum, vagal nerve activation, and by a direct action on the G-cells of the antrum and the duodenum. G-cells are unicellular endocrine glands for they respond to chemical changes by the release of the gastrointestinal hormone, gastrin.

Acetylcholine and cholinergic activation also produce gastrin release. High concentrations of epinephrine and calcium stimulate gastrin release, whereas hydrochloric acid, secretin, glucagon, calcitonin, and certain active gastrointestinal peptides inhibit its release.

At least three forms of gastrin act on the same receptor to cause release of hydrochloric acid and pepsinogen. The "little" gastrin that is secreted by the antrum has the most potent activity. "Big" gastrin, released from the duodenum, has a longer half-life. "Big-big" gastrin, released from the jejunum, is possibly responsible for basal acid secretion.

Gastrin-mediated hydrochloric acid and pepsinogen release occurs with histamine secretion. A sequential activation pattern is proposed where initial gastrin release induces histamine secretion; this action then causes the outflow of hydrochloric acid and pepsinogen.

Physiologic functions of gastrin (other than hydrochloric acid and pepsinogen release) include a protective function for the stomach mucosa by stimulating gastric mucosal cell proliferation and by tightening the gastric mucosal cell barrier. Gastrin also increases pancreatic enzyme secretions, bile flow, and gastric intestinal motility.

Histamine receptors that regulate hydrochloric acid secretion are H_2 receptors. Selective H_2 receptor blocking drugs effectively inhibit pentagastrin-induced gastric secretion, indicating that gastrin acts through histamine release.

The intestinal phase of gastric secretion involves both stimulation and inhibition. Partially digested food (chyme) in the intestine stimulates a weak, mediator-induced gastric secretion by the action of "big" gastrin, cholecystokinin, and pancreozymin.

Inhibition is mediated by ill-defined gastrointestinal hormones, which are collectively termed enterogastrones. An enterogastrone is any substance secreted from the small intestine that inhibits gastric secretion. The main stimulus for enterogastrone release is the presence of hydrochloric acid, fat, protein breakdown products, or hyperosmolar substances in the duodenum.

GASTRIC MOTILITY

The proximal stomach receives and stores the food mass from the esophagus. The contents then travel into the distal stomach where peristalsis mixes the chyme with gastric juice before passage into the duodenum through the pyloric valve. Gastric emptying into the duodenum depends upon the resistance of the pyloric sphincter. Gastric distention stimulates stomach emptying and increases the gastric emptying rate.

SMALL INTESTINE

The small intestine, about 6.5 m in length and tapering to about 2.5 cm at its lower end, is compactly wound into the abdomen. The duodenum, meaning "12 fingerbreadths long" (20 to 25 cm), begins where the pyloric sphincter disgorges partially digested spurts of material.

The duodenum makes a horseshoe curve so that its starting point and termination site are close together.

An alkaline environment exists in the duodenum, in contrast to the acid nature of the gastric region. The highly alkaline bile, pancreatic juice, and local intestinal wall secretions form the medium in which most of the digestion and absorption occurs. The common bile duct and pancreatic duct open into the duodenum at about the midpoint of the horseshoe curve.

The duodenum joins the jejunum (about 3 m long) and the jejunum connects to the ileum (about 3 to 3.5 m long), which comprises the rest of the small intestine. The mesentery, a flat membranous structure attached to the dorsal body wall, radiates outward like an open fan with the curved edge of the fan attaching to the intestine. Thus, the intestines are supported and propped up (like guy wires strung from a tentpole) with some freedom of movement. Another important role of the mesentery is to supply nerves and blood vessels to the small intestine.

The surface of cells facing the intestinal mucosa is composed of slender, closely packed, finger-shaped projections called microvilli (Figure 8.4). Estimated to number 5 million, the microvilli are like "velvet" carpet pile; these projections greatly increase the surface area available for absorption. In fact, the internal surface of the small intestine has more than five

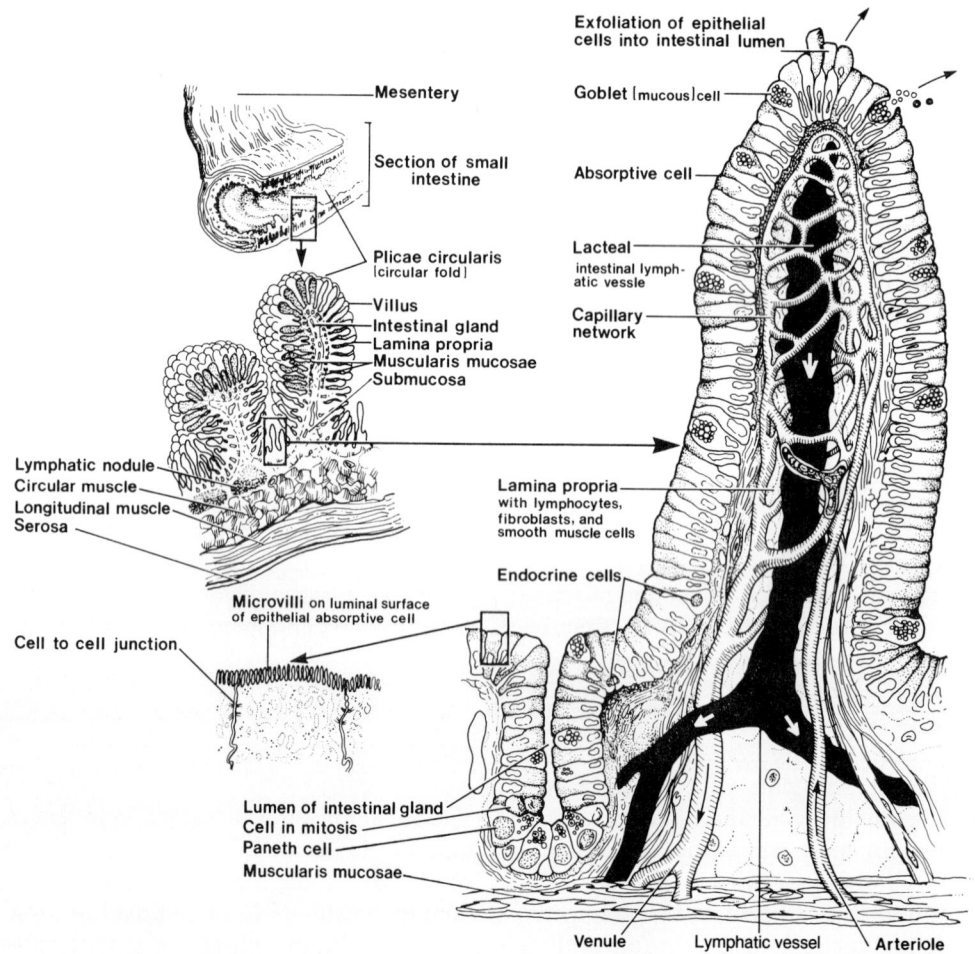

Fig. 8.4 Intestinal microvilli. (From Crouch, J.E.: Essential Human Anatomy. Philadelphia, Lea & Febiger, 1982.)

times the area of the body's skin surface. The microvilli are not inert, but they wave like wheat fields; they also lengthen and shorten, swell and shrink, and generally stir the partially digested luminal admixture.

Most nutrients are absorbed in the duodenum and jejunum; the rest of the small intestine remains available for reserve absorptive function. The ileum, however, plays an important, unique role in the active transport of vitamin B_{12} and bile acids. Additionally, there are differences in the handling of water and electrolytes between sections of the intestinal tube. The duodenum and upper jejunum contain a rapid and voluminous fluid circuit in which water and electrolytes enter the intestinal lumen about as fast as they leave it. Consequently, the luminal content volume remains fairly constant. In the ileum, however, the exchange is less voluminous and movement out of the lumen is more than the influx into the lumen. Therefore, the volume of luminal contents greatly decreases. In addition to the small intestine, the gallbladder and the colon are important in water and electrolyte absorption.

Carbohydrate, protein, and fat (lipid) absorption occurs in the small intestine following appropriate digestive mechanisms. The pancreas is the primary source of digestive enzymes that are active in the lumen of the small intestine. The pancreas synthesizes and secretes more protein than any other gland (except the lactating mammary gland) and produces the following enzymes: amylase, lipase, trypsin, chymotrypsin, carboxypeptidase, elastase, ribonuclease, and deoxyribonuclease.

The secretion of bile by the liver serves two important physiologic functions: to provide bile salts necessary for lipid absorption and to act as the excretory pathway for water soluble substances, such as cholesterol, steroid hormones, drugs, and bilirubin (the breakdown product of hemoglobin and other heme proteins). Bile is secreted continually, but because the gallbladder acts as a storage organ, bile is delivered intermittently to the small intestine.

The terminal ileal sphincter is analogous to the lower esophageal sphincter (LES) in that it prevents reflux of cecal contents into the distal ileum. The terminal ileal sphincter is located just proximal to the ileal-cecal junction. Distention in the ileum above the sphincter results in relaxation, whereas distention of the cecum leads to increased intrasphincter pressure.

COLON

The colon, the portion of the large intestine extending from the cecum to the rectum (Figure 8.1), consists of an ascending section which extends upward on the right side of the abdomen from the cecum to the hepatic flexure. The descending colon extends downward on the left side of the abdomen from the splenic flexure to the sigmoid colon (the S-shaped part of the colon in the pelvis between the descending colon and rectum). Stationary segmental muscle contractions predominate in the transverse colon, whereas a mass movement of the intestinal contents results when a strong caudal-directed contraction occurs in the transverse colon and descending colon.

The colon is primarily a storage and dehydrating organ where material enters in a liquid form and becomes semisolid as water is absorbed. The colon reduces the volume of the enteric contents delivered to it by absorbing water and electrolytes. Collection of the remaining chyme for excretion by defecation is another of the colon's functions.

The sigmoid flexure of the colon becomes the rectum and terminates in the anus. Two ringlike voluntary muscles (anal sphincters) terminate the digestive tract. The urge for a bowel movement results from intestinal nerve reflex signals.

ADDITIONAL ORGANS VITAL TO DIGESTION

The liver and the pancreas secrete enzymes and other factors that are required in the digestive process.

LIVER

The liver (the largest solid organ of the body) weighs about 1.8 kg and occupies the upper part of the abdomen beneath the diaphragm

(Figure 8.1). Most of the liver occupies the right side of the abdomen. The organ is divided by a fissure into a large right lobe and a smaller tapered left lobe, whose tip overlies the stomach near the esophageal junction.

The liver has several important physiologic functions, one of which is a critical detoxifying role in rendering ingested toxins harmless. Additionally, the liver acts as a blood reservoir and storage organ for oil-soluble vitamins and carbohydrates and serves as an enzyme synthesis powerplant and bile production site.

Bile (gall) is a complex fluid containing bile salts, bile pigments, and other constituents. Bile salts promote efficient fat digestion by a detergent action that emulsifies the lipid materials. Bile is stored in the gallbladder, a saclike organ about 7.5 cm long and located on the underside of the liver (Figure 8.1). The gallbladder modifies bile chemically and concentrates it about tenfold. The wall of the gallbladder has a muscle layer that contracts at intervals to squeeze the bile into the duodenum. A high-fat meal is a particularly powerful stimulant to gallbladder contraction. Gallstones sometimes form when the constituents of bile crystallize.

PANCREAS

About 15 cm long, the pancreas has a broad right end (head) that nestles into the curve of the duodenum (Figure 8.1). The pancreas has a dual role as an endocrine gland and as an exocrine organ; of these, the exocrine function is particularly important in digestive processes. Pancreatic digestive juice, containing amylase, lipase, and trypsin, is collected into a central pancreatic duct that joins the common bile duct to empty into the duodenum.

DISORDERS OF THE DIGESTIVE/GASTROINTESTINAL SYSTEM

Disorders of the digestive/gastrointestinal system include functional disease and infections.

DISORDERS OF THE MOUTH/SALIVARY GLANDS

Herpetic infections and other microorganism invasions of the oral cavity occur frequently.

STOMATITIS

Stomatitis results from either traumatic influence (irritant chemicals) or infection. Viral infection is especially common, particularly that caused by the herpes virus. Primary herpetic gingivostomatitis is an acute condition characterized by widespread lesions on the oral mucosa and skin, associated with involvement of the pharyngeal and regional lymph nodes. Recurrent herpetic stomatitis is a milder condition which consists of lip lesions ('"cold sores" or "fever blisters") or lesions in the mouth ("canker sores"). A worsening of the lesions often follows primary infection, fever, gastrointestinal upset, or onset of menstruation.

Less frequently occurring types of stomatitis infections include candidiasis (thrush) and actinomycosis. Whitish patches on the palate and other oral structures characterize candidiasis, a fungal infection. Actinomycosis, another fungal infection, affects the jaws and produces sores which drain into the oral cavity.

BENIGN TUMORS (GROWTHS)

Papilloma, fibromas, epulis lesions, torus lesions, and exostosis are benign oral tumors. Papillomas (raised, firm lesions which closely resemble warts) occur indiscriminately in the oral cavity. Fibromas are pale, firm, slowly growing lesions that occur most often in intraoral (buccal) areas. Epulis lesions (calculus caused by foreign material) result from chronic irritation below the gum line. Torus lesions and exostosis are bony lesions that are actually outgrowths of normal oral bone tissue.

MALIGNANT TUMORS

Many malignant tumors are preceded by the development of leukoplakia. The most common malignant oral tumor is squamous cell carcinoma. Its incidence is higher in men than in women. Squamous cell carcinoma may occur in most intraoral areas, as well as on the lower lip of smokers. The lesions are usually ragged, ulcerated, and whitish.

Adenocarcinoma, a less common oral malignancy, is characterized by a swelling of the affected area.

INFECTIOUS OR EPIDEMIC PAROTITIS (MUMPS)

Mumps is an acute contagious disease caused by a virus present in nasal discharges and saliva. Swelling of the parotid glands (one or both sides), fever, and malaise are symptoms of this condition. Complications of mumps usually involve the ovaries and testes, and sterility sometimes occurs in men.

ESOPHAGEAL DISORDERS

Esophageal disorders are often due to or aggravated by reflux of gastric contents.

ESOPHAGITIS

Severe pain below the sternum or a burning sensation upon swallowing characterize esophagitis. Reflux esophagitis is a diffuse inflammation of the distal esophagus caused by regurgitation of gastric or duodenal contents through an incompetent lower esophageal sphincter (LES). This condition is frequently associated with hiatal hernia or a duodenal ulcer.

ESOPHAGEAL ULCER

An esophageal ulcer occurs in the lower esophagus, apparently as the result of regurgitation of acidic gastric juice. Vomiting and hemorrhage are symptoms of this disorder.

HIATUS HERNIA

The protrusion of part of the stomach into or next to the esophagus is called a hiatus hernia. Although the condition may be asymptomatic, pain under the sternum, burning, or regurgitation of foods and liquids are often present. Symptoms may worsen after meals or during straining or stooping. The condition is often associated with chronic esophagitis.

ESOPHAGEAL TUMORS

Esophageal tumors vary from the size of a pea to that of a marble. Symptoms of a benign tumor include difficulty in swallowing and a feeling of fullness or pressure. The symptoms of esophageal carcinoma resemble those of a benign esophageal tumor. Generally, the symptoms progress and worsen, resulting in weight loss, hemorrhage, and perhaps perforation into the lung.

STOMACH DISORDERS

Symptoms related to stomach disorders (for example, "heartburn" and flatulence) constitute a large percentage of patient complaints.

GASTRITIS

Gastritis (i.e., inflammation of the gastric mucosa) involves a break in the normal gastric mucosal barrier, which allows hydrochloric acid to enter the mucosa, injure vessels, and cause inflammation, erosion, and hemorrhage. The symptoms are burning pain over the stomach, nausea, and vomiting.

Accounting for about one in three gastrointestinal bleeding episodes, acute gastritis may occur after the ingestion of aspirin or alcohol, in uremia, during infection, and as a complication of stress. With removal of the initiating cause, the process is self-limiting and the bleeding stops spontaneously in 2 to 5 days.

Chronic gastritis refers to a number of gastric lesions that do not heal over a period of time. Bleeding and symptoms of pernicious anemia may develop in such cases.

GASTRIC ULCERS

Gastric ulcers are a form of peptic ulcer (a lesion of the mucous membrane of the stomach or duodenum). Peptic ulcers are probably caused by an increase in hydrochloric acid and pepsin, a decrease in the mucosal resistance, or a combination of both these factors.

Although gastric ulcers occur most frequently as a single lesion along the lesser curvature and adjacent posterior wall of the antrum within 5 cm of the pyloric sphincter, they occasionally appear in the cardia, pyloric canal, and the greater curvature of the stomach body and fundus. In contrast to duodenal ulcers, hyperacidity is not a frequent finding in gastric ulcers. In fact, gastric ulcer patients may have low or normal hydrochloric acid secretion.

Gastric ulcers are sometimes associated with chronic gastritis, in which an increase in back diffusion of hydrogen ion (H^+) may break down the gastric mucosal barrier. Reflux of duodenal contents, especially bile acids, is often a related factor. Smoking (associated with an increased incidence of gastric ulcer) causes duodenogastric reflux. Additionally, bile salts occur more frequently and in higher concentrations in the stomachs of gastric ulcer patients than in normal persons or duodenal ulcer patients.

Common patient complaints are pain and gastrointestinal bleeding. Cramping or dull pain usually occurs within 30 to 60 minutes following eating and lasts for 60 to 90 minutes. Gastric ulcer patients may associate eating with the pain and stop regular meals, resulting in excessive weight loss which requires corrective measures. Radiating somatic pain into the back region sometimes indicates perforation and constitutes a medical emergency.

Five to ten percent of all gastric ulcers are carcinomas. The mortality from nonmalignant gastric ulcers is low, but the morbidity is high. Gastric ulcers are more resistant than duodenal ulcers to therapeutic measures and require surgery more often.

GASTRIC ADENOCARCINOMA

Gastric adenocarcinoma is most often located in the distal-third of the stomach in the antrum or pylorus. Sometimes found as cauliflower-like masses that protrude into the stomach cavity, the tumors may also diffusely infiltrate the stomach wall. Infiltrating tumors frequently ulcerate, making them difficult to distinguish from chronic gastric ulcer.

Symptoms of gastric adenocarcinoma are indefinite. Persistent abdominal discomfort with weight loss, anorexia, and other symptoms similar to benign gastric ulcer are common. Anemia and bloody stools also occur frequently.

There is a distinct relationship between atrophic gastritis (particularly that associated with pernicious anemia) and the development of gastric adenocarcinoma for approximately 50% of all gastric adenocarcinoma patients have achlorhydria.

INTESTINAL DISORDERS

Intestinal disorders include functional deficiencies of digestive factors, mucosal ulceration (benign or malignant), and infectious disease.

DUODENAL ULCERS

Duodenal ulcers are mucosal lesions which are usually located in the anterior wall of the duodenum's proximal end just beyond the pyloric channel through which gastric contents enter the duodenum. Ulcers also form distal to the duodenal bulb or spread back into the pyloric channel or antrum.

Duodenal ulcer disease probably represents a mixture of disorders with different etiologies but a common pathophysiologic expression. Excessive hydrochloric acid and pepsin apparently are causative factors. Several abnormalities may contribute to the increased quantities of hydrochloric acid and pepsin that reach the duodenum. A large parietal cell mass, increased sensitivity to gastric secretogogues, heightened vagal or hormone influence, defective secretory inhibition processes, and an increased gastric rate are all proposed causative factors in duodenal ulcers.

Also implicated in duodenal ulcer etiology are emotional and stress factors. Additionally, cigarette smokers are twice as likely as nonsmokers to develop duodenal ulcers.

Acid secretion during sleep is considered a key factor in peptic ulcer formation and healing. Acid suppression (by use of H_2 receptor blockers) during the nocturnal hours often effectively heals ulcers.

The primary symptoms of duodenal ulcers are pain and gastrointestinal bleeding. Epigastric pain (severe enough to awaken a sleeping individual) is a highly reliable indicator of peptic ulcer disease. Food relieves pain from a duodenal ulcer; however, the pain recurs approximately 1.5 to 3 hours following food ingestion and persists until the next meal.

Bleeding from a duodenal ulcer usually produces a change in stool color and consistency. Specifically, the blood present in the fecal mass results in black and tarry stools.

Major complications of duodenal ulcers involve bleeding, perforation, and obstruction. Iron deficiency anemia may result from excessive bleeding. Perforation is accompanied by sudden, explosive, generalized abdominal pain, prostration, and abdominal rigidity. Vomiting is the most common sign of gastric outlet obstruction. Both perforation and obstruction in duodenal ulcer disease are indications for acute surgical intervention.

SMALL INTESTINE ADENOCARCINOMA

Adenocarcinoma of the duodenum, jejunum, and ileum are uncommon. However, their incidence is higher in patients with Crohn's disease.

COLON CARCINOMA

Adenocarcinoma of the colon is a common form of cancer. Fifty percent of all colon carcinomas are located in the sigmoid flexure or rectum. The tumor usually assumes a napkin ring-like infiltration of the intestinal wall, which constricts the lumen. The manifestations include ulceration, obstruction, bleeding, and a sense of incomplete evacuation. Carcinomas in the cecum do not ordinarily result in obstruction. Occult bleeding sometimes results in progressive anemia.

DIARRHEA

Diarrhea is the frequent passage of loose or watery stools. A variety of infectious organisms that attack the small and large intestine frequently cause acute diarrhea.

Diarrhea Due to Infectious Agents.

Typhoid Fever. Salmonella typhi, a gram-negative microorganism, causes typhoid fever. Ulceration of the small intestine and a marked systemic reticuloendothelial hyperplasia characterize this disease.

Typhoid fever is usually transmitted by the fecal contamination of water or food. The incubation period for typhoid fever is from 10 to 14 days; during this time, the organisms are located within the lymphoid tissue (Peyer's patches) of the gastrointestinal tract. At this site, the microorganisms proliferate and cause marked hypertrophy of the lymphoid tissue. After about 10 days to 2 weeks, the microorganisms then flood the circulating blood and invade the reticuloendothelial (RE) system.

Symptomatology includes heptatosplenomegaly, fever, prostration, abdominal cramps, and bloody diarrhea. Bradycardia and leukopenia also occur commonly. A "rose spot" rash may occur and bacilli are found in the stools.

Important complications of typhoid fever are profuse hemorrhage of the intestine, perforation of the bowel wall, and rupture of the spleen. About 2% of all recovering patients become carriers of the disease ("Typhoid Mary") and continue to harbor Salmonella typhi in their biliary tract.

Bacillary Dysentery (Shigellosis). This gastrointestinal disease is caused by the Shigellae, a group of gram-negative organisms that include Shigella dysenteriae, Shigella flexneri, Shigella boydii, and Shigella sonnei. Transmitted by contaminated food or water, the disease has a short incubation period. Abrupt onset of symptoms sometimes occurs only a day after microorganism invasion.

In contrast to typhoid fever, the colon, rather than the small intestine, is the usual site of Shigella infection. Consequently, bacteremia rarely occurs and tissue damage is confined to the gastrointestinal tract. An endotoxin released by Shigella causes many effects, such as superficial ulceration of the colon mucosa. Abdominal pain and diarrhea precede fever, and stools frequently contain blood and mucus.

Cholera. Cholera, an acute diarrheal disease, is caused by food or water contaminated with Vibrio cholerae or Vibrio El Tor. The vibrios are curved gram-negative bacilli that act by release of a toxin that intensely irritates the intestinal wall.

The disease has an explosive onset after a relatively short incubation period of a few days. The epithelial tissue remains intact, but the underlying vasculature becomes engorged, resulting in a massive outflow of fluid and electrolytes into the intestinal lumen.

Cholera symptoms include severe vomiting, abdominal cramps, and profuse diarrhea. Fluid, yellowish stools are characterized by flecks of mucus ("rice water stools"). The complications of cholera result from profound dehydration and electrolyte imbalance.

Salmonellosis. Salmonella species, other than those responsible for typhoid fever, may produce an infectious diarrhea. The incubation period for this Salmonellae-induced condition is from 12 to 24 hours. Fever, malaise, muscle aching, epigastric or periumbilical pain, and anorexia characterize this infectious, inflammatory condition.

Traveler's Diarrhea. This acute diarrhea commonly afflicts visitors to foreign countries that have warm climates, lax sanitary measures, and nonexistent or ineffective water purification systems. Although difficult to trace to known pathogens, enterotoxigenic Escherichia coli are considered a prime cause of traveler's diarrhea. The condition probably results from a marked alteration in the intestinal microbial population. A sudden onset of loose stools, nausea, abdominal cramping, and occasional vomiting characterize traveler's diarrhea.

Giardiasis (Hiker's Diarrhea). Giardia lambia, a protozoal flagellate, causes an acute diarrhea which often results from ingestion of nontreated water, such as that found in mountain lakes and streams. After a 1 to 3 day incubation period, watery stools and abdominal cramps occur.

Amoebic Dysentery. Intestinal Entamoeba histolytica infection (amebiasis) occurs most often in individuals who live in institutions, migrant labor camps, or areas with poor sanitation. Abdominal cramps and diarrhea (within 3 to 10 days of incubation) characterize this condition.

Other Forms of Diarrheal Disease. Food allergies or excessive ingestion of irritating substances can cause acute diarrhea. Usually resulting from multiple factors, chronic diarrhea may be psychogenic, drug-induced, or malabsorptive.

Staphylococcal Food Poisoning. Staphylococci grow rapidly in food, especially in contaminated, nonrefrigerated products, such as meat, potato salad, and creamfilled pastries. A toxin produced by the staphylococci causes diarrhea within 1 to 2 hours after ingestion; this condition is literally a "food poisoning." Infection by the microorganism does not produce the inflammatory processes causing diarrhea but rather the toxin formed in the food product causes the diarrheal attack.

Botulism, another form of "food poisoning," occurs when Clostridium botulinum neurotoxin forms in improperly canned or processed food. This is a rare but potentially deadly occurrence.

CONSTIPATION

Constipation of organic origin should be differentiated from conditions where no organic lesion is present. Causes of chronic constipation (due to organic lesions) include obstructive tumors, hypothyroidism, anal and rectal disorders, and diseases of the liver and gallbladder. Laxatives and cathartics are contraindicated in these cases which require proper medical diagnosis and treatment.

Constipation that results from faulty diet and eating habits, insufficient exercise, or drugs (such as in hospitalized patients) can usually be alleviated by correcting these causative factors. For instance, an increase in fiber-containing food and a proper exercise schedule may reverse the constipation.

This condition primarily afflicts the elderly in part because of their restricted activity, dietary factors, and/or failure to drink enough water (1 to 2 L of fluid a day). Also affected by this condition are those who have a neurotic preoccupation with bowel habits and who routinely use laxatives to satisfy this psychologic dependency.

A healthy person should not ordinarily require a laxative or cathartic. However, conditions necessitating a cathartic include the preparation of abdominal viscera prior to roentgen examination and the production of soft stools to avoid irritation in rectal disorders, such as hemorrhoids.

HEMORRHOIDS (PILES)

Hemorrhoids are abnormally large varicose dilations of vessels, supporting tissues, and overlying mucous membrane or skin in the anorectal area. Symptoms of hemorrhoids include itching, burning, pain, inflammation, irritation, swelling, and discomfort. Bleeding, seepage, protrusion, prolapse, and thrombosis are more serious complications.

External hemorrhoids occur below the anorectal line and may be thrombotic. Some previously thrombosed external hemorrhoids evolve into "skin tags" in which the clot has become organized and replaced by connective tissue.

Internal hemorrhoids occur above the anorectal line. Sometimes, because of its size, an internal hemorrhoid descends below the anorectal line and outside the anal sphincter; it is then termed a prolapsed hemorrhoid.

Mixed hemorrhoids (external-internal) are either prolapsed or nonprolapsed. A strangulated hemorrhoid is one that has prolapsed to such a degree and for so long that its blood supply is occluded by the anal sphincter's constricting action. This painful type of hemorrhoid usually becomes thrombosed.

Hemorrhoids occur most commonly in those 20 to 50 years old. Predisposing etiologic factors include heredity, posture, occupation, and diet. Precipitating causes of hemorrhoids are constipation, diarrhea, pregnancy, anal infection, rectal carcinoma, pelvic tumors, cardiac failure, portal hypertension, coughing, sneezing, vomiting, and physical exertion.

ULCERATIVE COLITIS

Bloody diarrhea characterizes this inflammatory disease of the large intestine. The ulcerated lesions are usually restricted to the mucosa or submucosa and do not extend to the muscular layer. The cause of ulcerative colitis is unknown, although a cell-mediated immunologic mechanism of injury is probable.

Complications of ulcerative colitis are perforation, hemorrhage, anal fissures, and pararectal abscesses. Colon carcinoma is ten times more likely to occur in patients with ulcerative colitis.

CROHN'S DISEASE

Crohn's disease has been described as a disease of Western civilization. Clinical symptoms include diarrhea, abdominal pain, fever, weight loss, anemia, peritoneal abscesses, and perianal disease. Characteristically, the disease occurs in recurring episodes, often with extensive periods of remission. The ileum is the most frequently affected region of the intestines, although the colon is sometimes involved (granulomatous colitis).

Causes implicated as factors in Crohn's disease include infections, immunologic disorders, or emotional disturbances.

CELIAC SPRUE (GLUTEN-SENSITIVE ENTEROPATHY)

Celiac sprue is a malabsorption syndrome marked by extensive loss of mucosal villi in the entire small intestine. The genetic factor is unclear, but cell-mediated immunologic damage to the mucosal cells is probable. Diarrhea with bulky, frothy, fatty, fetid stools; abdominal distention; weight loss; asthenia; deficiencies of vitamins B, D, and K; and electrolyte depletion characterize celiac sprue, a syndrome which is precipitated by gluten-containing foods. Thus, a gluten-free diet dramatically reverses the disease process.

WHIPPLE'S DISEASE

Whipple's disease, intestinal lipodystrophy, is a rare malabsorptive disorder, which is characterized by diarrhea, steatorrhea, skin pigmentation, arthralgia, lymphadenopathy, and CNS lesions. Macrophages containing fragments of microorganisms distend the intestinal villi. Whipple's disease responds well to specific antibiotic therapy.

INTESTINAL HELMINTH INFESTATIONS

Ascariasis, enterobiasis, hookworm, trichuriasis, strongyloidiasis, trichinosis, and tapeworm constitute the most frequently occurring forms of intestinal helminthiasis, Helminthiasis, the most common disease in the world, affects more than 2 billion people.

Ascariasis (Large Roundworm). Ascaris lumbricoides is a parasitic nematode that causes colicky pains and diarrhea, especially in children. Approximately the size of an earthworm, Ascaris lumbricoides is the most common cause of helminth infestation. The first signs of the disease are respiratory symptoms due to larvae (which hatch in the intestine) invasion of the lungs. The larvae later migrate back to the stomach and intestine where they reach adult size. Intestinal obstruction is a complication of massive helminth infestation.

Enterobiasis (Pinworm). Enterobius vermicularis is an intestinal nematode that frequently infests children and causes intense itching in the anal region and occasionally in the vulva and vagina. Pinworm is spread by improper hygiene; contaminated sandboxes, doorknobs, and the like often cause helminthiasis to afflict an entire family.

Hookworm. Necator americanus or Ancylostoma duodenale produce hookworm infection. Hookworm larvae, which enter broken skin or are ingested with contaminated food, migrate to the small intestine. As adult helminths, they attach to the intestinal wall and ingest blood. Hookworm symptoms include abdominal pain, diarrhea, colic, and anemia.

Cutaneous larva migrans (ground itch) is another form of hookworm infestation.

Trichuriasis (Whipworm). Trichuris trichura, an intestinal nematode, causes colic and bloody diarrhea. The whip-shaped worm attaches itself to the colon wall; heavy infestations in children can result in iron deficiency anemia.

Strongyloidiasis (Threadworm). A parasitic nematode, Strongyloides stercoralis is found mainly in the tropics and subtropics. Symptoms of infestation include diarrhea and intestinal ulceration. The female worm lays eggs beneath the mucosa of the small intestine; the larvae may migrate to the lungs, liver, and heart. Bronchopneumonia and lung or liver abscesses are often fatal.

Trichinosis. Trichinosis results from the ingestion of Trichinella spiralis-contaminated undercooked meat. Adult Trichinella spiralis, which grow to maturity in the intestinal tract, do not enter the tissues; larvae deposited in the intestinal mucosa by the female, however, pass into the bloodstream and are then carried to skeletal muscles, the heart, and brain. Pneumonia, cardiac failure, and encephalitis may occur in severe trichinosis cases.

Symptoms include diarrhea, nausea, colic, and fever. Systemic helminthiasis or muscle invasion by the larvae causes muscle swelling, fever, sweating, circumorbital edema, and capillary hemorrhages in the eyes and nail bed.

Tapeworm (Taenia saginata-beef; Taenia solium-pork; Diphylobothrium latum-fish). The tapeworm parasite is a segmented cestode, which has a flat, band-like form. Its head or scolex attaches to the intestinal wall and the numerous segments absorb nutrients from the luminal contents. Beef tapeworms are from 3.5 to 7.5 m long and the pork tapeworm measures from 1.5 m to 3.5 m.

Mild abdominal symptoms and weight loss may accompany tapeworm infestation, which generally results from the ingestion of inadequately cooked, contaminated meat. Pork tapeworm, which rarely occurs in the United States, can cause cysticercosis (larval invasion of the skeletal muscles, lungs, liver, and/or brain).

LIVER DISORDERS

Disease reduces the liver's digestive and detoxification roles. Jaundice and cirrhosis adversely affect the digestive role of the liver by reducing bile formation. Tumors of the liver may develop, although primary malignancies are rare; most liver cancers have metastasized from another site.

Viral hepatitis can be contracted from contaminated food (especially from raw seafood) or by blood products containing the hepatitis B virus. Syringes used by IV drug users often transmit the hepatitis virus.

GALLBLADDER DISORDERS

The gallbladder, a sac-like structure, stores and concentrates bile. A primary symptom of gallbladder disease is severe pain in the upper right quadrant of the abdomen. A fatty meal usually precipitates or aggravates the pain.

CHRONIC CHOLECYSTITIS

This chronic inflammatory disease of the gallbladder is almost invariably associated with gallstones. Symptoms are episodic pain in the upper right quadrant of the abdomen, nausea, and vomiting. Gallstone formation probably results when bile concentration increases with precipitation of bile salts, cholesterol, or calcium; infection; and excessive ingestion of fat.

CHOLANGITIS

Cholangitis refers to an acute inflammation of the common bile duct that leads from the gallbladder to the duodenum. Bacterial invasion from the intestinal tract or bloodstream probably causes this condition. Chills, fever, and pain in the upper right quadrant of the abdomen characterize cholangitis.

PANCREATIC DISORDERS

Pancreatic disorders can result in endocrine deficiency (as in diabetes mellitus) or in reduced pancreatic exocrine function.

PANCREATITIS

Acute pancreatitis occurs as a sudden, severe inflammatory process in the pancreas. Pancreatic enzymes escape from the gland alveoli into the pancreas tissue. This condition usually results from an obstruction to pancreatic juice outflow. Adjacent biliary tract disease or obstructive stone formation may also produce this blockage. Islet cell destruction and diabetes mellitus sometimes result from chronic pancreatitis.

CARCINOMA OF THE PANCREAS

Pancreatic adenocarcinoma is often associated with chronic alcoholism and biliary disease. Also implicated are cigarette smoking and excessive ingestion of coffee. About two out of three pancreatic carcinomas arise in the head of the organ. Obstructive jaundice, abdominal pain, and anorexia are early symptoms. Carcinoma of the organ body and tail resist early diagnosis and are usually larger in size when detected.

DRUGS USED IN THE TREATMENT OF DIGESTIVE/ GASTROINTESTINAL DISORDERS

Antacids, antispasmodics, and histamine (H_2) receptor blockers are important drug classes used in the management of peptic ulcer disease. Laxatives, antidiarrheals, digestive aids, and antiemetics are drug classes effective in the treatment of functional and infectious gastrointestinal diseases. Antibiotics and antihelminthics are used to treat gastrointestinal infections and infestations.

DRUGS USED IN THE TREATMENT OF PEPTIC ULCER

Effective management of peptic ulcer disease often requires the use of antacids, antispasmodics, and/or histamine (H_2) blocking agents.

ANTACIDS

Gastric antacids (Table 8.1) represent one of the largest classes of medicinal substances used in current therapeutics. Neutralization of gastric hydrochloric acid is a primary aim in treating peptic ulcers, as the presence of the acid hinders ulcer healing and possibly contributes to the pain. The pH of gastric juice is normally between 1 and 2; the therapeutic goal is elevation of the pH to about 4. Complete neutralization is undesirable because of pepsin inactivation and an increased rebound secretion of gastric acid. Antacids are divided into two categories: systemic and nonsystemic drugs.

Sodium Bicarbonate (Baking Soda). Sodium bicarbonate is the only systemic antacid that is used medicinally. Although largely abandoned by physicians, the drug remains popular in some sectors of the lay public.

Mechanism of Action. Sodium bicarbonate effectively neutralizes gastric acid and by reaction with hydrochloric acid, liberates carbon dioxide (CO_2). Alkalosis occurs when the blood absorbs the sodium ion. This systemic alkalosis results in an exaggerated increase in gastric acid or "acid rebound."

Table 8.1. GASTRIC ANTACIDS.

Available products	Trade names	Daily dosage range
Aluminum compounds:		
Aluminum hydroxide gel	Amphojel; Dialume; others	600 mg 3–6 times daily
Aluminum carbonate gel	Basaljel	2 capsules or tablets as often as q. 2 hrs
Aluminum phosphate gel	Phosphaljel	15–30 ml undiluted q. 2 hrs
Dihydroxyaluminum aminoacetate	Robalate	1–2 g q.i.d.
Dihydroxyaluminum sodium carbonate	Rolaids Antacid	1 or 2 tablets as required
Calcium compounds:		
Calcium carbonate	Tums; Chooz; others	0.5–2 g
Calcium phosphate	—	1–4 gm
Magnesium compounds:		
Magnesium carbonate	—	0.5–2 g
Magnesia	Milk of Magnesia	5–10 ml q.i.d.
Magnesium oxide	Par-Mag; Maox; others	250–1000 mg
Magnesium phosphate	—	1–2 g
Magnesium trisilicate	—	1–14 g q.i.d.
Mixtures of aluminum and magnesium compounds:		
Aluminum hydroxide and magnesium hydroxide tablets	Aludrox; Gelusil; Mylanta; Di-Gel	300–600 mg
Aluminum hydroxide and magnesium carbonate liquid	Gaviscon	5–30 ml
Aluminum hydroxide and magnesium trisilicate tablets	Neutracomp; Magnatrel	300–600 mg
Magaldrate	Riopan	480–960 mg
Magnesia and alumina oral suspension	Maalox; others	5–30 ml; 200–400 mg tablets
Miscellaneous:		
Sodium bicarbonate	Soda Mint	0.3–2g 1–4 times daily

Clinical Indications. Sodium bicarbonate is employed as a gastric antacid.

Adverse Effects/Precautions. Sodium bicarbonate contains 27% sodium and a systemic alkalosis can develop with its chronic use. If taken with milk for extended periods, a milk-alkali syndrome results. Clinical symptoms of this milk-alkali (Burnett) syndrome include anorexia, weakness, mental confusion, hypercalcemia, and rarely, tetany. As kidney impairment may occur, renal insufficiency predisposes an individual to the milk-alkali syndrome.

Aluminum Hydroxide Gel. Aluminum hydroxide gel removes hydrogen ions from solution at the acid pH of the gastric contents.

Mechanism of Action. Aluminum hydroxide gel partially neutralizes and partially adsorbs gastric acid. The gel does not produce an alkaline reaction, and, hence, "acid rebound" does not result. The onset of action is fairly slow and the pH of the stomach contents is raised to about 4.

Aluminum hydroxide is converted to aluminum chloride in the stomach. The alkalinity of the small intestine produces a reformed aluminum hydroxide with concurrent chloride release and absorption into the blood. Consequently, no alteration in blood acid-base occurs.

Clinical Indications. Aluminum hydroxide gel is a local acting gastric antacid.

Adverse Effects/Precautions. The main side effect of aluminum hydroxide gel is its constipating tendency. Another possible reaction is excessive fecal phosphate loss due to the capacity of aluminum to bind and decrease the absorption of phosphate. Anorexia, malaise, and muscle weakness characterize this hypophosphatemia.

Elevated serum and bone levels of aluminum occur in some patients receiving chronic aluminum hydroxide therapy. Also reported is an aluminum system toxicity evidenced by encephalopathy. Decreased gastrointestinal absorption of fluoride may also occur with aluminum hydroxide therapy. The resorption of calcium and demineralization of bone that accompanies phosphate depletion may occur as early as the third week of aluminum hydroxide therapy, resulting in osteomalacia. Aluminum phosphate is less likely to cause phosphate loss; however, it has a lower capacity (50% less) than aluminum hydroxide to neutralize hydrocloric acid.

Magnesium Hydroxide. Magnesium hydroxide (hydrated magnesium), also called "milk of magnesia," is regarded as a popular antacid and cathartic by the lay public. Magnesium hydroxide is often combined with aluminum hydroxide in antacid preparations.

Mechanism of Action. Magnesium hydroxide has a prompt neutralizing effect on gastric hydrochloric acid. Soluble magnesium chloride is formed after interaction of the antacid with hydrochloric acid. Acid rebound following magnesium hydroxide is not clinically significant. The laxative effect of magnesium hydroxide counteracts the constipating effect of aluminum salts when they are combined in antacid preparations.

Clinical Indications. A nonsystemic antacid usually found in combination with aluminum antacids, magnesium hydroxide is effective in the treatment of peptic ulcer.

Adverse Effects/Precautions. A disadvantage of magnesium hydroxide in some patients is its cathartic effect. A small percentage of the magnesium in magnesium hydroxide (5 to 10%) is absorbed; extensive retention may result in neurologic, neuromuscular, and cardiovascular impairment. Chronic use of magnesium hydroxide has produced fecal stones composed of magnesium carbonate and magnesium hydroxide.

Magnesium Trisilicate. Magnesium trisilicate is a nonsystemic antacid that is often combined with aluminum hydroxide gel in antacid preparations.

Mechanism of Action. Magnesium trisilicate is converted to magnesium chloride and hydrated silicon dioxide. The value of the latter is that it coats the ulcer craters and protects the underlying tissue from hydrochloric acid and pepsin. Magnesium chloride is converted to magnesium carbonate in the alkalinity of the small intestine, making the chloride available for absorption. Chloride absorption helps maintain the blood acid-base balance.

Clinical Indications. Magnesium trisilicate is used as an antacid to treat peptic ulcer.

Adverse Effects/Precautions. Magnesium trisilicate produces diarrhea in some patients. Some silica is apparently absorbed since silicon-containing kidney stones have been reported (15 g/day magnesium trisilicate for 3 to 4 years).

Dihydroxyaluminum Sodium Carbonate. This compound combines in a single entity the properties of sodium bicarbonate and aluminum hydroxide.

Mechanism of Action. The sodium carbonate moiety reacts promptly with the hydrogen ion, resulting in the evolution of carbon dioxide (CO_2) and the formation of aluminum hydroxide. The latter then exerts a more sustained moderate buffering action.

Clinical Indications. Dihydroxyaluminum sodium carbonate is effective in treating gastric acidity (heartburn and gastrointestinal discomfort).

Adverse Effects/Precautions. Aluminum antacids may bind with phosphate ions in the intestine to form insoluble aluminum phosphate; therefore, prolonged use could result in hypophosphatemia. The aluminum ion inhibits spontaneous and induced smooth muscle contractions and consequently reduces gastric emptying. Thus, cautious use of aluminum-containing products is recommended in patients with gastric outlet obstruction.

Calcium Carbonate. Calcium carbonate, a prompt acting potent antacid, may produce acid rebound.

Mechanism of Action. Calcium carbonate and sodium bicarbonate have the greatest acid neutralizing capacity. Calcium carbonate reacts with hydrogen ions in the formation of carbon dioxide (CO_2), water, and calcium ions. The latter react in the alkaline of the small intestine to form calcium carbonate. The minimal absorption of calcium carbonate results in a minor degree of hypercalcemia; thus, chronic therapy is not advised.

Clinical Indications. Calcium carbonate is used for the symptomatic relief of upset stomach due to hyperacidity.

Adverse Effects/Precautions. Calcium carbonate causes a constipating effect in some patients. This reaction is reversible through the combination of calcium carbonate with magnesium oxide or magnesium hydroxide. Calcium carbonate is especially prone to produce acid rebound.

Magaldrate. Magaldrate is a chemical combination of aluminum hydroxide and magnesium hydroxide.

Mechanism of Action. Magaldrate has a greater acid neutralizing capacity than magnesium trisilicate but is less than that of magnesium hydroxide, aluminum hydroxide, or aluminum phosphate.

Clinical Indications. Magaldrate is indicated for the symptomatic treatment of heartburn, sour stomach, and indigestion associated with gastric hyperacidity. It is also used for symptomatic relief of hyperacidity associated with peptic ulcer, gastritis, peptic esophagitis, and hiatal hernia.

Adverse Effects/Precautions. Patients with kidney disease should avoid excessive magaldrate dosage.

Sucralfate. Sucralfate, a sulfated disaccharide which is minimally absorbed from the gastrointestinal tract, is an ulcer-coating drug.

Mechanism of Action. Sucralfate forms an ulcer-adherent complex with the proteinaceous exudate at the ulcer site. A sucralfate-albumen film acts as a barrier to hydrogen ions. Sucralfate's anti-ulcer activity apparently results from its protective action against acid, pepsin, and bile salts by the formation of an ulcer-adherent complex that coats the ulcer crater. Sucralfate absorbs pepsin and may inhibit pepsin activity up to 33% over a 30-minute period. By binding to bile salts, the drug has potential value in cases of gastric ulcer that have high bile salt concentrations. Sucralfate has almost no acid-neutralizing capacity.

Clinical Indications. Sucralfate, available as Carafate[R], is indicated for the short-term (up to 8 weeks) treatment of duodenal ulcer. The recommended dosage is 1 g q.i.d. (1 hour before meals and at bedtime) on an empty stomach.

Adverse Effects/Precautions. Constipation is the most frequently reported adverse effect.

HISTAMINE H_2 RECEPTOR BLOCKING DRUGS

Cimetidine and ranitidine (Table 8.2) prevent a histamine-triggered release of hydrochloric acid by blocking histamine receptors on acid secretory cells.

Cimetidine. Cimetidine was the first histamine H_2 receptor blocking drug to be introduced for the treatment of peptic ulcer.

Mechanism of Action. Cimetidine inhibits the action of histamine at the H_2 receptor site on gastric parietal cells. Both daytime and nocturnal basal gastric acid secretion, as well as chemically induced secretion, are blocked by cimetidine. The resultant decreased volume of gastric juice reduces total pepsin output.

Clinical Indications. Cimetidine is indicated in the prophylaxis and short-term treatment of both peptic ulcer and benign gastric ulcer. Hypersecretory conditions, such as Zollinger-Ellison (Z-E) syndrome, are also treated with cimetidine.

Adverse Effects/Precautions. Although cimetidine is generally well tolerated and side effects are infrequent, reports of central nervous system (CNS) side effects, including drowsiness, hyperactivity, delirium, and occasionally psychoses, have followed cimetidine administration. These adverse reactions are most likely to occur in patients with impaired renal function. Cimetidine has antiandrogen effects that become evident as gynecomastia and impotence; these reactions appear in the first few weeks of therapy and usually disappear with time. Cimetidine also increases serum creatinine in some patients.

Ranitidine. An H_2 receptor antagonist, ranitidine is chemically dissimilar from cimetidine as it contains a substituted furan ring instead of a substituted imidazole ring.

Mechanism of Action. Ranitidine is a reversible competitive inhibitor of histamine action at H_2 receptors, including those of the gastric parietal cells. Ranitidine inhibits both basal daytime and nocturnal acid secretion and acid secretion initiated by food and pentagastrin. Pepsin, gas-

Table 8.2. HISTAMINE H_2 RECEPTOR BLOCKERS.

Available products	Trade names	Daily dosage range
Cimetidine	Tagamet	300 mg q.i.d.
Famotidine	Pepcid	40 mg/day at bedtime
Ranitidine	Zantac	150 mg t.i.d.

trin, and intrinsic factor secretion are not significantly affected by ranitidine.

Clinical Indications. Ranitidine is used for the short-term treatment of active duodenal ulcer, as well as in Zollinger-Ellison (Z-E) syndrome treatment.

Adverse Effects/Precautions. Headache is the most frequently reported side effect of ranitidine. Malaise, dizziness, constipation, nausea, and rash are other adverse reactions. The decreased risk of CNS side effects is attributed to the furan ring in the ranitidine structure, rendering it less likely to cross the blood brain barrier.

Famotidine. Famotidine, a new histamine H_2 receptor blocker, is available in oral and intravenous forms.

Mechanism of Action. Famotidine is a reversible competitive inhibitor of histamine action at H_2 receptors.

Clinical Indications. Famotidine is used to treat duodenal ulcers and gastric acid hypersecretory states and to prevent duodenal ulcer recurrence. Once a day (at bedtime) dosage is recommended for treatment of duodenal ulcer.

Adverse Effects/Precautions. Adverse effects reported with famotidine include headache, dizziness, constipation, nausea, flatulence, anorexia, and diarrhea. Disorientation and hallucinations are CNS side reactions that have occurred with famotidine therapy.

ANTISPASMODICS/ANTICHOLINERGICS

The gastrointestinal anticholinergics (Table 8.3) decrease motility in the gastrointestinal and biliary tracts; some of these agents also have an antisecretory effect. These drugs exert their pharmacologic response by competitive antagonism of acetylcholine at postganglionic receptors on smooth muscle of the gastrointestinal tract. These are muscarinic sites in classical terminology (see Chapter 2); hence, the term antimuscarinic agents is often applied to these drugs.

Mechanism of Action. Appropriate doses of these drugs block the muscarinic actions of acetylcholine on gastrointestinal smooth muscle and secretory sites. Only larger doses of these drugs (which often cause adverse effects) ordinarily inhibit gastrointestinal secretions. Some of these agents inhibit CNS muscarinic receptors. Large doses may also block nicotinic receptors at the autonomic ganglia and at the neuromuscular junction of voluntary skeletal muscles.

Clinical Indications. The antispasmodic/anticholinergics are used as adjunctive therapy together with diet, antacids, and possibly a histamine H_2 receptor blocker in the treatment of peptic ulcer. In general, gastric acid secretion can be inhibited only at dosage levels that produce clinically significant side effects.

Other functional disorders that respond well to these drugs include spastic gastrointestinal conditions, general gastrointestinal hypermotility, mild ulcerative colitis, acute pancreatitis, gastritis, and gastroenteritis. Spastic disorders of the biliary tract (biliary colic, biliary dyskinesia) are treated with these agents, usually in conjunction with a narcotic analgesic.

Adverse Effects/Precautions. The adverse effects are dose-related and ordinarily pertain to muscarinic receptor blockade. These reactions include dry mouth, tachycardia, urinary retention, and blurred vision. Central nervous system reactions, such as headaches, flushing, and nervousness, may also occur. High doses are associated with CNS stimulation.

LAXATIVES

Laxatives (Table 8.4) are useful in the short-term treatment of constipation. Oftentimes, however, laxatives are misused because of the mistaken belief that a voluminous daily bowel movement is essential to good health. Several different classes of laxatives are available, in-

Table 8.3. ANTISPASMODIC DRUGS.

Available products	Trade names	Daily dosage range
Naturally occurring:		
Atropine sulfate	—	0.4–0.6 mg
Belladonna	Belladonna Extract; Belladonna Tincture	15 mg t.i.d.–q.i.d.; 0.6–1.0 ml t.i.d.–q.i.d.
Levorotatory Alkaloids of Belladonna	Bellafoline	0.25–0.5 mg t.i.d.
Hyoscyamine sulfate	Anaspaz; Levsin; others	0.125–0.25 mg q. 3–4 hrs orally
Methscopolamine bromide	Pamine	2.5–5 mg
Scopolamine HBr	—	Oral, 0.4–0.8 mg
Synthetic anticholinergics:		
Anisotropine methylbromide	Valpin 50	50 mg t.i.d.
Clidinium bromide	Quarzan	2.5–5 mg t.i.d. or q.i.d.
Glycopyrrolate	Robinul	1 mg b.i.d.
Hexocyclium methylsulfate	Tral	25 mg q.i.d.
Isopropamide iodide	Darbid	5 mg q. 12 hrs
Mepenzolate bromide	Cantil	25–50 mg q.i.d.
Methantheline bromide	Banthine	50–100 mg q. 6 hrs
Methixene HCl	Trest	1–2 mg t.i.d.
Oxyphencyclimine HCl	Daricon	10 mg
Oxyphenonium bromide	Antrenyl Bromide	10 mg q.i.d.
Propantheline bromide	Pro-Banthine; others	7.5 mg t.i.d.
Tridihexethyl Cl	Pathilon	25–50 mg t.i.d. or q.i.d.
Synthetic antispasmodics with limited anticholinergic activity:		
Dicyclomine HCl	Bentyl; others	10–20 mg t.i.d. or q.i.d.
Thiphenamil HCl	Trocinate	100–400 mg

cluding stimulant, lubricant, bulk, saline, and fecal softening agents.

STIMULANT (IRRITANT) LAXATIVES

Stimulant laxatives increase intestinal motor activity by a direct action. Prolonged use of stimulant (irritant) laxatives can lead to dependence and loss of normal bowel function.

Phenolphthalein. Phenolphthalein is a tasteless, rather mild stimulant laxative.

Mechanism of Action. Phenolphthalein exerts its stimulating effect on the colon, usually within 6 to 8 hours. First dissolved by the bile salts and alkaline intestinal secretions and absorbed, phenolphthalein is then excreted back into the intestinal tract in the bile. The enterohepatic cycle prolongs the phenolphthalein activity.

Clinical Indications. Phenolphthalein is used for the short-term treatment of constipation.

Adverse Effects/Precautions. Idiosyncratic reactions to phenolphthalein include a polychromatic skin eruption that is characterized by macular plaques of different sizes. These lesions are dark pink or purple and may persist for several months, accompanied by itching and burning. Reports of cardiac and respiratory distress have followed administration of this laxative. Also, phenolphthalein causes pink or red discoloration of sufficiently alkaline urine. Osteomalacia may result from excessive use of phenolphthalein due to impaired absorption of vitamin D and calcium. Abuse of this laxative also produces renal juxtaglomerular cell hyperplasia and resultant secondary aldosteronism.

Bisacodyl. Chemically related to phenolphthalein, bisacodyl is a stimulant laxative.

Table 8.4. LAXATIVES.

Available products	Trade names	Daily dosage range
Irritant:		
Bisacodyl	Dulcolax; Deficol	10–15 mg
Casanthranol	In Peri-Colace	30 mg
Cascara sagrada	—	325–650 mg
Cascara sagrada, aromatic fluid extract	—	5 ml
Cascara sagrada, fluid extract	—	1 ml
Castor oil	Castor Oil; others	15–60 ml
Danthron	Dorbane; Modane	37.5–150 mg
Phenolphthalein	Phenolax; Ex-Lax; others	30–195 mg
Senna	Senokot Syrup; others	10–15 ml
Senna fluid extract	—	2 ml
Calcium Salts of Sennocides A and B	Glysennid; Nytilax	12 mg
Bulk/Osmotic:		
Magnesium sulfate	Epsom salts	variable
Magnesia magma	Milk of Magnesia; others	15–30 ml
Indigestible Fiber-type—Agar	In Agoral	7.5–30 ml
Psyllium	Metamucil; Mucilose; others	1 tsp 1–3 times daily
Softening:		
Lubricants—Mineral oil	Nujol; others	5–30 ml
Fecal softeners—Docusate calcium	Surfak; others	50–150 mg
Docusate potassium	Dialose; Kasof	100–300 mg
Docusate sodium	Colace; Doxinate; others	50–240 mg
Lactulose	Chronulac	15–30 ml
Poloxalkol	Magcyl; Polykol	200 mg
Poloxamer	Alaxin	480 mg

Mechanism of Action. Bisacodyl has a direct action on the colon mucosa. Parasympathetic reflexes are activated by the contact action of bisacodyl with the mucosal nerve plexus (Auerbach's plexus).

Clinical Indications. Used for the short-term treatment of constipation, bisacodyl is also recommended for cleaning the colon before and after surgery and before x-ray examination. Another of its uses is to evacuate the colon before proctologic examination.

Adverse Effects/Precautions. Abdominal cramps are occasionally noted with bisacodyl. Bisacodyl tablets are enteric coated to prevent gastric irritation and should not be broken up or chewed before swallowing.

Senna and Sennocides. Senna, an anthracene-type laxative, is obtained from the dried leaves or pods of Cassia acutifolia or Cassia augustifolia.

Mechanism of Action. Emodin glycosides that are present in senna (sennocides) are hydrolyzed by colonic bacteria to emodin in the intestine. By stimulating the colon, emodin induces a cathartic activity. As such, sennocides also have a purgative action. The site of action is Auerbach's plexus in the wall of the colon.

Clinical Indications. Senna preparations are effective in functional constipation (chronic, geriatric, antepartum, postpartum, drug-induced, and pediatric), as well as in functional constipation that is concurrent with heart disease or anorectal surgery.

Adverse Effects/Precautions. At recommended dosage levels, senna preparations are virtually free of adverse effects. However, loose stools or abdominal discomfort may accompany senna use. Following ingestion of a senna laxative, postpartum women have noted a discoloration in their breast milk. Chrysophanic acid, a component of senna, colors acidic urine brownish and alkaline urine reddish-violet.

Danthron. Danthron (1,8 dihydroxyanthraquinone) is a breakdown product of senna glycosides whose properties and site of action resemble those of the senna glycosides. An important difference, however, is that danthron is partially absorbed in the small intestine and undergoes hepatic biotransformation. Danthron, which tends to produce fecal dehydration, is commonly combined with docusate in laxative preparations.

Cascara Segrada ("Sacred Bark"). Cascara segrada is the dried bark of the buckthorn tree, Rhamnus purshiana. Called the "All-American" laxative, cascara segrada was originally used by the Native Americans of California.

Mechanism of Action. Cascara segrada contains emodin which acts on the colon to increase peristalsis and evacuation. In ordinary doses, cascara segrada is the mildest anthraquinone laxative.

Clinical Indications. Cascara segrada is used in the short-term treatment of constipation. Liquid preparations of cascara segrada have a more reliable laxative action than the solid dosage forms.

Adverse Effects/Precautions. Prolonged use (4 to 15 months) of cascara segrada can cause melanotic pigmentation of the colon mucosa (melanosis coli). This melanosis disappears within several months after discontinuation of the drug.

Casanthranol. Casanthranol, a proprietary preparation of the cascara segrada glycosides, is present with docusate in combination laxative products.

Castor Oil. An irritant laxative, castor oil is extracted from the seed of Ricinus communis (castor bean).

Mechanism of Action. Castor oil is a triglyceride of the unsaturated fatty acid ricinoleic acid. In the alkaline juices of the small intestine, it is hydrolyzed to ricinolic acid by pancreatic lipase; ricinolic acid and sodium ricinolate cause the laxative action. The mechanism of the laxative effect apparently relates to adenosine 3', 5'-monophosphate (cyclic AMP)-induced fluid secretion.

The increased motility is along the entire gastrointestinal tract, including the small intestine, so that excessive loss of fluid, electrolytes, and nutrients may occur. Castor oil produces a fluid stool in 2 to 6 hours.

Clinical Indications. Usually administered on an empty stomach, castor oil is effective in the short-term treatment of constipation, as well as prior to x-ray examination of the gastrointestinal tract and before bowel surgery.

Adverse Effects/Precautions. Depending upon the degree of irritation, castor oil may be contraindicated during menstruation or pregnancy. This laxative should not be used if nausea, vomiting, or abdominal pain (possible appendicitis) are present.

LUBRICANT LAXATIVES

Lubricant laxatives are bland, pharmacologically inert oils, such as mineral oil and olive oil.

Mineral Oil. Mineral oil (liquid petrolatum) is a mixture of indigestible liquid hydrocarbons obtained from petroleum.

Mechanism of Action. Mineral oil penetrates and softens the fecal contents by coating them, thus inhibiting colonic absorption of water. Emulsified preparations of mineral oil are more effective in penetrating the fecal mass.

Clinical Indications. Mineral oil is used for the short-term treatment of constipation, especially when straining during defecation is a hazard. Mineral oil enemas soften and lubricate hard stools, easing their passage without irritating the mucosa.

Adverse Effects/Precautions. Adverse effects usually result from prolonged and repeated use of mineral oil. These reactions include significant absorption where parafinnomas have been noted in the mesenteric lymph ducts. Lipid pneumonia, due to aspiration of the oil, is possible, especially if the liquid is taken before bedtime. The intestinal absorption of calcium, phosphates, and oil-soluble vitamins (A, D, E, and K) is possibly inhibited. Finally, leakage through the anal sphincter is another potential problem. Because of their greater penetration properties, emulsified preparations of mineral oil are possibly less likely to produce this adverse effect.

BULK LAXATIVES

Bulk-forming laxatives most closely approximate the physiologic mechanism in promoting evacuation. This laxative class consists of natural and semi-synthetic polysaccharides and cellulose derivatives that dissolve or swell in the intestinal fluids. Emollient gels are formed that facilitate passage of the fecal mass and stimulate peristalsis. Bulk laxatives should be taken with a full glass of water, followed by additional fluid intake. Although these laxatives usually act in 12 to 24 hours, they may require as long as 3 days.

Psyllium (Plantago Seed). Psyllium seeds contain a mucilagenous material; in the presence of moisture, these seeds swell to form a jelly-like indigestible mass. Psyllium hydrophillic muciloid, a refined dietary fiber, is derived from the husk of Plantago ovata.

Mechanism of Action. Psyllium hydrophillic muciloid forms a bland, non-irritating bulky mass to promote normal intestinal evacuation.

Clinical Indications. Psyllium seed products are indicated in the management of chronic constipation, as adjunctive therapy in the constipation of duodenal ulcer and diverticulitis, and in the bowel management of patients with hemorrhoids.

Adverse Effects/Precautions. Ingested or inhaled psyllium powder may cause allergic reactions in hypersensitive patients. Psyllium products are contraindicated in intestinal obstruction and fecal impaction.

Agar (Japanese Seaweed). Agar, a mucilaginous substance, is extracted from marine algae growing along the eastern coast of Asia.

Mechanism of Action. Consisting mainly of an indigestible hemicellulose which forms a gelatinous mass in contact with water, agar adds bulk to the intestinal contents.

Clinical Indications. Agar is effective, usually in laxative combinations, as a mild laxative.

Adverse Effects/Precautions. The use of a bulk-forming laxative can cause intestinal obstruction, especially if stimulant laxative abuse has compromised colon motility.

Other Natural Bulk Laxatives. Alginates (derived from sea kelp) and plant gums, such as tragacanth, chondrus, and karaya are additional bulk-forming laxatives used to manage constipation.

SYNTHETIC CELLULOSE DERIVATIVES

Methylcellulose and carboxymethyl cellulose are often present in combination laxative products that also contain stimulant and/or fecal-softening laxatives.

Calcium polycarbophil is the calcium salt of a hydrophilic polyacrylic resin indicated for the treatment of constipation.

SALINE LAXATIVES

Saline laxatives contain nonabsorbable cations and anions that act to provide osmotic retention of water in the intestinal lumen.

Magnesium Sulfate (Epsom Salts) Magnesium sulfate is a prototype isomotic laxative that draws water into the intestinal lumen.

Mechanism of Action. The increased intraluminal pressure, resulting from osmotic water retention in the intestinal lumen, exerts a mechanical stimulus which increases intestinal motility. This laxative produces liquid stools.

Clinical Indications. Magnesium sulfate is generally indicated for use in acute evacuation of the bowel in preparation for endoscopic examination and for elimination of drugs in suspected poisoning. The drug is not medically accepted in the long-term management of constipation.

Adverse Effects/Precautions. Prolonged intestinal retention of magnesium sulfate can cause significant magnesium absorption, renal impairment, and systemic effects, including CNS depression. Hypotension, muscle weakness, and electrocardiogram changes may signal magnesium toxicity.

Other Osmotic Laxatives. Glycerin suppositories induce an osmotic effect; this together with the local irritant effect of the sodium stearate base, usually produces a bowel movement within 30 minutes.

Dibasic sodium phosphate, monobasic sodium phosphate, sodium sulfate, and sodium biphosphate are other examples of saline laxatives.

FECAL SOFTENERS

Docusate, formerly known as dioctyl sodium sulfosuccinate, is a prototype surface-active agent that facilitates admixture of aqueous and fatty substances. The formation of oil in water emulsions softens the fecal mass.

Docusate Sodium. Docusate, a nonabsorbable, nontoxic surfactant, is used as a fecal softening agent.

Mechanism of Action. Docusate, an anionic surfactant, promotes water retention in the fecal mass, thus softening the stool. Although most effective as a laxative when the feces are hard and dry, docusate is also useful in anorectal conditions in which passage of a firm stool is painful.

Clinical Indications. Docusate is indicated in the management of constipation in which maximum ease of stool passage is desirable and when peristaltic stimulation is contraindicated.

Adverse Effects/Precautions. Bitter taste, throat irritation, and nausea are the primary side effects reported with docusate use. Docusate calcium and docusate potassium are alternates to docusate sodium when sodium is contraindicated. Poloxamer 188, a nonionic surfactant, is also used as a fecal softener.

Lactulose. Lactulose, a synthetic disaccharide analog of lactose, produces stool softening.

Mechanism of Action. Oral doses of lactulose pass to the colon virtually unchanged. Colonic bacteria (such as lactobacilli, Escherichia coli, and Streptococcus faecalis) break down lactulose to lactic acid, formic acid, acetic acid, and carbon dioxide. These degradation products increase osmotic pressure and acidify the colonic fecal mass. The result is a fecal softening effect and an increase in stool water.

Clinical Indications. Lactulose is used to manage constipation.

Adverse Effects/Precautions. Reports of transient flatulence, nausea, and intestinal cramps have followed lactulose use. Diarrhea may also occur with excessive dosage.

Bile Salts. Bile salts are absorbed orally and exhibit choleretic action.

Mechanism of Action. Choleretics increase bile flow and aid fat digestion and absorption.

Clinical Indications. Bile salts are used as a laxative in the symptomatic treatment of uncomplicated constipation.

Adverse Effects/Precautions. Excessive dosage may result in loose stools and cramping. Bile salts are contraindicated in the presence of abdominal pain, nausea, and vomiting.

DIGESTIVE AIDS

These agents (Table 8.5) are often replacement drugs used to correct defective digestive processes resulting from deficient gastrointestinal

Table 8.5. DIGESTIVE AIDS.

Available products	Trade names	Daily dosage range
Chenodiol	Chenix	13–16 mg/kg in 2 divided doses
Dehydrocholic acid	Decholin; Cholan-DH	240–500 mg t.i.d
Glutamic acid HCl	Acidulin; Muripsin	300–600 mg
Bile salts	Ox Bile Extract; Bilron	150–600 mg
Pancreatin	Pancreatin; Viokase	500–1000 mg
Pancrelipase	Cotazyme; Ilozyme; others	150–300 mg

secretions. Some drugs stimulate a hypofunctional gland or secretory cells to release necessary digestive factors.

PANCREATIC ENZYMES

Pancreatin and pancrelipase are enzymes that are used in replacement therapy for patients with deficient pancreatic exocrine function. These drugs are of bovine or porcine origin.

Mechanism of Action. These enzymes aid in the digestion of fats, triglycerides, and carbohydrates. Pancreatin and pancrelipase exert their effect in the duodenum and upper jejunum. The use of enteric coatings to protect the enzymes, although theoretically sound, may partially inhibit delivery of the enzymes to the duodenum. Histamine H_2 receptor blockers and antacids may increase the availability of pancreatin in the duodenum. Pancrelipase has greater lipase activity than pancreatin and is effective in lower doses to control steatorrhea.

Clinical Indications. These enzymes are used as replacement therapy in chronic pancreatitis, ductal obstruction in pancreatic carcinoma, cystic fibrosis, pancreatic insufficiency, and for steatorrhea in malabsorption syndrome.

Adverse Effects/Precautions. High doses may produce nausea, abdominal cramps, and/or diarrhea. Hyperuricosuria and hyperuricemia have followed administration of extremely high doses of these enzymes.

OTHER DIGESTANTS

Miscellaneous digestants include pepsin (an aid in protein digestion), diastase (an enzyme that facilitates starch digestion), and cellulase (to break down dietary cellulose). Bile extracts activate lipase and facilitate the emulsification of fats. Glutamic acid HCl and betaine HCl are useful as acidifiers in the lack of sufficient endogenous gastric hydrochloric acid.

Dehydrocholic Acid. A derivative of cholic acid, dehydrocholic acid acts as a hydrocholeretic by increasing bile secretion and by aiding fat digestion.

Mechanism of Action. Dehydrocholic acid increases the production of bile with a low viscosity and high water content.

Clinical Indications. Dehydrocholic acid is used as an adjunct in various clinical conditions involving the biliary tract (cholecystitis, biliary dyskinesia, and bile duct obstruction). This drug is also used in the treatment of uncomplicated constipation.

Adverse Effects/Precautions. Dehydrocholic acid should not be used when abdominal pain, nausea, or vomiting are present.

Chenodiol (Chenodeoxycholic Acid). Chenodiol is the only purified, naturally occurring human bile acid that is available commercially.

Mechanism of Action. Chenodiol suppresses synthesis of hepatic cholesterol and cholic acid. Chenodiol eventually replaces cholic acid and its metabolite, deoxycholic acid, in an expanded bile acid pool. These events lead to biliary cholesterol desaturation and gradual dissolution of radiolucent cholesterol gallstones.

Clinical Indications. Chenodiol is used when surgery for cholesterol gallstones is not feasible. Chenodiol therapy is reserved for carefully selected patients.

Adverse Effects/Precautions. Monitoring liver function is necessary due to increased incidences of intrahepatic cholestasis following chenodiol therapy. Serum aminotransferase (SGPT) elevations occur in about 30% of the patients receiving chenodiol. Those who develop chenodiol-induced serum aminotransferase elevation are poor inactivators (sulfate conjugation) of lithocholic acid, a known hepatotoxin. Active hepatitis is therefore a distinct possibility, especially in patients with pre-existing liver disease. Mild and transient diarrhea (dose-related) may also occur in about 30 to 40% of the patients receiving chenodiol therapy.

ANTIDIARRHEALS

Antidiarrheals (Table 8.6) include gastrointestinal adsorbents, lactobacillus cultures, and antiperistaltic drugs. Oral electrolyte concentrate is also used to treat diarrhea. Although controversial opinions surround the effectiveness of antidiarrheals in controlling diarrhea, the adsorbents are the most frequently used nonprescription antidiarrheals.

Kaolin. Kaolin is hydrated aluminum silicate.

Mechanism of Action. Kaolin acts locally in the gastrointestinal lumen to adsorb toxins, bacteria, and various noxious substances. It also adds solid matter to the colonic contents and improves fecal consistency.

Clinical Indications. Kaolin is used in combination with pectin or other antidiarrheal drugs to treat nonspecific mild diarrhea.

Adverse Effects/Precautions. No clinically significant side effects are noted with kaolin.

Pectin. Pectin, a complex carbohydrate present in many fruits, is extracted from citrus rinds and apple pomace.

Mechanism of Action. Pectin provides a protective coating on the irritated gastric mucosa, as well as acting as a gastrointestinal adsorbent.

Table 8.6. ANTIDIARRHEALS.

Available products	Trade names	Daily dosage range
Locally acting:		
Activated attapulgite	In Polymagma Plain	4 tablets
Bismuth subgallate	In Devron	1 or 2 tablets
Bismuth subsalicylate	In Pepto-Bismol	30 ml
Carboxymethylcellulose sodium	In Kaodene Non-Narcotic	45 ml
Kaolin mixture with pectin	Kaopectate	60–120 ml
Zinc phenolsulfonate	In Diastay	2–6 tablets
Systemically active:		
Antiperistaltic opiates—		
Opium, powdered	In Diabismul	1 or 2 tablets q.i.d.
Opium, tincture,	In Parelixir	15–30 ml t.i.d.–q.i.d.
Paregoric	In Corrective Mixture with Paregoric	30 ml
Antiperistalic opiate derivatives—		
Diphenoxylate HCl with atropine sulfate	Lomotil; Diphenatol; others	5 mg q.i.d.
Loperamide HCl	Imodium	2 mg

Clinical Indications. Pectin is often combined with kaolin and other antidiarrheal agents to treat mild, uncomplicated diarrhea.

Adverse Effects/Precautions. As with kaolin, no clinically significant adverse reactions occur with this antidiarrheal.

Attapulgite. A hydrous magnesium aluminum silicate, attapulgite is activated by thermal treatment and is employed as a fine powder.

Mechanism of Action. Attapulgite consists of finely divided particles that have adsorptive properties because of their high surface area. This drug probably acts by adsorbing toxins that are responsible for the diarrhea. Furthermore, attapulgite adds bulk to the intestinal contents to improve their consistency.

Clinical Indications. Attapulgite is used in combination with other antidiarrheals to treat mild, uncomplicated diarrhea.

Adverse Effects/Precautions. Attapulgite, like the other antidiarrheals, produces no known side effects.

Other Gastrointestinal Adsorbents. Activated charcoal is rarely used as an antidiarrheal, but it possesses excellent adsorbent properties. Bismuth subnitrate and bismuth subsalicylate are employed in antidiarrheal preparations as adsorbent astringents and protectives. Bismuth subnitrate is contraindicated in infants under the age of 2. Hypotension and methemoglobemia may result if gastrointestinal absorption of the nitrate (from the subnitrate) ion occurs. Bismuth compounds tend to color stools a dark color.

Lactobacillus Cultures. The seeding of the intestinal tract with viable Lactobacillus acidophilus and Lactobacillus bulgaricus is a controversial method of treating diarrhea. The bacterial flora of the gastrointestinal tract helps maintain bowel function. Certain situations, such as antibiotic therapy, may upset the microorganism balance in the intestinal tract, resulting in diarrhea.

Mechanism of Action. Lactobacillus acidophilus and Lactobacillus bulgaricus apparently suppress the growth of intestinal pathogens and restore a normal intestinal flora. No controlled studies document the effectiveness of lactobacilli in managing diarrhea by favorably modifying the intestinal flora.

Clinical Indications. Lactobacillus preparations have been used to control diarrhea that results from disruption of the normal bacterial flora.

Adverse Effects/Precautions. Recommended doses of Lactobacillus preparations produce no serious adverse reactions.

ANTIPERISTALTIC DRUGS

Several antiperistaltic preparations are widely used as effective antidiarrheal preparations.

Diphenoxylate with Atropine Sulfate. Diphenoxylate, a meperidine congener, has constipating properties, but it lacks any analgesic activity. A subtherapeutic dose of atropine is included in diphenoxylate preparations to discourage abuse.

Mechanism of Action. Diphenoxylate, an opiate-like drug which has a relatively selective action on the bowel, depresses gastrointestinal motility, especially propulsive movements. These actions may result from stimulation of cholinergic, tryptaminergic, and enkephalinergic receptors on the mesenteric plexus of the intestine. Additionally, a central mechanism may also contribute to the antidiarrheal effect.

High doses of diphenoxylate cause typical opiate-like activity, including euphoria, suppression of the morphine abstinence syndrome, and physical dependence after chronic administration.

Clinical Indications. Diphenoxylate is used as adjunctive therapy in acute or chronic diarrhea.

Adverse Effects/Precautions. Diphenoxylate may prolong or aggravate infectious diarrhea associated with intestinal mucosal invasion, such as that caused by salmonellae, shigellae, and toxigenic Escherichia coli. Diphenoxylate is contraindicated for use in these conditions. Since atropine sulfate is included in diphenoxylate preparations, excessive dosage may cause anticholinergic toxicity. These side effects, including dryness of the skin and mucous membranes, flushing, hyperthermia, tachycardia, and urinary retention, occur more frequently in children than in adults.

Loperamide. Loperamide, a chemical relative of diphenoxylate, has specific antidiarrheal activity.

Mechanism of Action. By binding to opiate receptors in the intestinal musculature, loperamide elicits a constipating effect. Inhibition of intestinal motility and effects on water and electrolyte movement in the bowel are mechanisms responsible for the antidiarrheal effect of loperamide. This drug prolongs the transit time, reduces the volume, and increases the bulk density/volume of the fecal mass, as well as diminishing the loss of blood and electrolytes. Tolerance to the constipating effects is not clinically significant.

Clinical Indications. Loperamide is used to treat nonspecific acute diarrhea and chronic diarrhea associated with inflammatory intestinal disorders. It also reduces the volume of discharge from ileostomies.

Adverse Effects/Precautions. Hypersensitivity reactions are the most serious adverse consequence of loperamide use. Abdominal pain and/or distention, nausea, and vomiting are other side effects that frequently occur with this drug; these reactions are similar to the symptoms of the diarrheal condition being treated.
Loperamide should not be used in acute infectious diarrhea in which the microorganisms commonly invade the intestinal mucosa (enteroinvasive Escherichia coli, salmonellae, shigellae). In some acute ulcerative colitis patients, the delay in transit time and decrease in intestinal motility relates to the development of toxic megacolon.

ORAL ELECTROLYTE CONCENTRATE (GASTROLYTE)

Oral rehydration is a simple and safe treatment for acute watery diarrhea, regardless of the causative factor.

MISCELLANEOUS GASTROINTESTINAL DRUGS

Miscellaneous gastrointestinal drugs include polycarbophil, simethicone, metoclopramide, dexpanthenol, and live yeast cell derivative.

COMBINATION LAXATIVE/ ANTIDIARRHEALS

A hydrophilic agent may exhibit dual action as a gastrointestinal drug.

Polycarbophil. A hydrophilic substance, calcium polycarbophil acts as a bulk laxative or as an antidiarrheal.

Mechanism of Action. Polycarbophil acts as a bulk laxative by retaining free water within the intestinal lumen. Diarrhea characterized by insufficient water absorption by the intestinal mucosa is controlled because of the absorption of free fecal water by polycarbophil with resultant gel formation and a formed stool.

Clinical Indications. Polycarbophil is used to treat constipation or diarrhea associated with irritable bowel syndrome and diverticulitis. The drug is also effective in nonspecific acute diarrhea.

Adverse Effects/Precautions. Polycarbophil is relatively free of side effects, but abdominal fullness may occur occasionally.

ANTIFLATULENT

Relieving flatulence often benefits patients with indigestion and gastric hyperacidity with gas.

Simethicone. Simethicone, an off-white translucent liquid, has antifoaming properties and is often present in combination products with antacids.

Mechanism of Action. The defoaming action of simethicone relieves flatulence by dispersing and preventing formation of mucus-encircled gas pockets in the gastrointestinal tract. Simethicone reduces the surface tension of the gas bubbles, allowing them to coalesce and free the gas. The gas is then eliminated more easily by passing flatus (belching).

Clinical Indications. Simethicone relieves excessive gas in the gastrointestinal tract in conditions such as peptic ulcer, spastic or irritable colon, postoperative gas distention, or diverticulitis.

Adverse Effects/Precautions. No significant adverse reactions occur with simethicone.

GASTROINTESTINAL MUSCULATURE STIMULANTS

In addition to the cholinergic (muscarinic) stimulants, such as urecholine (see Chapter 2), several drugs are used to stimulate gastrointestinal motility in selected clinical situations.

Metoclopramide (Reglan^R). Metoclopramide stimulates motility in the upper gastrointestinal tract without activating gastric, biliary, or pancreatic secretions.

Mechanism of Action. Metoclopramide sensitizes the gastrointestinal musculature to the muscarinic action of acetylcholine. Although the action of metoclopramide does not depend upon vagal innervation, it can be abolished with muscarinic blocking drugs.

Metoclopramide increases the tone and amplitude of antral contractions, relaxes the pyloric sphincter, and increases peristalsis in the duodenum and jejunum. These effects accelerate gastric emptying and increase intestinal transit.

Clinical Indications. Metoclopramide is used to relieve symptoms associated with acute and recurrent diabetic gastroparesis (diabetic gastric stasis). The clinical manifestations of delayed gastric emptying, such as nausea, fullness after meals, and anorexia, are relieved by metoclopramide.

Adverse Effects/Precautions. Adverse effects occur in 20 to 30% of patients receiving metoclopramide. CNS side effects, such as drowsiness, extrapyramidal reactions, and parkinsonism-like symptoms, are also frequently reported. Nausea and diarrhea occur in fewer than 10% of the patients receiving this drug.

Dexpanthenol (Dextro Pantothenyl Alcohol, Panol^R, Ilopan^R). Dexpanthenol is the alcohol analog of the vitamin pantothenic acid.

Mechanism of Action. The mechanism of action is unknown. Pantothenic acid, an integral component of coenzyme A, functions in the synthesis of acetylcholine. As the neurotransmitter at parasympathetic postganglionic fibers (Chapter 2), acetylcholine contributes to the maintenance of normal gastrointestinal motility. If acetylcholine content is lower in decreased peristalsis or adyamic ileus, then increasing its levels would theoretically counteract these conditions.

Clinical Indications. Dexpanthenol is indicated for prophylactic use after major surgery to minimize the possibility of intestinal atony or paralytic ileus.

Adverse Effects/Precautions. Although adverse reactions to dexpanthenol are infrequent, itching, tingling, and breathing difficulty may occur.

ANTIHEMORRHOID PREPARATIONS

Local anesthetics (see Chapter 10) and live yeast cell derivative are used to relieve hemorrhoidal symptoms. Live yeast cell derivative (Preparation H^R) apparently acts by increasing the oxygen uptake of dermal tissue and by promoting collagen formation.

ANTIEMETICS

Antiemetic activity results from several classes of pharmacologic agents (Table 8.7). These include sedative-hypnotics (agents that reduce anxiety), anticholinergics (drugs that reduce the excitability receptors in the labyrinthine apparatus), antihistamines (H_2 receptor blockers that act on the vestibular apparatus and are effective in motion sickness), phenothiazines (compounds that depress the medullary chemoreceptive trigger zone), and a miscellaneous group (agents that act directly on the hyperactive gut to relieve emesis).

Sedative-hypnotics, like phenobarbital, allay anxiety, a frequent precipitating factor in emesis. Anticholinergics, represented by scopolamine, block cholinergic receptors in the labyrinthine apparatus of the inner ear to reduce emesis. Antihistamines, such as dimenhydrinate and meclizine, which act on the vestibular apparatus, are commonly used as antimotion sickness drugs. Phenothiazines depress the chemoreceptive trigger zone in the medulla oblongata.

Chapters 1, 2, and 7 contain complete discussions of the preceding classes of drugs. In this section, we will discuss only antiemetics that act directly or locally.

DIRECT OR LOCAL ACTING ANTIEMETICS

Phosphorylated Carbohydrate Solution (Emetrol[R]). Phosphorylated carbohydrate solution is a mixture of fructose (levulose) and glucose (dextrose) with phosphoric acid added to adjust the pH of the solution. A "physiologic antiemetic action" is attributed to the liquid.

Mechanism of Action. Phosphorylated carbohydrate solution, which apparently has a direct relaxant effect on rapidly contracting smooth muscle, may prevent the transmission of impulses to the medullary emetic center by a direct effect on the hyperactive intestinal tract. The antiemetic activity may relate to a delay in gastric emptying because of the osmotic pressure of the solution.

Clinical Indications. Phosphorylated carbohydrate solution is used to treat problem regurgitation in children, the nausea and vomiting of morning sickness, and functional emesis (as that which occurs in anxiety).

Adverse Effects/Precautions. Although phosphorylated carbohydrate solution has no reported significant adverse reactions, large doses of fructose cause abdominal pain and diarrhea. Hypouricemia and hyperuricemia occur

Table 8.7. ANTIEMETICS.

Available products	Trade names	Daily dosage range
Benzquinamide HCl	Emete-con	50 mg IM; 25 mg IV
Buclizine HCl	Bucladin-S	50 mg
Chlorcyclizine HCl	Diparalene; Perazil	50 mg
Chlorpromazine HCl	Thorazine; others	10–25 mg q. 4–6 hrs
Cyclizine HCl	Marezine	50 mg
Dimenhydrinate	Dramamine; others	50–100 mg q. 4–6 hrs
Diphenhydramine HCl	Benadryl; others	50 mg
Diphenidol	Vontrol	25 mg q. 4 hrs
Meclizine HCl	Bonine; Antivert	25–50 mg
Perphenazine	Trilafon	8–16 mg
Prochlorperazine	Compazine	5–10 mg t.i.d. or q.i.d.
Promethazine HCl	Phenergan	25–50 mg
Scopolamine HBr	Triptone	0.25–0.8 mg
Thiethylperazine maleate	Torecan	10–30 mg
Triflupromazine HCl	Vesprin	20–30 mg
Trimethobenzamide HCl	Tigan; Tegamide	250 mg t.i.d. or q.i.d.

with high (500 mg/kg) oral doses of fructose. Diabetics should be forewarned of the high glucose content of this drug.

Bismuth Compounds. Bismuth preparations are promoted for the relief of nausea, vomiting, and upper gastrointestinal distress.

Mechanism of Action. Bismuth subsalicylate and bismuth subnitrate may coat the gastric mucosa to relieve nausea and heartburn.

Clinical Indications. Bismuth sub-salts (subsalicylate and subnitrate) may reduce the subjective complaints of nausea and abdominal cramping associated with certain types of intestinal disorders, such as excessive food and drink discomfort and gastroenteritis.

Adverse Effects/Precautions. Bismuth subnitrate introduces a risk of methemoglobinemia, especially in children under the age of 2. In adults, the tongue, dentures, and stools may darken with the use of bismuth compounds.

ANTIBIOTICS/ANTI-INFECTIVES USED IN GASTROINTESTINAL INFECTIONS

Many forms of gastrointestinal infectious disease are amenable to therapy with antibiotics/anti-infectives (Table 8.8).

ANTIBIOTICS

Several potentially fatal gastrointestinal diseases are effectively treated with antibiotics.

Chloramphenicol. Chloramphenicol is the antibiotic of choice in acute infections caused by Salmonella typhi. It is now mainly prepared synthetically after its initial isolation from Streptomyces venezuelae.

Mechanism of Action. Chloramphenicol inhibits bacterial protein synthesis by an action on the ribosomes. Specifically, chloramphenicol acts on the larger 50S subunit of the bacterial ribosome to inhibit its function.

Clinical Indications. The use of chloramphenicol is restricted primarily to the treatment of acute fever caused by Salmonella typhi (typhoid fever).

Adverse Effects/Precautions. Serious and fatal blood dyscrasias may occur after chloramphenicol administration. This drug must not be used for trivial infections or for infections in which other less potentially dangerous drugs are effective. Gray syndrome in infants and premature newborns (usually in the first 2 days of life) has occurred after chloramphenicol use; abdominal distention, progressive pallid cyanosis, and vasomotor collapse characterize this possibly fatal condition.

Neomycin. Neomycin, an aminoglycoside antibiotic, is produced by Streptomyces fradiae.

Mechanism of Action. Neomycin inhibits bacterial protein synthesis by an action of the 30S subunit of the ribosome.

Clinical Indications. Neomycin is effective in the treatment of gastrointestinal infections especially those due to enteropathogenic Escherichia coli. It is also indicated for suppression of the normal bacterial flora, such as in preoperative preparation.

Adverse Effects/Precautions. Oral administration of neomycin can result in intestinal malabsorption and superinfection.

Colistin (Polymyxin E). Colistin is a polypeptide antibiotic produced by strains of Bacillus polymyxa.

Mechanism of Action. By binding to the plasma membranes of sensitive bacteria, colistin causes leakage of small molecules, such as phosphates and nucleosides, from the cell interior. Colistin acts as a cationic surfactant to selectively alter susceptible bacterial plasma membranes.

Clinical Indications. Indicated in gastroenteritis due to Shigella organisms, colistin is also used as a pediatric treatment for diarrhea

Table 8.8. ANTIBIOTICS/ANTI-INFECTIVES.

Available products	Trade names	Daily dosage range
Antibiotics:		
Chloramphenicol	Chloromycetin; Mychel	50 mg/kg divided q. 6 hrs
Colistin sulfate	Coly-Mycin S	5–15 mg/kg in 3 divided doses
Neomycin sulfate	Neomycin Sulfate; Mycifradin Sulfate; Neobiotic	3 g
Tetracycline	(see Chapter 7, Table 7.2)	
Anti-infectives:		
Metronidazole	Flagyl; Metryl; others	750 mg t.i.d. for 5–10 days
Sulfamethoxazole	Ganatol; Urobak	2 g
Trimethoprim	Proloprim; Trimpex	100 mg q. 12 hrs

caused by susceptible strains of enteropathogenic Escherichia coli.

Adverse Effects/Precautions. Therapeutic doses do not produce adverse reactions. However, prolonged or repeated colistin therapy may result in suprainfection with bacterial or fungal overgrowth.

Tetracycline. Tetracycline is a broad-spectrum antibiotic isolated from Streptomyces aurefaciens.

Mechanism of Action. Tetracycline is primarily bacteriostatic and binds to both mRNA and the 30S subunit of the ribosome to inhibit protein synthesis.

Clinical Indications. Tetracycline is the drug of choice for both classical and El-tor cholera. Fluid and electrolyte replacement, urgently needed in such conditions, forms the basis for therapy.

Adverse Effects/Precautions. The toxic effects of tetracycline include gastrointestinal irritation, hypersensitivity reactions, photosensitivity, and superinfections by resistant organisms. Tetracycline chelates various metallic ions and forms insoluble, nonabsorbable complexes with Ca^{++}, Mg^{++}, AL^{+++}, and Fe^{++}-Fe^{+++}.

ANTI-INFECTIVES

Anti-infectives that are used to treat gastrointestinal disease include trimethoprim, sulfamethoxazole, and metronidazole.

Trimethoprim. Trimethoprim is chemically similar to part of the folic acid molecule.

Mechanism of Action. Trimethoprim impairs the synthesis of deoxyribonucleic acid (DNA). By inhibiting dihydrofolate reductase, trimethoprim blocks the conversion of dihydrofolic acid to tetrahydrofolic acid. The sensitivities of the enzymes in bacteria and certain protozoa to trimethoprim are many thousand times greater than that of mammalian enzymes. Thus, the host toxicity is minimal, and the bacterial biosynthesis of nucleic acids and proteins is preferentially blocked.

Clinical Indications. Trimethoprim in combination with sulfamethoxazole is indicated in acute gastroenteritis caused by sensitive strains of Salmonella and Shigella species.

Adverse Effects/Precautions. Dermatologic reactions, including rash, pruritus, and enfoliative dermatitis, are frequent adverse effects of trimethoprim. Epigastric distress, nausea, vomiting, and glossitis may also occur.

Sulfamethoxazole. Sulfamethoxazole, a "sulfa-drug," is a competitive inhibitor of para-aminobenzoic acid (PABA) in bacterial metabolism.

Mechanism of Action. Sulfamethoxazole is a structural analog and a competitive antagonist of para-aminobenzoic acid (PABA). The drug inhibits the incorporation of PABA into dihydropteroic acid, the immediate precursor of folic acid. Sulfamethoxazole does not affect mammalian cells by this mechanism since they require preformed folic acid and cannot synthesize it. Thus, a combination of sulfamethoxazole and trimethoprim provides a sequential block in bacterial folic acid and metabolism. Sulfamethoxazole inhibits the biosynthetic pathway of folic acid and trimethoprim blocks the utilization of folic acid once it is formed by the bacteria. The synergistic interaction is thus predictable from the drugs' respective mechanisms. A ratio of 20 parts/sulfamethoxazole to 1 part/trimethoprim is an optimal therapeutic combination.

Clinical Indications. Sulfamethoxazole, in combination with trimethoprim, is indicated in acute gastroenteritis caused by sensitive strains of Salmonella and Shigella species.

Adverse Effects/Precautions. Hematologic abnormalities, hypersensitivity reactions, gastrointestinal distress, and CNS toxicity are possible with sulfamethoxazole therapy.

Metronidazole. A nitroimidazole compound, metronidazole acts against certain anaerobic bacteria and protozoa.

Mechanism of Action. The nitro group of metronidazole acts as an electron acceptor for electron transport proteins to produce a reduced form of the drug. The chemically reactive reduced form of the drug apparently induces lethal biochemical lesions in the bacterial cell. For instance, reduced metronidazole disrupts the helical structure of DNA with strand breakage, thus impairing its function.

Clinical Indications. Metronidazole is used to treat amebic dysentery (acute amebic colitis). Reports of good cure rates for severe intestinal amebiasis and liver abscess have followed metronidazole therapy.

Adverse Effects/Precautions. Although side effects are relatively rare with metronidazole, the most serious adverse reactions are convulsive seizures and peripheral neuropathy. Gastrointestinal symptoms include anorexia, nausea, vomiting, and diarrhea.

Patients on metronidazole therapy should avoid alcoholic beverages since metronidazole interferes with alcohol metabolism to produce unpleasant sensations (such as palpitations and dizziness).

Sulfasalazine. A poorly absorbed sulfonamide, sulfasalazine is used in the treatment of ulcerative colitis and regional enteritis. Sulfasalazine has an unexplained benefit in ulcerative colitis that is not dependent upon the drug's antibacterial action. A metabolite produced, 5-aminosalicylate, may be the effective moiety in inflammatory intestinal disease.

ANTINEOPLASTICS

Certain antineoplastics (Table 8.9) have limited use in the palliative management of gastrointestinal carcinomas.

Streptozocin. Streptozocin, a nitrosourea compound, acts as an alkylating agent in the treatment of certain neoplasms.

Mechanism of Action. Streptozocin inhibits DNA synthesis in mammalian cells, probably by inducing DNA alkylation and causing cross-linking. The drug is cell cycle nonspecific (see Chapter 4).

Clinical Indications. Streptozocin is indicated in metastatic islet cell carcinoma of the pancreas.

Adverse Effects/Precautions. Renal toxicity occurs in about 67% of all patients treated with streptozocin. Nausea and vomiting occur in nine out of ten patients. Hematologic toxicity is rare.

Fluorouracil (5-FU) and Floxuridine. Fluorouracil and floxuridine are antimetabolites used as antineoplastic agents. Floxuridine is rapidly converted to fluorouracil so the two drugs have the same antimetabolic and toxic effects.

Mechanism of Action. Fluorouracil is a competitive inhibitor of thymidylate synthetase, resulting in impairment of DNA synthesis; these effects are most pronounced on rapidly dividing cells.

Clinical Indications. Fluorouracil is indicated for IV administration in the palliative management of carcinoma of the colon, rectum, stomach, and pancreas in selected patients who are considered incurable by surgical procedures or other means.

Floxuridine is used in the palliative management of gastrointestinal adenocarcinoma metastatic to the liver. The drug is given by continuous arterial infusion to patients considered incurable by surgical procedures or other means.

Adverse Effects/Precautions. Cardiovascular and gastrointestinal adverse reactions may occur with these drugs. Myocardial ischemia and angina are possible, and diarrhea, anorexia, vomiting, and cramps occur frequently. Hematologic toxicity, as evidenced by leukopenia and thrombocytopenia, are also possible. Alopecia is another frequently occurring adverse effect.

Bleomycin. Bleomycin sulfate is a mixture of glycopeptide antibiotics isolated from Streptomyces verticillus.

Mechanism of Action. Bleomycin inhibits DNA synthesis with lesser impairment of RNA and protein synthesis. Bleomycin is cell cycle phase specific, having pronounced effects in the G_2 and M phases.

Clinical Indications. Bleomycin is indicated in squamous cell carcinoma of the mouth, tongue, tonsil, nasopharynx, oropharynx, sinus, palate, lip, buccal mucosa, gingiva, epiglottis, skin, and larynx.

Table 8.9. ANTICANCER DRUGS.

Available products	Trade names
Bleomycin sulfate	Blenoxane
Floxuridine	FUDR
Fluorouracil	Fluorouracil; Adrucil
Mitomycin	Mutamycin
Streptozocin	Zanosar

Adverse Effects/Precautions. Pulmonary fibrosis is the most severe reaction that occurs with bleomycin therapy. Toxicity is commonly noted as pneumonitis, which may progress to pulmonary fibrosis. About 50% of the patients receiving bleomycin have adverse reactions of the integument and mucous membranes, including erythema, rash, hyperpigmentation, and skin tenderness. Hyperkeratosis, nail changes, alopecia, pruritus, and stomatitis may also occur.

Mitomycin (Mitomycin-C; MTC). Mitomycin is a urethane derivative that contains a quinone moiety and aziridine ring in its structure. The antibiotic is isolated from Streptomyces caespitosus.

Mechanism of Action. Mitomycin selectively inhibits DNA synthesis. The degree of cytotoxicity related to DNA cross-linking correlates with the guanine and cytosine content.

Clinical Indications. In combination with other antineoplastics, mitomycin is indicated in the treatment of disseminated adenocarcinoma of the stomach or pancreas. Mitomycin is used, in combination with fluorouracil and doxorubicin (see Chapter 4), for advanced gastric or pancreatic carcinoma.

Adverse Effects/Precautions. Bone marrow suppression, particularly thrombocytopenia and leukopenia, occurs in about two out of three patients receiving mitomycin. Renal toxicity is also possible with mitomycin therapy.

ANTHELMINTICS

Intestinal anthelmintics and their clinical indications are listed in Table 8.10.

DRUG INTERACTIONS

Antacids and antidiarrheals may inhibit the absorption of several concurrently administered drugs. Histamine (H_2) receptor blockers inhibit hepatic microsomal enzymes and may alter the metabolism of other drugs.

ORAL ANTACIDS

Benzodiazepines. Magnesium-aluminum hydroxide apparently reduces the rate of chlordiazepoxide absorption, but not the total amount absorbed.

Cimetidine. Antacids evidently inhibit the gastrointestinal absorption of cimetidine and ranitidine, necessitating administration of separate doses.

Iron Preparations. Since magnesium trisilicate may form poorly soluble substances with the oral iron, decreased iron absorption results. Carbonate-containing antacids may have a similar effect.

Sodium Polystyrene Sulfonate Resin (SPSR). Systemic alkalosis may result from impairment of the normally occurring combination of magnesium or calcium with bicarbonate ions in the small intestine which generally balances the neutralization of gastric acid by the antacid.

H_2 RECEPTOR BLOCKERS

Cimetidine.

Narcotic Analgesics. Cimetidine may inhibit both the hepatic metabolism of certain narcotic analgesics and the histamine released in response to narcotic analgesics. Enhanced respiratory and CNS depression may result when cimetidine and narcotic analgesics are used in combination therapy.

Oral Anticoagulants. Cimetidine may inhibit the metabolism of warfarin.

Theophylline. Since cimetidine inhibits the hepatic metabolism of theophylline, adjustment of theophylline dosage is usually necessary with either initiation or discontinuation of cimetidine therapy. As ranitidine does not evidently produce this adverse interaction with theophylline, it is preferred to cimetidine in patients receiving theophylline.

ANTIDIARRHEALS

Kaolin.

Pseudoephedrine. Through its adsorption ability, kaolin inhibits the gastrointestinal absorption of pseudoephedrine.

LAXATIVES

Mineral Oil.

Vitamin A. Since mineral oil may impair the gastrointestinal absorption of vitamin A, separate doses of vitamin A and mineral oil are recommended.

Table 8.10. INTESTINAL ANTHELMINTICS.

Available products	Trade names	Clinical indications
Mebendazole	Vermox	Whipworm; Ascariasis; Enterobiasis; Hookworm
Niclosamide	Niclocide	Taeniasis
Piperazine	Antepar; Vermizine	Ascariasis; Enterobiasis
Praziquantel	Biltricide	Taeniasis; Cysticercosis
Pyrantel pamoate	Antiminth	Ascariasis; Enterobiasis
Pyrvinium pamoate	Povan	Enterobiasis
Thiabendazole	Mintezol	Trichinosis; Strongyloidiasis; Cutaneous Larvae Migrans

SUMMARY

The site of action of gastrointestinal drugs is usually on receptors on the muscle or lining of the gastrointestinal tract or locally within the gastrointestinal space or lumen. In certain cases, however, such as antiemetics, the primary activity may occur on distant structures (for example, the medulla oblongata, inner ear, or the cerebral cortex).

Replacement of a missing element in the metabolic scheme of digestive processes is an important approach in treating some gastrointestinal disorders. Stimulation or inhibition of gastrointestinal physiologic processes offer another pharmacologic approach. To illustrate, stimulant laxatives act to increase peristalsis, whereas histamine H_2 receptor blockers are used to treat gastric gland overactivity (hyperacidity).

Gastrointestinal bacterial and/or protozoal infections usually respond to antibiotic/anti-infective drugs. However, correction of fluid and electrolyte imbalance that results from diarrhea must accompany administration of these drugs.

Common medical problems relating to the gastrointestinal tract are the management of peptic ulcer, constipation, diarrhea, and deficiencies of digestive factors. Many drugs effective in these conditions are OTC products; consequently, the pharmacist is often asked to recommend patient therapy. For instance, the pharmacist's role in monitoring peptic ulcer disease may include a critique of drug efficacy, patient compliance, and potential adverse effects of therapy. Referral of patients to physicians for accurate diagnosis is often an initial step as many patients with chronic abdominal pain are sometimes reluctant to consult a physician.

It is important for the pharmacist to keep abreast of current concepts in the pathophysiology of gastrointestinal disease. For example, stress is no longer viewed as a specific cause for peptic ulcer, but smoking, the use of nonsteroidal anti-inflammatory drugs and aspirin, age, and family history are currently targeted as contributing factors. Additionally, nocturnal acid secretion has surfaced as a key factor in the development of peptic ulcer.

Research on gastrointestinal hormones and the role of endogenous opiate-like receptors in intestinal function is significant to our understanding of normal and disease processes. The development of new pharmacologic agents with greater specificity and efficacy in treating gastrointestinal disease seems probable with continued advancements in medical science.

SUGGESTED READINGS

David, R.L.: Non-drug considerations in treating constipation. Am Col Apoth Profess Pract Newsletter, 5:1, 1984.
Famotidine. Med Lett Drugs Ther, 29:17, 1987.
Garnett, W.R.: Update on upper GI disorders. Optimal therapy. Wellcome Trends in Pharmacy, 7:8, 1985.
Gilman, A.G., et al. (eds.): The Pharmacological Basis of Therapeutics. 7th Ed. New York, Macmillan Publishing Co., Inc., 1985.
Hansten, P.D.: Drug Interactions. 5th Ed. Philadelphia, Lea & Febiger, 1985.
Immunizations and chemoprophylaxis for travelers. Med Lett Drugs Ther, 27:33, 1985.
Kastrup, E.K., and Boyd, J.R. (eds.): Drug Facts and Comparisons. Philadelphia, J.B. Lippincott Co., 1985.
Kinsella, J.M.: Anthelmintic Products. In Handbook of Nonprescription Drugs. Vol. 8. Washington, American Pharmaceutical Association, 1986.
Pastewski, B.M.: Peptic ulcer disease and its medical management. Am Druggist, 182:35, 1980.
Roth, H.P., and Shapiro, I.: What's new in drugs used to treat digestive diseases. Pharmacy Times, 49:38, 1983.
Sucralfate for peptic ulcer. A reappraisal. Med Lett Drugs Ther, 26:43, 1984.
Wizwer, P.I.: Management of constipation. A Practical Approach. NARD J, 106:77, 1984.

CHAPTER EXAMINATION

A middle-aged male sees his physician for a burning epigastric pain in the right upper abdominal area. The pain is more frequent in the morning, but also occasionally awakens him during sleep. The physician prescribes an aluminum hydroxide/magnesium hydroxide combination liquid.

1. The medication prescribed is best described as
   a. a systemic antacid
   b. a nonsystemic combination antacid that neutralizes gastric acid and prevents the conversion of pepsinogen to pepsin
   c. a histamine (H_2) receptor blocking drug
   d. an anticholinergic drug
2. The patient tells his pharmacist that food relieves the pain briefly, but it returns in a couple of hours after eating. Additionally, the medication relieves the pain almost always. This information suggests
   a. esophageal tumor
   b. ulcerative colitis
   c. acute pancreatitis
   d. duodenal ulcer
3. Magnesium salts are sometimes added to aluminum antacids to
   a. counteract the astringent and constipating effects of aluminum antacids
   b. prevent diarrhea
   c. disperse gas bubbles in the gastric contents
   d. prevent systemic absorption of the aluminum ion
4. The patient develops an infection that requires a tetracycline antibiotic. The antacid dose should be taken
   a. at the same time as the tetracycline
   b. at appropriate intervals between the tetracycline dosing
   c. only once daily at noon
   d. with milk at the same time as the tetracycline

A 63-year-old female goes to a gastroenterologist who determines, after x-rays, that she has a duodenal ulcer. Cimetidine is prescribed for a 6- to 8-week regimen.

---

5. During this period, the patient should be monitored for
   a. serum creatinine
   b. blood pressure
   c. pulmonary function
   d. intraluminal pancreatic lipase

6. The patient complains of drowsiness and "weird feelings" after a week of cimetidine therapy. Her medication history indicates the intermittent occurrence of kidney problems. An alternate drug less likely to cause her reported side effects without sacrificing the therapeutic benefit is
   a. calcium polycarbophil
   b. dehydrocholic acid
   c. ranitidine
   d. sucralfate
7. Cimetidine may elevate patient prolactin levels resulting in
   a. agranulocytosis
   b. galactorrhea
   c. encephalopathy
   d. cholestasis
8. Anticholinergics, in low doses, are sometimes combined with cimetidine in the treatment of duodenal ulcer. Propantheline is added to this patient's regimen; side effects which may occur with propantheline include
   a. diarrhea and CNS depression
   b. bradycardia and urinary incontinence
   c. nasal stuffiness and blepharospasm
   d. xerostomia, blurred vision, tachycardia, and urinary retention
9. Cimetidine inhibits metabolism of several drugs that are metabolized by the hepatic cytochrome P-450 system. A clinically significant drug interaction occurs when
   a. warfarin is taken concurrently
   b. dicyclomine is added to the patient's regimen
   c. the patient begins OTC antacid therapy
   d. sucralfate is prescribed
10. The mechanism of action of cimetidine is based upon
    a. inhibition of histamine synthesis
    b. activation of histidine decarboxylase
    c. blockade of histamine (H_2) receptors
    d. its reaction with gastric acid

When asked to recommend a mild OTC laxative for an elderly male's periodic constipation, the pharmacist suggests a preparation that contains a naturally occurring hydrophilic fiber.

11. This type of laxative preparation is referred to as a
    a. stimulant laxative
    b. saline laxative
    c. surfactant laxative
    d. bulk laxative
12. The most physiologic-type of laxative product is a
    a. bulk producer
    b. peristaltic stimulant that produces activation of Auerbach's plexus
    c. product containing castor oil
    d. mineral oil preparation
13. This same patient returns and requests a more forceful and rapidly acting (over-night) laxative. An alternate laxative is a
    a. phenophthalein containing product
    b. docusate-casanthanol combination
    c. combination containing sennosides A and B
    d. all of the above
14. Mineral oil was not considered because of the possibility of
    a. lipid pneumonia
    b. loss of fat-soluble vitamins
    c. leakage from the anal sphincter
    d. all of the above
15. Phenophthalein
    a. may discolor an alkaline urine
    b. is a naturally occurring bile salt
    c. is a surfactant laxative
    d. is never taken internally

A college student comes into your pharmacy after a trip "south of the border" and complains only of diarrhea and cramps.

16. The patient should be advised
    a. that he has typhoid fever
    b. that he should take a kaolin-pectin mixture and see a physician if his condition doesn't improve
    c. to request antibiotics from his physician
    d. to take a dose of castor oil and go to bed

17. The student returns to your pharmacy the next day feeling a lot better, but he still has diarrhea. After you contact his doctor, the physician prescribes diphenoxylate. This drug is
    a. an effective anti-infective against bacterial gastroenteritis
    b. a constipating opiate-like drug
    c. a specific against giardiasis
    d. likely to increase intestinal peristalsis
18. Diphenoxylate
    a. and kaolin have identical mechanisms of action
    b. is a local acting antacid
    c. acts on specific receptors in the intestinal musculature
    d. is combined with atropine sulfate to reduce the acidity of diphenoxylate
19. If a gastroenteritis is tentatively diagnosed as shigellosis or salmonellosis, the initial recommended treatment is
    a. chloramphenicol
    b. trimethroprim-sulfamethoxazole
    c. mitomycin
    d. bleomycin
20. If diarrhea continues for several days, the most serious potential consequence is
    a. fluid-electrolyte imbalance
    b. CNS stimulation
    c. gastric hyperacidity
    d. angina pectoris

ANSWER KEY

1.	b	11.	d
2.	d	12.	a
3.	a	13.	d
4.	b	14.	d
5.	a	15.	a
6.	c	16.	b
7.	b	17.	b
8.	d	18.	c
9.	a	19.	b
10.	c	20.	a

chapter 9

REPRODUCTIVE/ GENITOURINARY SYSTEM

CHAPTER OBJECTIVES

After studying this chapter, you should be able to:
1. Describe the anatomic and physiologic characteristics of the female and male genitourinary systems.
2. Discuss the incidence and treatment of urinary tract infections (UTIs).
3. Name several venereal diseases that are presently prevalent.
4. Describe the drug treatment of gonorrhea, syphilis, and genital herpes.
5. List several synthetic antimicrobial drugs that are valuable in the treatment of genitourinary tract infections.
6. Discuss the mechanisms of antimicrobial activity for penicillin G, trimethoprim, tetracycline, sulfamethoxazole, and methenamine.
7. Outline the biosynthesis of the prostaglandins.
8. Discuss the incidence and morbidity/mortality profile of several types of carcinomas of the genitourinary tract and breast cancer.
9. Describe the mechanism of action of several antineoplastic drugs that are valuable in the treatment of carcinomas of the genitourinary tract.
10. Name several classes of drugs that affect uterine contractility, and comment on their clinical efficacy and therapeutic application.

INTRODUCTION

The reproductive/genitourinary system is closely interrelated with the endocrine system. See Chapter 6 for a complete discussion of the influence of the endocrine system on the reproductive/genitourinary system (hypergonadal, hypogonadal, and birth control implications).

Infectious disease of the reproductive/genitourinary system is a major cause of morbidity. Antimicrobial agents, including the antiviral drug acyclovir, are often effective against many causative organisms. However, clinical problems, including resistant pathogen strains and superinfection, pose therapeutic dilemmas. Knowledge in chemotherapeutics is rapidly expanding, especially with significant advances in elucidating microbial cellular metabolic processes. Thus, the broad spectrum antibiotics extend cytotoxicity to formerly resistant gram-negative organisms.

Malignancies of the reproductive/genitourinary system constitute a major health problem in both morbidity and mortality. Cancer chemotherapy, especially the utilization of combination antineoplastic agents, has supplemented surgery and radiation to reduce death rates in some reproductive/genitourinary malignancies. In these instances, the knowledge garnered from molecular biology has contributed to the development of drug combinations that have different cytotoxic mechanisms; this combination therapy often results in synergistic toxicity toward neoplastic cells and an accrued benefit of reduced cytotoxicity to normal cells.

Certain other drugs, by virtue of their activity on the uterus, are useful in obstetrics and gynecology. For example, prostaglandins were first introduced into medicine because of their effects on uterine smooth muscle.

ANATOMY AND PHYSIOLOGY OF THE REPRODUCTIVE/GENITOURINARY SYSTEM

The female and male reproductive/genitourinary systems (Figures 9.1 and 9.2) contrast markedly in anatomy; however, their physiologic functions are similar and complement each other in the reproductive process.

FEMALE GENITAL SYSTEM

Ovulation from an ovary results in the egg entering the oviduct (fallopian tube) where cilia move it along toward the uterus. About the size of a fist, the uterus (womb) lies in the lower portion of the abdominal cavity just behind the bladder. If an egg is fertilized in the oviduct, it becomes implanted in the uterine wall where the embryo develops until the time of birth.

The uterus connects to the vagina, a muscular tube that serves as the receptacle for the penis during copulation (coitus). The walls of the vagina are elastic to allow not only penis entrance but also the passage of the baby during childbirth. Situated at the opening of the uterus is the cervix, a muscular ring of tissue which protrudes into the vagina. In young females, the opening of the vagina is partly closed by the hymen, a thin membrane also called the "maidenhead."

The vulva comprise the external female genitalia. The vulvar area is bounded by two folds of skin: the labia minor and labia major which enclose the vestibule. The vagina opens at the rear of the vestibule, and the urethra opens into the midportion of the vestibule. In the female, there is no interconnection between the reproductive and urinary systems. In contrast to males in whom the urethra delivers both semen

REPRODUCTIVE/GENITOURINARY SYSTEM **417**

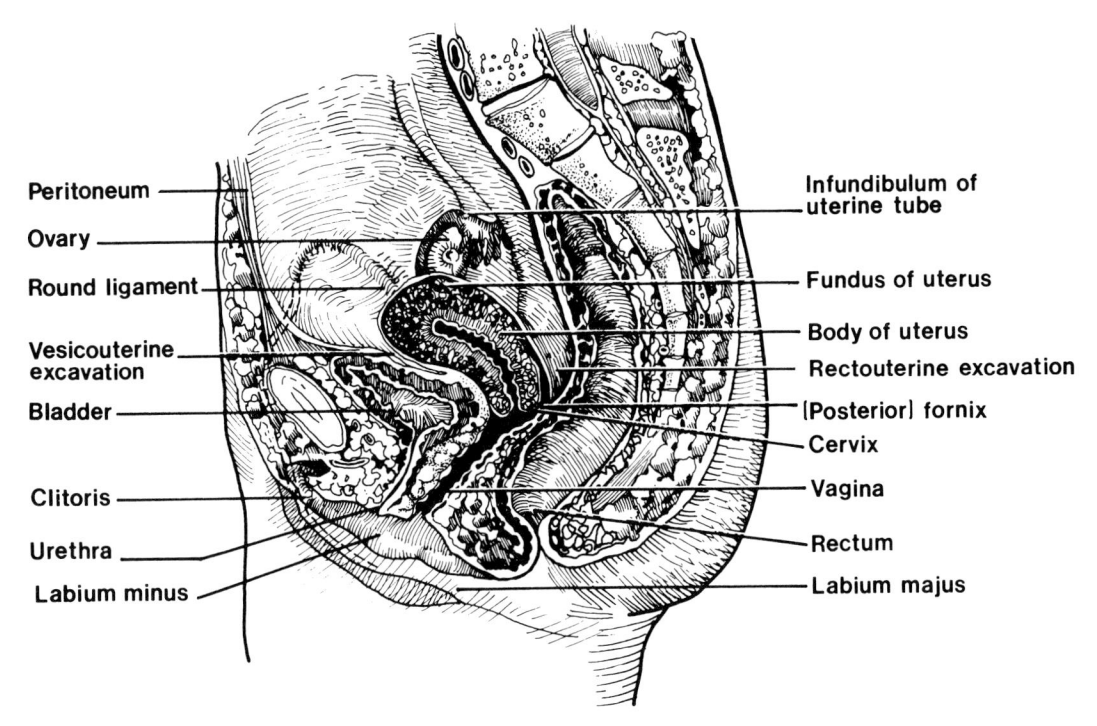

Fig. 9.1 Female pelvis, median sagittal section. (From Crouch, J.E.: Essential Human Anatomy. Philadelphia, Lea & Febiger, 1982.)

(sperm and seminal fluid) and urine to the outside of the body, the female urethral tract functions in only urine excretion.

The front anterior portion of the vestibule contains the clitoris, a small erectile organ. Composed of the same embryonic tissues as the male penis, the clitoris becomes engorged with blood during copulation.

MALE GENITAL SYSTEM

The testes descend, about the time of birth, from the abdomen into the scrotum, a pouch whose cavity is continuous with the abdominal cavity via the inguinal canal. This passageway closes with connective tissue after the testes have descended.

Each testis has two functional components: the seminiferous tubules in which sperm cells are produced and the interstitial cells which synthesize and secrete testosterone. If the testes do not descend (cryptorchidism), the abdominal temperature is not supportive for development of the seminiferous tubules, causing their eventual degeneration. The cooler temperature in the external scrotal sac supports seminiferous tubule activity which begins at the time of puberty.

Mature sperm cells pass via ducts from the seminiferous tubules into the epididymis, a coiled tube on the testes' surface. Sperm cells, which are stored in the epididymis, attain motility by epididymal activation. A lengthy sperm duct, the vas deferens, passes from each epididymis through the inguinal canal and into the abdominal cavity. At this site, it loops over the bladder and joins with the urethra just beyond where the urethra emerges from the bladder. The urethra passes through the penis and empties to the outside of the body.

Seminal fluid from the seminal vesicles, prostate gland, and Cowper's glands is added to the sperm as it travels through the vas deferens and urethra to form semen. Besides serving as a vehicle for sperm, seminal fluid also lubricates the

418 THERAPEUTIC PHARMACOLOGY

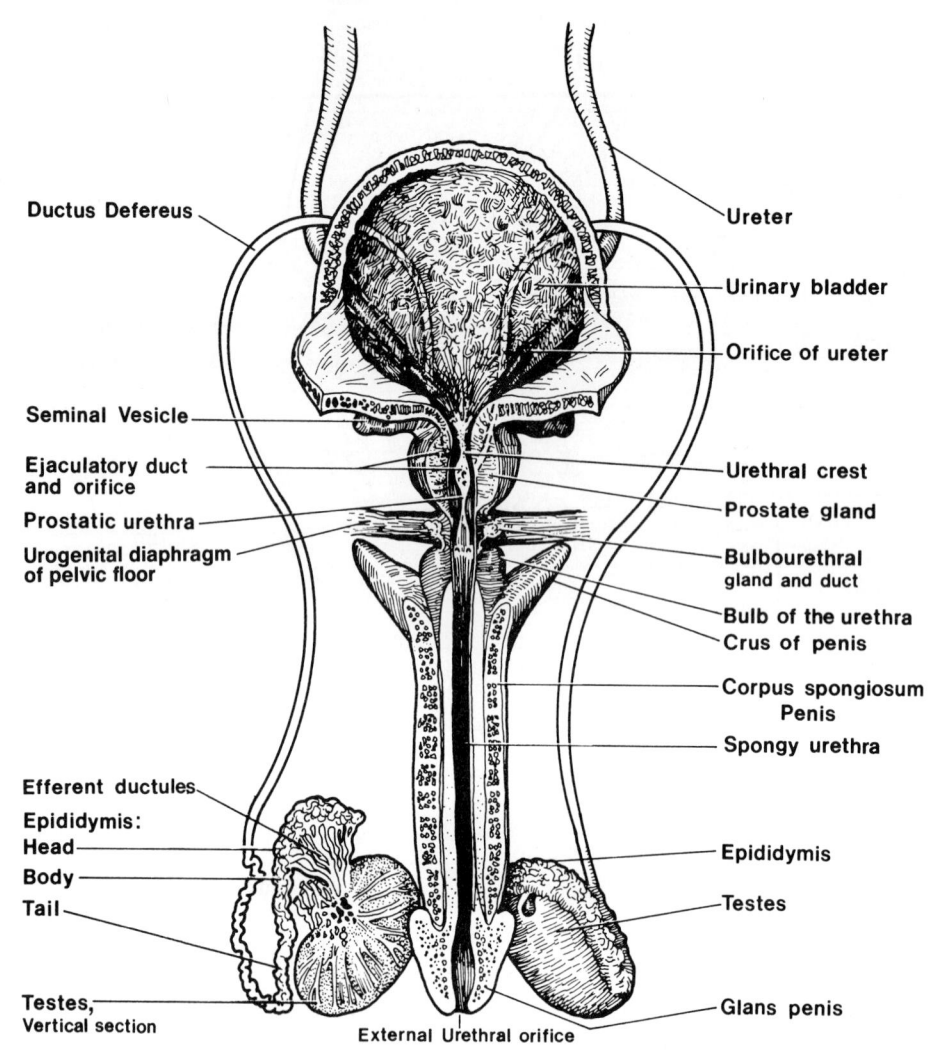

Fig. 9.2 Male reproductive system, anterior view. (From Crouch, J.E.: Essential Human Anatomy. Philadelphia, Lea & Febiger, 1982.)

passages through which sperm cells travel. The seminal fluid contains a high concentration of fructose (for sperm cell energy processes) and is buffered to protect the sperm from the acid of the female genital tract.

Arteries to the penis dilate during sexual excitement, and activation of the autonomic nervous system (ANS) causes constriction of the veins. The penis, engorged with blood, becomes hard and erect to better prepare it for insertion into the vagina during copulation.

During coitus, friction-induced sympathetic nervous system reflexes move the sperm to mix with the seminal fluid and eventually expel the semen. These contractions result in waves of muscle contraction in the genital passages (orgasm).

RENAL/URINARY EXCRETION SYSTEM

Chapter 5 contains a detailed discussion of the renal/urinary excretion systems.

DISEASES AND DISORDERS OF THE GENITOURINARY SYSTEM

Most genitourinary system illnesses are either venereal diseases or urinary tract infections (UTIs).

VENEREAL INFECTIONS (SEXUALLY TRANSMITTED DISEASES)

Venus, the goddess of love, is the namesake of the term "venereal," as venereal diseases are infections transmitted by sexual contact. Chlamydial infection, herpes infection, gonorrhea, and syphilis are examples of venereal diseases.

CHLAMYDIAL INFECTION

Chlamydiae are nonmotile, gram-negative intracellular parasites that may be pathogenic to humans. Chlamydia trachomatis is the probable pathogen in many cases. Non-gonococcal urethritis, a type of chlamydial infection, is a common form of sexually transmitted disease.

The clinical symptoms of dysuria (painful or difficult urination) and urethritis usually occur from 6 days to 3 weeks following intercourse. The urethral discharge is less profuse and tends to be watery or mucoid (rather than purulent), compared to gonococcal disease. Recurrence and multiple attacks are also characteristic of chlamydial infection. Additionally, non-gonococcal urethritis causes an arthritis in 0.5 to 1% of all chlamydial infection cases.

GENITAL HERPES

Following an incubation period of a few days, infections by herpes simplex virus (Types I and II) are evident as genital ulcers in women and as blisters or ulcers in men. First starting as typical vesicles, genital herpes forms single or mutiple ulcers in moist areas; these ulcers can progress to erosive sores in females. Characterized by painful lesions and tender adenitis, genital herpes is a frequently occurring venereal disease.

GONORRHEA

The causative agent of this sexually transmitted disease is Neisseria gonorrhoeae, a gram-negative diplococcus. Gonorrhea, the most common venereal disease (300 cases per 100,000 people in 1980) primarily affects males and females in the 15- to 29-year old age group. Following an incubation period from 2 to 10 days, gonorrhea results in urethritis, dysuria, urethral pain, and a yellow, creamy discharge in males. Untreated infection may spread to the prostate, seminal vesicles, and vas deferens. Chronic inflammation sometimes leads to fibrosis and blockade of sperm transport.

Although often asymptomatic, infected females may have urethritis, dysuria, yellowish discharge, and urinary frequency and urgency. Also, as this infection commonly spreads to the fallopian tubes and ovaries, gonococcal salpingitis may result in ectopic pregnancy with the fertilized ovum becoming embedded and growing in the fallopian tube.

Another consequence of this disease is that gonococcal arthritis occurs in 1 to 3% of all gonorrhea cases. Neonatal morbidity is evidenced by ophthalmia neonatorum, at one time a leading cause of blindness.

SYPHILIS

Treponema pallidum is the causative agent for syphilis. The incubation period is from 2 to 3 weeks, and the first sign of the infection is a chancre (painless venereal lesion) in the genital area.

Syphilis is usually described as progressing in three stages. The primary stage is characterized by both a local lesion that contains the causative organism and an enlargement of the regional lymph glands. Also, in about one in three untreated cases, the chancre ulcerates and heals by scar formation, terminating the disease process.

Secondary syphilis often occurs weeks or months after the primary lesion heals in about two out of three untreated patients. A widespread rash on the skin and mucous membrane indicates disease progression to the second stage. These external lesions can infect other contacts.

Tertiary syphilis is the final stage of the infection; one in three of the initial untreated cases progress to this state. Sometimes latent for years, the disease can manifest as lesions develop in the cardiovascular system, central nervous system (CNS), bone, and other body tissues. Syphilis is sometimes called the "great mimic" because during this last stage, it often attacks various body tissues and resembles a multitude of organic diseases.

NONVENEREAL INFECTIONS

Included in this category are the various inflammatory disorders of the female genital tract and the urinary tract infections (UTIs).

VAGINITIS

Evidenced by a pale, cloudy, or mucoid discharge, vaginitis primarily results from either hormonal imbalance (atropic vaginitis) or infections, although it is sometimes transmitted by sexual contact. Common infectious causes of vaginitis include Trichomonas vaginalis and Candida albicans. Trichomonas organisms are found in the secretions of the vagina and cervix, as well as in the male urethra where it may be asymptomatic. Fungal infection, most commonly caused by Candida albicans and indicated by a thick yellowish urethral discharge and severe itching, is especially prevalent in pregnant and diabetic patients.

CERVICITIS

Commonly caused by pyogenic bacteria, acute cervicitis (inflammation of uterine cervix) frequently occurs after childbirth or in association with gonorrhea. Herpes virus II is possibly another causative agent of this acute cervicitis.

ENDOMETRITIS

The most common infectious causes of this inflammation of the uterine lining are pyogenic bacteria that produce postpartum inflammation and Myobacterium tuberculosis, which results in granulomatous endometritis.

SALPINGITIS

Multiple infectious causes of this inflammation of the fallopian tubes include Escherichia coli or various pyogenic bacteria; gonococcal infection also commonly causes this disease. The infection frequently originates from a uterine focus; acute salpingitis results from tuberculosis that spreads from a pulmonary focus.

URINARY TRACT INFECTIONS

Occurring frequently in both community and hospital environments, urinary tract infections (UTIs) are the most common human bacterial infections. Approximately 20% of all women in the general population will have at least one UTI during their lifetime and many will experience multiple episodes. In older males, prostatic obstruction accounts for many UTIs. The frequency of incidence in females may result from the shorter urethra and anatomic proximity of the anus and urethral opening, allowing fecal intestinal bacteria to enter the urethra and invade the bladder.

Escherichia coli, an enteric bacteria, accounts for four out of five UTI cases. Enteric Escherichia coli can readily colonize the vaginal and periurethral areas, which is the initial occurrence site in UTI development. Proteus species, the next most common infectious agent in UTI, appears frequently following instrumental examination of the urinary tract.

Predisposing factors to UTI include female gender, age (disease incidence increases with age), pregnancy, instrumental examination of the genitourinary tract, urinary tract obstruction, neurologic dysfunction, and renal disease. The bladder is most often the focus of infection (cystitis). In more widespread infection, the renal pelvic area is affected (pyelonephritis).

Accounting for more than 30% of all surgical infections, UTIs are the most common type of infection seen in surgical patients. The development of gram-negative bacteremia and sepsis often increases the severity and complications of postsurgical urinary tract infections (a frequent major source of morbidity).

Lower abdominal pain, dysuria and urinary frequency and/or urgency are common signs of

UTI. Nausea, vomiting, low back pain, and headache indicate renal involvement. If the infection becomes systemic, fever, chills, and weakness occur.

ENDOMETRIOSIS

Endometriosis describes the aberrant occurrence of tissue, resembling the endometrium, in various locations in the pelvic cavity. Internal endometriosis (adenomyosis) is the presence of endometrial glands and stroma within the myometrium. External endometriosis consists of endometrial tissue implants at sites distant from the uterus.

Frequent locations of extrauterine endometrial tissue include the ovaries, broad ligaments, rectovaginal septum, and sites in the peritoneal cavity represented by the appendix, intestines, and umbilicus. Responsive to hormones (endogenous or exogenous), extrauterine implants of endometrial tissue may undergo cyclic maturation and bleeding. Cyst formation and scarring sometimes occur and many symptoms of external endometriosis (pain, abnormal bleeding from organ sites other than the uterus, and infertility) relate to these deposits.

CARCINOMAS OF THE FEMALE REPRODUCTIVE SYSTEM

Neoplasms of the female reproductive system, including the breast, are among the most prevalent forms of cancer.

VULVAR CARCINOMA

Squamous cell carcinoma occurs most frequently in postmenopausal patients. Vulvar carcinoma metastasizes first to the regional lymph glands.

VAGINAL CARCINOMA

Vaginal clear cell adenocarcinoma, an unusual type of malignancy, occurs in some young females whose mothers received diethylstilbestrol (DES) during pregnancy. The prognosis for this neoplasm is poor.

CERVICAL CARCINOMA

Squamous dysplasia represents an initial stage of neoplastic disease in the cervical epithelium. Invasive squamous carcinoma may develop from a full epithelial cell thickness alteration, although the time interval in the invasive process is sometimes as long as 10 to 20 years.

Cervical carcinoma spreads to the regional lymph nodes and may metastasize to other sites, including the pelvic wall, bladder, and rectum. The Pap smear is valuable in the early diagnosis of this disease.

UTERINE CARCINOMA

Endometrial adenocarcinoma is the malignancy that occurs most frequently in the female genital tract. Generally regarded as a disease of postmenopausal women, this carcinoma primarily affects those in their 60s. Abnormal estrogen stimulation of the endothelium is a potential risk factor of this disease which is also associated with exogenous estrogen therapy. Approximately 37,000 new cases of endometrial adenocarcinoma are diagnosed each year in the United States alone, and the annual death rate is 3,500.

CHORIOCARCINOMA

Choriocarcinoma is a rare malignancy of the trophoblast (tissue formed by the developing embryo as a means of anchoring the fetus to the endometrium). Thus, the trophoblast, although generally well-tolerated, is foreign tissue to the maternal host. Occurring in only 1 of every 100,000 pregnancies, this tumor arises in the uterus following pregnancy.

OVARIAN CANCER

Of all strictly gynecologic malignancies, ovarian cancer is the leading cause of death, possibly due to late diagnosis of the disease. Although there are several types of ovarian cancers, the most common involves epithelial tissue.

Germ cell tumors of the ovary occur mainly in postmenopausal patients, but they may also affect children and young adults. These neoplasms probably arise from primitive undifferentiated germ cells that have not fully developed into oocytes (eggs). Teratomas, the most common germ cell neoplasms found in the ovary, are usually cystic tumors which consist of many different types of mature adult-appearing tissues composed of skin and skin appendages (dermoid cysts).

Stromal ovarian tumors are ordinarily benign or of low malignant potential. Metastatic ovarian carcinoma, usually from breast carcinoma sites, is fairly common.

BREAST CARCINOMA

The hormonal and functional involvement of the female breasts in the human reproductive process are understood. Breast carcinoma, although not strictly a genital neoplasm, is probably best discussed with these cancers.

Occurring in 1 of 11 women, breast cancer is the leading cause of female cancer deaths in the United States and Western European countries. Carcinomas of duct origin, comprising about 85% of all breast carcinomas, are the most common type; lobular carcinoma occurs less frequently.

The most important risk factor is a family history of breast carcinoma; women whose mothers had breast cancer are five times more likely to develop the disease than are women with no family history of breast cancer. Other risk factors are endocrine-associated and include first full pregnancy after age 30, early menarche and late menopause, and low parity. Also implicated are diet factors—specifically, high animal fat diets.

Breast carcinoma metastasizes initially to the regional lymph nodes. Although it may also spread to any organ of the body, it often affects the liver, bone, brain, and lung. Breast carcinoma is an unusual cancer in that metastases may appear relatively late in the course of the disease, possibly 10 to even 20 years after the original diagnosis.

CARCINOMAS OF THE MALE REPRODUCTIVE SYSTEM

Carcinomas of the prostate gland and testes are representative of this neoplasm group.

PROSTATE CARCINOMA

A common malignancy, prostate adenocarcinoma affects primarily older males in the United States. Posterior lobe involvement is the most common form and early metastasis to pelvic lymph nodes and to the lumbar vertebrae is possible. Rarely affecting those younger than age 40, this carcinoma is androgen-dependent as it does not occur in the absence of testes.

TESTICULAR CARCINOMA

Testicular neoplasms account for only 1% of tumors in males, but they represent a significant proportion of malignancies in the 15- to 35-year old age group. Most of these cancers are germ cell malignancies.

Germ cell tumors include: seminomas, the most common type being characterized by clear cells; embryonal carcinoma, composed of anaplastic cells arranged in glandular patterns; and teratomas, a form which may contain cartilage, neural tissue, and epithelial material.

BREAST CARCINOMA

Male breast carcinoma is an extremely rare disease. Always of the ductal variety (the male breast does not develop lobules), the tumors often reach a large size before diagnosis. Consequently, the prognosis is usually unfavorable.

CARCINOMA OF THE URINARY BLADDER

Bladder carcinoma is one of the leading causes of death in men over the age of 75. Also, there is a marked male predominance of urinary bladder cancer with a frequency rate of 3:1. Transitional cell carcinomas constitute 90% of all bladder cases, most of which are found in the trigone area.

Identified risk factors include cigarette smoking, exposure to industrial carcinogens, analgesic drug abuse, pelvic irradiation, and antimetabolite drug therapy (e.g., cyclophosphamide). The role of saccharin use, often implicated with increased risk, remains debatable as an associated contributing factor.

DRUGS USED IN THE TREATMENT OF GENITOURINARY DISEASES AND INFECTIONS

Anti-infectives constitute a majority of the drugs used to treat reproductive/genitourinary diseases.

DRUGS USED TO TREAT INFECTIONS

Sulfonamides, urinary tract antiseptics, and antifungal agents represent the major drug classes of useful anti-infectives.

ANTIMICROBIAL DRUGS

Antimicrobial drugs may act as antimetabolites or may otherwise disrupt microorganism function to have a cytotoxic effect.

Sulfonamides. In the 1930s, the sulfonamides (Table 9.1) became the first effective antibacterial drugs to be employed clinically in nontoxic doses. Additionally, the studies on their mechanism of action facilitated the further introduction of active antimetabolic compounds. Although antibiotics have generally replaced the sulfonamides in the treatment of many infectious diseases, certain sulfonamides remain clinically valuable, especially in urinary tract infections (UTIs).

Mechanism of Action. Sulfonamides are bacteriostatic and act by competitive inhibition of the participation of para-aminobenzoic acid (PABA) in bacterial folic acid synthesis (Figure 9.3). Since folic acid is necessary for DNA and RNA synthesis, it is required for bacterial growth and multiplication.

Bacteria usually synthesize their own folic acid rather than obtaining it from an exogenous source, as is the case in humans. Thus, sulfonamides block an important metabolic step specific for bacteria growth. Organisms that do not synthesize folic acid are not susceptible to the actions of sulfonamides.

Clinical Indications. Sulfonamides are used to treat UTIs. A sulfonamide in conjunction with a penicillin is a recommended treatment for epidemic cerebrospinal meningitis caused by infection with Neiserria meningitidis. Chanchroid, inclusion conjunctivitis, trachoma, and nocardiosis are other clinical indications for the sulfonamides.

Adverse Effects/Precautions. Sulfonamides may produce transient nausea, vomiting, malaise, headache, and mental depression. Cyanosis (due to methemoglobin formation) occurs occasionally. Serious adverse effects in-

Table 9.1. SULFONAMIDES.

Available products	Trade names	Daily dosage range*
Sulfacytine	Renoquid	250 mg q.i.d.
Sulfadiazine	Microsulfon	2–4 g
Sulfamethizole	Thiosulfil; Microsul; others	0.5–1 g t.i.d. or q.i.d.
Sulfamethoxazole	Gantanol; Urobak	1 g morning and evening
Sulfisoxazole	Gantrisin; SK-Soxazole; others	Oral, 4–8 g in 4–6 divided doses
Multiple Sulfonamides	Triple Sulfa; Neotrizine; others	2–4 g initially, then 2–4 g daily in 3–6 divided doses

* Maintenance dosage

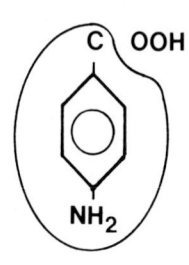

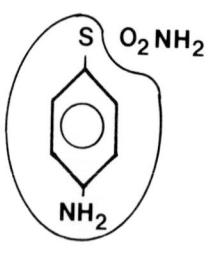

Fig. 9.3 Sulfonamide-PABA relation to folic acid.

clude diarrhea, hypersensitivity reactions, and crystalluria.

The latter results from precipitation of less soluble sulfonamides in the tubular urine, especially when the urine is acid. The possibility of crystalluria is lessened by administering moderate doses of three sulfonamides: the "triple sulfas"—sulfadiazine, sulfamerazine, and sulfamethazine. The presence of one sulfonamide does not influence the solubility of others, but their antimicrobial effects are additive. The maintenance of an alkaline urine (via sodium citrate orally or sodium bicarbonate, either orally or intravenously) or the use of a highly water soluble sulfonamide reduces the possibility of crystalluria.

Hypersensitivity reactions include rashes, photosensitivity, fever, hepatitis, agranulocytosis, purpura, aplastic anemia, peripheral neuritis, polyarteritis nodosa, and, rarely, Stevens-Johnson syndrome (a fatal type of erythema mutiforme).

Local Acting Sulfonamides. Vaginal creams and intravaginal tablets that contain sulfonamides are useful in the treatment of vaginitis caused by Hemophilus vaginalis. Sulfonamides in these products exert a bacteriostatic action by competitive inhibition of PABA, an essential component of folic acid synthesis. Adverse reactions to these local acting products include irritation and, rarely, allergic reactions (pruritus, urticaria, and vulvitis).

Trimethoprim. Originally developed as an antimalarial drug, trimethoprim is chemically similar to pyrimethamine and to part of the folic acid molecule. Some UTI cases respond well to a trimethoprim/sulfamethoxazole combination.

Mechanism of Action. Trimethoprim is a selective inhibitor of dihydrofolate reductase in lower microorganisms. By blocking bacterial nucleic acid and protein synthesis, this action retards their growth and multiplication.

The antimicrobial activity of the combination of trimethoprim and sulfamethoxazole results from its action on two steps in the tetrahydrofolic acid biosynthetic pathway. Sulfamethoxazole inhibits the incorporation of PABA into folic acid and trimethoprim prevents the reaction of dihydrofolate to tetrahydrofolate.

Clinical Indications. Trimethoprim and the trimethoprim/sulfamethoxazole combination are indicated in the treatment of initial uncomplicated UTIs caused by susceptible strains of Escherichia coli, Proteus mirabilis, Klebsiella pneumoniae, and Enterobacter species.

Adverse Effects/Precautions. Rash, pruritus, exfoliative dermatitis, epigastric distress, glossitis, and stomatitis are relatively common adverse reactions to trimethoprim. Thrombocytopenia, leukopenia, and megaloblastic anemia may also occur, possibly due to prior folate deficiency in the host.

Sulfamethoxazole produces the same adverse reactions as the other sulfonamides. A combination of trimethoprim and sulfamethoxazole causes about three times more dermatologic reactions than the sulfonamide alone.

URINARY TRACT ANTISEPTICS

The urinary tract antiseptics (Table 9.2) effectively inhibit bacterial growth in the urinary tract. These drugs do not achieve significant blood or tissue levels in safe doses, so they are ineffective as therapeutic agents in treating systemic infections. However, the urinary tract antiseptics are concentrated in the renal tubules and thus are valuable in the treatment of UTIs via a local action.

Methenamine. Methenamine (hexamethylenetetramine) is a urinary tract antiseptic used to treat chronic UTIs.

Mechanism of Action. Methenamine decomposes to formaldehyde, accounting for the drug's antibacterial action. Acidification of the urine promotes the formation of formaldehyde from methenamine and thus enhances the antibacterial activity. All bacteria are not sensitive to formaldehyde at the concentrations produced in therapeutic doses. Furthermore, Proteus and Pseudomonas species tend to elevate the pH of the urine to inhibit formaldehyde formation. The mandelate and hippurate salts of methenamine help maintain a low urine pH, as do vitamin C and acid-producing foods (such as cranberry juice).

Clinical Indications. Methenamine is indicated for suppression or elimination of bacteriuria associated with pyelonephritis, cystitis, and other chronic UTIs.

Adverse Effects/Precautions. Gastrointestinal distress and difficulty in micturation occur, especially with high doses. Ammonia produced as a result of methenamine breakdown worsens hepatic insufficiency.

Nalidixic Acid. Nalidixic acid, an effective urinary tract antiseptic, is bactericidal to most gram-negative bacteria that cause UTIs.

Mechanism of Action. Nalidixic acid interferes with DNA polymerization in the bacterial cell and may also inhibit bacterial RNA synthesis.

Clinical Indications. Nalidixic acid is used to treat UTIs that are caused by susceptible gram-negative organisms, including the majority of Proteus strains, Escherichia coli, Klebsiella species, and Enterobacter species.

Adverse Effects/Precautions. Nausea, vomiting, and abdominal distress may occur. Drowsiness, weakness, headache, dizziness, and vertigo are infrequent. Toxic psychoses or brief convulsions are rare and usually occur in

Table 9.2. URINARY TRACT ANTISEPTICS.

Available products	Trade names	Daily dosage range
Cinoxacin	Cinobac	1 g in 2 or 4 divided doses
Methenamine	Methenamine	1 g q.i.d.
Methenamine hippurate	Hiprex; Urex	1 g b.i.d.
Methenamine mandelate	Mandelamine	1 g q.i.d.
Methylene blue	Urolene Blue	65–130 mg t.i.d.
Nalidixic acid	NegGram	4 g
Nitrofurantoin	Furadantin; Furan; others	50–100 mg q.i.d. orally
Nitrofurantoin macrocrystals	Macrodantin	50–100 mg q.i.d.
Norfloxacin	Noroxin	400 mg b.i.d.

patients with predisposing factors such as parkinsonism, cerebral vascular insufficiency, or epilepsy. Excessive dosage in children has resulted in CNS toxicity. Photosensitivity reactions are also possible with this drug.

Cinoxacin. A synthetic quinolone derivative, cinoxacin is chemically related to nalidixic acid.

Mechanism of Action. Cinoxacin inhibits bacterial DNA replication.

Clinical Indications. Indicated in initial and recurrent UTIs in adults, cinoxacin is effective against most strains of Escherichia coli, Proteus mirabilis, Proteus vulgaris, Klebsiella pneumoniae, Klebsiella species, and Enterobacter species.

Adverse Effects/Precautions. Common adverse reactions to cinoxacin are nausea and abdominal cramps.

Other Quinolones. Several newer quinolone derivatives (norfloxacin, ciprofloxacin, and pefloxacin) appear promising for the treatment of UTIs. Additionally, these newer drugs may have a broader clinical application for systemic infections.

Norfloxacin. A fluoroquinolone derivative which is structurally related to nalidixic acid and cinoxacin, norfloxacin has an unusually broad spectrum of activity.

Mechanism of Action. Norfloxacin inhibits the activity of DNA gyrase which results in an interference with bacterial DNA replication.

Clinical Indications. Norfloxacin is used for oral antibacterial therapy of complicated UTIs, especially with resistant Enterobacter species, Pseudomonas aeruginosa, and enterococci. Development of bacterial resistance occurs less frequently with norfloxacin than with nalidixic acid and cinoxacin.

Adverse Effects/Precautions. Nausea, headache, dizziness, fatigue, rash, vulvar irritation, abdominal pain, dyspepsia, insomnia, diarrhea, tendonitis, and joint swelling are infrequent adverse reactions to norfloxacin. Increased blood levels of warfarin (Coumadin[R]) and theophylline have occurred with concurrent norfloxacin therapy. The effect of norfloxacin on human DNA is unknown, and the drug is not recommended for children or for pregnant or nursing females.

Nitrofurantoin. Nitrofurantoin, a synthetic nitrofuran, is used to prevent and treat UTIs.

Mechanism of Action. Nitrofurantoin inhibits acetylcoenzyme A (acetyl CoA), which disrupts bacterial carbohydrate metabolism. Bacterial cell wall formation may be blocked by this drug. Also, the antibacterial activity of nitrofurantoin is greater in an acidic urine.

Clinical Indications. Nitrofurantoin is indicated in the treatment of UTIs resultant from susceptible strains of Escherichia coli, enterococci, Staphylococcus aureus, and certain strains of Klebsiella, Enterobacter, and Proteus species. Parenteral nitrofurantoin should be used in patients with more serious UTIs when oral therapy is not possible.

Adverse Effects/Precautions. Nausea, vomiting, and diarrhea are frequent adverse reactions to this drug. Other reported effects include pulmonary sensitivity reactions. The hepatotoxicity that sometimes occurs is not dose-related and usually reverses upon discontinuation of nitrofurantoin therapy.

AMEBICIDES

Amebic infections of the genitourinary tract primarily involve Trichomonas vaginalis.

Metronidazole. Metronidazole is a trichomonacidal agent that also displays antibacterial activity against all anaerobic cocci and both anaerobic gram-negative bacilli (including Bacteroides species) and anaerobic spore-forming gram-positive bacilli.

Mechanism of Action. The nitro group of metronidazole accepts electrons from ferredoxins or equivalent electron-transport proteins in microorganisms. The reduced form of metronidazole thus produced is chemically reactive and induces biochemical lesions that promote the death of the ameba or bacteria. Metronidazole also inhibits amebic and bacterial DNA synthesis and may disrupt its helical structure.

Clinical Indications. Metronidazole is indicated in the treatment of trichomoniasis in both females and males, even if the conditions are asymptomatic in either sex. Another of its uses is in gynecologic infections caused by Bacteroides species, Clostridium species, Peptococcus species, and Peptostreptococcus species; these conditions include endometritis, endomyometritis, tubo-ovarian abscess, and postsurgical vaginal cuff infection.

Adverse Effects/Precautions. The most common side effects are nausea, anorexia, diarrhea, epigastric distress, and abdominal cramping. Serious adverse reactions include convulsive seizures and peripheral neuropathy.

ANTIVIRAL DRUGS

In contrast to most other infectious agents, viruses require the active participation of the host cell; therefore, achieving selective toxicity is difficult with the antiviral agents. Consequently, medical scientists often encounter complex problems in their search for antiviral drugs.

Acyclovir (Zovirax^R). Acylovir is a synthetic acyclic purine nucleoside analog of the naturally occurring guanosine.

Mechanism of Action. Acyclovir is converted to acyclovir monophosphate (acyclo-GMP) in virus-infected cells. The biotransformation proceeds to acyclo-GDP and acyclo-GTP in these cells. The affinity of the viral enzymes for acyclovir is about 200 times that of the mammalian enzymes and the amount of acyclo-GTP formed in herpes virus-infected cells is 40 to 100 times that present in uninfected cells. The acyclo-GTP thus formed acts as a potent inhibitor of viral DNA polymerase. Additionally, when acyclo-GTP is incorporated into viral DNA, termination of the biosynthesis of the viral DNA strand occurs. A 300 to 3000-fold greater toxicity exists for herpes viruses compared to that of mammalian cells.

Clinical Indications. Acyclovir is effective in the treatment of initial and recurrent mucosal and cutaneous Herpes simplex (HSV-1 and HSV-2) infections in immunologically impaired hosts (children and adults). The drug is also indicated for severe clinical episodes of genital herpes in patients who are not immunocompromised.

Adverse Effects/Precautions. Topical acyclovir preparations may produce irritation and transient burning. Reports of occasional nausea, amnesia, or headaches have followed acyclovir administration. Also, inflammation or phlebitis at the intravenous injection site occurs in some patients. Transient renal impairment may result in elevated serum creatinine levels, and rash and/or hives occur fairly often.

ANTIFUNGALS

Treatment of vaginal candidiasis (moniliasis) is complicated by a high recurrence rate that results from the ubiquitous presence of Candida albicans and predisposing factors, including diabetes mellitus, pregnancy, and the use of antibiotics, corticosteroids, and/or oral contraceptives.

Nystatin. Nystatin (topical) is used for the local treatment of vulvovaginal candidiasis.

Mechanism of Action. Nystatin binds to sterols in the fungal cell membrane, changing the permeability and causing leakage of intracellular components.

Clinical Indications. Nystatin is administered intravaginally in the treatment of moniliasis (vulvovaginal candidiasis).

Adverse Effects/Precautions. Local irritation, sensitization, or vulvovaginal burning rarely occur with nystatin use.

Miconazole. A fungicidal agent, miconazole (topical) is used to treat moniliasis.

Mechanism of Action. Miconazole permeates the chitin of the fungal cell wall to increase the leakage of essential intracellular substances.

Clinical Indications. Miconazole is used to treat vulvovaginal candidiasis.

Adverse Effects/Precautions. Reports of vulvovaginal symptoms (irritation and burning), pelvic cramps, hives, skin rash, and headache have followed miconazole use.

Clotrimazole. Topical clotrimazole is used to treat vulvovaginal candidiasis.

Mechanism of Action. When clotrimazole enters the chitin of the fungal cell wall, leakage of intracellular substances results.

Clinical Indications. Clotrimazole is used in the treatment of moniliasis.

Adverse Effects/Precautions. Skin rash, lower abdominal cramps, bloating, and slight urinary frequency are reported side effects of clotrimazole therapy. Burning and/or irritation in the sexual partner occur rarely.

Flucytosine (5-fluorocytosine; 5-FC). Flucytosine acts as an antimetabolite in fungal cell metabolism.

Mechanism of Action. After entering the fungal cell, flucytosine is converted to 5-fluorouracil (5-FU) by cytosine deaminase. 5-FU acts as a competitive inhibitor of nucleic acid biosynthesis. Human cells lack cytosine deaminase so they are not capable of the bioconversion of 5-FC to 5-FU.

Clinical Indications. Flucytosine is indicated in the treatment of UTIs caused by Candida species.

Adverse Effects/Precautions. Nausea, vomiting, diarrhea, rash, anemia, leukopenia, thrombocytopenia, and elevation of hepatic enzymes have been reported.

Amphotericin B. Amphotericin B (see Chapter 7) is used as a bladder irrigant in the treatment of UTIs caused by Candida species.

Ketoconazole. Ketoconazole is used orally in the treatment of selected Candida infections.

Mechanism of Action. Ketoconazole impairs synthesis of ergosterol, the main sterol in fungal cell membranes, allowing increased permeability and leakage of cellular substances.

Clinical Indications. Ketoconazole is used to treat vaginitis caused by Candida species.

Adverse Effects/Precautions. Gastrointestinal complaints, including nausea and vomiting, are the most common side effects of ketoconazole therapy. Abdominal pain, pruritus, and gynecomastia are less frequent reactions.

PENICILLINS (SEE CHAPTER 7)

A single intramuscular (IM) dose of procaine penicillin G with concurrent administration of probenecid is the usual initial treatment of uncomplicated gonorrhea. Alternative drugs to procaine penicillin G are ampicillin or amoxicillin. Patients with a history of penicillin allergy are treated with either tetracyclines or spectinomycin. If the disease results from penicillinase-producing gonococci, cephalosporins, including cefuroxime and cefoxitin, are indicated.

Penicillin (benzathine or procaine penicillin G) is the drug of choice in the treatment of syphilis. Hetacillin and bacampicillin are indicated in UTIs (cystitis, pyelonephritis, and prostatitis/urethritis) caused by Escherichia coli, Proteus mirabilis, and Streptococcus faecalis (enterococci).

UTIs that are caused by susceptible organisms (including Escherichia coli, Proteus mirabilis, and Streptococcus faecalis) respond to the extended spectrum penicillins: carbenicillin, ticarcillin, mezlocillin, piperacillin, and azlocillin.

Amdinocillin (Coactin[R]; Mecillinam) is a new semisynthetic penicillin that is used parenterally for serious UTIs. Amdinocillin, which acts synergistically with other beta-lactam antibiotics, may be useful in multiple-antibiotic resistant gram-negative enteric infections, especially Enterobacteriaceae, but it has minimal activity against gram-positive microorganisms and Pseudomonas. Amdinocillin's synergistic activity with other beta-lactams may be explained by its binding to sites that differ from those of other penicillins.

CEPHALOSPORINS (SEE CHAPTER 7)

The cephalosporins are effective in treating UTIs caused by gram-negative bacteria, including Escherichia coli, Proteus mirabilis, and Klebsiella species. In combination with doxycycline, cefoxitin is especially valuable in treating acute pelvic inflammatory disease (endometritis, salpingitis, parametritis, or peritonitis).

TETRACYCLINES (SEE CHAPTER 7)

The tetracyclines are used in gonorrhea or syphilis patients who are allergic to penicillin. Because of the risk of hepatotoxicity, pregnant women with either gonorrhea or syphilis should not receive tetracyclines. Having less antitreponemal activity than penicillin, tetracyclines are considered as alternate drugs in syphilis treatment.

Tetracyclines are the drugs of choice in the treatment of non-gonococcal urethritis (Chlamydia infection). Acute pelvic inflammatory disease (endometritis, salpingitis, parametritis, and peritonitis) responds to doxycycline in combination with cefoxitin or metronidazole.

AMINOGLYCOSIDES (SEE CHAPTER 7)

Aminoglycosides, e.g., gentamicin, tobramycin, amikacin, and netilmicin, are used to treat serious UTIs that are caused by gram-negative bacilli, including Pseudomonas aeruginosa, Enterobacter, Klebsiella, Serratia, and other species resistant to less toxic antibiotics.

OTHER ANTIBIOTICS

Erythromycin and spectinomycin are structurally related antibiotics that are used to treat gonorrhea.

Erythromycin. The various uses of erythromycin include the treatment of urethritis in adult males; uncomplicated urethral, endocervical, or rectal infections in which tetracyclines are contraindicated; conjunctivitis in the newborn caused by Chlamydia trachomata; and acute pelvic inflammatory disease caused by Neisseria gonorrhoeae. Although it is an alternate drug and a less efficient antitreponemal drug than penicillin, erythromycin is sometimes used to treat primary syphilis.

Spectinomycin. Related to the aminoglycosides, spectinomycin is an aminocyclitol antibiotic that is derived from Streptomyces spectabilis.

Mechanism of Action. Spectinomycin inhibits bacterial protein synthesis by binding the 30S ribosomal subunit.

Clinical Indications. Spectinomycin is used to treat acute gonorrheal urethritis and prostatitis in the male. It is also effective in the treatment of acute gonorrheal cervicitis and proctitis (due to susceptible strains of Neisseria gonorrhoeae) in the female.

Adverse Effects/Precautions. Soreness of the injection site, urticaria, dizziness, nausea, chills, fever, and insomnia are reported side effects.

DRUGS THAT AFFECT UTERINE MUSCULATURE

The myometrium is the thick, smooth muscle which forms the middle layer of the uterine wall. Alpha-adrenergic innervation to the human uterus mediates stimulation, as do cholinergic (muscarinic) receptors. Beta-adrenergic receptor activation results in uterine inhibition. The uterus is susceptible to hormone influence as estrogens enhance responsiveness and progesterone decreases activity.

Certain agents that alter uterine contractility (Table 9.3) are valuable in obstetrics. Commonly used drugs for enhancing contractions of the uterus are prostaglandins, oxytocin, and ergot alkaloids, especially ergonovine. Other

Table 9.3. DRUGS THAT AFFECT UTERINE MUSCULATURE.

Available products	Trade names	Daily dosage range
Oxytocic agents:		
Carboprost tromethamine	Prostin/15 M	Initial dose: IM, 1 ml
Dinoprost tromethamine	Prostin F₂ alpha	40 mg by slow inject. into the amniotic sac
Dinoprostone	Prostin E₂	20 mg
Ergonovine maleate	Ergotrate	IM, 0.2 mg
Methylergonovine maleate	Methergine	IM, 0.2 mg
Oxytocin, parenteral	Pitocin; Syntocinon	Variable
Uterine muscle relaxant:		
Ritodrine HCl	Yutopar	Oral maintenance: 10–20 mg q. 4–6 hrs

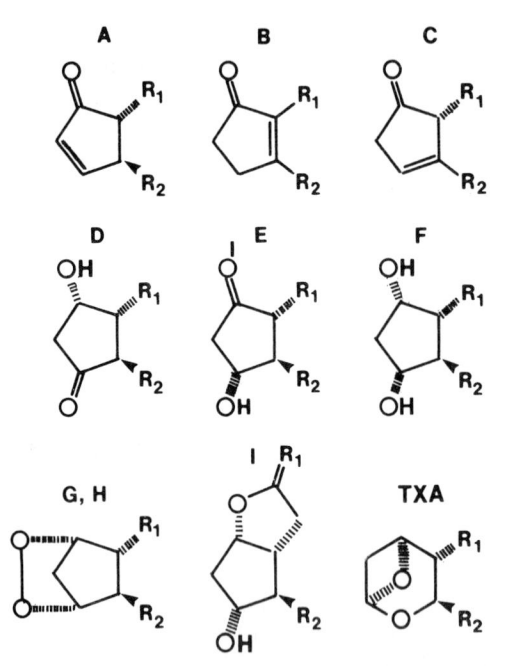

Fig. 9.4 Prostaglandin types. (From Gilman, A.G., et al. [eds.]: The Pharmacological Basis of Therapeutics. 7th Ed. New York, Macmillan Publishing Co., Inc., 1985.)

uterine relaxants (such as ritodrine) also have important clinical application.

PROSTAGLANDINS

Originally isolated from seminal fluid, prostaglandin compounds (Figure 9.4) are a series of acidic lipids which possess various pharmacologic effects. Specifically, they influence blood pressure, body temperature, inflammation, pain, and uterine muscle contractility. The four major prostaglandin groups are termed E, F, A, and B on the basis of their ring structure; numeral subscripts designate the degree of unsaturation in the side chains. Prostaglandins of the E and F series are sometimes referred to as "primary" prostaglandins, whereas the A and B prostaglandins are actually derivatives of the E group.

Biosynthesis of the primary prostaglandins occurs in a sequential manner catalyzed by a complex of microsomal enzymes (Figure 9.5). The fatty acid precursors for prostaglandin synthesis are dihomo-gamma-linolenic acid and arachidonic acid. These fatty acids are released from their esterified form in cell membranes by phospholipases. Arachidonic acid is converted to cyclic endoperoxides (Prostaglandin G_2 or H_2) by prostaglandin synthetase (fatty acid cyclooxygenase). These cyclic endoperoxides are unstable and have a short half-life. Their further biotransformation results in either the formation of prostaglandin E_2, $F_{2\,alpha}$, and D_2; thromboxane A_2; or prostacyclin (Figure 9.5).

A lipoxygenase pathway also exists in arachidonic acid metabolism in which case hydroxy acids (HETE—*h*ydroxyperoxy*e*icosa*t*etra*e*naic acids) and leukotrienes are produced (Figure 9.6). A leukotriene mixture is apparently the material referred to as slow-reacting substance of anaphylaxis or SRS-A.

Prostaglandins stimulate intracellular adenosine 3′, 5′-monophosphate (cyclic AMP) production and Ca^{++} utilization. Whereas prosta-

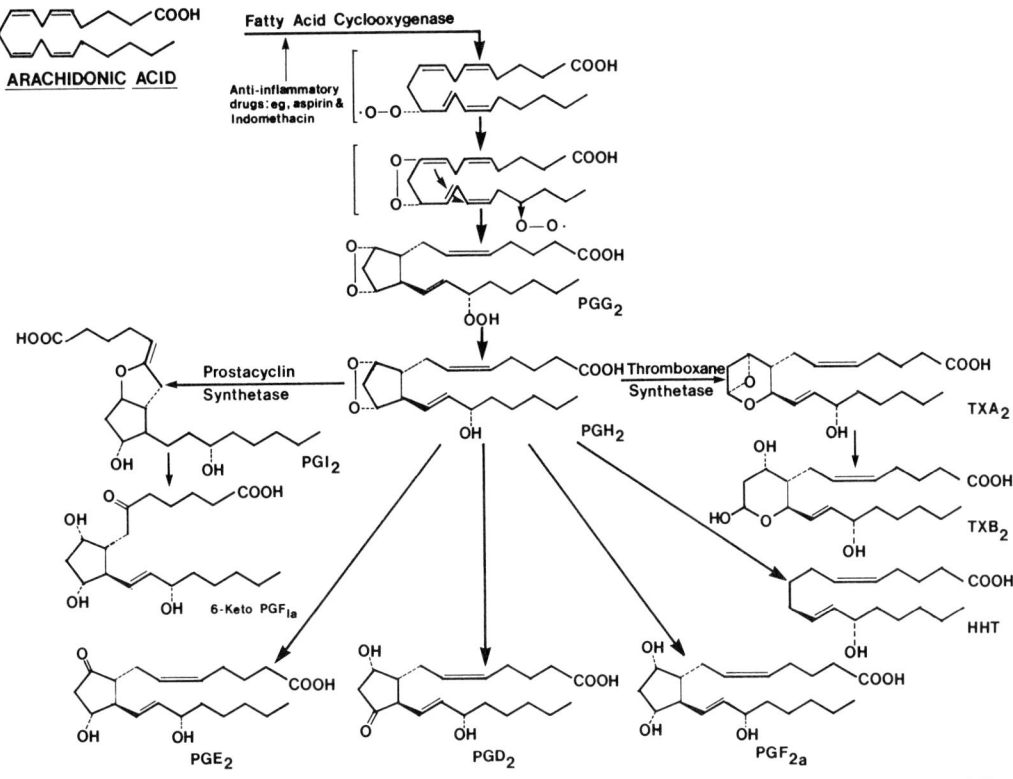

Fig. 9.5 Prostaglandin synthesis. (Modified from Gilman, A.G., et al. [eds.]: The Pharmacological Basis of Therapeutics. 7th Ed. New York, Macmillan Publishing Co., Inc., 1985.)

glandin E relaxes the nonpregnant uterus but contracts the pregnant uterus, prostaglandin F contracts both the pregnant and nonpregnant uterus.

Dinoprost Trometamine (Prostaglandin F$_{2\ alpha}$). Dinoprost tromethamine was introduced as an abortifacient for use in the second trimester of pregnancy.

Mechanism of Action. Dinoprost causes strong uterine contractions during the last two trimesters of pregnancy and induces delivery of the fetus in most cases. This drug stimulates the myometrium of the gravid (pregnant) uterus to contract in a manner similar to that seen at term (during labor).

Clinical Indications. Dinoprost is administered intra-amniotically to induce abortion and to evacuate the uterus in the management of missed abortion. This drug is also a potential alternative to oxytocin for labor induction.

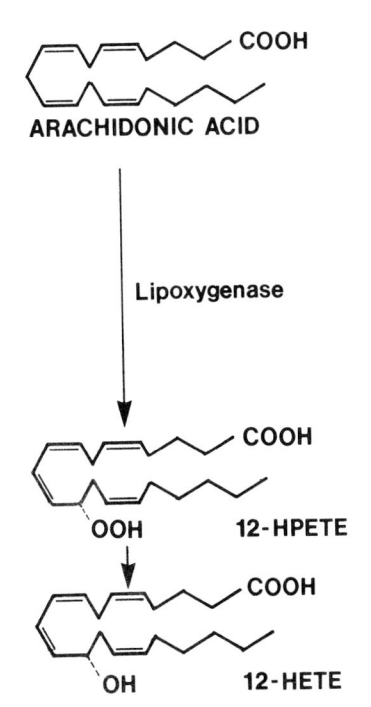

Fig. 9.6 Arachidonic acid—lipoxygenase pathway.

Adverse Effects/Precautions. Adverse reactions include nausea, vomiting, diarrhea, hypertension, allergic reactions, bronchospasm, hypotension, syncope, and uterine lacerations. The gastrointestinal reactions probably relate to the capacity of dinoprost to stimulate the smooth muscle of the gut.

Dinoprostone (Prostaglandin E_2). Administered intravaginally, dinoprostone is an abortifacient.

Mechanism of Action. Dinoprostone stimulates the myometrium of the gravid uterus to contract in a manner like that which occurs during labor.

Clinical Indications. Dinoprostone is indicted for inducing therapeutic abortion from the twelfth to the twentieth gestational week as calculated from the last menstrual period. Another of the drug's uses is evacuation of the uterine contents in the management of missed abortion or intrauterine fetal death up to 28 weeks' gestational time. Dinoprostone is also used in the management of nonmetaplastic gestational trophoblastic disease (benign hydatidiform mole).

Adverse Effects/Precautions. The most commonly noted adverse reactions to dinoprostone relate to smooth muscle stimulation; these side effects include nausea, vomiting, and diarrhea. Temperature elevation, headache, and shivering and chills, as well as hypotension (transient diastolic decreases), may also occur with dinoprostone use.

Carboprost Tromethamine (Prostaglandin 15-methyl $F_{2\,alpha}$). Carboprost is used as an abortifacient.

Mechanism of Action. Carboprost, a prostaglandin, stimulates the myometrium in a manner similar to labor contractions that occur at term.

Clinical Indications. Carboprost is used to abort pregnancy between the thirteenth and twentieth gestational week as calculated from the first day of the last regular menstrual period. It is also employed to expel the uterine contents after a missed abortion with another method.

Adverse Effects/Precautions. Pyrexia over 2°F is a frequent adverse reaction. The commonly occurring side effects of nausea, vomiting, and diarrhea are transient and disappear upon cessation of therapy with carboprost.

OXYTOCIN

Oxytocin, an endogenous posterior pituitary hormone, is indicated for the medical induction of labor. See Chapter 6 for a discussion of the actions of oxytocin.

ERGOT ALKALOIDS

The ergot alkaloids have diverse pharmacologic activity including adrenergic blocking action; see Chapter 2. Ergonovine is an ergot alkaloid with pronounced oxytocic action.

Ergonovine Maleate. Ergonovine, an amino alcohol derivative of lysergic acid, belongs to the ergobasine group of ergot alkaloids.

Mechanism of Action. Ergonovine differs from oxytocin in that it increases the activity of the cervix, whereas oxytocin decreases it. The frequency of uterine contractions is also greater with ergonovine than with oxytocin. With this increased frequency, the relaxation period is shortened, thereby increasing uterine tone.

Larger doses of ergonovine produce short contractions of higher frequency that are superimposed upon the elevated tone of the uterus, creating an even higher tone. This action further interferes with uterine relaxation. Ergonovine, therefore, is not useful prior to delivery because of these characteristics which are potentially dangerous to the baby and mother.

The ergonovine contraction profile provides strong sustained contractions of the postpartum uterus and effectively reduces and controls postpartum bleeding. To illustrate, the blood vessels are clamped shut since they are located between the myometrial latticework matrix, and as the muscle filaments contract, bleeding decreases.

Although earlier studies determined that ergonovine acted directly on the myometrial receptor substance, recent evidence shows that ergonovine exerts its effects as a partial agonist or antagonist at alpha-adrenergic, dopaminergic, and trypaminergic receptors.

Clinical Indications. Ergonovine is effective in the prevention and treatment of postpartum and postabortal hemorrhage.

Adverse Effects/Precautions. Although nausea, vomiting, and diarrhea may occur, the incidence of these reactions is infrequent. Allergic reactions have also been reported.

Methylergonovine Maleate. Methylergonovine maleate, an ergonovine derivative, is used as an oxytocic.

Mechanism of Action. Methylergonovine increases the strength, duration, and frequency of uterine contractions and reduces uterine bleeding following the delivery of the placenta. Methylergonovine shortens the third stage of labor and reduces blood loss by inducing rapid and sustained tetanic uterine contractions.

Clinical Indications. Methylergonovine is effective in the management of postpartum myometrial atony and hemorrhage. In selected cases and under full obstetric supervision, methylergonovine is administered in the second stage of labor following delivery of the anterior shoulder.

Adverse Effects/Precautions. Reported adverse reactions include nausea, vomiting, transient hypertension, headache, tinnitus, sweating, palpitations, and breathing difficulty.

UTERINE MUSCLE RELAXANTS

Uterine muscle relaxants are beneficial in the control of premature labor.

Ritodrine. A beta-adrenergic agonist, ritodrine exerts a specific effect on beta$_2$-adrenergic receptors in the myometrium.

Mechanism of Action. Activation of the beta$_2$-adrenergic receptors in uterine muscle results in a decrease in contractility. The mechanism of myometrial inhibition involves stimulation of adenyl cyclase with the resultant increase in intracellular cyclic AMP. An alteration of intracellular Ca^{++} (i.e., reduction of free Ca^{++}) inhibits the myometrial contraction. Ritodrine also inhibits myosin light-chain kinase, thereby affecting the interaction between myometrial actin and myosin.

Clinical Indications. Ritodrine is used to treat premature labor.

Adverse Effects/Precautions. Adrenergic effects, including tachycardia (maternal and fetal), nervousness, tremor, nausea, and vomiting, are usually controllable through dosage adjustment.

Ethanol. Intravenous ethanol has sometimes been used to treat premature labor. A 10% ethanol solution is administered by IV infusion for up to 10 hours. Ethanol is useful in cases (such as cardiac disease) where ritodrine is contraindicated.

Magnesium Sulfate. Given by IV injection, magnesium sulfate inhibits uterine contractions. This drug is effective in patients who have normal kidney function and in whom ritodrine is contraindicated.

ANTINEOPLASTIC DRUGS

Combination chemotherapy is often used to treat neoplastic disease of the genitourinary tract and breast.

Triethylenethiophosphoramide (TSPA; TESPA). TESTPA is a cell cycle nonspecific alkylating agent.

Mechanism of Action. Release of ethyleneamine radicals by TESPA disrupts the bonds of deoxyribonucleic acid (DNA).

Clinical Indications. Although largely replaced by other antineoplastics, TESPA is sometimes used to treat breast adenocarcinoma, ovarian adenocarcinoma, and superficial papillary carcinoma of the urinary bladder.

Adverse Effects/Precautions. Highly toxic to the hematopoietic system, TESPA commonly causes leukopenia, thrombocytopenia, and anemia. Nausea, vomiting, anorexia, amenorrhea, dizziness, and headache are other reported adverse reactions.

Cisplatin. Cisplatin, an inorganic heavy metal coordination complex which acts as a nonspecific alkylating agent, contains a central platinum ion surrounded by two chloride atoms and two ammonia molecules in the cis position.

Mechanism of Action. Cisplatin produces interstrand and intrastrand cross-linking of DNA.

Clinical Indications. Cisplatin is used in combination therapy with bleomycin and vinblastine (VBP) in metastatic testicular tumors in patients who have received appropriate surgery or radiotherapy. In combination with doxorubicin, cisplatin is also used in metastatic ovarian tumors. Combination therapy with cyclophosphamide and doxorubicin (CISCA) is sometimes used to treat metastatic urinary tract disease. As a single agent, cisplatin is used as secondary therapy in patients with disseminated ovarian cancer who are unresponsive to standard chemotherapy and in those with transitional cell bladder cancer that is no longer amenable to surgery or radiotherapy.

Adverse Effects/Precautions. Nephrotoxicity, usually resulting in electrolyte imbalance, is the major dose-limiting toxicity. Ototoxicity (manifested by tinnitus or hearing loss) occurs in more than 30% of the patients receiving cisplatin therapy. In addition to possible anaphylaxis, other reactions include hematologic abnormalities and gastrointestinal distress.

Estramustine Phosphate Sodium. Estramustine is a combined form of estradiol and non-nitrogen mustard.

Mechanism of Action. Estramustine is a weak alkylating agent with minimal estrogenic activity. The estrogenic portion of the molecule acts as a carrier to impart selective uptake of the drug into estrogen receptor-positive cells.

Clinical Indications. Estramustine is used in the palliative treatment of metastatic or progressive prostatic carcinoma.

Adverse Effects/Precautions. Thrombosis, including myocardial infarction, occurs frequently in men receiving estrogens for prostatic cancer. Hematologic, gastrointestinal, and dermatologic adverse reactions are also common. Caution is advised in the administration of estramustine in patients with hepatic insufficiency.

Methotrexate (See Chapter 4). Methotrexate is used in the treatment of gestational choriocarcinoma, chorioadenoma destruens, and hydatidiform mole. The drug is also used alone or in combination with other antineoplastic drugs, for example, with cyclophosphamide and fluoruracil (CMF), in the treatment of breast cancer.

Doxorubicin (See Chapter 4). Doxorubicin is used in combination with other antineoplastic drugs to produce regression in breast carcinoma, ovarian carcinoma, and transitional cell bladder carcinoma.

Cyclophosphamide (See Chapter 4). Cyclophosphamide is often used in combination therapy (i.e., doxorubicin — AC; methotrexate, fluoruracil — CMF; methotrexate, fluoruracil, prednisone — CMFP; CMFP + vincristine — CMFVP; fluoruracil, doxorubicin — FAC).

Fluorouracil; 5-FU (See Chapter 4). Fluorouracil is used in combination therapy for the palliative management of breast cancer in selected patients.

Prednisone (See Chapters 4 and 6). A synthetic adrenocorticosteroid, prednisone is sometimes added to antineoplastic combination regimens.

Hormones (See Chapter 6). Androgens are used in the palliative treatment of advanced inoperable or metastatic breast carcinoma in postmenopausal women. Drugs that block estrogen receptors (e.g., tamoxifen) in estrogen-sensitive tumors are used in the palliative management of breast carcinoma. Progestins are effective in the palliative treatment of advanced carcinoma of the breast or endometrium. Estrogens are used for inoperable, progressive prostatic carcinoma.

Leuprolide (Lupron^R), a synthetic analog of gonadotropin releasing hormone (LH-RH), is indicated in the palliative treatment of advanced prostatic cancer. An LH-RH agonist, leuprolide inhibits (after an initial increase) gonadotropin secretion by the adenohypophysis. During continuous daily administration, a transient increase in gonadal steroids is followed by a decrease; in males, testosterone is reduced to castrate levels.

Antiemetics Used as Adjunctive Agents in Cancer Chemotherapy. In addition to conventional antiemetics, such as prochlorperazine (see Chapter 1), particular drugs are specifically indicated to counteract the nausea and vomiting which occurs with cancer chemotherapy. For example, metoclopramide (see Chapters 2 and 8), administered intravenously, often effectively relieves the nausea and vomiting that is almost invariably present in cisplatin therapy.

Dronabinol (delta-9-tetrahydrocannibanol; Marinol^R) is a synthetic marijuana derivative that is sometimes used as an alternate drug in patients who fail to respond to conventional antiemetic treatments. Given orally, dronabibol, which apparently acts centrally to depress the vomiting center in the medulla oblongata, is generally reserved for resistant cases because of the possibility of behavioral changes, including detachment, anxiety, depression, panic, distortions in time perception, and hallucinations. Psychologic and physical dependence are additional potential adverse reactions to dronabinol therapy.

DRUG INTERACTIONS*

Drug interactions, with the exception of those that occur with methenamine compounds and metronidazole, are discussed in previous chapters.

Methenamine Compounds.

Acetazolamide. Acetazolamide, an effective urinary alkalinizer, antagonizes the action of methenamine compounds. Proper conversion of methenamine to free formaldehyde in the urine requires maintenance of a urinary pH of 5.5 or lower.

Sodium Bicarbonate. As with acetazolamide, sodium bicarbonate renders the urine alkaline. Thus, the same situation requiring maintenance of a urinary pH of 5.5 or lower also applies.

Sulfonamides. Formation of a precipitate (crystalluria) in the urine frequently results from concomitant administration of methenamine compounds and sulfamethazole.

Metronidazole.

Disulfiram. Since some patients receiving the combination therapy of metronidazole and disulfiram have experienced psychotic episodes and confusion, concomitant use of these drugs is discouraged.

Ethanol. The combined use of ethanol and metronidazole in some patients produces possible "disulfiram reactions." Thus, patients on metronidazole therapy should be advised of potential adverse reactions following ethanol ingestion.

SUMMARY

Organisms that cause infectious disease and drugs that aid hosts to combat them remain in constant flux. Although some resourceful orga-

---

* See Chapter 7 for the drug interactions of the penicillins, cephalosporins, and tetracyclines.

nisms have developed metabolic bypasses and other novel means to circumvent a drug's cytotoxic effect and survive as resistant strains, medical science continually introduces drugs which are effective against such resistant organisms. Recently developed antiviral drugs are now capable of killing viruses that formerly resisted all attempts toward their demise. Acyclovir, for example, is an important addition to the physician's resources against genital herpes. An expanded knowledge of bacterial metabolism permits drug combinations (such as trimethoprim/sulfamethoxazole) which act synergistically at different sites in bacterial metabolic processes.

Chemotherapy is mainly palliative for the neoplastic diseases of the genitourinary tract. Thus, early diagnosis, surgical procedures, and radiation therapy remain the mainstays of curing these malignancies.

Certain current research areas are undergoing considerable expansion. One such focus is on the prostaglandins which have emerged as one of the most interesting classes of active endogenous substances, both from their role in disease causation and from a therapeutic standpoint. Additionally, advances in interferon research will undoubtedly present exciting new approaches in the treatment of both neoplastic disease and infections.

SUGGESTED READINGS

Amdinocillin. Med Lett Drugs Ther, 27:30, 1985.
Fendler, K.: Postsurgical urinary tract infections. Therapeutics. New York, Biomedical Information Corporation and Smith Kline Beckman Corporation, 1986.
Gilman, A.G., et al. (eds.): The Pharmacological Basis of Therapeutics. 7th Ed. New York, Macmillan Publishing Co., Inc., 1985.
Hansten, P.D.: Drug Interactions. 5th Ed. Philadelphia, Lea & Febiger, 1985.
Kastrup, E.K., and Boyd, J.R. (eds.): Drug Facts and Comparisons. Philadelphia, J.B. Lippincott Co., 1985.
Leuprolide for prostate cancer. Med Lett Drugs Ther, 27:69, 1985.
Norfloxacin. Med Lett Drugs Ther, 29:25, 1987.
Ogburn, P.L., Jr., and Brenner, W.E.: The physiologic actions and effects of prostaglandins. Current Concepts. Kalamazoo, MI, UpJohn Company, 1981.
Oral acyclovir for genital herpes simplex infection. Med Lett Drugs Ther, 27:41, 1985.
Rubin, R., and Swartz, M.N.: Trimethoprim-sulfamethoxazole. N Engl J Med, 303:426, 1980.
Sethi, M.L.: Viral diseases and drug therapy. U S Pharmacist, 10:42, 1985.

CHAPTER EXAMINATION

A young male confides in you that his street friends told him that although he may have a "dose of clap," he shouldn't worry because they think gonorrhea is no worse than a common cold and a "shot" will clear it up. You advise him to see a physician immediately.

1. The drug used initially in gonorrhea treatment is a form of
   a. metronidazole
   b. cisplatin
   c. penicillin
   d. tetracycline

2. The organism that causes gonorrhea is a
   a. gram-negative diplococcus
   b. virus
   c. fungus
   d. gram-positive streptococcus

3. A drug that could be used concurrently to maintain therapeutic blood levels of penicillin is
   a. erythromycin
   b. spectinomycin
   c. trimethoprim
   d. probenecid

4. Since the initial drug therapy has not been successful, resistant strains of the gonorrhea organism may have infected the young male. Drugs indicated in resistant gonorrhea cases include
   a. sulfamethoxazole and metronidazole
   b. tetracycline and spectinomycin
   c. probenecid and chloramphenicol
   d. methenamine and miconazole

5. Penicillin G
   a. inhibits bacterial cell wall biosynthesis
   b. binds the 50S ribosomal subunit
   c. binds the 30S ribosomal subunit
   d. changes the permeability of the bacterial plasma membrane, resulting in leakage of intracellular nutrients

A young female with symptoms of painful urination and urinary urgency receives a prescription for a trimethoprim-sulfamethoxazole combination.

6. The patient has probably developed
   a. ovarian cancer
   b. a urinary tract infection (UTI)
   c. endometriosis
   d. prostatitis
7. Trimethoprim
   a. binds bacterial dihydrofolate reductase
   b. competes with para-aminobenzoic acid (PABA) in bacterial enzymatic processes
   c. binds to the 30S ribosomal subunit to inhibit bacterial protein synthesis
   d. blocks sterol metabolism in the bacterial cell wall
8. Sulfamethoxazole
   a. competes with PABA in bacterial metabolism
   b. may produce adverse reactions, including hematologic abnormalities, erythema multiforme, and crystalluria
   c. interferes with the formation of bacterial folic acid
   d. all of the above
9. The organisms most prevalent in producing infections in the genitourinary tract are
   a. Escherichia coli and Proteus mirabilis
   b. Staphylococcus aureus and Clostridia species
   c. Herpes 1 virus and Cryptococcus imitis
   d. Hemophilus species and Enterobacter species
10. An antibiotic often indicated in the treatment of serious gram-negative infections of the genitourinary tract is
    a. colistin
    b. miconazole
    c. gentamicin
    d. amphotericin

Genital herpes is a prevalent venereal disease in young adults. The local nurses' association invites you to address them on the current drug therapy of this disease.

11. Genital herpes is best treated with
    a. tetracycline
    b. oxytetracycline
    c. acyclovir
    d. penicillin G
12. The causative organism in genital herpes is a
    a. virus
    b. fungus
    c. bacterium
    d. gram-negative diplococcus
13. Your remarks on prevention and treatment are especially germane since
    a. almost any antibiotic kills the causative organism
    b. the disease is not communicable
    c. the treatment is specific and recurrent infections are common
    d. no effective treatment is currently available

An elderly male patient complains of having to get up several times during the night to urinate. Difficulty in urination is an additional problem.

14. A problem suspected in this case is
    a. tertiary syphilis
    b. prostatic hyperplasia
    c. endometriosis
    d. testicular carcinoma
15. In addition to making a positive diagnosis of one of the above conditions (#14), the physician prescribes methenamine and sodium biphosphate. This patient probably has a concurrent
    a. chronic UTI
    b. hypergonadal condition
    c. hypogonadal syndrome
    d. herpes infection
16. The bactericidal effectiveness of methenamine depends upon
    a. the liberation of formaldehyde
    b. an acid urine

c. the duration that the urine is retained in the bladder
d. all of the above

17. Although the patient's biopsy confirms carcinoma, major surgery is not feasible. An antineoplastic agent possibly indicated for this patient is
    a. testosterone
    b. busulfan
    c. leuprolide
    d. prednisone

18. Several newer products in your hospital pharmacy are in the prostaglandin classification. Prostaglandins are
    a. endogenous acid lipids
    b. primary estrogenic substances
    c. biproducts of antibiotic synthesis
    d. antiviral agents of choice in the treatment of genital herpes

19. The main clinical application of dinoprost (PG $F_{2\,alpha}$), dinoprostone (PG E_2), and carboprost (15-methyl PG $F_{2\,alpha}$) is
    a. postpartum hemorrhage
    b. counteracting preterm uterine contraction
    c. treating UTIs
    d. therapeutic abortion

20. Prostaglandin E_2 and ergonovine maleate both induce myometrial contractions. In addition, ergonovine maleate is
    a. valuable in the control of postpartum hemorrhage
    b. a useful antineoplastic drug
    c. a potent inhibitor of gonadotropin release
    d. a $beta_2$-adrenergic receptor agonist

ANSWER KEY

1. c	11. c
2. a	12. a
3. d	13. c
4. b	14. b
5. a	15. a
6. b	16. d
7. a	17. c
8. d	18. a
9. a	19. d
10. c	20. a

chapter 10

INTEGUMENTARY/ CONNECTIVE TISSUE SYSTEM

CHAPTER OBJECTIVES

After studying this chapter, you should be able to:
1. Discuss the anatomic and physiologic characteristics of the skin and connective tissue.
2. Describe several common infectious dermatoses.
3. List examples of drugs in several dermatologic categories.
4. Name three drugs that are employed orally to treat skin diseases and describe their mechanism of action.
5. Explain the mechanism of the anti-inflammatory activity of acetylsalicyclic acid.
6. Delineate the clinical advantages of the newer nonsteroidal anti-inflammatory drugs (NSAIDs) over the salicylates.
7. Name the major forms of arthritis and describe the symptomatology of each.
8. Discuss the incidence and treatment of tinea infections.
9. Evaluate the role of gold compounds in the treatment of rheumatoid arthritis.
10. Compare the hypouricemic mechanism of allopurinol to that of probenecid.

INTRODUCTION

The skin acts as a barrier between a potentially dangerous external environment and the internal body structures and organs. The alive human skin, moistened by salt water and lubricated by a film of oil, continually renews itself and sheds dead cells.

Protection of the body from harmful agents, such as pathogens and irritant substances, is a function of the skin. Additional roles include sensory experience, temperature control, development of pigment, and vitamin D synthesis. The skin is also important in body water regulation as it controls both water loss from the body and moisture penetration into the body. Thus, the "sea within us" is prevented from evaporating and our metabolic fires do not produce lethal internal overheating.

The skin, aptly called "the mirror of the body," often functions as an early alarm system for potential problems originating in underlying organs; it also indicates emotional reactions. To illustrate, facial blushing represents an emotional reponse to a stimulus, as well as the intimate association that exists between the brain and skin.

Consisting of many types of complex tissue, the skin is subject to various disorders including infections, inflammations, and neoplasms. Many skin disorders respond to various drugs employed in the prevention and treatment of such conditions.

Connective tissue serves as the body's supporting system. The structural elements and matrix of the connective system include fibrous tissue, bones, and cartilage. Anti-inflammatory drugs with analgesic action find extensive clinical use in the treatment of connective tissue disorders, such as rheumatoid arthritis.

ANATOMY AND PHYSIOLOGY OF THE INTEGUMENTARY/CONNECTIVE TISSUE SYSTEM

The largest organ of the body, the skin wraps around the adult body, representing about 1.8 m^2 of tissue and constituting about 17% of the body weight. The normal skin thickness is 3 to 5 mm; the thickest skin is located on the hand palms and feet soles and the thinnest is found on the eyelids and genitals.

The skin is divided into three layers (Figure 10.1). Of these, the compact and nonvascular epidermis (the outermost skin layer) is comprised of several distinct sublayers consisting of squamous epithelial cells. Dead epithelial cells, shed from the epidermal surface, are rapidly replaced by new cells generated by mitotic activity in the lower strata of the epidermis.

The dermis (corium), the second skin layer, supports the epidermis and separates it from the lower fatty layer. The dermis consists mainly of collagen and elastin embedded in a mucopolysaccharide substance. Dermal nerves and capillaries exist in close proximity to hair follicles, sebaceous glands, and sweat glands.

The hypodermis, the third and lowest skin layer, consists of loose connective tissue and provides for skin pliability. Adipose tissue, present in the hypodermis of most body areas, aids in thermal control, food reserve, and cushioning or padding.

Millions of minute and intricate structures dot and penetrate the skin (Figure 10.1). For example, hair follicles have their roots in the skin. Whereas coiled sweat glands generally open directly to the skin surface, sebaceous glands secrete oil (sebum) into the hair follicles where it eventually reaches the epidermal surface.

INTEGUMENTARY/CONNECTIVE TISSUE SYSTEM **441**

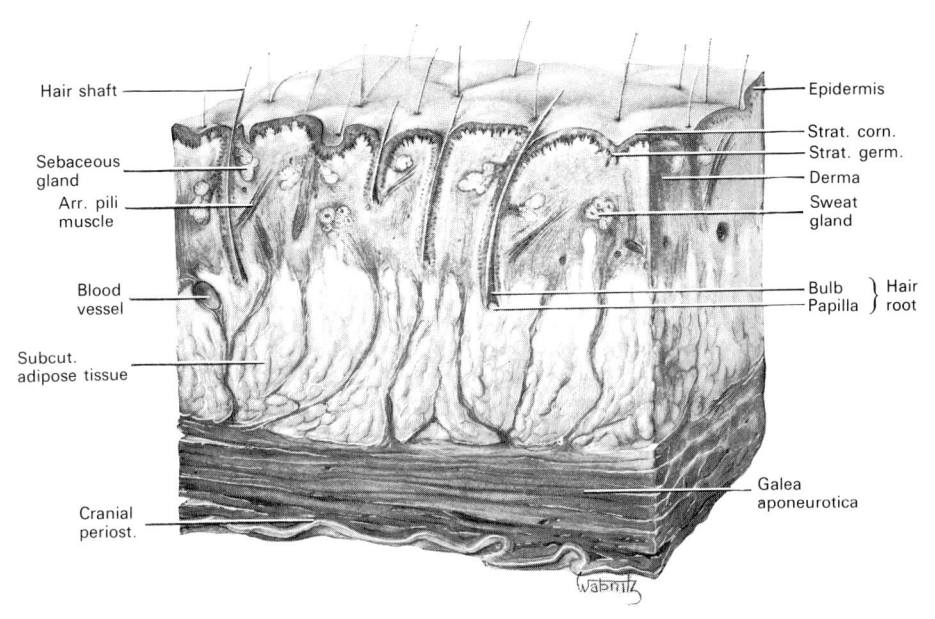

Fig. 10.1 Section through scalp of adult cadaver. 5X. (From Clemente, C.D., ed.: Gray's Anatomy. 30th Ed. Philadelphia, Lea & Febiger, 1985.)

CONNECTIVE TISSUE

The human skeleton contains an axial skeleton, essential to life, that includes the skull, spinal column and ribs, and an appendicular skeleton represented by the arms and legs. Muscles of the abdomen and spine hold the axial skeleton in an upright position. Since the movement in the spine is greatest in the lower back, degeneration changes are more pronounced in this region.

Joints are structures that permit one bone to glide over another. The matrix of connective tissue supplies lubricating elements of the joint fluids, allowing smooth, reduced-friction contact between different bones. The hip, a ball-and-socket joint that is subject to a weight-bearing burden, is susceptible to structural changes with the continual thrust of body weight. As a hinge in the middle of a long limb, the knee (the largest joint in the body) is continually exposed to injury. The wrist, elbow, ankle, and foot represent other joint sites.

Skeletal muscles move bones by contracting; in many instances, they serve as levers. The termination of muscles are tendons, fibrous cords that attach the muscle to a bone. Tears in tendons and muscles around joints are frequent causes of pain. Tendonitis usually results from strain or injury of a muscle (often sports-related as in "tennis elbow"). Lumbago is a special tendonitis involving the attachments of the muscles of the lumbar region.

Inflammatory changes in connective tissue often produce lesions in muscle, skin, blood vessels, heart, and other internal organs. As "collagen" designates connective tissue, the term "collagen disease" usually describes arthritis or other connective tissue disease.

Skeletal muscles contain pain receptors that, upon stimulation, send sensory impulses to the brain where pain perception occurs (see Chapter 1). Muscle pain and soreness may follow strenuous exercise or result from prolonged, fixed, and/or stressful positions (such as bending over for extended periods or driving a car long distances).

The shoulder area, because of its location and structure, is subject to pronounced stress and strain. Its pendulum structure makes it especially susceptible to gravitational forces. Thus, certain occupations (for example, house painting) may predispose a person to shoulder pain.

Bursae are closed sacs that are lined with cellular membranes which contain viscid fluid. Usually present over bony prominences, between and beneath tendons, and between certain movable structures (subdeltoid bursae), a bursa facilitates movement by diminishing friction. Bursitis is a common cause of joint pain.

FUNCTIONS OF THE SKIN

A major function of the skin is protection of the underlying organ systems from trauma, temperature changes, harmful penetrations, moisture, humidity, radiation, and invasion by microorganisms. The skin contains nerve endings that provide the sense of touch and send electrical messages of pain, cold, or heat to the brain which interprets their significance.

Secretions (sebum and sweat) from the skin waterproof the skin and prevent excessive internal body temperature by an evaporative cooling system. An important function of sebum is lubrication of the skin surface to promote both suppleness and dermal hydration by preventing moisture loss. Sebum also prevents penetration by other substances and possesses antiseptic and antifungal properties.

The skin acid mantle (pH 4.5 to 5.5), supplied by sebum and sweat, has a protective role because microorganisms tend to reproduce better at a near neutral pH (6 to 7.5). Additionally, several fatty acids (proprionic, caproic, and caprylic) have bacteriostatic and fungistatic activity. Lastly, the normal skin flora that reside in the skin secretion environ are often antagonistic to potential pathogenic microorganisms.

The skin also participates in carbohydrate, protein, fat, and (with the aid of sunshine) vitamin D metabolism, as well as producing antibodies against foreign bodies. Delayed hypersensitivity reactions also occur in the skin.

SWEAT GLANDS

There are two types of sweat glands: eccrine and apocrine. Cholinergic neurons, although anatomically sympathetic, innervate the eccrine glands. The volume of sweat produced (several L/day) by the eccrine glands is much greater than that produced by apocrine glands. Emotional stress and anxiety often trigger eccrine sweating; eccrine sweat contains no fats, carbohydrates, or proteins and has a pH of approximately 5. Found over almost all of the body except for the genital region and legs, the eccrine sweat glands are especially numerous on the palms of the hands and soles of the feet.

Apocrine sweat glands, found mainly in the anogenital area, the axillae, and the nipples, are attached to hair follicles by a duct. Apocrine glands do not function in body temperature regulation, and their onset of activity is puberty-related as they respond to hormone influence. Adrenergic activation (as in stress) produces a milky secretion which contains fats, sugars, and proteins. Apocrine sweat is odorless until bacterial action produces the characteristic pungent, musky odor of apocrine sweat.

SKIN APPENDAGES

The hair which emerges from each follicle is a fiber of keratinized epithelial cells. Hair growth results from cell multiplication in the hair germ at the base of the follicle. Although possibly genetically related, hair loss occurs as a side effect from ingestion of certain drugs (especially with the antineoplastic agents). Finger and toe nails are modifications of the keratinized layer of the epidermis.

DISEASES AND DISORDERS OF THE INTEGUMENTARY/ CONNECTIVE TISSUE SYSTEM

SKIN INFECTIONS

Staphylococcal and tinea skin infections occur frequently, especially if there is a break or superficial injury to the dermis. Viral infections and cutaneous candidiasis often depend upon multiple etiologic factors.

IMPETIGO, ERYSIPELAS, AND FURUNCLES

A superficial infection, impetigo is caused by staphylococci, a mixture of staphylococci and streptococci, or, infrequently, by streptococci alone. Vesicles or bullae become pustular, rupture, and form yellow crusts.

Erysipelas, caused by Streptococcus pyogenes, is an infection of the skin and superficial parts of subcutaneous tissues. The invading bacteria usually enter through a break in the skin and constitutional symptoms accompany the redness and swelling in the affected area. Vesicular and bullous lesions are also characteristic of this infection.

A furuncle (boil) is an acute infection of a hair follicle. A painful nodule with a central "core" or slough forms in the skin by circumscribed inflammation of the dermis and subcutaneous tissue. Most often found in otherwise healthy persons, furuncles also commonly accompany diabetes mellitus, uremia, and cases of immunologic abnormality. "Carrier" sites (i.e., nose, throat, and perineum) are probable factors in recurrent infection.

LUPUS VULGARIS (TUBERCULOSIS OF THE SKIN)

Lupus vulgaris, a low grade infection, is marked by the formation of brownish nodules in the dermis, chronic ulceration, and severe scarring. The course of the skin lesion is often chronic with a tendency toward self-healing. The presence of tuberculosis at other sites is uncommon and the dermatologic infection rarely spreads to other organs.

WARTS

This common infection is caused by a deoxyribonucleic acid (DNA)-containing wart virus. Most warts undergo spontaneous regression. Warts sometimes spread rapidly in those who lack immunity to the virus (especially children).

HERPES SIMPLEX

Groups of vesicles on the skin characterize herpes simplex, an infection also caused by a DNA-containing virus. These lesions often occur on the borders of the lips, nostrils, or genitals. Herpes simplex sometimes accompanies fever, hence the descriptive term "fever blister."

HERPES ZOSTER (SHINGLES)

Herpes zoster is an acute, self-limited inflammatory disease of cerebral ganglia and the ganglia of posterior nerve roots and peripheral nerves in a segmented distribution. Herpes zoster is caused by the DNA-containing chicken pox virus. Groups of small vesicles in the cutaneous area along the course of affected nerves and neuralgic pain characterize this disease.

CANDIDIASIS

Candida dermal infections commonly occur in patients who have been treated with immunosuppressive drugs, antibiotics, and oral contraceptives. Patients with diabetes mellitus, hypoparathyroidism, and other underlying systemic diseases also frequently develop candidiasis.

RINGWORM (TINEA INFECTIONS)

Ringworm, a fungal skin disease that appears in circular patches, is caused by species in the genera Epidermophyton, Microsporum, and Trichophyton. Tinea infections develop on the skin in various areas of the body including the scalp (tinea capitus); the crural or perineal folds, extending to the upper inside of the thighs (tinea cruris, "jock-itch"); and the skin of the feet, especially between the toes and on the soles (tinea pedis, "athlete's foot"). Lesions may become deep inflammatory areas.

Spread either by direct contact, a comb or headgear of an infected person, or infected pets, tinea capitis particularly affects children before puberty. Loosening and partial loss of scalp hair in patches and breaking off of the infected hair characterize this infection.

Tinea cruris, a skin infection which is usually spread by contaminated athletic supporters or clothing, requires warmth, moisture, and friction for its development.

Affecting 90% of the persons in the United States one or more times during their lives, tinea pedis occurs most commonly in males in the summer months. Excessive perspiration of the feet is a frequent predisposing factor in the development of tinea pedis; thus, good foot care can help prevent this infection.

SKIN INFESTATIONS

Scabies and pediculosis are frequently found in those who lack adequate personal hygiene.

SCABIES

Caused by the itch mite, Sarcoptes scabei var. hominis, scabies is a contagious skin disease evidenced by intense itching and eczema (a result of scratching). The female mite lays eggs in the skin (stratum corneum) that form burrows (cuniculi). These lesions are particularly common in the finger webs and on the wrist flexures.

PEDICULOSIS

Pediculosis is infestation with the louse, Pediculus humanus, a species that feeds on human blood. Lice infest the body and hair areas, including the scalp and pubic area (Phthirus pubis, crab louse). Exudative lesions and secondary infection may result from infestation by lice—major vectors of typhus, relapsing fever, and trench fever.

MISCELLANEOUS SKIN DISORDERS

Occurring most frequently in teenagers, acne often resists treatment. Some skin disorders, such as psoriasis and discoid lupus erythematosus are chronic and often present clinical dilemmas.

ACNE

An eruption of papules or pustules characterizes acne, an inflammatory skin disease. Chronic acne (acne vulgaris), evidenced by comedones, papules, nodules, and pustules on the face, neck, and upper part of the body trunk, usually affects adolescents. Most teenagers have acne to some extent, but the condition usually regresses with time. Disfiguration and scarring may result from severe acne cases.

Contributing factors to acne development include an excessively greasy skin, bacterial conversion of sebum fat to irritant fatty acids, blockage of sebaceous gland ducts, and increased sensitivity of skin end organs to androgens.

PSORIASIS

Psoriasis, a chronic recurrent and strongly hereditary dermatosis, is characterized by discrete bright red macules, papules, or plaques covered with silvery lamellated scales. Trigger factors include localized trauma (for example, sunburn, operation incision) and streptococcal infections.

Increases in epidermal cell mitosis represent a fundamental metabolic lesion in this condition. Psoriasis lesions have ten times the "normal" epidermal cell turnover rate.

ECZEMA

Redness, itching, minute papules and vesicles, weeping, oozing, and crusting characterize eczema, a superficial inflammation of the epidermis. Subsequent scaling, lichenification, and pigmentation may also occur with this disease, which possibly results from either an external irritant/allergen or an unknown cause. Atopic dermatitis is a form of eczema associated with circulating IgE antibodies to one or more of a wide variety of antigens.

URTICARIA (HIVES)

Urticaria is a vascular reaction of the skin characterized by transient appearance of slightly elevated wheals. Severe itching is also usually present. Urticaria may be acute or chronic; although clinical patterns vary, there is always a degree of whealing and some erythematous flare. In this way, the basic lesion resembles that produced by experimental intradermal injection of histamine (triple reaction of Lewis, "wheal and flare" reaction). Factors in the development of urticaria include dermatographia, heat, cold, ingestion of food allergens, and drugs.

DISCOID LUPUS ERYTHEMATOSUS (DLE)

Discoid lupus erythematosus, a chronic skin disease, is characterized by red, circular, scaly macules which often occur after exposure to sunlight. Limited to cutaneous manifestations, the lesions of DLE typically form a butterfly pattern over the bridge of the nose and cheeks.

SKIN CANCERS

Skin cancer, the most commonly occurring form of malignancy, is usually curable, especially with early diagnosis and adequate medical treatment. The two common types of skin cancer are the basal cell variety and squamous cell cancer.

The basal cell variety originates as a small fleshy nodule, often located in the facial region. These growths typically look like a translucent knob and have "pearly" borders. Ulceration occurs after a varying time period and bleeding then follows. Specifically, a crusted lesion periodically opens and bleeding ensues. Basal cell cancers do not metastasize although underlying skin areas are sometimes affected.

Squamous cell cancer usually appears on pre-existent, precancerous lesions found on any area of the skin or mucous membranes; the lips, mouth, and genitalia are frequent sites of skin cancer development. Often appearing as a lump with a scaly surface, squamous cell lesions increase in size; also, the formation of a large fungoid mass is possible. Metastases usually occur in the later course of squamous cell cancer. Predisposing factors in squamous cell cancer include leukoplakia of the tongue and mouth, smoking, and excessive exposure to sunlight (the latter is especially applicable to those with blond hair and/or blue eyes).

Malignant melanoma is a highly dangerous skin cancer which tends to spread rapidly. Generally beginning as a mottled brown to black patch with irregular borders, the tumor arises either from an existing mole or as a new growth. Common brown moles are frequently present in large numbers. Asymmetry, border irregularity, color variegation, and a fairly large diameter (0.5 cm) that is often wider than a pencil eraser tip are characteristics which suggest the possibility of a melanoma.

DISORDERS OF THE JOINTS AND CONNECTIVE TISSUES

The arthritides frequently cause painful disability in many adults, especially the elderly.

ARTHRITIS

Arthritis, literally meaning inflammation of a joint, refers to approximately 100 different conditions which involve pain in joints and connective tissue. The term applies to a variety of disorders that develop and progress in different ways (Table 10.1). Major forms of arthritis include rheumatoid arthritis and osteoarthritis.

Rheumatoid Arthritis. A chronic inflammatory disease, rheumatoid arthritis afflicts an estimated 7 million Americans. The disease usually begins between the ages of 20 and 45 and affects women three times more frequently than men. Rheumatoid arthritis occurs in multiple joints, especially in the hands and feet (Figure 10.2). The polyarticular involvement is characterized by inflammatory changes in the

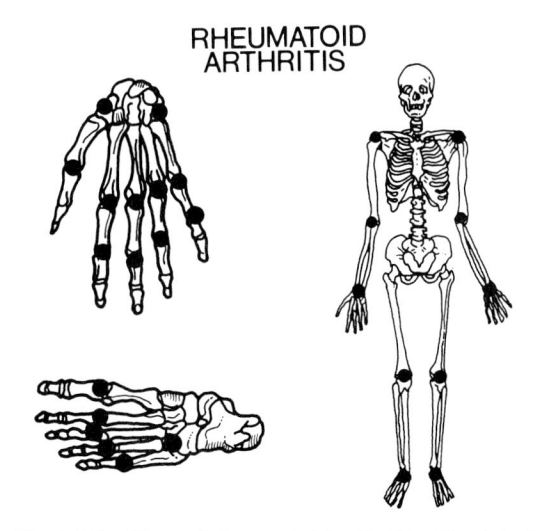

Fig. 10.2 Sites of rheumatoid arthritis. (Reprinted with permission of Drug Topics, Medical Economics Co., July 21, 1986.)

Table 10.1. MAJOR FORMS OF ARTHRITIS.*

Type	Symptoms
Osteoarthritis	Pain
	Loss of mobility in one or more joints
Rheumatoid Arthritis	Symmetric joint pain, swelling, and possible deformity
	Morning stiffness
	Fatigue
	Weight loss
Juvenile Rheumatoid Arthritis	Knee or other joint pain and stiffness
	Can begin with high fever, rash, and no joint symptoms
Ankylosing Spondylosis	Pain and stiffness in spine
Gout	Sudden onset of acute pain and inflammation usually in a single joint (often the big toe)
Scleroderma	Tightness or hardening of skin
	Often affects joints and internal organs
Systemic Lupus Erythematosus (SLE)	Sometimes starts with fever, weakness, weight loss, and rash (particularly on the arms, neck, and face)
	Joint pain and symptoms of organ damage may follow

* Modified from White, J.P.: New nonsteroidals coming to the rescue. Drug Topics, **130**:40, 1986.

synovial membranes and joint structures with bone rarefaction and atrophy. Deformity is common if the disease process is not interrupted. Rheumatoid arthritis is now considered as an autoimmune disease.

The inflammatory response in patients with rheumatoid arthritis is apparently initiated by the combination of gamma globulin (antigen) with rheumatoid factor (antibody). A subsequent local release of leukocyte-attracting (chemotactic) factors occurs. Phagocytosis of the antigen-antibody complex follows with the release of lysosomal enzymes. The liberated lysosomal enzymes cause inflammation and damage to cartilage and surrounding tissue.

Cell-mediated immune reactions and prostaglandin release also characterize the inflammatory reaction in rheumatoid arthritis. Prostaglandins are closely related to the inflammatory process and the pain associated with it. Additionally, leukotriene B, formed via the lipoxygenase pathway in arachidonic acid metabolism, promotes leukocyte migration and furthers the inflammatory response.

Osteoarthritis. A degenerative joint disease, osteoarthritis is characterized by deterioration of the articular cartilage, bone hypertrophy at the margins, and changes in the synovial membrane. Commonly involved sites include the hip joints, spine, and finger articulations (Figure 10.3).

The incidence of osteoarthritis increases with age and affects about 17 million Americans, mainly the elderly. This condition also sometimes develops in younger individuals following joint injuries, such as those sustained in athletic events.

SYSTEMIC LUPUS ERYTHEMATOSUS (SLE)

Systemic lupus erythematosus is a collagen vascular disease with pronounced skin manifestations; symptoms include skin eruptions, arthralgia, fever, leukopenia, visceral lesions, and autoimmune phenomena. This condition is a chronic generalized connective tissue disorder that ranges from mild to fulminating. Nonspecific rashes often appear in light exposed areas.

DRUGS USED IN THE TREATMENT OF INTEGUMENTARY/CONNECTIVE TISSUE DISORDERS

The nonsteroidal anti-inflammatory drugs (NSAIDs) represent one of the largest classes of current drugs. Several of these agents are among the most frequently prescribed drugs in medical practice; they are also contained in immense numbers of over-the-counter products for the treatment of integumentary/connective tissue diseases.

DRUGS USED TO TREAT SKIN DISEASES

Various drugs control the symptoms of skin disease, as well as being an actual curative factor in skin infections.

LOCAL ANESTHETICS

Classified according to their chemical type, local anesthetics are usually designated as amides or esters (Chapter 1). Amides that are commonly used in topical preparations for skin disorders are dibucaine and lidocaine; benzocaine, butamben, and tetracaine are ester-type anesthetics. Cyclomethycaine and pramoxine are other topical local anesthetics that do not fit either the amide or the ester classification.

Mechanism of Action. Local anesthetics block the generation and conduction of nerve impulses from sensory nerves. The nerve cell membrane is the main site of action where local anesthetics alter the permeability to ions. These drugs inhibit the sodium influx following depolarization of the nerve cell membrane by inactivation of the sodium channels.

The receptor for local anesthetics is apparently on the inner surface; therefore, for effective conduction blockade, the drugs must first cross the membrane in an uncharged, nonionized form and then react in their charged, ionized form to the binding site. Electrophysiologic evidence indicates that the local anesthetic receptor is situated about halfway down the sodium channel. Calcium ion (Ca^{++}) alters the reactivity of the sodium channel receptor to local anesthetics and may either attentuate or intensify local anesthetic action.

Clinical Indications. Local anesthetics alleviate pruritus, pain, and discomfort in skin disorders, including minor burns or scalds, fungus infections, prickly heat, diaper rash, eczema, sunburn, and skin manifestations of systemic disease (such as chicken pox).

Adverse Effects/Precautions. Allergic reactions, including urticaria, edema, contact dermatitis, and anaphylactoid reactions, are possible. If an extensive skin area is being treated, the possibility of significant systemic absorption exists.

OSTEOARTHRITIS

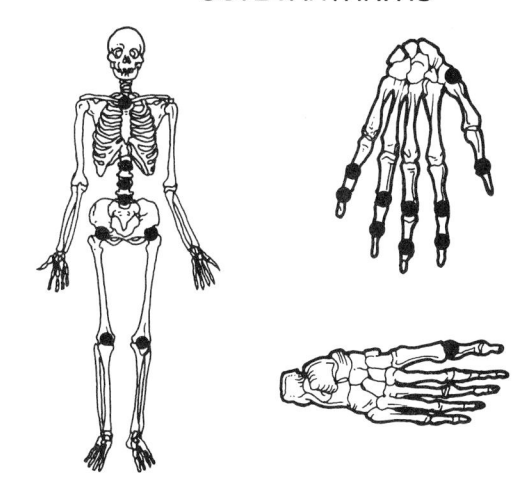

Fig. 10.3 Sites of osteoarthritis. (Reprinted with permission of Drug Topics, Medical Economics Co., July 21, 1986.)

ANTIBIOTICS

Antibiotics (Table 10.2) are used topically and systemically in the treatment of skin diseases.

General Skin Anti-infectives. Antibiotics are used to treat superficial infections of the skin that are caused by susceptible organisms. Topical antibiotics are also used for infection prophylaxis in minor skin abrasions.

Mechanism of Action. Chloramphenicol and tetracycline-type (oxytetracycline, tetracycline, chlortetracycline) and aminoglycoside (neomycin, gentamicin) antibiotics act by inhibiting bacterial protein synthesis (see Chapter 7). Polymyxin B disrupts the structure of bacterial plasma membranes and alters their permeability. Bacitracin inhibits bacterial cell wall synthesis.

Clinical Indications. Antibiotics are used for the prophylaxis and treatment of skin infections caused by susceptible organisms.

Table 10.2. TOPICAL ANTI-INFECTIVE AGENTS.

Available products	Trade names	Forms
Antibiotics:		
Bacitracin	Baciguent	Ointment
Chloramphenicol	Chloromycetin	Cream
Chlortetracycline HCl	Aureomycin	Ointment
Erythromycin	Ilotycin	Ointment
Gentamicin	Garamycin	Ointment, Cream
Neomycin sulfate	Neomycin; Myciguent	Ointment, Cream
Tetracycline	Achromycin	Ointment
Burn preparations:		
Mafenide	Sulfamylon	Cream
Silver sulfadiazine	Silvadene	Cream
Nitrofurazone	Furacin	Soluble dressing, Topical cream
Tannic Acid Compound	Amertan	Jelly
Antifungal agents:		
Acrisorcin	Akrinol	Cream
Amphotericin B	Fungizone	Cream, Lotion, Ointment
Ciclopirox olamine	Loprox	Cream
Clotrimazole	Lotrimin; Mycelex	Cream, Solution, Lotion
Econazole nitrate	Spectazole	Cream
Haloprogin	Halotex	Cream, Solution
Iodochlorhydroxyquin	Vioform; Quin III; Torofor	Cream, Ointment
Miconazole nitrate	Micatin; Monistat-Derm	Cream, Lotion, Powder
Nystatin	Mycostatin; Nilstat; Candex	Cream, Ointment, Lotion, Powder
Tolnaftate	Tinactin; Aftate	Cream, Powder, Liquid, Solution
Triacetin	Enzactin; Fungoid; Fungacetin	Cream, Ointment, Solution
Undecylenic acid	in Desenex; in NP-27; in others	Liquid, Solution, Foam, Soap, Ointment, Powder, Cream
Zinc undecylenate	in Cruex; Pedi-Dri; in others	Cream, Powder
Scabicides and/or pediculicides:		
Crotamiton	Eurax	Cream, Lotion
Lindane	Kwell; Scabene	Cream, Lotion, Shampoo
Malathion	Prioderm	Lotion

Adverse Effects/Precautions. Severe infections may require systemic antibiotic therapy. Potential problems of particular antibiotics include possible nephrotoxicity and ototoxicity of neomycin, requiring caution if extensive skin areas are treated (no more than 20% of the body surface in burn cases); overgrowth of nonsusceptible organisms, especially fungi, may result from prolonged use of topical antibiotic preparations. Blood dyscrasias have followed chloramphenicol therapy, photosensitization has been reported in topical gentamicin use, and allergic contact dermatitis has occurred in patients treated with bacitracin ointment.

Tetracycline. By decreasing the amount of free fatty acids present in acne lesions, oral tetracycline reduces irritation. Topical tetracycline apparently has a local effect, although the precise mechanism whereby acne improves is unknown.

Erythromycin. Topical erythromycin reduces the inflammation in acne vulgaris, probably as a result of the drug's antibiotic action.

Clindamycin. Clindamycin inhibits the growth of Corynebacterium (Propionibacterium) acnes, an organism commonly associated with

Table 10.3. ACNE PRODUCTS.

Available products	Trade names	Forms
Benzoyl Peroxide, cleanser	Desquam-X Wash; Benzac W Wash; PanOxyl; Fostex 10%	Liquid, Bar
Benzoyl Peroxide, lotions	Clearasil; Oxy-5; others	Lotion
Benzoyl Peroxide, creams	Cuticura Medicated Acne; Persadox; others	Cream
Benzoyl Peroxide, sticks and pads	Propa P.H. Acne	Pads, Sticks
Benzoyl Peroxide Combinations	Sulfoxyl; Vanoxide	Lotion
Benzoyl Peroxide, gels	Clear By Design; others	Gel
Clindamycin, topical	Cleocin T	Topical solution
Erythromycin, topical	A/T/S; Eryderm; others	Topical solution
Meclocycline sulfosalicylate	Meclan	Cream
Sulfur Preparations	Xerac; Acne Aid; Bensulfoid; others	Gel, Lotion, Powder
Tetracycline HCl	Topicycline	Topical solution
Tretinoin	Retin-A	Cream, Gel, Liquid

acne vulgaris. The reduction of free fatty acids in the acne lesions by clindamycin suggests a reduction in lipolysis of sebum fat to the irritant fatty acids.

ANTI-INFECTIVES

Several anti-infectives (Table 10.3) find clinical usefulness in treating acne and seborrhea.

Benzoyl Peroxide. Benzoyl peroxide is an antibacterial agent used in topical preparations.

Mechanism of Action. The antibacterial action of benzoyl peroxide releases active or free-radical oxygen, resulting in oxidation of bacterial proteins. Reduction in Corynebacterium (Propionibacterium) acnes population occurs in acne lesions together with a lower level of free fatty acids.

Clinical Indications. Mild to moderate acne responds to benzoyl peroxide treatment.

Adverse Effects/Precautions. Adverse reactions include peeling and erythema due to an excessive drying effect of benzoyl peroxide. Allergic contact sensitization is also possible with this anti-infective.

Sulfacetamide Sodium. Sulfacetamide is a topical antibacterial agent.

Mechanism of Action. Sulfacetamide exerts a bacteriostatic action by competing with para-aminobenzoic acid (PABA) in biochemical reactions that involve bacterial synthesis of folic acid (see Chapter 9). Sulfacetamide is effective against gram-positive and gram-negative organisms which are commonly present in secondary cutaneous pyogenic infections.

Clinical Indications. Sulfacetamide is used in the treatment of seborrhea sicca (dandruff) and in secondary bacterial skin infections.

Adverse Effects/Precautions. Systemic absorption of topical sulfacetamide may occur following application to large or denuded skin areas. Prolonged use of sulfacetamide may result in overgrowth of bacteria or fungi.

ANTIFUNGALS

Numerous topical agents are used in cutaneous fungal infections. Griseofulvin is an orally effective drug used to treat tinea infections.

Topical Antifungals. Several antifungal agents (Table 10.2) are available for topical use; these include undecylenic acid, iodochlorhydroxyquin, miconazole, econazole, ciclopirox, clotrimazole, acrisorcin, triacetin, haloprogin, tolnafate, nystatin, and amphotericin B.

Mechanism of Action. Many of the antifungal agents (e.g., miconazole, nystatin, and amphotericin B) bind to components in the plasma membrane of the fungus, thus producing a change in permeability. This action results in a leakage of essential intracellular components and a fungistatic or fungicidal activity. Undecylenic acid and derivatives, iodochlorhydroxyquin, and acrisorcin have antibacterial activity in addition to their antifungal action.

Clinical Indications. The antifungal dermatologicals are used to treat tinea (ringworm) infections caused by Trichophyton, Microsporin, and Epidermophyton species. Topical preparations of nystatin and amphotericin B are used principally for cutaneous or mucocutaneous mycotic infections that are caused by Candida albicans. Acrisorcin is used only in the treatment of tinea versicolor, a superficial mycosis caused by Malassezia furfur.

Adverse Effects/Precautions. Local irritation, erythema, stinging, blistering, and related topical reactions may occur with the antifungal dermatologicals.

Griseofulvin (Fulvicin[R]). Obtained from a species of Penicillium, griseofulvin is an orally effective antifungal drug that is used in mycoses caused by Epidermophyton, Microsporin, and Trichophyton species (tinea infections).

Mechanism of Action. Griseofulvin is deposited in the keratin precursor cells, especially in diseased or fungal infected tissue. The infected tissue is gradually exfoliated and griseofulvin binds to the newly formed keratin. This drug/keratin complex is highly resistant to fungal invasion. Fungistatic only against the tinea causing genera (i.e., Trichophyton, Epidermophyton, and Microsporin), griseofulvin has no effect on other fungi or bacteria.

Clinical Indications. Griseofulvin is used to treat ringworm infections of the skin, hair, and nails.

Adverse Effects/Precautions. Patients on prolonged oral antifungal therapy should undergo periodic monitoring of renal, hepatic, and hematopoietic functions. The possibility of cross-sensitivity to penicillin exists, although some patients with known sensitivity to penicillin have taken griseofulvin without incident. A lupus erythematosus-like syndrome occurs in some patients receiving griseofulvin. As photosensitivity reactions are possible, patients should avoid natural or artificial sunlight.

ANTISEPTICS

Many antiseptic agents are used externally for their broad antimicrobial activity. These include iodine, povidone-iodine, thimerosal, merbromin, hexachlorophene, chlorhexidene, benzalkonium chloride, and oxychlorosene.

EMOLLIENTS

Emollients are used in several topical preparations to soften or soothe the skin. Emollient compounds, including anhydrous lanolin (wool fat), cocoa butter, beeswax, and white petrolatum, are often used as ointment bases or vehicles for other drugs.

EPITHELIAL STIMULANTS

Tretinoin (trans-Retinoic acid) is an irritant that stimulates turnover of epithelial cells and peeling. This agent is indicated in the treatment of acne vulgaris. Dexpanthenol stimulates epithelization and aids in healing skin lesions.

ORAL VITAMIN A PREPARATION FOR ACNE

Isotretinoin (13 cis-Retinoic acid; Accutane[R]). Isotretinoin is an isomer of retinoic acid, a metabolite of retinol (vitamin A).

Mechanism of Action. By an unknown mechanism, isotretinoin apparently reduces sebum secretion. The decrease in sebum secretion is related to the dose and duration of treatment.

Clinical Indications. Isotretinoin is only indicated in severe cystic acne where other drug treatment or conventional therapy (including antibiotics) has failed. The known teratogenic effects of isotretinoin limit its use.

Adverse Effects/Precautions. Symptoms of hypervitaminosis A may occur, and cheilitis has been reported in 9 out of 10 patients receiving isotretinoin. Other frequent adverse effects include eye irritation (50% of patients), conjunctivitis (40% of patients), pruritis (80% of patients), and dry mouth (80% of patients). Muscle pain, lethargy, and gastrointestinal symptoms (e.g., nausea, vomiting, abdominal pain) may occur. Isotretinoin therapy has also been associated with several cases of pseudotumor cerebri.

Pregnant women must not take isotretinoin because of the drug's teratogenic effects. Hydrocephalus, microcephalus, absent external ear canals, and cardiac abnormalities have occurred in offspring of women who had taken isotretinoin during pregnancy; thus, a serious risk exists if pregnancy develops during isotretinoin therapy.

ENZYME PREPARATIONS

Sutilains and collagenase digest necrotic soft tissue and aid in the removal of detritus thus assisting granulation and subsequent epithelization of dermal lesions. Enzyme preparations are used in the debridement of skin lesions, including burns and dermal ulcers (such as bedsores).

KERATOLYTICS

Salicylate acid, benzoic acid, and resorcinol are examples of agents that loosen and separate the horny layer of the epithelium. Salicylic acid produces desquamation by solubilizing the intercellular cement that binds scales in the stratum corneum and is effective in the removal of excessive keratin in hyperkeratotic skin disorders.

HAIR GROWTH STIMULANTS

In a topical dosage form, minoxidil (Regaine[R]) is presently marketed in Canada and Europe for hair growth stimulation. Noted to cause hair growth when used as an antihypertensive drug, minoxidil is undergoing clinical trials for alopecia areata. Another antihypertensive drug, diazoxide, shows promise in this area.

ANTISEBORRHEICS

Selenium sulfide, zinc pyrithione, and tar derivatives are used to treat seborrheic dermatitis of the scalp. These agents apparently reduce the turnover of epidermal cells, thereby correcting abnormalities in keratinization.

SCABICIDES AND/OR PEDICULOCIDES

Lindane (gamma benzene hexachloride) and crotamiton are indicated for the topical treatment of scabies. Lindane, pyrethrins, and malathion (see Table 10.2) are used externally to treat lice infestation.

ANTIPSORIATICS

Anthralin, ammoniated mercury, coal tar, corticosteroids, and salicylic acid are dermatologicals that are used to treat psoriasis. Anthralin reduces the metabolic rate and proliferation of epidermal cells by inhibiting the synthesis of nucleic protein.

Methotrexate (see Chapter 4) inhibits DNA synthesis and cell replication. Since epithelial cell replication is excessive in psoriasis, methotrexate reduces the psoriatic process. Methotrexate is used only in the symptomatic control of severe, recalcitrant, disabling psoriasis that is refractory to other treatment.

Psoralen-ultraviolet light A (PUVA) is also used to treat psoriasis. Compared to other treatments, PUVA therapy more effectively controls the disease and is less expensive than hospitalization.

Etretinate (Tegison[R]). Etretinate, a retinoid related to vitamin A, is similar to isotretinoin.

Mechanism of Action. By an unknown mechanism, etretinate normalizes the histology of skin cells in the epidermis, dermis, and stratum corneum. Decreased cutaneous inflammation and scaling are noted with etretinate therapy.

Clinical Indications. Effective by oral administration, etretinate is used to treat severe psoriasis not responsive to other types of therapy.

Adverse Effects/Precautions. Toxic effects of etretinate resemble hypervitaminosis A and include mucous membrane dryness, chapped lips, alopecia, joint pain, and peeling of the skin from the palms, soles, and fingertips. Eye irritation occurs frequently (50% of patients).

Calcification of extraspinal tendons and ligaments (ankles, knees, and pelvis), hepatic toxicity, and elevation of serum triglycerides and cholesterol are additional serious adverse reactions to etretinate. Also, pseudotumor cerebri has been reported with etretinate use.

Teratogenic effects, such as CNS abnormalities, extremity malformations, and multiple synostoses, limit use of the drug in young girls or women who desire to have children. Etretinate's teratogenic effect may persist for years.

CORTICOSTEROIDS

Topical corticosteroids (Table 10.4) possess anti-inflammatory, antipruritic, and vasoconstrictive action. These dermatologicals relieve the inflammation and itching of corticosteroid-responsive dermatoses. Corticosteroids are contraindicated in fungal infections, viral infections (such as herpes simplex and varicella), and tuberculosis of the skin. Systemic absorption of topical steroids must be considered as a possible adverse effect when the preparation is used over a large surface area, especially with prolonged use of a potent corticosteroid.

SUNSCREEN PRODUCTS

Excessive exposure to the sun can cause both acute and chronic skin injury. Sunscreen products reduce the amount of ultraviolet radiation

Table 10.4. TOPICALLY APPLIED CORTICOSTEROIDS.

Available products	Trade names	Forms
Amcinonide	Cyclocort	Ointment, Cream
Betamethasone	Celestone	Cream
Betamethasone benzoate	Benisone; Uticort	Gel, Cream, Lotion, Gel
Betamethasone valerate	Valisone; Betatrex; Beta-Val	Lotion, Cream, Ointment
Betamethasone dipropionate	Diprosone; Diprolene	Cream, Ointment, Lotion, Aerosol
Clocortolone pivalate	Cloderm	Cream
Desonide	Tridesilon	Cream, Ointment
Desoximetasone	Topicort	Cream, Gel
Dexamethasone	Decadron; Hexadrol; Aeroseb-Dex	Cream, Gel, Aerosol
Diflorasone diacetate	Florone; Maxiflor	Cream, Ointment
Flumethasone pivalate	Locorten	Cream
Fluocinolone acetonide	Fluonid; Synemol; Synalar	Cream, Ointment, Solution
Fluocinonide	Lidex; Topsyn	Ointment, Cream, Gel, Solution
Fluorometholone	Oxylone	Cream
Flurandrenolide	Cordran	Cream, Ointment, Lotion, Tape
Halcinonide	Halog; Halciderm	Cream, Ointment, Solution
Hydrocortisone	Hytone; Eldecort; Aeroseb-HC; Cortril; others	Cream, Ointment, Lotion, Aerosol
Hydrocortisone acetate	Cort-Dome; Epifoam; Cortef Acetate; others	Ointment, Foam
Methylprenisolone acetate	Medrol Acetate	Ointment
Prednisolone	Meti-Derm	Cream
Triamcinolone acetonide	Aristocort; Kenalog; Kenac; others	Cream, Ointment, Lotion, Aerosol

skin damage upon exposure to the sun. Because of this protection, use of these products reduces the risk of burning and skin cancer. The most common adverse effects of topical sunscreen preparations are photosensitivity reactions, contact dermatitis, and allergic responses to vehicle ingredients.

Para-aminobenzoic acid (PABA) and its esters are popular chemical sunscreens; others include benzophenones, cinnamates, salicylates, and anthranilates. Physical sunscreens, such as zinc oxide preparations, scatter light and prevent sun rays from reaching the skin.

Chemical sunscreens have their peak UV absorption in the range where sunburn occurs (UVB). In temperate climates only a small amount of UVB radiation reaches the earth's surface before 10 a.m. or after 3 p.m. The sun protection factor (SPF), indicated on most sunscreens, specifies the ratio of the time required to produce erythema (skin redness) through a chemical sunscreen to the time required to produce the same degree of erythema without the sunscreen. The SPF values range from 2 (minimal protection) to 15 or more (maximal protection).

The intensity of erythema-producing sunlight is greater at higher altitudes (an approximate 300 m increase in altitude adds 4% to intensity). Reflected sunlight from sand, snow, and water are additional contributors to erythema.

DRUGS USED TO TREAT DISEASES OF THE JOINTS AND CONNECTIVE TISSUES

The nonsteroidal anti-inflammatory drugs are used for the symptomatic treatment of diseases of the joints and connective tissues.

NONSTEROIDAL ANTI-INFLAMMATORY DRUGS (NSAIDS)

The NSAIDs include aspirin and related salicylates, derivatives of both pyrazolone and methylated indole or related compounds, and propionic acid.

Aspirin (Acetylsalicylic Acid; ASA). Aspirin remains the most widely prescribed and popular analgesic, antipyretic, and anti-inflammatory drug.

Mechanism of Action. The analgesic action of aspirin is most pronounced in conditions such as headache, arthralgia, myalgia, and in pain that emanates from integumental structures rather than from the viscera. The analgesic activity results from inhibition of prostaglandin synthesis at peripheral sites. In addition to sensitizing pain receptors to mechanical and chemical stimuli, prostaglandins are associated with the pain caused by injury or inflammation. A direct depressant effect in the thalamic region of the brain is another proposed site for aspirin activity.

The antipyretic activity of aspirin is also based upon inhibition of prostaglandin synthesis. Prostaglandin release occurs in the hypothalamic nuclei, a site associated with fever production.

The anti-inflammatory activity of aspirin relates to cyclooxygenase inhibition and subsequent inhibition of prostaglandin synthesis (see Chapter 9).

Clinical Indications. Aspirin is used as an analgesic in mild to moderate pain and as an anti-inflammatory in the treatment of rheumatoid arthritis and osteoarthritis.

Adverse Effects/Precautions. Gastrointestinal side effects, including heartburn, gastric irritation, and bleeding, are often limiting factors when aspirin is used in arthritis treatment. Gastric damage beyond the drug's known local irritant effects may involve inhibition of the synthesis of mucosal protective prostaglandins (PGI_2 and PGE_2). Allergic reactions, such as bronchospasm or hives, may occur in susceptible individuals. Dizziness, tinnitus aurium, nausea, vomiting, diarrhea, and mental confusion are characteristics of mild salicylism, which usually follows prolonged use of higher doses. Aspirin use in children, as in influenza, has been associated with Reye syndrome.

Other Nonsteroidal Anti-inflammatory Drugs. Fenamates, indole derivatives, and derivatives of proprionic acid comprise the remainder of the nonsteroidal anti-inflammatory drugs (Table 10.5). Their pharmacologic activity and toxicity profile are essentially the same as those of aspirin, although some may produce less gastrointestinal irritation.

Pyrazolone Derivatives. The pyrazolone derivatives (Table 10.5), phenylbutazone and oxyphenbutazone, possess analgesic, antipyretic, anti-inflammatory, and mild uricosuric activity.

Mechanism of Action. Phenylbutazone and oxyphenbutazone inhibit prostaglandin synthesis (see Chapter 9), leukocyte migration, and the activity and release of lysosomal enzymes; all these effects reduce the inflammatory response.

Clinical Indications. Phenylbutazone and oxyphenbutazone are used primarily in the treatment of acute gouty arthritis, rheumatoid arthritis, ankylosing spondylitis, and painful shoulder conditions (such as bursitis).

Adverse Effects/Precautions. Gastrointestinal distress, edema, and rash are common adverse reactions to the pyrazolone derivatives. Due to extensive plasma protein binding by these agents, they often displace concurrently administered drugs, which usually results in an increase in the activity and toxicity of the drug being given with phenylbutazone or oxyphenbutazone. See Chapters 1, 3, 4, and 5 for de-

Table 10.5. ANALGESICS, ANTIPYRETICS, AND ANTI-INFLAMMATORY DRUGS.

Available products	Trade names	Daily dosage range
Salicylates and related drugs:		
Aluminum aspirin	Aluminum acetylsalicylate	670 mg
Aspirin	various	Variable
Choline salicylate	Arthropan	870 mg
Diflunisal	Dolobid	500–1000 mg
Enteric coated aspirin	Ecotrin	Variable (325 unit dose)
Magnesium salicylate	Durasal; Magan; others	500–600 mg t.i.d. or q.i.d.
Salicylamide	Uromide	325–650 mg t.i.d. or q.i.d.
Salsalate	Disalcid	3000 mg in divided doses
Sodium salicylate	Uracel 5	325–650 mg q. 4–8 hrs
Sodium thiosalicylate	Anthrolate; Nalate	50–100 mg
Pyrazolone derivatives:		
Phenylbutazone	Phenylbutazone; Azolid; Butazolidin	400 mg
Oxyphenbutazone	Oxalid; Tandearil	400 mg
Para-aminophenol derivative:		
Acetaminophen	in Tylenol and others	300–650 mg q. 4 hrs
New nonsteroidal anti-inflammatory drugs (NSAIDs):		
Carprofen	Rimadyl	Variable
Diclofenac	Voltaren	Variable
Etodolac	Ultradol	Variable
Fenoprofen	Nalfon	3200 mg*
Ibuprofen	Motrin; Advil; Nuprin; Rufen	2400 mg*
Indomethacin	Indocin; Indocin SR	Variable
Ketoprofen	Orudis	Variable
Meclofenamate	Meclomen	200–400 mg
Naproxen	Anaprox; Naprosyn	1250 mg*
Piroxicam	Feldene	20 mg
Sulindac	Clinoril	400 mg*
Tolmetin	Tolectin; Tolectin DS	Variable

* Maximum daily dosage; varies according to clinical situation

scriptions of the numerous drug interactions that occur with phenylbutazone.

MISCELLANEOUS DRUGS USED IN ARTHRITIS TREATMENT

Several miscellaneous drugs are sometimes effective in arthritis therapy when standard treatment fails.

Hydroxychloroquine Sulfate (Plaquenil^R). Hydroxychloroquine is used to treat some collagen diseases.

Mechanism of Action. Hydroxychloroquine suppresses the formation of antigens involved in the hypersensitivity reactions that are responsible for the collagen disease process.

Clinical Indications. Hydroxychloroquine is used to treat chronic discoid and systemic lupus erythematosus and acute or chronic rheumatoid arthritis.

Adverse Effects/Precautions. Patients with psoriasis, hepatic disease, or alcoholism should use hydroxychloroquine with caution. Ocular adverse reactions include physical changes in the cornea and retina. Irritability, nervousness, vertigo, nystagmus, and neuromuscular side effects are also possible with hydroxychloroquine use.

Gold Compounds. Gold compounds suppress or prevent the the symptoms of arthritis and synovitis.

Mechanism of Action. Gold compounds accumulate in Kupffer cell and synoviocyte lysosomes and inhibit lysosomal enzyme activity. This action decreases the phagocytic activity of macrophages and reduces the inflammatory process.

Clinical Indications. Gold compounds are indicated in the adjunctive treatment of selected cases of rheumatoid arthritis. Auranofin (Ridaura^R) is an oral dosage form of gold which has been approved for some patients with rheumatoid arthritis. Its use, generally, is in refractory cases treated with one or more NSAIDs or if patient intolerance (adverse reactions) to usual therapy exists. The oral gold form is apparently comparable in antiarthritic activity to injectable gold preparations.

Adverse Effects/Precautions. Adverse reactions may occur at any time during gold therapy. The toxicity is apparently unrelated to plasma gold levels, but may correlate with total gold accumulation in the body. The most serious adverse reactions to oral gold (i.e., thrombocytopenia, leukopenia, anemia, and proteinuria) are attributed to the gold ion. Commonly noted adverse effects involve the gastrointestinal tract; for example, diarrhea occurs in 40 to 50% of patients receiving oral gold. Auranofin is contraindicated in patients with a history of necrotizing enterocolitis, pulmonary fibrosis, exfoliative dermatitis, or bone marrow aplasia.

DRUGS USED IN THE TREATMENT OF GOUTY ARTHRITIS

Acute gouty arthritis attacks are usually best managed with colchicine, an alkaloid that is obtained from the meadow saffron (Colchicum autumnale). Alternate drugs for acute episodes include phenylbutazone, oxyphenbutazone, indomethacin, and adrenal glucocorticoids.

Although uricosuric drugs, such as probenecid or sulfinpyrazone (see Chapter 5), control chronic gouty arthritis by reducing the uric acid levels in the body, allopurinol is often used in the long-term management of the disease.

Colchicine. Colchicine, used medicinally for hundreds of years, relieves the pain of acute gout attacks.

Mechanism of Action. Although the mechanism of action of colchicine is unknown, the drug inhibits leukocyte migration and reduces phagocytosis. Colchicine inhibits lactic acid production by leukocytes, which results in a decreased urate crystal deposition in the affected joints. A reduction in the inflammatory response accrues, apparently as a consequence of several interactions of colchicine with leukocytes.

Clinical Indications. Given orally in the treatment of acute gouty arthritis, colchicine is also occasionally used in the chronic management of the disease to prevent the development of an acute attack. For example, after the initiation of allopurinol therapy, the incidence of acute attacks is greater; thus colchicine is given concurrently for several days.

Adverse Effects/Precautions. Vomiting, diarrhea, and abdominal pain often occur at the doses required to relieve the acute attack. Long-term colchicine therapy has produced bone marrow depression.

Allopurinol. Allopurinol is a potent inhibitor of xanthine oxidase, which consequently reduces the formation of uric acid.

Mechanism of Action. Allopurinol, and its metabolite oxypurinol, inhibits xanthine oxidase, thereby reducing the hypoxanthine to xanthine and xanthine to uric acid reactions in the body. Allopurinol acts to reduce the production of uric acid without affecting the synthesis of essential purines.

Clinical Indications. Allopurinol is used primarily in the management of chronic gouty arthritis.

Adverse Effects/Precautions. Acute attacks of gout may increase during the early stages of allopurinol treatment. Skin rash, hematopoietic disturbances, and gastrointestinal upset occur frequently with allopurinol.

PARA-AMINOPHENOL DERIVATIVE

Acetaminophen (Table 10.5), a para-aminophenol derivative, is present in several OTC preparations, such as Tylenol[R], as an analgesic-antipyretic.

Acetaminophen (N-Acetyl-P-Aminophenol; APAP). Acetaminophen is chemically related to phenacetin and acetanilid.

Mechanism of Action. Acetaminophen inhibits prostaglandin synthetase (fatty and cyclooxygenase) in the CNS but has minimal effects on this enzyme at peripheral sites. Although it lacks a clinically useful anti-inflammatory action, acetaminophen is an effective central acting analgesic-antipyretic that reduces fever by a direct action on thermoregulatory centers in the hypothalamus. Acetaminophen does not inhibit platelet aggregation and is preferred over aspirin if prothrombin-reducing anticoagulants are being taken concurrently; aspirin is undoubtedly the more highly efficacious anti-inflammatory drug.

Clinical Indications. Acetaminophen is used as an analgesic in various arthritides and rheumatic conditions, especially if aspirin use is contraindicated or not tolerated by the patient.

Adverse Effects/Precautions. When used in recommended dosage ranges, acetaminophen is relatively free of side effects; however, chronic use has resulted in blood dyscrasias and allergic reactions. Hepatotoxicity is characteristic of acetaminophen poisoning.

DRUG INTERACTIONS

Drug interactions involving griseofulvin or tetracycline may be clinically significant, as are those that occur with indomethacin, a frequently prescribed NSAID which interacts with several drugs. Since drugs in the NSAID category are used as standard treatment in inflammatory conditions, their drug interactions are significant.

Griseofulvin.

Barbiturates. Phenobarbital inhibits the absorption of griseofulvin.

Oral Anticoagulants. Altered anticoagulant effect is possible since griseofulvin may induce hepatic microsomal enzymes, enhancing the metabolism of oral anticoagulants.

Tetracycline. Specific interactions with tetracycline are described in Chapter 7.

Indomethacin.

Bumetanide. Concurrent administration may reduce the diuretic and natriuretic response to bumetanide since indomethacin inhibits prostaglandin synthesis, resulting in sodium retention by the patient.

Captopril. By inhibiting prostaglandin synthesis, indomethacin blocks the antihypertensive response to captopril.

Corticosteroids. Increased incidence and/or severity of gastrointestinal ulceration are possible from the combined effects of indomethacin and corticosteroids.

Furosemide. By inhibiting prostaglandin synthesis, indomethacin evidently blocks the antihypertensive and diuretic effects of furosemide.

Lithium Carbonate. Indomethacin reduces renal lithium excretion and increases plasma lithium levels. The latter effect causes lithium toxicity in some patients.

Oral Anticoagulants. Since indomethacin is ulcerogenic and possibly inhibits platelet function, patients receiving both drugs should be watched for bleeding, especially of the gastrointestinal tract.

Triamterene. Concurrent administration may result in triamterene-induced nephrotoxicity.

Piroxicam.

Lithium Carbonate. Piroxicam, by inhibiting prostaglandin synthesis, apparently blocks renal lithium clearance.

Sulindac.

Oral Anticoagulants. Concurrent use may result in enhanced hypoprothrombinemia and bleeding.

Allopurinol.

Mercaptopurine. Allopurinol inhibits the catabolism of mercaptopurine to 6-thiouric acid. Adding allopurinol to a mercaptopurine regimen may necessitate reducing the mercaptopurine dose to 25 to 30% of the pre-allopurinol dose. Allopurinol also inhibits the metabolism of azathioprine, an imidazolyl derivative of 6-mercaptopurine.

Iron Salts. Iron salts should not be given simultaneously with allopurinol since the latter may increase hepatic iron concentrations.

SUMMARY

The dermatologic medications comprise a highly varied and extensive pharmacologic classification. These drugs range from topical antiseptics and germicides to oral drugs which are eventually deposited in target skin tissue. Some skin disorders are relatively mild and amenable to quick resolution (for example, prickly heat, diaper rash); others (such as psoriasis) resist all forms of therapy. Additionally, diseases of the joints and connective tissues, such as rheumatoid arthritis and osteoarthritis, represent challenges to modern medicine. Newer NSAIDs are designed to surpass the standby aspirin in potency and efficacy without aspirin's toxicity, but they have yet to emerge as a panacea in arthritis treatment. Current active research efforts may provide safe, potent, antiinflammatory medications to control the debilitating diseases of the integumentary/connective tissue system.

SUGGESTED READINGS

Anderson, T.F., and Voorhees, J.J.: Psoralen photochemotherapy of cutaneous disorders. Annu Rev Pharmacol Toxicol, 20:235, 1980.
DeSimone, E.M., II: Sunscreen and suntan products. In Handbook of Nonprescription Drugs. Vol. 8. Washington, American Pharmaceutical Association, 1986.
Drugs for rheumatoid arthritis. Med Lett Drugs Ther, 27:25, 1985.
Drugs, ultraviolet light found effective for severe psoriasis. Wellcome Trends in Pharmacy, 8:15, 1986.
Etretinate for psoriasis. Med Lett Drugs Ther, 29:9, 1987.
Gilman, A.G., et al. (eds.): The Pharmacological Basis of Therapeutics. 7th Ed. New York, Macmillan Publishing Co., Inc., 1985.
Hansten, P.D.: Drug Interactions. 5th Ed. Philadelphia, Lea & Febiger, 1985.
Kastrup, E.K., and Boyd. J.R. (eds.): Drug Facts and Comparisons. Philadelphia, J.B. Lippincott Co., 1985.
Sunscreens. Med Lett Drugs Ther, 26:56, 1984.
White, J.P.: New nonsteroidals coming to the rescue. Drug Topics, 130:38, 1986.

CHAPTER EXAMINATION

A middle-aged male patient has been using a topical coal tar preparation for several years to treat his psoriasis. Since the lesions recently began spreading, the patient's physician considers methotrexate therapy.

1. Methotrexate
   a. is only effective by IV injection
   b. inhibits DNA synthesis
   c. preferentially acetylates cyclooxygenase
   d. therapy is ordinarily used in an initial treatment regimen for psoriasis
2. Psoriasis
   a. responds favorably to oral tetracycline
   b. invariably progresses to systemic lupus erythematosus
   c. is a form of fungal infection
   d. none of the above
3. The patient develops a recurrence of acute rheumatoid arthritis. Since he cannot tolerate ASA or steroids, he receives a prescription for hydroxychloroquine in a long-term treatment program. The choice of hydroxychloroquine is
   a. contraindicated
   b. excellent because it will also effectively control psoriasis
   c. always an initial drug choice in acute recurring rheumatoid arthritis
   d. none of the above
4. Hydroxychloroquine is used clinically to treat
   a. malaria
   b. discoid lupus erythematosus
   c. systemic lupus erythematosus
   d. all of the above

Rheumatoid arthritis has recently been diagnosed in a 30-year-old female. She has multiarticular inflammation in her hands and experiences mild to moderate pain.

5. The drug of first choice is
   a. triamcinolone
   b. acetylsalicylic acid
   c. griseofulvin
   d. phenylbutazone
6. Aspirin
   a. inhibits prostaglandin synthesis by acetylating cyclooxygenase
   b. activates thromboxane A_2
   c. markedly inhibits lipooxygenase
   d. stimulates the formation of prostacyclin
7. Lipooxygenase and cyclooxygenase are enzymes that function in the initial steps of
   a. sebum lipolysis
   b. thromboxane A_2 catabolism
   c. prostacyclin catabolism
   d. arachidonic acid metabolism
8. In the early stage of her therapy, the patient informs her physician that she experiences heartburn and epigastric pain. An alternate anti-inflammatory drug to replace her initial medication is
   a. naproxen
   b. oxyphenbutazone
   c. phenylbutazone
   d. acetaminophen
9. Examples of newer NSAIDs include
   a. sodium salicylate, ibuprofen, and prednisone
   b. choline magnesium salicylate, dexamethasone, and indomethacin
   c. piroxacam, etretinate, and triamcinolone
   d. carprofen, etodolac, and diclofenac
10. Rheumatoid arthritis is
    a. most often caused by viruses
    b. a systemic fungal disease
    c. apparently an autoimmune disease
    d. an acute disorder that usually resolves itself in 2 weeks

A teenage girl with severe acne takes oral tetracycline and also uses a topical benzoyl peroxide/combination preparation. She informs you that she is planning to vacation at the beach and will "live in the sun for 2 weeks."

11. You should warn her about the possibility of increased photosensitivity because

a. acne patients are more susceptible to UV rays
b. benzoyl peroxide reacts with UV rays to produce a carcinogenic moiety
c. of the tetracycline in her treatment regimen
d. none of the above

12. Benzoyl peroxide
    a. releases free oxygen radicals
    b. competes with PABA in Corynebacterium acnes metabolism
    c. decreases epithelization of dermal cells
    d. inhibits DNA synthesis

13. Oral tetracycline is effective in acne vulgaris because it
    a. reduces sebum production
    b. inhibits DNA synthesis in Epidermophyton species
    c. increases lipolysis of sebum
    d. decreases the concentration of free fatty acids in acne lesions

14. Acne vulgaris is characterized by
    a. an excessively greasy skin
    b. lipolysis of sebum to irritant fatty acids
    c. increased skin and organ receptivity to androgens
    d. all of the above

A young college student takes oral griseofulvin for ringworm of the fingernails.

15. Griseofulvin
    a. should also be administered in a topical form
    b. concentrates in fungal infected tissue and binds to newly formed keratin at the junction of diseased cells
    c. should only be used until the "white nails" begin to fade
    d. has wide antifungal activity

16. Drug interactions with griseofulvin may occur with
    a. diazepam and tetracycline
    b. phenobarbital and warfarin
    c. aspirin and acetaminophen
    d. digoxin and clonidine

Indomethacin has been prescribed for an acute gout episode in a 50-year-old male who was previously asymptomatic.

17. A common adverse effect of indomethacin is
    a. diarrhea
    b. tinnitus aurium
    c. xerostomia
    d. renal impairment

18. The patient does not tolerate the indomethacin therapy. An alternate drug for an acute gouty arthritis attack is
    a. acetaminophen
    b. hydroxychloroquine
    c. phenylbutazone
    d. methotrexate

19. This patient also has a family history of "the gout." A blood screen indicates elevated uric acid levels and an otherwise normal blood profile. A drug that will prevent further attacks by inhibiting the formation of uric acid is
    a. probenecid
    b. colchicine
    c. allopurinol
    d. sulfinpyrazone

20. Secondary hyperuricemia may occur in
    a. certain forms of leukemia
    b. polycythemia vera
    c. tertiary syphilis
    d. pancreatic carcinoma

ANSWER KEY

1. b	11. c
2. d	12. a
3. a	13. d
4. d	14. d
5. b	15. b
6. a	16. b
7. d	17. a
8. a	18. c
9. d	19. c
10. c	20. a

APPENDICES

Appendix A. OCULAR ANTI-INFLAMMATIVES AND ANTI-INFECTIVES.

Available products	Trade names	Forms
Corticosteroids for topical ophthalmic use:		
Dexamethasone	Maxidex	Suspension
Dexamethasone phosphate	Decadron; in AK-Dex	Solution
Fluorometholone	FML Liquifilm	Suspension
Hydrocortisone acetate	in Hydrocortone Acetate	Ointment
Medrysone	HMS Liquifilm	Suspension
Prednisolone acetate	in Pred Mild; in Econopred; others	Suspension
Prednisolone phosphate	in Metreton	Solution
Prednisolone sodium phosphate	in Inflamase; in AK-Pred	Solution
Topical ophthalmic anti-infective agents:		
Bacitracin	in Baciguent	Ointment
Chloramphenicol	in Chloromycetin	Ointment, Powder
Chlortetracycline	in Aureomycin	Ointment
Erythromycin	in Ilotycin	Ointment
Gentamicin	in Garamycin; Genoptic; Gentacidin	Solution, Ointment
Neomycin sulfate	in Myciguent; Neotal	Ointment
Oxytetracycline	in Terramycin	Ointment
Polymyxin B sulfate	in Statrol; Neosporin; others	Solution, Ointment
Sulfacetamide sodium	Sulamyd; Sulf-10; others	Solution, Ointment
Sulfisoxazole	Gantrisin	Solution, Ointment
Tetracycline	in Achromycin	Suspension, Ointment
Tobramycin	in Tobrex	Solution, Ointment

462 THERAPEUTIC PHARMACOLOGY

Appendix B. FLUID-ELECTROLYTE AND NUTRITIONAL REPLENISHERS.

Available agents

Agents used in the treatment of abnormal hydration states:

Dehydration treatments—
Dextrose injection (5% in H_2O)
Dextrose and sodium chloride injection
Sodium chloride injection (isotonic 0.9%)
Sodium chloride injection (3%; 5%)
Combined electrolyte solutions (Isolyte; Normosol; Plasma-Lyte; others)
Other electrolytre depletion treatments—
Potassium chloride (Kaochlor; Klorvess; Kay Ciel; Cena-K; others)
Potassium gluconate (Kaon; Bayon; others)
Potassium bicarbonate; potassium citrate (in Potassium Trikates; Tri-K; K-Lyte; others)
Calcium gluconate
Magnesium sulfate
Ringer's injection
Lactated Ringer's Injection
Lactated potassic saline injection

Acidosis treatment:

Sodium acetate
Sodium bicarbonate (tablets and injections)
Sodium lactate injection (⅙ molar solution)
Tromethamine (Tham)

Alkalosis treatment:

Ammonium chloride
Potassium chloride, sodium chloride, others

Nutritional deficiency treatment:

Amino acids (L-Tryptophan; L-Lysine)
Hypertonic dextrose injection
Fructose and sodium chloride injection
Fructose injection
Invert sugar injection (Travert)
High calorie solution for injection (Isolyte H 900; Normosol M 900)
Protein hydrolysates (A/G-Pro; Pro-Mix; others)

Appendix C. VITAMINS.

Available products	Trade names	RDA*
Water-soluble vitamins:		
Ascorbic acid	Cevalin; Cecon; others	Approx. 60 mg
Choline dihydrogen citrate and other salts of choline	Choline chloride	Unknown**
Cyanocobalamin	Redisol; Kaybovite	5 μg
Folic acid	Folvite	0.4 mg
Inositol	Inositol	Unknown**
Nicotinic acid	Nicobid; Nico-400; others	13–20 mg equiv.
Nicotinamide	Nicotinamide; Vitamin B$_3$	As above, based upon caloric intake and tryptophan
Para-aminobenzoic acid	Potaba	Unknown**
Calcium pantothenate	Pantholin; Durasil	5–10 mg
Pantothenyl alcohol	Panthenol	—
Pyridoxine HCl	Hexa-Betalin; Pyroxine; others	2 mg/100 g of protein intake
Riboflavin	Riboflavin; Riobin-50	1.5–2.0 mg
Thiamine HCl	Betalin S; Bewon; Biamine	1.0–1.5 mg
Fat-soluble vitamins:		
Vitamin A	Aquasol A; Alphalin	5,000 units
Vitamin D	—	400 units
Cholecalciferol calcitriol	Rocaltrol	—
Ergocalciferol	Deltalin; Drisdol	—
Calcifediol	Calderol	—
Dihydrotachysterol	DHT; Hytakerol	—
Vitamin E	Aquasol E; Eprolin; others	25–30 units
Vitamin K	—	0.3 μg/kg of body weight
Phytonadione	AquaMEPHYTON; Mephyton; Konakion	—
Menadione	Menadione	—
Medadiol sodium diphosphate	Synkayvite	—

* Recommended Daily Dietary Allowance
** Possibly not a true vitamin

Appendix D. IMMUNOLOGIC AGENTS.

Disease	Products used for prevention/treatment
Botulism	Botulism Equine Antitoxin (ABE)
Chicken Pox	Chicken Pox Virus Vaccine, Live (Experimental Vaccine)
Cholera	Cholera Vaccine
Diphtheria	Diphtheria Antitoxin; Diphtheria Toxoid; Adsorbed Diphtheria Toxoid; Diagnostic Diphtheria Toxin
Diphtheria, Tetanus, Pertussis	Adsorbed DTP Vaccine (Tri-Immunol; Ultrafined Triple Antigen)
Hemophilus Influenzae, Invasive (Meningitis)	b-Capsa I
Hepatitis	Hepatitis B Immune Globulin (H-BIG); Hepatitis B Vaccine (Heptavax-B)
Influenza	Influenza Virus Vaccine (Fluogen; Fluzone)
Measles	Measles Virus Vaccine, Live, Attenuated (Attenuvax); Measles Virus, Inactivated; Measles Immune Glubulin; Immune Serum Globulin
Measles, Mumps, and Rubella Virus	Measles, Mumps, and Rubella Virus, Live (M-M-R II)
Meningitis	Meningitis Polysaccharide Vaccine (Groups A; C; A and C; and A,C, Y, and W-135)
Mumps	Mumps Virus Vaccine, Live, (Mumpsvax); Mumps Vaccine; Inactivated Virus for Active Prophylaxis; Mumps Immune Globulin Human
Pertussis	Pertussis Vaccine; Pertussis Immune Globulin
Plague	Plague Vaccine
Pneumonia	Pneumococcal Vaccine, Polyvalent (Pneumovax 23; Pnu-Imune 23)
Poliomyelitis	Poliomyletis Vaccine (Salk Vaccine); Live Oral Poliovirus Vaccine, Trivalent (Orimune)
Rabies	Rabies Vaccine (Imovax; WYVAC)
Smallpox	Smallpox Vaccine
Tetanus	Tetanus Toxoid, Fluid; Adsorbed Tetanus Toxoid; Tetanus Antitoxin; Tetanus Immune Globulin (Hyper-Tet)
Tuberculosis	BCG Vaccine; Old Tuberculin Tine Test (diagnostic aid); Purified Protein Derivative of Tuberculin diagnostic aid (Aplisol; Tubersol)
Typhoid	Typhoid Vaccine
Yellow Fever	Yellow Fever Vaccine (YF-Vax)

Appendix E. RADIOPAQUE AGENTS AND RADIOGRAPHIC ADJUNCTS.

Available products	Trade names	Dosage/administration
Barium sulfate	Fleet Oral Barium; Oratest	See manufacturer's directions
Diatrizoate meglumine	Cardiografin; Gastrografin; Reno-M-60; Angiovist	Variable
Diatrizoate sodium	Hypaque Sodium; Urovist Sodium	Variable
Ethiodized oil	Ethiodol	0.5–20 ml intracavitary
Iocetamic acid	Cholebrine	3 or 4.5 g
Iodipamide meglumine 10.3%	Cholografin Meglumine	100 ml by slow IV infusion
Iopanoic acid	Telepaque	3 g
Iothalamate meglumine	Conray	Variable
Iothalamate sodium 66.8%	Conray-400	Variable
Ipodate calcium	Oragrafin calcium	3–6 g
Ipodate sodium	Oragrafin Sodium; Bilivest	3–6 g
Isosulfan Blue	Lymphazine 1%	0.5 ml SC into 3 interdigital spaces
Metrizamide	Amipaque	Variable
Potassium perchlorate	Perschloracap	200–400 mg
Tyropanoate sodium	Bilopaque	3 g

Appendix F. IMMUNOSUPPRESSIVE DRUGS.

Available products	Trade names	Clinical indications
Azathioprine	Immuran	Renal homotransplantation; Adult rheumatoid arthritis not amenable to conventional treatment (severe, active, erosive disease)
Cyclosporine (Cyclosporin A)	Sandimmune	Prophylaxis of organ rejection (kidney, liver, and heart) allogenic transplants
Immune Globulin Intravenous	Sandoglobulin	Immunodeficiency
Rh_o (D) Immune Globulin (Human)	Rh_oGAM; HypRho-D	Indicated* whenever it is known or suspected that fetal red cells have entered the circulation of an Rh negative mother, unless the fetus or the father can be shown conclusively to be Rh negative
Rh_o (D) Immune	MICRh$_o$GAM; HypRho-D; Mini-Dose	Indicated* for Rh negative women following spontaneous or induced abortion or termination of ectopic pregnancy up to and including 12 weeks' gestation, unless the father is shown conclusively to be Rh negative

* See manufacturer's literature for specific indications

INDEX

Page numbers in *italics* indicate figures; page numbers followed by "t" indicate tables.

Abbokinase, 240
Abdominal distention, cirrhotic, 272
Abortion, agents producing, 431–432
　prevention of, progestins in, 322
Abraham, penicillin and, 355
Absence seizure(s), defined, 19
　treatment of, 38–43
Absorbable gelatin, 235–236
Accutane, 450–451
Acebutolol, 142
　as antihypertensive agent, 197
Aceclidine, 114
Acetaminophen, in arthritis treatment, 456
　interaction of, with cholestyramine, 254
Acetazolamide, as anticonvulsant agent, 43
　as diuretic, 276
　interaction of, with methenamine, 283, 435
Acetyl coenzyme A, synthesis of acetylcholine from, 96, *96*
Acetylcholine, acetylcholinesterase and, 114–116
　adverse effects of, 112
　atropine versus, 120
　clinical indications for, 112
　digitalis and, 182
　in autonomic nervous system, 94–100, *96–99*
　in central nervous system, 12, *13*
　in digestion, 379
　mechanism of action of, 112
　narcotics and, 47
　neuromuscular blocking agents and, 126–128
　nicotinic blocking agents and, 124–128
　parkinsonism and, 24
　receptors of. *See* Acetylcholine receptor(s)
　storage forms of, 96
　synthesis of, 96, *96*
Acetylcholine receptor(s), 97–100, *97–99*
　activity of, 111
　cholinergic agents and, 111–112, 118–120
　in myasthenia gravis, 107
　muscarinic, 98–100, *100*
　nicotinic, 98–99, *98–99*
Acetylcholinesterase, binding sites of, 114, *115*
　inhibition of, 115, *115*
　interaction of, with neostigmine, 115–116, *115*
　　with physostigmine, 115–116
　pralidoxime and, 129, *129*

Acetylcysteine, as mucolytic agent, 368
N-Acetylprocainamide, 172
Acetylsalicylic acid. *See* Aspirin
Achlorhydria, in gastric cancer, 384
Acid(s). *See* specific entities
Acid-base balance, renal system in, 268–269, *269*
Acidosis, from asthma, 109
　treatment of, 462t
Acne, 444
　treatment of, 448–449, 449t
　　vitamin A in, 450–451
Acquired immune deficiency syndrome, 226
Acrisorcin, 450
Acromegaly, 304
Actin-myosin, digitalis and, 180, *180*
Actinomycosis, oral, 382
　pulmonary, 346
Action potential(s), cardiac, 157–158, *156–158*
Acyclovir, 427
Addison's disease, 306–307
　treatment of, 320
Addisonian anemia, 221–222
Adenocarcinoma, gastric, 384
　small intestine, 385
Adenohypophysis. *See* Pituitary gland, anterior
Adenoidectomy, controversy over, 342
Adenosine, caffeine and, 55
　dipyridamole and, 187
Adenosine diphosphate, in hemostasis, 217
Adenosine monophosphate, adrenergic receptors and, 104–105, *105*
　asthma and, 109
　hormones and, 290, *292, 294*
　prazosin and, 197
Adenosine triphosphatase, digitalis and, 179–180
Adenosine triphosphate, adrenergic receptors and, 104, *105*
Adenyl cyclase, acetylcholine receptor and, 100
　calcitonin and, 298–299
　hormones and, 290, *292*
　parathyroid preparations and, 318
Adrenal cortex, hormones produced by, 299
Adrenal gland(s), anatomy and physiology of, 299–300
　hyperfunction of, 307
　hypofunction of, 306–307
　preparations of, 318–320, 319t
　　drug interactions with, 328–329
Adrenal medulla, hormones produced by, 299–300

467

Adrenal steroid(s), etomidate and, 29
  in adrenal hypofunction, 306
  storage of, 303
Adrenaline. *See* Epinephrine
Adrenergic agent(s), 129–144
  anorexiant, 134
  bronchodilatory, 129t, 130–133, 135–137
  decongestant, 130t, 130–133
  disorders treated with, 109–110
  drug interactions with, 145–146
  endogenous, 130–132, *132*
  in treatment, of congestive heart failure, 184–185
  monoamine oxidase inhibitors as, 144
  vasoconstrictive, 131–134
  See also specific agents and types of agents
Adrenergic blocking agent(s), 137–143
  as antihypertensive agent(s), regimen for, 199
  disorders treated with, 110–111
  neuronal, 143
  See also specific agents and types of agents
Adrenergic fiber(s), defined, 94
Adrenergic neurotransmission, 100–105, *100–105*
Adrenergic receptor(s), 102–105, *103–105*
  alpha, 103–104, *103–104*
  antihypertensive agents and, 191–192, 196–198, *197*
  beta, 103–105, *104–105*
  propranolol and, 175
Adrenocorticotropic hormone, adverse effects of, 311
  clinical indications for, 311
  diurnal patterns and, 303
  function of, 297, 298t
  in adrenal hypofunction, 306–307
  mechanism of action of, 311
Adrenogenital syndrome, treatment of, 320
Adynamic ileus, 107–108
Affective disorder(s), 20–21
Agar, as bulk laxative, 398
Aglycone, cardiac glycoside, 179
Agranulocytosis, from chlorpromazine, 68
  from propylthiouracil, 317
Ahlquist classification of adrenergic receptors, 102–103
Akathisia, from chlorpromazine, 69
  treatment of, propranolol in, 76
D-Alanine, cycloserine and, 359
Albumen, plasma lipids and, 213
Albuterol, 136
Alcohol, in obstetrics, 433
  interaction of, with amitriptyline, 61
    with antihistamines, 371
    with benzodiazepines, 31, 83
    with chloral hydrate, 79
    with ethchlorvynol, 79
    with ethinamate, 80
    with flurazepam, 80
    with glutethimide, 79
    with methyprylon, 79
    with metronidazole, 408, 435
    with monoamine oxidase inhibitors, 82
    with nitrates, 203
    with phenytoin, 81
    with procarbazine, 255
    with sulfonylureas, 330
    with temazepam, 80
    with triazolam, 80
  withdrawal from, benzodiazepines in, 74–75
Alcoholism, anemia in, 222

Aldosterone, in cirrhosis, 272
  in renal physiology, 266–267, *266*, 270, *271*
Aldosterone antagonist(s), 279–280
Alfalfa, vitamin K and, 220
Alginate(s), as bulk laxative, 398
Aliphatic phenothiazine(s), 68–69
Alkalosis, from diuretics, 281
  from sodium bicarbonate, 390–391
  treatment of, 462t
Alkylamine antihistamine(s), 349
Alkylating agent(s), in cancer treatment, 246–248
Allergen(s), in allergy pathophysiology, 340
Allergic rhinitis, 342
  treatment of, 369
Allergy, pathophysiology of, 340–341, *341*
  to aspirin, 453
  to erythromycin, 364
  to local anesthetics, 29, 447
  to pentobarbital, 33
  treatment of, 347–350
  See also Hypersensitivity; Anaphylaxis
Allopurinol, in gout, 274, 456
  interaction of, with cyclophosphamide, 255
    with iron salts, 457
    with mercaptopurine, 255, 457
n-Allylnormorphine, formation of, 46
Alopecia, from anticancer agents, 247, 409
Alpha-adrenergic blocking agent(s), 137t, 137–140, *138*
  as antihypertensive agents, 196
  drug interactions with, 146
Alpha-adrenergic receptor(s), 103–104, *103–104*
Alphaprodine, 51
Alprazolam, 73
Altitude, erythrocyte count and, 211–212
  sunlight and, 453
Aluminum hydroxide gel, as antacid, 391
Aluminum phosphate, as antacid, 391
Aluminum silicate, as antidiarrheal, 401
Alveolus(i), anatomy of, 336, *338*
Alzheimer's disease, 23–24
  treatment of, 70–72
Amantidine, 79
Ambenonium, 117
Amdinocillin, clinical indications for, 428–429
Amebic dysentery, 386
  treatment of, 408
Amebicide(s), 426–427
Amenorrhea, treatment of, 322
Amikacin, 362
Amiloride, interaction of, with digitalis, 201–202
  mechanism of action of, 279
Amino acid(s), in neurotransmission, 13
  nicotinic receptor and, 98
Aminocaproic acid, in treatment, of hemorrhage, 233–234
  interaction of, with oral contraceptives, 253
Aminoglycoside antibiotic(s), 361–362
  clinical indications for, genitourinary, 429
  drug interactions with, 370–371
  interaction of, with loop diuretics, 284
    with vitamin B_{12}, 253
  See also specific agents
Aminophylline, adverse effects of, 368
  as diuretic, 280
  clinical indications for, 368
Aminosalicylic acid, clinical indications for, 365
  interaction of, with vitamin B_{12}, 253

Aminotransferase, chenodiol and, 401
Amiodarone, as antiarrhythmic agent, 176
　interaction of, with anticoagulants, 200
　　with digitalis, 200
Amitriptyline, 61
　catecholamines and, 60–61
Amobarbital, 34
　barbital versus, 32
Amoxapine, 62
d-Amphetamine. *See* Dextroamphetamine
Amphetamine(s), clinical indications for, 54
　interaction of, with haloperidol, 83
　　with monoamine oxidase inhibitors, 81–82
　　with phenothiazines, 82
　　with tricyclic antidepressants, 82
Amphotericin B, clinical indications for, antifungal, 428
　respiratory, 366
　interaction of, with digitalis, 371
　　with gentamicin, 370
　topical, 450
Ampicillin, 358
Amrinone, 185
Amyl nitrite, 186t, 186–187
Anabolic steroid(s), drug interactions with, 253, 329
　See also Androgen(s); Testosterone
Anal sphincter(s), anatomy of, 381
Analgesia, in anesthesia, 25
　narcotics in, 44–52
Analgesic(s), in arthritis treatment, 453–455, 454t
　See also specific agents and types of agents
Anaphylaxis, from asparaginase, 22
　from iron dextran, 230
　from penicillin, 37
Androgen(s), 323–325, 324t
　clinical indications for, 435
　danazol as, 310
　drug interactions with, 329
　function of, 301
Androsterone, clofibrate and, 243
Anemia, 220–224
　causes of, 216–217
　drug-induced, 222–223
　folic acid deficiency, 222–223
　iron deficiency, 221, 228t–229t, 228–230
　pernicious. *See* Pernicious anemia
　pyridoxine-responsive, 223
　sickle cell, 216–217
　symptoms of, 220–221
　treatment of, 228–232, 228t–229t
　　drug interactions in, 253
Anesthesia, forms of, 25
　induction of, 25
　nitrous oxide in, 26–27
　neuromuscular blocking agents in, 126–128
　stages of, 25–26, 25
Anesthetic agent(s), general. *See* General anesthetic agent(s); specific agents
　interaction of, with barbiturates, 80
　local, 29, 447
Angina pectoris, in coronary artery disease, 167
　treatment of, 185–189
Angiotensin, captopril and, 199
　enalapril and, 199
　in renal physiology, 270–271, 271
Anisindione, 239

Anorexia, from adrenergic agents, 134
Antacid(s), 390–393, 390t
　interaction of, with anticholinergics, 144
　　with benzodiazepines, 410
　　with cimetidine, 410
　　with corticosteroids, 328
　　with digitalis, 202
　　with iron, 253, 410
　　with phenytoin, 81
　　with quinidine, 201
　　with sodium polystyrene sulfonate resin, 410
　　with tetracylcines, 371–372
Anthralin, 451
Anthraquinone, morphine and, 48
Antianginal agent(s), 185–189, 186t
Antianxiety agent(s), 58t, 72–76
　butabarbital as, 34
　dosages of, 58t
　drug interactions with, 83
　mephobarbital as, 35
　See also specific agents
Antiarrhythmic agent(s), 169–178, 169t–170t, 178t, 170, 173, 175–177
　classification of, 169–170, 170t
　digitalis glycosides as, 177–178
　dosages of, 169t, 178t
　therapeutic range of, 169
　type I, 170–175
　type II, 175–176
　type III, 176
　type IV, 177
　See also specific agents
Antibacterial agent(s). *See* Antibiotic(s); Antituberculosis agent(s)
Antibiotic(s), 350–366
　affecting cell wall synthesis, 354–360
　affecting protein synthesis, 360–364
　altering plasma membrane permeability, 365–366
　aminoglycoside. *See* Aminoglycoside antibiotic(s); specific agents
　as antimetabolites, 365
　bactericidal, 354
　bacteriostatic, 354
　beta-lactam, 359
　　See also Cephalosporin(s)
　broad spectrum, defined, 354
　drug interactions with, 145, 255, 284, 370–372
　in treatment, of bacterial meningitis, 24
　　of endocarditis, 199
　　of gastrointestinal infections, 406–408
　　of hematologic cancer, 250–251
　　of otorhinolaryngeal disorders, 353t
　　of respiratory infections, 336, 352t, 357–365
　　of skin infections, 447–449, 448t
　macrolide, 363–364
　mechanism of action of, 353–354, 354
　ocular, 461t
　topical, 447–449, 448t
　See also specific agents and types of agents
Antibody(ies), in hypersensitivity reactions, 340
Anticancer agent(s), antiemetics and, 435
　breast, 433–435
　drug interactions with, 255
　gastrointestinal, 408–409, 409t
　genitourinary, 433–435
　hematologic, 244t–245t, 244, 246–252

Anticholinergic agent(s), 76–78, 77t
  in treatment, of peptic ulcers, 394
  interaction of, with antacids, 144
    with antihistamines, 144
    with benzodiazepines, 144
    with cholinesterase inhibitors, 144
    with corticosteroids, 144
    with glutethimide, 79
    with guanethidine, 144
    with histamine, 144
    with monoamine oxidase inhibitors, 145
    with phenothiazines, 82
    with reserpine, 144
    with sympathomimetic agents, 145
    with tricyclic antidepressants, 82, 144
  See also Muscarinic blocking agent(s); Nicotinic blocking agent(s); specific agents
Anticholinergic effect(s), of chlorpromazine, 68–69
  of disopyramide, 172
  of tricyclic antidepressants, 62–64
Anticholinesterase agent(s), 115–118, 115
  drug interactions with, 144
  irreversible, 118
  pilocarpine and, 113–114
  reversible, 115–118
Anticoagulant(s), 237–239, 237t
  interaction of, with amiodarone, 200
    with anabolic steroids, 253
    with antidiabetics, 253
    with barbiturates, 80, 253
    with chloral hydrate, 79
    with cholestyramine, 254
    with cimetidine, 253, 410
    with clofibrate, 253, 255
    with dextrothyroxine, 253–254
    with diazepam, 254
    with disulfiram, 254
    with ethchlorvynol, 80
    with glutethimide, 79, 254
    with griseofulvin, 456
    with heparin, 254
    with indomethacin, 457
    with oral contraceptives, 329
    with phenylbutazone, 254
    with phenytoin, 81
    with quinidine, 201
    with rifampin, 254
    with salicylates, 254
    with sulfinpyrazone, 254, 285
    with sulfonamides, 254
    with sulindac, 457
    with thiazide diuretics, 283
    with thyroid preparations, 254
Anticonvulsant agent(s), 37–43, 37t, 37
  acetazolamide as, 43
  anemia from, 222–223
  barbiturates as, 83–39
  carbamazepine as, 42
  classes of, 37, 37
  clonazepam as, 42–43
  dosage of, 37t
  drug interactions with, 80–81
  hydantoins as, 39–40
  mephobarbital as, 35
  oxazolidinediones as, 41–42
  phenacemide as, 43

primidone as, 43
succinimides as, 40–41
valproic acid as, 42
Antidepressant agent(s), 57t, 57–66, 59–60
  dosages of, 57t
  drug interactions with, 81–82
  efficacy of, 59
  miscellaneous, 57t, 65–66
  monoamine oxidase inhibitors as. See Monoamine oxidase inhibitor(s)
  tricyclic. See Tricyclic antidepressant(s)
  types of, 57
Antidiabetic agent(s), 327–328, 327t
  drug interactions with, 329–330
  interaction of, with anticoagulants, 253
    with beta-adrenergic blocking agents, 203
    with clofibrate, 254
    with sulfinpyrazone, 285
    with thiazide diuretics, 283
  See also Insulin; other agents
Antidiarrheal agent(s), 401–403, 401t
  drug interactions with, 410
Antidiarrheal/laxative(s), 403
Antidiuretic hormone. See Vasopressin
Antiemetic agent(s), 405–406, 405t
  in cancer chemotherapy, 435
Antiestrogen(s), clomiphene citrate as, 310
Antiflatulent agent(s), 403–404
Antifungal agent(s), 354t
  in genitourinary infections, 427–428
  in respiratory infections, 366
  topical, 448t, 449–450
Antihelminthic agent(s), 410t
Antihemophilia factor, 220, 236
Antihemophilic agent(s), 236–237
Antihemorrhoidal agent(s), 404
Antihistamine(s), 347–350, 348t
  adverse effects of, 347
  alkylamine, 349
  drug interactions with, 371
  ethanolamine, 348
  ethylenediamine, 349
  interaction of, with anticholinergics, 144
    with carbazochrome, 253
    with triazolam, 80
  mechanism of action of, 347
  phenothiazine, 349–350
  piperazine, 350
  piperidine, 350
  types of, 348
Antihyperlipidemic agent(s), drug interactions with, 254–255
Antihypertensive agent(s), 190–199, 191t
  adrenergic blocking, 196–198
  autonomic ganglionic, 193
  central nervous system, 190–193
  diuretics and, in combined therapy, 273–274
  dosages of, 191t
  future, 199
  ideal, 190
  interaction of, with bronchodilators, 145
  regimen for, 199, 199
  renin-angiotensin, 199
  vascular muscular, 194–196
Anti-infective agent(s). See Antibiotic(s)

Anti-inflammatory agent(s), corticosteroids as, 452
  glucocorticoids as, 318–320
  in arthritis treatment, 453–455, 454t
  nonsteroidal, 453–455, 454t
  ocular, 461t
Anti-inhibitor coagulant complex, 236
Antimania agent(s), drug interactions with, 83
Antimetabolite(s), antibiotics as, 353–354, 365
  drug interactions with, 255
  gastrointestinal, 409
  in cancer treatment, 248–250
Antimicrobial agent(s). *See* Antibiotic(s)
Antimuscarinic agent(s), 118–123, 119t
Antineoplastic agent(s). *See* Anticancer agent(s)
Antiparkinsonism agent(s), 76–79, 77t
  drug interactions with, 83
  See also specific agents
Antiperistaltic agent(s), antidiarrheal, 402–403
Antipernicious anemia factor, defined, 216
Antipsoriatic agent(s), 451–452
Antipsychotic agent(s), 67–72
  dosages of, 58t
  drug interactions with, 82
  See also specific agents
Antipyretic agent(s), in arthritis treatment, 453, 454t
Antiseborrheic agent(s), 451
Antiseptic(s), topical, 450
  urinary tract, 425–426, 425t
Antispasmodic agent(s), dosages of, 395t
  in treatment, of peptic ulcers, 394
Antithrombin III, heparin and, 239
Antithrombotic agent(s), 240
Antithyroid agent(s), 316–317, 316t
Antituberculosis agent(s), 353t
  anemia from, 223
  cycloserine as, 359
  ethambutol as, 365
  isoniazid as, 360
  rifampin as, 364
  streptomycin as, 361–362
Antitussive agent(s), 367t, 369–370
Antiviral agent(s), 427
Anxiety, defined, 72
  from morphine, 47
  in psychoneurosis, 21
  treatment of, 72–76. *See also* Antianxiety agent(s); specific agents
Aortic depressor reflex, 154, *155*
Apnea, from morphine, 48
  from succinylcholine, 128
  sleep, 18
Appestat, hypothalamus and, 8
Appetite suppression, from adrenergic agents, 134
  from amphetamines, 54
Aprobarbital, 34
Arachidonic acid, in hemostasis, 217
  pain and, 14
  prostaglandin synthesis and, 430, *431*
Arachnoid, defined, 5
Arrhythmia(s), cardiac. *See* Cardiac arrhythmia(s); specific arrhythmias
Arteriosclerosis, in congestive heart failure, 166
Artery(ies), anatomy of, 158–159, *159*
  hypertension and, 168
  in coronary artery disease, 166–167
  See also Coronary artery disease

Arthritis, 445–446, *445, 446, 447*
  gonococcal, 419
  gouty, treatment of, 274, 280–281, 454–456
  rheumatoid, 445–446, *445*, 453–456
  types of, 446t
  See also Osteoarthritis
Asbestosis, bronchogenic cancer and, 347
Ascariasis, 388
Ascending reticular activating system, anatomy and physiology of, 6–7, *6*
  in autonomic nervous system, 94
  sleep and, 17
Ascites, treatment of, 272
Asparaginase, in cancer treatment, 252
Asparagine, cancer cells and, 252
Aspergillosis, pulmonary, 346
Aspirin, adverse effects of, 453
  as antithrombotic agent, 240
  clinical indications for, 453
  interaction of, with probenecid, 284–285
    with sulfinpyrazone, 285
    with vitamin K, 220
  mechanism of action of, 453
Association, in schizophrenia, 21
Asthma, 109
  as chronic obstructive pulmonary disease, 343–344
  as hypersensitivity reaction, 340
  morphine and, 48
  pilocarpine and, 114
  thiopental use in, 28
  treatment of, adrenergic agents in, 130–132, 135–136
    bronchodilators in, 366–368
    ephedrine in, 132
    epinephrine in, 131
    isoproterenol in, 135
    mucolytic agents in, 369
Atenolol, as antihypertensive agent, 142, 197
Atherosclerosis, in coronary artery disease, 167
Athlete's foot, 443
Atony, gastrointestinal, 107–108
  urinary bladder, 108
Atracurium, 127–128
Atrial arrhythmia(s), 161–164, *162–164*
Atrial fibrillation, 162–163, *162*
  treatment of, antiarrhythmic agents in, 171–172
    digitalis in, 178
Atrial flutter, 162, *162*
  treatment of, 178
Atrial naturetic factor, 199
Atrioventricular disorder(s), 164
  verapamil and, 177
Atrium(a), anatomy of, 150, *151–152, 152*
Atropa belladonna, defined, 118–119
Atropine, adverse effects of, 121
  clinical indications for, 120–121
  diphenoxylate and, as antidiarrheal, 402–403
  in cholinergic neurotransmission, 95, 99–100, *100*
  in treatment, of digitalis toxicity, 184
  interaction of, with acetylcholine, 97
  mechanism of action of, 119–120
Atropine-like quaternary ammonium compound(s), 123
Atropine-like tertiary amine(s), 123
Atrovent, 368
Attapulgite, as antidiarrheal, 402
Attention deficit disorder, 23
  treatment of, 54, 56

Aura, epileptic, 19
Auranofin, 455
Autism, in schizophrenia, 22
Autoimmune disease(s), 446
Autonomic agent(s), 111–144
  as antihypertensive agents, 193–198
  disorders treated with, 105–111
  drug interactions with, 144–146
  types of, 111
  See also specific agents
Autonomic nervous system, agents in, 89–146. *See also* specific agents
  anatomy and physiology of, 91–95, *91, 92t, 93*
  biofeedback and, 3
  central nervous system and, 3, 4
  characteristics of, 94–95
  digitalis and, 182
  hypothalamus in, 7–8
  in digestion, 378–379
  introduction to, 90
  neurotransmission in, drug action on, 95–105
  parasympathetic, 91, *91, 92t, 93*
  summary of, 146
  sympathetic, 91, *91, 92t, 93,* 93–94

B lymphocyte(s), anatomy of, 212
Bacampicillin, clinical indications for, 428
Bacillary dysentery, 385
Bacitracin, 360
Bacterial infection(s). *See* Infection(s); specific disorders
Bacterial meningitis, 24
Bacterial pneumonia, 344
Bacterium(a), antibiotic site of action in, 351, *351*
  biology of, 350–351
  pathogenicity of, 351, 353
  phagocytosis of, 212–213
  protein synthesis in, 360–361, *361*
  resistance to antibiotics of, 354
  types of, 350–351
Bainbridge reflex, 154, *154*
Baking soda. *See* Sodium bicarbonate
Band(s), defined, 212
Barbital, amobarbital versus, 32
  duration of action of, 32
  metharbital and, 39
Barbiturate(s), 31–35, *32–33*
  as anticonvulsant agents, 38–39
  as sedative and hypnotic agents, 32–33
  benzodiazepines versus, 30–31, 33, *33*
  dosages of, 30, 30t
  interaction of, with anesthetic agents, 80
    with anticoagulants, 80, 253
    with chloramphenicol, 80
    with corticosteroids, 80, 328
    with cyclophosphamide, 255
    with digitalis, 80, 202
    with doxorubicin, 255
    with doxycycline, 80
    with estradiol, 80
    with ethchlorvynol, 79
    with furosemide, 81
    with griseofulvin, 456
    with monoamine oxidase inhibitors, 80
    with oral contraceptives, 329
    with phenytoin, 81
    with quinidine, 80–81, 201
    with tricyclic antidepressants, 80, 82

    with valproic acid, 80
  lipid solubility and, 32
  onset of action of, 32
  structure of, 37
  synthesis of, 32, *32*
  withdrawal of, 33
  See also Specific agents
Basal cell carcinoma, 445
Basal ganglia, function of, 6
  in parkinsonism, 24
Bedsore(s), treatment of, 451
Belladonna alkaloid(s), levorotatory, 121–122
Belladonna extract, 122
Benzathine, clinical indications for, 428
Benzodiazepine receptor, 32
Benzodiazepine(s), 72–75
  barbiturates versus, 30–31, 33
  clinical indications for, 30
  compared, 72–73
  drug interactions with, 83
  interaction of, with alcohol, 31, 83
    with antacids, 410
    with anticholinergics, 144
    with cimetidine, 83
    with disulfiram, 83
    with levodopa, 83
    with oral contraceptives, 329
  mechanism of action of, 73
  parenteral effects of, 74–75
  See also specific agents
Benzothiadiazide(s). *See* Thiazide diuretic(s)
Benzoyl peroxide, 449, 449t
Benztropine, 77
Benzylpenicillin, 356–357
Beta cell(s), pancreatic, 302, 327
Beta-adrenergic blocking agent(s), 140t, 140–143
  as antianginal agents, 187–188
  as antiarrhythmic agents, 175–176
  as antihypertensive agents, 197–198, *197–198*
  interaction of, with antidiabetic agents, 203
    with cimetidine, 203
    with decongestants, 145
    with epinephrine, 203
    with insulin, 329
    with rifampin, 203
    with sulfonylureas, 330
    with theophylline, 203
    with verapamil, 203
  nonselective, 140–142
  postmyocardial infarction, 190
  selective, 142–143
  with alpha-adrenergic activity, 143
  withdrawal of, adverse effects of, 140–141
Beta-adrenergic receptor(s), 104–105, *104–105*
Bethanechol, 113
Bicarbonate, renal system and, 268–269, *269,* 275–276
Bicarbonate-carbonic acid system, 268–269, *269*
Bile, in digestion, 381–382
Bile acid(s), cholestyramine and, 241
Bile salt(s), as digestive aids, 400
  laxative, 399
Biofeedback, research into, 3
Biological clock(s), 303–304
Biperidin, 77
Bipolar depression, defined, 20
Bipyridine agent(s), in heart failure treatment, 185
Birth defect(s). *See* Teratogenicity

Bisacodyl, 395–396
Bishydroxycoumarin. *See* Dicumarol
Bismuth preparation(s), antidiarrheal, 402
 antiemetic, 406
Bladder, anatomy of, 417, *418*
 cancer of, 422–423
  treatment of, 434
 cyclophosphamide and, 247
Blastomycosis, pulmonary, 346
Bleomycin, clinical indications for, gastrointestinal, 409
 hematologic, 250–251
Bleuler, schizophrenia description of, 21
Blood, components of, 211–213
 disorders of, 220–228
 formation of, 215–216
 function of, 210
 renal flow of, 261, *261*, 263–264, *263*, 265
 renal volume of, 260
Blood cell(s), red. *See* Erythrocyte(s)
 white. *See* Leukocyte(s)
Blood clot(s), formation of, 217–218, 220
Blood clotting, 217–218, 217t–218, *218*, 220
 anticoagulants and, 237–239
 disorders of, 226–227
 drugs affecting, 232–241, *232, 234,* 233t, 237t
 drugs promoting, 232–233, *232*
 factors in, 217, 217t–218t, *218*
 in multiple myeloma, 225
 prevention of, heparin in, 239
Blood dyscrasia(s), from carbamazepine, 42
 from chloramphenicol, 406
 from phenacemide, 43
 from propylthiouracil, 317
 from quinidine, 171
 from trimethadione, 41
Blood gas exchange, 336, 338
Blood platelet(s). *See* Thrombocyte(s)
Blood pressure, components of, 159
 determinants of, 190, *190–191*
 in hypertension, 167–168
 influences on, 159
Blood vessel(s), anatomy and physiology, 158–160, *159*
 See also specific types of vessels
Blood-forming organ(s), anatomy of, 215–217, *217, 219,* 218t–219t, 220
Boil(s), nasal, 342
Bone disorder(s), from hypoparathyroidism, 306
 See also specific disorders
Bone marrow, in blood formation, 215–216
 types of, 215
Bone marrow disorder(s), from antineoplastic agents, 246–251
 from chlorambucil, 246
 from gold compounds, 455
 from mitomycin, 409
Botulism, 386
Bowman's capsule, 263–264
Bradycardia, defined, 153
 sinus, 161, *161*
Bradykinin, as cause of pain, 14
 in allergy, 340
Brain, anatomy and physiology of, 3–9, *3, 6–8*
 embryology of, 4
 functions of, 3
 gray matter of, 5
 weight of, 3
 white matter of, 5

Brain stem, formation of, 4
 in neurotransmission, 10, *11*
Breast, cancer of, 422
 treatment of, 433–435
Bretylium tosylate, as adrenergic blocking agent, 143
 as antiarrhythmic agent, 176, *176*
 interaction of, with norepinephrine, 176
Broad spectrum antibiotic(s), defined, 354
Broad-beta disease, 227t, 228
Bromide, intoxication with, 274
 thiazide diuretics and, 277
Bromocryptine, 79
Bronchial asthma. *See* Asthma
Bronchiole(s), anatomy of, 336, *337–338*
 in asthma, 343–344
Bronchitis, as chronic obstructive pulmonary disease, 343
 treatment of, 368
Bronchoconstriction, in cough reflex, 339
Bronchodilation, physiology of, 336
Bronchodilator(s), 366–368, 367t
 adrenergic, 129t, 130–133, 135–137
 drug interactions with, 145
 in treatment, of asthma, 109
Bronchogenic carcinoma, 346–347
 treatment of, 370
Bronchopneumonia, 344
Bronchospasm, from propranolol, 176
 treatment of, epinephrine in, 131
Bronchus(i), in asthma, 343–344
Buerger's disease, 110
Bumetanide, interaction of, with indomethacin, 456–457
Bungarotoxin, acetylcholine receptor and, 97
Burkitt's lymphoma, 224
Burn(s), treatment of, 451
Burnett syndrome, 391
Bursa(e), defined, 441–442
Bursitis, 442
Buspirone, effects of, 76
Busulfan, in cancer treatment, 247–248
Butabarbital, 34
Butorphanol, 52
Butyrophenone(s), 71
 See also specific agents

Caffeine, adverse effects of, 55
 clinical indications for, 55, 280
 structure of, *55*
Calcitonin, function of, 298–299
Calcitonin-salmon, 317–318
Calcitriol, parathormone and, 299
Calcium, calcitonin-salmon and, 317
 calcium channel blocking agents and, 188–189, *188–189*
 digitalis and, 179–180, *179–181*
 histamine and, 341
 in cardiac electrophysiology, 157–158, *157*
 in hemostasis, 217, 218t
 in norepinephrine synthesis, 101–102
 in parathyroid dysfunction, 305–306
 injections of, clinical indications for, 318
 interaction of, with digitalis, 202
 parathormone and, 299
 parathyroid preparations and, 318
 thiazide diuretics and, 277
 thyroid hormones and, 298
Calcium carbonate, as antacid, 392

Calcium channel blocking agent(s), as antianginal agents, 188–189, *188–189*
　as antiarrythmic agents, 177
Calcium polycarbophil, as laxative, 398
Cancer, bladder, 422–423
　breast, 324, 422, 433–435
　bronchogenic, 346–347
　cervical, 421
　colon, 385
　endometrial, 321
　esophageal, 383
　gastric, 384
　gastric ulcers and, 384
　gastrointestinal, 384–385
　　treatment of, 408–409, 409*t*
　genitourinary, 421–423
　hematologic, survival rates in, 244
　　treatment of, 244*t*–245*t*, 244, 246–252
　hepatic, 389
　　from androgens, 325
　laryngeal, 347
　oral, 382–383, 409
　ovarian, 421–422, 434
　pancreatic, 389
　prostatic, 422
　skin, 445
　small intestinal, 385
　testicular, 422, 434–435
　thyroid, 317
　treatment of, 408–409, 433–435
　　antiemetics in, 435
　　doxorubicin in, 251
　　prednisone in, 319
　uterine, 421, 434–435
　vaginal, 421
　vulvar, 421
Candida albicans, drugs against, 427–428
Candidiasis, as superinfection, 354
　dermal, 443
　genitourinary, 427–428
　oral, 382
　pulmonary, 345–346
　vaginal, 420
Canker sore(s), defined, 382
Canrenone, 279
Capillary(ies), adenohypophyseal, 296
　anatomy of, 159
　nephron and, 263–264, *263*
　vitamin C and, 217
Captopril, as antihypertensive agent, 199
　interaction of, with indomethacin, 203, 457
Carafate, 393
Carbachol, 113
Carbamate, interaction of, with cholinesterase inhibitors, 144
Carbamazepine, as anticonvulsant agent, 42, *42*
　interaction of, with phenytoin, 81
　　with posterior pituitary injection, 328
　　with vasopressin, 328
Carbazochrome, interaction of, with antihistamines, 253
Carbazochrome salicylate, 234
Carbenicillin, 358–359
Carbidopa, 78–79
Carbohydrate metabolism, diuretics and, 281
　in diabetes mellitus, 307–308
　in digestion, 381

Carbohydrate solution, phosphorylated, 405–406
Carbon dioxide, in circulatory system, 210–211
　in respiratory physiology, 336–338
Carbonic acid-bicarbonate system, 268–269, *269*
Carbonic anhydrase, renal system and, 268–269, 275–276
Carbonic anhydrase inhibitor(s), 275–276, 275*t*
　adverse effects of, 276
　clinical indications for, 276
　interaction of, with methenamine, 283
　mechanism of action of, 275–276
Carbonyl oxygen, in acetylcholine receptor, 98, *99*
Carboprost tromethamine, 432
Carcinoma, bronchogenic, 346–347
　laryngeal, 347
　squamous cell. *See* Squamous cell carcinoma
Cardia, anatomy of, 377, *378*
Cardiac action potential, bretylium tosylate and, 176
Cardiac afterdepolarization(s), digitalis and, 181–182, *182*
Cardiac arrhythmia(s), 160–165
　atrial, 161–163
　atrioventricular, 164
　from digitalis, 183–184
　from halothane, 26
　sinoatrial, 160–161
　supraventricular, 175–178
　treatment of, 169–178
　　See also Antiarrhythmic agent(s); specific agent(s)
　types of, 160
　ventricular, 164–165
　See also specific arrhythmias
Cardiac depolarization(s), antiarrhythmic agents and, 170–175, 181
Cardiac disorder(s), 160–168
　asthma and, 109
　from amphetamines, 54
　from antineoplastic antibiotics, 251
　from atropine, 120–121
　from beta-adrenergic blocking agents, 140–143
　from chlorpromazine, 68
　from chronic obstructive pulmonary disease, 343
　from desipramine, 62
　from diuretics, 281–282
　from fluorouracil, 409
　from propranolol, 176
　from quinidine, 171
　in diabetes mellitus, 308
　morphine in, 48
　pentazocine and, 52
　treatment of, beta-adrenergic blocking agents in, 140–143
Cardiac effect(s), autonomic, 92, 92*t*
　of adrenergic receptors, 104
　of alpha-adrenergic blocking agents, 137–138
　of antiarrhythmic agents, 170–178
　of antihypertensive agents, 190–199
　of caffeine, 55
　of digitalis glycosides, 179–184
　of diuretics, 271–272
　of local anesthetic agents, 29
　of morphine, 48
　of narcotics, 47
　of nicotine, 125
　of potassium, 270
　of thyroid preparations, 315
Cardiac electrophysiology, 155–158, *156–158*
Cardiac excitation, digitalis and, 179–182, *181*
Cardiac extrasystole(s), 161

Cardiac glycoside(s), 178t, 178–184
  interaction of, with insulin, 329
  See also Digitalis entries
Cardiac infection(s), 168
  treatment of, 199
Cardiac nerve(s), 153, 153
Cardiac pacemaker, in cardiac electrophysiology, 155
Cardiac reflex(es), 153–155, 154–155
Cardiac valve(s), anatomy of, 151, 152
  infection in, 168
Cardiovascular system, 149–205
  anatomy and physiology of, 150, 151–159, 152–160
  diseases of, 160–168, 160–165, 204–205
    See also Cardiac disorder(s); specific disorders
    treatment of, 168–199
  introduction to, 150
  summary of, 204–205
Carmustine, as antineoplastic agent, hematologic, 247
  interaction of, with cimetidine, 255
Carotid artery, in carotid sinus reflex, 155, 155
Carotid sinus reflex, 155, 155
Casanthranol, as stimulant laxative, 397
Cascara segrada, as stimulant laxative, 397
Castle's hypothesis, 221
Castor oil, as stimulant laxative, 397
Castration, gonadal hypofunction from, 307
Cataplexy, in narcolepsy, 18
Catatonia, in schizophrenia, 22
Catecholamine hypothesis of depression, 20
Catecholamine(s), adrenergic receptors and, 104–105, 104
  as adrenergic agents, 130–132, 135
  biosynthesis of, 100–101, 100
    agents inhibiting, 144
  depression and, 20–21
  hypersensitivity to, propranolol and, 140
  lithium carbonate and, 66
  migraine and, 110
  monoamine oxidase inhibitors and, 64–65
  nicotine and, 125
  schizophrenia and, 22–23
  tricyclic antidepressants and, 60–61
Catechol-O-methyltransferase, in catecholamine catabolism, 101–102
Cavitation, in tuberculosis, 345
Cecum, in digestion, 381
Cefoxitin, 359
Celiac sprue, 387
Cell cycle, cancer therapy and, 244, 245
Cell membrane(s), phenobarbital and, 38
Cell mitosis inhibitor(s), in cancer treatment, 250
Cell(s), beta, 302, 327
  cardiac, 156–157
  Leydig, 301
  Reed-Sternberg, 225
  sperm, 417–418
Cell wall, antibiotics affecting, 354–360
Cellulose, in hemostasis, 236
Cellulose derivative(s), as laxatives, 398
Central nervous system, 1–87
  adrenergic receptors in, 103
  agents in, drug interactions of, 79–83
  anatomy and physiology of, 3–13, 3, 4, 6–8, 10–13
  disorders of, 13–24. See also specific disorders
    amenable to drug therapy, 13
  hypothyroidism and, 305
  infections of, 24
  neurotransmission in, 9–13, 10–13
  stimulants of. See also specific agents
    cortical, 53t, 54–56, 55
    medullary, 53t, 56–57
  stimulants of, 53t, 53–57, 55
  synopsis of, 2–3
  therapeutic drugs in, 24–79. See also specific agents
    interactions of, 79–83
Central nervous system depressant(s), interaction of, with antihistamines, 371
  with barbiturates, 80
  with chloral hydrate, 79
  with ethchlorvynol, 79
  with ethinamate, 80
  with flurazepam, 80
  with glutethimide, 79
  with methyprylon, 79
  with phenytoin, 81
  with temazepam, 80
  with triazolam, 80
Central nervous system disorder(s), from cimetidine, 393
  from nalidixic acid, 425–426
Central nervous system stimulant(s), 53t, 53–57, 55
  dosages of, 53t
  drug interactions with, 83
  mechanism of action of, 53–54
Centrilobular emphysema, 343
Cephaloridine, interaction of, with loop diuretics, 284
Cephalosporin(s), adverse effects of, 359
  clinical indications for, 359
    genitourinary, 429
  interaction of, with gentamicin, 371
  mechanism of action of, 359
Cerebellum, anatomy of, 5
Cerebral cortex, anatomy of, 5
  ascending reticular activating system and, 6–7
  sleep and, 6–7, 17
Cervical cancer, 421
Cervicitis, 420
Cestode infestation, 388–389
Chancre(s), syphilitic, 419
Charcoal, antidiarrheal, 402
Chemical toxin(s), in organic brain psychosis, 21
Chemoreceptor reflex(es), in respiratory physiology, 338
Chemotherapy, cancer. See Anticancer agent(s)
Chenodiol, as digestive aid, 400–401
Chenodyoxycholic acid, as digestive aid, 400–401
Cheyne-Stokes respiration, from morphine, 48
Chicken pox virus, shingles from, 443
Chlamydial infection(s), 419
  treatment of, 429
Chloral hydrate, 35
  adverse effects of, 35
  clinical indications for, 35
  interaction of, with alcohol and depressants, 79
    with anticoagulants, 79
    with furosemide, 79
    with loop diuretics, 284
Chlorambucil, in cancer treatment, 246
Chloramphenicol, clinical indications for, gastrointestinal, 406
  interaction of, with barbiturates, 80
    with iron, 253
    with penicillin, 371
    with phenytoin, 81
    with vitamin B_{12}, 253

Chlordiazepoxide, adverse effects of, 73
　clinical indications for, 73
　interaction of, with antacids, 410
　mechanism of action of, 73
Chloride, diuretics and, 282
　renal reabsorption of, 265–266, 266, 268
　thiazide diuretics and, 277
Chlorpheniramine, 349
Chlorpromazine, adverse effects of, 68–70
　as adrenergic blocking agents, 140
　clinical indications for, 68
　history of, 67
　mechanism of action of, 68
　structure of, *59*
Chlorpropamide, interaction of, with alcohol, 330
　　with posterior pituitary injection, 328
　　with rifampin, 330
　　with vasopressin, 328
Chlorprothixene, 70–71
Cholangitis, 389
Cholecystitis, chronic, 389
Cholera, 386
　treatment of, 407
Cholesterol, drugs lowering levels of, 241–243, 241*t*
　function of, 213
　guanabenz and, 192
Cholestyramine, adverse effects of, 242
　interaction of, with acetaminophen, 254
　　with anticoagulants, 254
　　with corticosteroids, 254
　　with digitalis, 202, 254
　　with hydrocortisone, 328
　　with thyroid hormones, 254
　　with thyroid preparations, 328
　mechanism of action of, 241–242
Choline, in acetylcholine synthesis, 96, *96*
Cholinergic agent(s), 111–118, 111*t*
　disorders treated with, 105–108
　drug interactions with, 144–145, 200
　ganglionic blocking, 123*t*–124*t*, 124–126
　ganglionic stimulant, 124
　muscarinic blocking, 118–123, 119*t*
　　See also Muscarinic blocking agent(s); specific agents
　nicotinic blocking, 123–128, 123*t*–124*t*
Cholinergic blocking agent(s), disorders treated with, 108–109
　drug interactions with, 144–145
　See also Anticholinergic agent(s); specific agents
Cholinergic fiber(s), defined, 94
Cholinergic neurotransmission, in autonomic nervous system, 96–100, *96–100*
　in central nervous system, 12, *13*
Cholinergic receptor(s), cholinergic agents and, 111–112, 118–120
Cholinesterase, acetylcholine and, 96
　regenerators of, 129
Choriocarcinoma, 421
Chromatopsia, from digitalis, 184
Chromosome 21, Alzheimer's disease and, 23
Chronic bronchitis, defined, 343
Chronic obstructive pulmonary disease, 343–344
　treatment of, 56
Chronotropism, defined, 153
Chrysophanic acid, in senna laxatives, 396–397
Chylomicron(s), formation of, 213
　in hyperlipoproteinemia, 228

Chyme, defined, 379
Cigarette smoking, bladder cancer and, 423
　bronchogenic cancer and, 346–347
　chronic obstructive pulmonary disease from, 343
　gastrointestinal ulcers and, 384
　hypertension and, 168
　insulin and, 330
　oral contraceptives and, 323, 329
　withdrawal from, 125
Cilium(a), nasal, 339
Cimetidine, in peptic ulcer treatment, 393
　interaction of, with antacids, 410
　　with anticoagulants, 253, 410
　　with benzodiazepines, 83
　　with beta-adrenergic blocking agents, 203
　　with carmustine, 255
　　with narcotics, 410
　　with phenytoin, 81
　　with procainamide, 200–201
　　with quinidine, 201
　　with theophylline, 410
　　with tricyclic antidepressants, 82
Cinchonism, from quinidine, 171
Cinoxacin, as urinary tract antiseptic, 426
Circulatory/reticuloendothelial system, 209–256
　anatomy and physiology of, 211–217, *211*, *214–215*, *219*, 218*t*–219*t*, *220*
　disorders of, 220–228, *223*, 227*t*
　drug interactions in, 252–255
　drugs affecting, 228–255. See also specific agents
　introduction to, 210
　summary of, 255–256
Cirrhosis, hepatic. See Hepatic cirrhosis
Cisplatin, in cancer treatment, 434
Claudication, intermittent, 241
Climacteric syndrome, 307
Clindamycin, adverse effects of, 364
　clinical indications for, 364
　topical, 448–449
Clitoris, anatomy of, 417, *417*
Clofibrate, as antihyperlipidemic agent, 243
　interaction of, with anticoagulants, 253, 255
　　with antidiabetics, 254
　　with furosemide, 255
　　with loop diuretics, 284
　　with posterior pituitary injection, 328
　　with vasopressin, 328
Clomiphene citrate, 310
Clonazepam, as anticonvulsant agent, 42–43
Clonic seizure(s), defined, 19
Clonidine, adrenergic receptors and, 103
　as adrenergic inhibitor, 143
　as antihypertensive agent, 191–192
　interaction of, with tricyclic antidepressants, 203–204
　neurotransmission and, 95–96
Clorazepate, 73–74
Clostridium botulinum, 386
Clotrimazole, 428
Cluster headache, 111
Coactin, 428–429
Coagulation, blood, 217–218, 217*t*–218*t*, *218*, 220
　See also Blood clotting
　disseminated intravascular, 227
Coccidioidomycosis, pulmonary, 346
Cochlea, 339, *340*
Codeine, 48–49

adverse effects of, 49
antitussive effects of, 47
clinical indications for, 49
Coitus, anatomic factors in, 416–418
Colchicine, in gout treatment, 455–456
Cold, common, 347
Cold sore(s), defined, 382
Colestipol, as cholesterol-lowering agent, 242
  interaction of, with digitalis, 255
    with diuretics, 255
    with thiazide diuretics, 284
Colistin, clinical indications for, 406–407
Colitis, from clindamycin, 364
  ulcerative, 387, 403
Collagen disease, defined, 441
Collagenase, topical preparations of, 451
Colon, anatomy of, 377, 381
  cancer of, ulcerative colitis and, 387
Coma, hepatic, 272
Commensal(s), bacterial, 351
Common cold, antihistamines in, 347
Conduction block, atrioventricular, 164
Congestive heart failure, 165–166
  antiarrhythmic agents and, 172–174
  beta-adrenergic blocking agents and, 198
  treatment of, adrenergic agents in, 184–185
    bipyridines in, 185
    diuretics in, 261, 271–272
    drugs in, 178–185
    principles of, 178
Connective tissue, anatomy and physiology of, 440–442
Connective tissue disorder(s), 445–446, 446t, 445–447
  from etretinate, 452
  treatment of, 453–456
  See also Arthritis entries
Consciousness, in anesthesia, 25–26
Constipation, causes of, 385–387
  from antacids, 391–393
  from morphine, 47–48
  from verapamil, 177
Contraceptive(s), oral. See Oral contraceptive(s)
Convulsion(s). See Seizure(s)
Copper, iron and, 215
Coronary artery disease, 166–167
  treatment of, 185–190
    antianginal agents in, 185–189
    postmyocardial infarction, 189–190
Corpus luteum, hormones in, 300–301
Corti, organ of, 340
Corticospinal fiber(s), defined, 5
Corticosteroid(s), edema from, 273
  in treatment, of allergic rhinitis, 367t, 369
  interaction of, with antacids, 328
    with anticholinergics, 144
    with barbiturates, 80, 328
    with cholestyramine, 254
    with cyclophosphamide, 255
    with diuretics, 284
    with estrogen, 329
    with indomethacin, 329, 457
    with methandrostenolone, 329
    with phenylbutazone, 329
    with phenytoin, 81
    with salicylates, 329
    with vitamin A, 329
  ophthalmic, 461t

topical, 452, 452t
Corticotropin. See Adrenocorticotropic hormone
Cortisol. See Hydrocortisone
Corynebacterium, drugs against, 448–449
Cosyntropin, 311
Cough, codeine and, 47
  in chronic bronchitis, 343
  morphine and, 48
  treatment of, 369–370
    See also Antitussive agent(s)
    codeine in, 49
    hydrocodone in, 50
Cough receptor(s), 339
Cough reflex, in respiratory physiology, 339
Coumadin. See Warfarin
Coumarin, 237–238, 237t
  interaction of, with barbiturates, 80
    with ethchlorvynol, 80
    with glutethimide, 79
    with phenytoin, 81
  mechanism of action of, 232
Countercurrent-multiplier model, 266, 267
Cranial nerve(s), classification of, 5
Cranium, defined, 3
Cretinism, 305
  treatment of, 315–316
Crohn's disease, 387
Crotamiton, 451
Cryptococcosis, pulmonary, 346
Cryptorchidism, anatomic factors in, 417
  in gonadal hypofunction, 307
Crystalluria, from sulfonamides, 424
Curare, history of, 126
Curare alkaloid(s), 126–128
Cushingoid syndrome, 307
Cushing's syndrome, 307
  iatrogenic, 320
Cutaneous larva migrans, 388
Cyanocobalamin, function of, 216, 222
  in pernicious anemia treatment, 230–231
Cyclizine, 350
Cyclomethycaine, 447
Cyclo-oxygenase, aspirin and, 240
Cyclopentolate, 122–123
Cyclophosphamide, clinical indications for, genitourinary, 434
  hematologic, 247
  drug interactions with, 255
Cycloplegia, from atropine, 120
Cycloserine, in tuberculosis treatment, 359
Cystic fibrosis, treatment of, 368
Cystitis, 420–421
Cytarabine, in cancer treatment, 249–250
Cytarabine syndrome, 250
Cytosine arabinoside, 249–250

Dam, vitamin K and, 220
Danazol, 310
  interaction of, with warfarin, 328
Danthron, as stimulant laxative, 397
Datura stramonium, 118–119
Daunorubicin, in cancer treatment, 251
Deafness, from otitis media, 343
  See also Ototoxicity
Death, from clindamycin, 364
  from coronary artery disease, 167

Death, *(continued)*
  from diabetes mellitus, 308
  from lithium carbonate, 67
  from morphine, 48
  from phenacemide, 43
  from phenobarbital, 35
  from propoxyphene, 51
  sudden cardiac, 164
Decamethonium, 129
Decongestant(s), 130*t*, 130–133, 369
  drug interactions with, 145–146
Degradation enzyme(s), in neurotransmission, 9–10
Dehydration, treatment of, 462*t*
Dehydrocholic acid, as digestive aid, 400
Delirium tremens, treatment of, 35
Demecarium, 117–118
Demeclocyline, 362–363
Dementia, senile, 23–24, 70–72
Dendrite(s), hypothalamic, 8
Dental abnormality(ies), from tetracyclines, 363
Deoxycorticosterone, 320
Deoxyuridylate, in anemia, 230–231, *230*
Dependence, drug. *See* Drug dependence
Depolarization, in neurotransmission, 95
Depressant(s), central nervous system. *See* Central nervous system depressant(s); specific agents
Depression, psychologic, 20–21
  respiratory. *See* Respiratory depression
Dermatologic disorder(s), as signs of illness, 440
  from glutethimide, 36
  from penicillin, 357–358
  from pentazocine, 52
  from phenolphthalein, 395
  from syphilis, 419
  from trimethoprim, 407, 424
  infectious, 442–443. *See also* specific disorders
  malignant, 445
  miscellaneous, 444–445
  parasitic, 444
  treatment of, bacitracin in, 360
    glucocorticoids in, 319
Dermis, anatomy of, 440, *441*
Desipramine, adverse effects of, 62
  catecholamines and, 60–62
  clinical indications for, 62
Deslanoside, clinical indications for, 182
Desmethyldiazepam, 74
Desmopressin acetate, 314
Dexamethasone, clinical indications for, 320, 369
  interaction of, with ephedrine, 328
    with phenytoin, 81
Dexpanthenol, as gastrointestinal stimulant, 404, 450
Dextro panthothenyl alcohol, as gastrointestinal stimulant, 404
Dextroamphetamine, 54
Dextromethorphan, abuse of, 370
Dextrose, in hypoglycemia treatment, 326
Dextrothyroxine, as cholesterol-lowering agent, 242–243
  interaction of, with anticoagulants, 253–254
Dezocine, morphine versus, 53
Diabetes insipidus, causes of, 304–305
  thiazide diuretics in, 276–277
  treatment of, 312–314
Diabetes mellitus, defined, 307
  treatment of, insulin in, 325
    metoclopramide in, 404
  sulfonylureas in, 326–327
  types of, 308
Diacetylmorphine, 45
Diaphragm, anatomy of, 337–338, *337*
Diarrhea, defined, 385
  in celiac sprue, 387
  in colitis, 387
  in helminth infestations, 388
  in Whipple's disease, 388
  infectious, 385–386
  noninfectious, 386
  treatment of, 401–403, 401*t*
    antiperistaltics in, 402–403
    paregoric in, 47
Diastole, defined, 152
Diastolic pressure, defined, 159
Diazepam, adverse effects of, 74
  clinical indications for, 74
  interaction of, with anticoagulants, 254
    with neuromuscular blocking agents, 145
  mechanism of action of, 74
  metabolism of, 73
Diazoxide, as antihypertensive agent, 194–195
  interaction of, with sulfonylureas, 330
    with thiazide diuretics, 204
Dibenoxapine(s), 72
Dicumarol, adverse effects of, 238
  clinical indications for, 238
  drug interactions with, 253–254
  history of, 237
  interaction of, with phenytoin, 81
    with vitamin K, 220
  mechanism of action of, 237–238
Dicyclomine, 123
Diencephalon, anatomy of, 4, 7–8
Diet, folic acid in, 216
  iron and, 215–216, *216*
  plasma lipids and, 213
  vitamin B_{12} in, 216
Diethylstilbestrol, as synthetic estrogen, 321
  postcoital, 322–323
  vaginal cancer and, 421
Digestion, 376–382
  pharmacologic aids to, 399–401, 400*t*
Digestive/gastrointestinal system, 375–411
  anatomy and physiology of, 376–382, *377–378*, *380*
  disorders of, 382–389
    See also Gastrointestinal disorder(s)
    drug interactions in, 410
    treatment of, 389–410
  introduction to, 376
  summary of, 411
Digitalis glycoside(s), adverse effects of, 183–184, *184*
  clinical indications for, 177–178, *177*, 178*t*, 182–183, *183*
  composition of, 178–179
  dosages of, 178*t*
  interaction of, with amiloride, 201–202
    with amiodarone, 200
    with amphotericin B, 371
    with antacids, 202
    with barbiturates, 202
    with bronchodilators, 145
    with calcium, 202
    with cholestyramine, 202, 254
    with colestipol, 255

with diuretics, 202, 283–284
  with kaolin-pectin, 202
  with metoclopramide, 202
  with neuromuscular blocking agents, 145
  with phenytoin, 174, 180, 184
  with propantheline, 202
  with propranolol, 175
  with quinidine, 171, 201
  with rifampin, 371
  with spironolactone, 202
  with sympathomimetics, 202
  with verapamil, 202–203
 mechanism of action of, 153, 177–178, *177*, 179–182, *179–182*
 regimen for, 183, *183*
 toxicity of, 183–184, *183*
 See also Digoxin; Digitoxin
Digitoxin, interaction of, with barbiturates, 80
  with sulfonylureas, 330
 metabolism of, 182
Digitoxose, cardiac glycoside, 179
Digoxin, adverse effects of, 178
 clinical indications for, 178
 interaction of, with phenylpropanolamine, 205
  with quinidine, 201
 mechanism of action of, 177–178, *177*
 metabolism of, 182
 route of administration of, 182
Dihydrocodeinone, 50
Dihydroergotamine, 139
Dihydroindolone derivative(s), 71–72
Dihydromorphine, 49
Dihydromorphinone, formation of, 46
 history of, 45
Dihydrotestosterone, 324
Dihydroxyaluminum sodium carbonate, 392
Dihydroxyphenylalanine, synthesis of, 100–101, *100*
Diltiazem, as antianginal agent, 188–189
Dimethylethanolamine, 112
Dinoprost tromethamine, 431–432
Dinoprostone, 432
Diphenhydramine, 348
Diphenoxylate, atropine and, 402–403
Diphenylbutylpiperidine(s), 71
Diphenylhydantoin. *See* Phenytoin
Diphtheria, treatment of, 357, 363
Dipyridamole, as antianginal agent, 187
 as antithrombotic agent, 240
Discoid lupus erythematosus, 445
Disease(s). *See* specific diseases and types of disease
Disodium edetate, in digitalis toxicity, 184
Disopyramide, adverse effects of, 172
 clinical indications for, 172
 interaction of, with lidocaine, 200
  with phenytoin, 81, 200
  with quinidine, 200
  with rifampin, 200
 mechanism of action of, 172
Disorder(s). *See* specific disorders and types of disorder
Disseminated intravascular coagulation, 227
 aminocaproic acid and, 234
Disulfiram, interaction of, with anticoagulants, 254
  with benzodiazepines, 83
  with metronidazole, 435
  with phenytoin, 81
Disulfiram reaction, from alcohol and sulfonylureas, 330

Diuresis, diuretic course and, 285
 influences on, 267–268
Diuretic(s), adverse effects of, 261–262
  in cirrhosis, 272
  in heart failure, 272
 age of patient and, 282
 as antihypertensive agents, 196, *196*
 caffeine as, 55
 carbonic anhydrase inhibitors as, 275–276, 275t
 clinical indications for, 260–261
 drug interactions with, 283–285
 electrolyte imbalances from, 281–282
 in treatment, of edematous disorders, 271–273
  of nonedematous disorders, 273–274
 loop. *See* Loop diuretic(s)
 mechanism of action of, 260–262
 osmotic, 274–275
 potassium-sparing, 279–280, 279t
 refractory edema and, 282
 regimen for, 262–263
 route of administration of, 282
 selection of, 282–283, 285–286
 thiazide. *See* Thiazide diuretic(s)
 types of, 262
  as antihypertensives, 273–274
  in heart failure treatment, 271
  in renal disorder treatment, 272–273
 See also specific agents
Dobutamine, 132
 in heart failure treatment, 184–185
Docusate, in laxative preparations, 397
Docusate sodium, 399
Dopamine, adverse effects of, 132
 amoxapine and, 62
 antiparkinsonism agents and, 78–79
 clinical indications for, 131–132, 185
 haloperidol and, 71
 in central nervous system, 11, *12*
 mechanism of action of, 131
 narcotics and, 47
 parkinsonism and, 24
 phenothiazines and, 67–68, 70
 pimozide and, 71
 schizophrenia and, 22–23
 synthesis of, 100–101, *100*
Dopamine-beta-hydroxylase, in neurotransmission, 9–10
 schizophrenia and, 22–23
Dopaminergic agent(s), 77, 78–79
Dopaminergic pathway(s), central nervous system, 11, *12*
Dopaminergic receptor(s), hormone release and, 295
Doxapram, 56
Doxepin, 62
Doxorubicin, clinical indications for, genitourinary, 434
  hematologic, 251
 interaction of, with barbiturates, 255
Doxycycline, 362–363
 clinical indications for, 363, 429
 interaction of, with barbiturates, 80
Dronabinol, in cancer treatment, 435
Droperidol, fentanyl and, 29
Drug(s). *See* specific agents and types of agents
Drug dependence, on antitussive agents, 370
 on barbiturates, 33
 on benzodiazepines, 31
 on glutethimide, 36
 on meperidine, 50

Drug dependence, *(continued)*
  on methadone, 51
  on morphine, 48
  on paraldehyde, 35
  on pentobarbital, 33
  on secobarbital, 34
Drug interaction(s), with antianginal agents, 203
  with antiarrhythmic agents, 200–201
  with antihypertensive agents, 203–204
  with autonomic agents, 144–146
  with cardiac glycosides, 201–203
  with central nervous system agents, 79–83
  with circulatory/reticuloendothelial agents, 252–255
  with diuretics, 283–285
  with endocrine drugs, 328–330
  with gastrointestinal agents, 410
  with genitourinary drugs, 435
  with integumentary drugs, 456–457
  with respiratory agents, 370–372
  with sedative and hypnotic agents, 79–81
  See also specific agents
Drug overdosage, bromide, treatment of, 274
  digitalis, 183–184
  treatment of, naloxone in, 53
    pralidoxime in, 129
Drug toxicity, digitalis, 183–184
  nitrate, 187
Drug withdrawal, of barbiturates, 33
Duodenum, anatomy of, 378, 379–380
  ulcers of, 108, 384–385
Dura mater, defined, 5
Dwarfism, pituitary, 304
  treatment of, 311
Dyphylline, 368
Dyscrasia(s), blood. *See* Blood dyscrasia(s)
  plasma cell, 225
Dysentery, amebic, 386
  treatment of, 408
  bacillary, 385
Dyskinesia, from chlorpromazine, 69
Dysmenorrhea, treatment of, 322
Dysproteinosis(es), 225
Dystonia, from chlorpromazine, 69
Dysuria, from sexually transmitted disorders, 419
  in urinary tract infection, 420
  postoperative, 108

Ear, anatomy and physiology of, 339–340, *339*
  disorders of, 342–343. *See also* Ototoxicity
Ecchymosis(es), defined, 217
  in hemorrhagic disorders, 226–227
Echothiophate, 118
Ectodermal disorder(s), from hypoparathyroidism, 306
Eczema, 444
Edema, defined, 260
  disorders associated with, 271–273
  drug-induced, 273
  from androgens, 325
  from hypothyroidism, 305
  in congestive heart failure, 166
  of pregnancy, 273
  premenstrual, 273
  treatment of, diuretics in, 261–263, 271–273
Edrophonium, adverse effects of, 117
  clinical indications for, 107, 117
  interaction of, with neuromuscular blocking agents, 117
  mechanism of action of, 117

Electrocardiography, 156–158, *156*
Electroconvulsive shock therapy, neuromuscular blocking agents in, 126–128
Electroencephalographic sleep wave(s), 17–18, *17*
Electrolyte(s), acetylcholine receptor and, 98–100
  adrenergic receptors and, 103–104
  antidiarrheal, 403
  balance of, renal system in, 269–270
  glucocorticoids and, 318
  imbalance of, from diuretics, 281–282
    treatment of, 274
  lithium carbonate and, 66
  replenishers of, 462*t*
Electrolyte/water balance, renal system in, 260, *261, 264–267, 266–267, 269–270*
Embolism, formation of, 217–218, 220
Embryonal carcinoma, 422
Emetrol, 405–406
Emodin, action of, 396
Emollient(s), 450
Emotion(s), central nervous system and, 6–8
  skin and, 440
  smell and, 7
  sweat and, 442
Emphysema, treatment of, 368
  types of, 343
Enalapril, as antihypertensive agent, 199
Encainide, 175
Encephalitis, 24
Endocarditis, 168
Endocrine disorder(s), 304–309
  from chlorpromazine, 69
  See also specific disorders
Endocrine gland(s), anatomy and physiology of, *291, 293–302, 296*
  dysfunction of, 304–309
  embryology of, 302
  in neuroendocrine system, 290, *290*
  interrelationship among, 291–293, *294–295*
  special aspects of, 303–304
  See also specific entities
Endocrine system, 289–331
  anatomy and physiology of, *291–292, 294–297, 293t, 298t,* 293–304
  central nervous system and, 4
  drugs affecting, 309–328
    drug interactions with, 328–330
  dysfunction of, 304–309
  hypothalamus and, 8
  in schizophrenia, 22
  introduction to, 290–293, *290–292, 294–295*
  summary of, 330–331
Endogenous depression, defined, 21
  treatment of, monoamine oxidase inhibitors in, 64–65
    tricyclic antidepressants in, 61–64
Endometrial adenocarcinoma, 421
Endometriosis, 421
  treatment of, 310, 322
    androgens in, 324
Endometritis, 420
Endometrium, hormones and, 300–301
Endoperoxide(s), in prostaglandin synthesis, 430
Endorphin(s), function of, 46
Endotoxin(s), defined, 353
Enflurane, 27
Enkephalin(s), function of, 16, 46
Entamoeba histolytica, 386

Enterococcus(i), endocarditis from, 199
Enterogastrone(s), in digestion, 379
Enteroglucagon, 302
Enteroniasis, 388
Enteropathy, gluten-sensitive, 387
Enuresis, nocturnal, 18
Environmental factor(s), in depression, 20
  in schizophrenia, 22
Enzyme(s), hepatic, barbiturates and, 33
  in neurotransmission, 9–10
  pain and, 14
  pancreatic, as digestive aids, 400
  schizophrenia and, 22–23
  streptomycin and, 362
  topical preparations of, 451
Eosinophil(s), anatomy of, 212
Ephedrine, 132–133
  interaction of, with dexamethasone, 328
    with monoamine oxidase inhibitors, 82
Epidermis, anatomy of, 440, 441
Epididymis, anatomy of, 417, 418
Epilepsy, 19–20
  grand mal, 19, 38–40, 43
  petit mal, 19, 38–43
  treatment of, 37–43. See also Anticonvulsant agent(s); specific agents
  See also Seizure(s)
Epinephrine, adverse effects of, 131
  biosynthesis of, 100, 100, 101
  blood pressure and, 167
  clinical indications for, 131
  function of, 299–300
  glucocorticoids and, 302–303
  in treatment, of asthma, 109
  insulin and, 308
  interaction of, with antihistamines, 371
    with beta-adrenergic blocking agents, 203
    with phenoxybenzamine, 138
  mechanism of action of, 130–131
    cardiac, 153
Epithelial stimulant(s), 450
Epsom salts, as laxative, 398–399
Epulis lesion(s), 382
Equilibrium, physiology of, 340
Ergonovine maleate, 432–433
Ergot alkaloid(s), 139, 432–433
  interaction of, with nitrates, 203
Ergotamine, 139
Erysipelas, 443
Erythrityl tetranitrate, 186–187
Erythrocyte(s), anatomy of, 211–212
  disorders of, 220–224
  formation of, 215–217
  pentoxifylline and, 240–241
Erythromycin, adverse effects of, 364
  clinical indications for, 363
    genitourinary, 429
  interaction of, with theophylline, 371
  mechanism of action of, 363
  topical, 448
Escherichia coli, antibiotics against, 406–407
  diarrhea from, 386
  urinary tract infection from, 419
    treatment of, 424–426, 428
Eserine. See Physostigmine
Esophageal ulcer, 108–109
Esophagitis, 383

Esophagus, anatomy of, 376–377, 378
  disorders of, 108–109, 383
Essential hypertension, defined, 168
Estradiol, 321t, 321
  interaction of, with barbiturates, 80
  See also Estrogen(s)
Estradiol, 321t, 321
Estramustine phosphate sodium, 434
Estrogen(s), clinical indications for, 307, 435
  drug interactions with, 329
  function of, 300–301
  preparations of, 320–321, 321t
  types of, 321
Ethacrynic acid, adverse effects of, 279
  clinical indications for, 278–279
  interaction of, with aminoglycosides, 371
Ethambutol, in tuberculosis treatment, 365
Ethanol. See Alcohol
Ethanolamine antihistamine(s), 348
Ethchlorvynol, adverse effects of, 36
  clinical indications for, 36
  interaction of, with alcohol and depressants, 79
    with coumarin anticoagulants, 80
    with tricyclic antidepressants, 80
  mechanism of action of, 36
Ethinamate, adverse effects of, 36–37
  clinical indications for, 36
  interaction of, with alcohol and depressants, 80
  mechanism of action of, 36
Ethosuximide, as anticonvulsant agent, 38, 40
Ethotoin, as anticonvulsant agent, 40
Ethylenediamine antihistamine(s), 349
Ethylnorepinephrine, 136
Etomidate, 29
Etretinate, 451–452
Eustachian tube, anatomy of, 339, 339
Exercise, cardiac reflexes in, 154, 154
  erythrocyte count and, 212
Exocytosis, in adrenergic neurotransmission, 101, 102
Exogenous depression, defined, 21
Exophthalmos, defined, 305
Exostosis, oral, 382
Exotoxin(s), defined, 353
Expectorant(s), 367t, 368–369
Extrapyramidal effect(s), of phenothiazines, 67–70
  of pimozide, 71
Extrasystole(s), 161
Eye, anatomy of, 106
  disorders of. See Ocular disorder(s); Visual disturbance(s); specific disorders

Factor VIII, in hemophilia treatment, 236
Factor IX complex, in hemophilia treatment, 237
Fallopian tube(s), anatomy of, 300
  disorders of, 419–420
Familial hyperchylomicroanemia, 227t, 227–228
Famotidine, in peptic ulcer treatment, 394
Fat metabolism, in diabetes mellitus, 307–308
  in digestion, 381
Fecal softener(s), 399
Feces, gastrointestinal ulcers and, 385
  in cholera, 386
Fentanyl, adverse effects of, 51
  clinical indications for, 51
  droperidol and, 29
Ferrous salt(s), in anemia treatment, 228t, 228–229

Fetal effect(s), of oxytocin, 314
    See also Teratogenicity
Fever, aspirin and, 453
    from carboprost tromethamine, 432
    in tuberculosis, 345
    San Joaquin, 346
Fever blister(s), defined, 382
Fibrillation, atrial, 162–163, *162*
    treatment of, 178
    ventricular, 165, *165*
    treatment of, 176
Fibrinogen, in hemostasis, 217, 218*t*
    pentoxifylline and, 241
Fibrinolytic system, 234, *234*
Fibroma(s), oral, 382
Fingernail(s), growth of, 442
First-dose syncope, from prazosin, 197
Flecainide, 174–175
Fleming, penicillin and, 355
Flight or fight reaction, defined, 300
Flory, penicillin and, 355
Floxuridine, clinical indications for, 409
Flucytosine, antifungal, 428
Fludrocortisone, 320
Fluid(s), replenishers of, 462*t*
5-Fluorocytosine, 428
Fluorouracil, clinical indications for, gastrointestinal, 409
    genitourinary, 434
Fluphenazine, 70
Flurazepam, adverse effects of, 31
    clinical indications for, 31
    interaction of, with alcohol, 31
        with alcohol and depressants, 80
Flushing, from nicotinic acid, 243
Focal seizure(s), defined, 19
Folic acid, deficiency of, anemia from, 222–223
        treatment of, 231–232
    dietary requirement of, 216
    in treatment, of anemia, 231–232
    interaction of, with phenytoin, 81, 253
        with pyrimethamine, 253
    sulfonamides and, 423, *424*
    vitamin B$_{12}$ and, 230–231, *230*
Folinic acid, 222
    interaction of, with methotrexate, 248
Follicle(s), graafian, 300
Follicle stimulating hormone, function of, 300–301
    mechanism of action of, 309
Food poisoning, staphylococcal, 386
Forebrain, anatomy of, 4
Formaldehyde, in urinary tract antiseptics, 425
Free fatty acid(s), function of, 213
Fructose, antiemetic, 405–406
    seminal, 418
Fulvicin, 450, 456
Fungal infection(s), dermatologic, 443
    respiratory, 345–346
        treatment of, 366
    stomatitis from, 382
Furosemide, adverse effects of, 279
    clinical importance of, 260
    clinical indications for, 278–279
    interaction of, with barbiturates, 81
        with chloral hydrate, 79
        with clofibrate, 255
        with indomethacin, 457
        with neuromuscular blocking agents, 145
        with phenytoin, 81
Furuncle(s), 443
    nasal, 342

Galactorrhea, dopaminergic receptors and, 295
Gallamine, 127
Gallbladder, disorders of, 389
    treatment of, 400–401
    in digestion, 381–382
Gallstone(s), formation of, 382, 389
    treatment of, 401
Gamma globulin, in rheumatoid arthritis, 446
Gamma-aminobutyric acid, barbiturates and, 32–33, *33*, 38
    benzodiazepines and, 31, 72–75
    in central nervous system, 13
    seizures and, 20
    thiopental and, 28
Ganglion(ganglia), autonomic, 93, 93–94
    receptors in, 124, *124*
    basal, 6
Ganglionic blocking agent(s), 123*t*–124*t*, 124–126
    as antihypertensive agents, 193
    drug interactions with, 145
Ganglionic stimulant(s), 124
Gastric motility, 379
Gastric secretion, 378–379
Gastric ulcer, 108
Gastrin, in digestion, 379
Gastritis, 383–384
Gastroesophageal reflux, 377
Gastrointestinal cancer, treatment of, 408–409, 409*t*
Gastrointestinal disorder(s), 382–389
    from amebicides, 427
    from antiarthritic agents, 453–456
    from anticancer agents, 246–250, 252, 434
        treatment of, 435
    from antifungal agents, 428
    from antihyperlipidemic agents, 242–244
    from anti-inflammatory agents, 453–454
    from antiparkinsonism agents, 78
    from aspirin, 453
    from clindamycin, 364
    from colchicine, 456
    from digitalis, 184
    from estrogens, 321
    from ethchlorvynol, 36
    from fluorouracil, 409
    from glucagon, 328
    from glucocorticoids, 320
    from iron, 229
    from morphine, 47–48
    from mucolytic agents, 368–369
    from narcotics, 47
    from pentoxifylline, 241
    from phensuximide, 41
    from phenytoin, 39
    from quinidine, 171
    from streptozocin, 408
    from tocainide, 174
    from trimethoprim, 424
    from uricosuric agents, 281
    from urinary antiseptics, 425–426
    from uterine-stimulating agents, 432–433
    from valproic acid, 42

from verapamil, 177
from vitamin K, 233
postoperative atony as, 107–108
treatment of, 389–410
atropine in, 120
drug interactions in, 410
glucocorticoids in, 319
muscarinic blocking agents in, 122–123
ulcers as, 108–109
Gastrointestinal effect(s), of parathormone, 299
Gastrointestinal muscle stimulant(s), 404
Gastrointestinal system. See Digestive/gastrointestinal system
Gastrolyte, antidiarrheal, 403
Gastroparesis, treatment of, 404
Gate theory of pain, 15, 16
G-cell(s), defined, 379
Gelatin, absorbable, 235–236
Gemfibrozil, as antihyperlipidemic agent, 244
General anesthetic agent(s), 25–29, 25t, 25
intravenous, 28–29
volatile, 26–28
See also specific agents
Genetic factor(s), in Alzheimer's disease, 23
in breast cancer, 422
in diabetes mellitus, 308
in schizophrenia, 22
Genetic mutation(s), from antineoplastic agents, 246–247
Genital disorder(s), 419–423
from cimetidine, 393
from mumps, 383
treatment of, estrogen in, 321
See also specific disorders
Genitourinary system. See Reproductive/genitourinary system
Gentamicin, adverse effects of, 362
clinical indications for, 362
interaction of, with amphotericin B, 370
with cephalothin, 371
Germ cell tumor(s), 422
Ghon focus, in tuberculosis, 345
Giardiasis, 386
Gigantism, pituitary, 304
Gingival hyperplasia, from phenytoin, 39
Gingivostomatitis, herpetic, 382
Gland(s), adrenal. See Adrenal gland(s)
endocrine. See Endocrine gland(s); specific entities
mammary. See Mammary gland(s)
parathyroid. See Parathyroid gland(s)
pituitary. See Pituitary gland
salivary, 376, 378, 382–383
sweat, 442
thyroid. See Thyroid gland(s)
Glare phenomenon, from trimethadione, 41
Glaucoma, 106–107
diazepam and, 74
treatment of, carbonic anhydrase inhibitors in, 276
cholinergic agents in, 112–118
timolol in, 141
tricyclic antidepressants in, 62
Globin, synthesis of, 216
Glomerular filtration, 264
Glomerular filtration rate, defined, 264
thiazide diuretics and, 277
xanthines and, 280
Glomerulonephritis, treatment of, 272–273

Glucagon, adverse effects of, 328
clinical indications for, 326–328
function of, 302
mechanism of action of, 327
Glucocorticoid(s), as antineoplastic agents, 252
epinephrine and, 302–303
function of, 299
interaction of, with somatotropin, 328
preparations of, adverse effects of, 320
clinical indications for, 318–320
dosages of, 319t
mechanism of action of, 318
risk-to-benefit ratio and, 320
Gluconeogenesis, epinephrine and, 300
in diabetes mellitus, 308
Glucose, antiemetic, 405–406
function of, 302
hormonal mechanisms and, 290–291
in hypoglycemia treatment, 326
insulin and, 325
Glue ear, defined, 343
Glutamic acid, in blood clotting, 237
Gluten-sensitive enteropathy, 387
Glutethimide, adverse effects of, 36
clinical indications for, 36
interaction of, with alcohol and depressants, 79
with anticoagulants, 254
with coumarin anticoagulants, 79
with other anticholinergic agents, 79
mechanism of action of, 36
Glycerin, as laxative, 399
dosage of, 275t
Glyceryl guiacolate, 368–369
Glycine pathway(s), central nervous system, 13
Glycinexylidide, 173
Glycogen, adrenergic receptors and, 105
Glycoside(s), cardiac, 178t, 178–184
See also Digitalis glycoside(s)
Gold compound(s), in arthritis treatment, 455
Gonad(s), anatomy and physiology of, 300–301
function of, abnormal, 307
Gonadotropin(s), chronologic patterns and, 303–304
function of, 301
human menopausal, 309–310
Gonorrhea, 419
Gout, treatment of, 274, 454–456
uricosuric agents in, 280–281
Graafian follicle, 300
Gram stain, bacteria classification by, 351
Grand mal seizure(s), defined, 19
treatment of, 38–40, 43
Granulocyte(s), anatomy of, 212
Graves' disease, 305
Gray syndrome, from chloramphenicol, 406
Griseofulvin, 450
interaction of, with anticoagulants, 456
with barbiturates, 456
Growth hormone, adverse effects of, 311
clinical indications for, 311
dysfunctional, 304
genetically engineered, 312
in diabetes mellitus, 308
mechanism of action of, 311
Guaifenesin, as mucolytic agent, 368–369
Guanabenz, as antihypertensive agent, 192
Guanadrel, as antihypertensive agent, 193–194

Guanethidine, as adrenergic blocking agent, 143
  as antihypertensive agent, 194
  interaction of, with anticholinergics, 144
    with tricyclic antidepressants, 204
  neurotransmission and, 95
Guanfacine, as antihypertensive agent, 192
Gynecomastia, from digitalis, 184

Hair, anatomy of, 440, *441*
  follicles of, *441*, 442–443
  growth of, 442
    stimulants of, 451
  minoxidil and, 196
Halazepam, 74
Hallucination(s), in schizophrenia, 22
Haloalkylamine(s), 137–138, *138*
Haloperidol, adverse effects of, 71
  as adrenergic blocking agents, 140
  clinical indications for, 71
  interaction of, with amphetamine, 83
    with lithium carbonate, 82
  mechanism of action of, 71
Halothane, adverse effects of, 26–27
  clinical indications for, 26
  interaction of, with bronchodilators, 145
  mechanism of action of, 26
Harvey, vascular anatomy and, 158
Hay fever, 340
Head injury(ies), morphine and, 48
  pentazocine and, 52
Headache(s), cluster, 111
  migraine, 110–111
  treatment of, 139
Hearing, disordered. See Ototoxicity
  physiology of, 339–340
Heart, anatomy and physiology of, 150, *151–158*, 152–158
  calcium channels in, 188–189, *188–189*
  disorders of. See Cardiac disorder(s); specific disorders
  electrophysiology of, 155–158, *156–158*
  nerves of, 153, *153*
  reflexes of, 153–155, *153–155*
Heart attack, symptoms of, 167
Heart failure, congestive. See Congestive heart failure
Heart rate, digitalis and, 182
Heartbeat(s), normal, 152
Heavy chain disease, 225
Helminthiasis, 376, 388–389
  treatment of, 410*t*
Hematologic disorder(s), 220–228
  from anticancer agents, 434
  treatment of, glucocorticoids in, 319
    malignant, 244*t*–245*t*, 244, 246–252
Hemoglobin, function of, 215–216
  in anemia, 220
    sickle cell, 216
Hemophilia, desmopressin in, 314
  genetic factor in, 220
  treatment of, 236–237
Hemophilus influenzae, antibiotics against, 358–359, 363, 365
Hemoptysis, in respiratory cancer, 347
  in tuberculosis, 345
Hemorrhage, from anticoagulants, 238–239
  from oxytocin, 314
  in gastrointestinal ulcers, 383–385
  in typhoid fever, 385

  postpartum, 433
  treatment of, 234–236
  urinary tract, 234
Hemorrhagic disorder(s), 226–227
Hemorrheologic agent(s), 240–241
Hemorrhoid(s), 387
  treatment of, 404
Hemostasis, defined, 217
  drugs promoting, drug interactions with, 253
  drugs promoting, 233–236, 233*t*, 234
Hemostat, microfibrillar collagen, 235
Hemostatic agent(s), 232–239, 233*t*, 237*t*, 232–234
Henle's loop, 264–266, *265*
  loop diuretics and, 278
Heparin, adverse effects of, 239
  antagonist of, 239–240
  clinical indications for, 239
  interaction of, with anticoagulants, 254
  mechanism of action of, 220, 239
Hepatic carcinoma, 325, 389
Hepatic cirrhosis, digestion and, 389
  potassium-sparing diuretics in, 280
  treatment of, 272
Hepatic coma, from diuretics, 272, 278
Hepatic disorder(s), benzodiazepines and, 73
  clomiphene and, 310
  digestive, 389
  from acetaminophen, 456
  from asparaginase, 252
  from ketoconazole, 366
  from nitrofurantoin, 426
  loop diuretics in, 279
  malignant, 325, 389
  methyldopa in, 193
  thiazide diuretics and, 278
  See also specific disorders
Hepatic enzyme(s), barbiturates and, 33
Hepatic failure, from valproic acid, 42
  in acquired immune deficiency syndrome, 226
Hepatitis, from halothane, 27
  from isoniazid, 360
  from paraldehyde, 35
  from phenacemide, 43
  viral, 389
Hepatosplenomegaly, in leukemia, 224
Hernia, hiatus, 383
Heroin, history of, 45
Herpes simplex virus infection(s), 443
  dermatologic, 443
  genital, 419
  stomatitis from, 382
  treatment of, 427
Herpes zoster virus infection(s), 443
Hetacillin, 428
Hexamethonium, 125
Hexamethylenetetramine, 425
Hiatus hernia, 383
Hiker's diarrhea, 386
Hindbrain, anatomy of, 4
Hirsutism, from androgens, 324–325
  from phenytoin, 40
His bundle, digitalis and, 181–182
  in cardiac electrophysiology, 155–156, *156*
Histamine, antihistamines and, 347
  asthma and, 109
  biosynthesis of, 341, *341*

in allergy, 340–341
  interaction of, with anticholinergics, 144
  migraine and, 110–111
  pain and, 14
Histamine receptor blocking agent(s). See Antihistamine(s); specific agents
Histamine receptor(s), in allergy, 340–341, 341
  in digestion, 379
Histidine, in histamine synthesis, 341, 341
Histoplasmosis, pulmonary, 346
Hive(s), 444
Hodgkin's disease, 225–226
  treatment of, 246–247, 250–252
Homatropine, 122
Homeostasis, hypothalamus and, 8
Hookworm infestation, 388
Hormone release factor(s), 293t
Hormone(s), adrenal cortical stimulating. See Adrenocorticostimulating hormone
  alterations in, in depression and, 21
  anterior pituitary, 296–297, 298t
  antidiuretic. See Vasopressin
  biological clock and, 303–304
  clinical indications for, in genitourinary cancer, 435
    rationale for, 304
  defined, 290
  follicle stimulating, 300–301, 309
  gastrointestinal, 379
  hypothalamus and, 8
  in schizophrenia, 22
  interaction of, with insulin, 329
  interrelationship among, 291–293, 294–295
  interstitial cell-stimulating, 300–301, 309
  luteinizing, 300–301, 309
  mechanism of action of, 290–293, 291–292, 294–295, 293t
  melanocyte-stimulating, 294
  pancreatic. See Pancreatic hormone(s); specific hormones
  pituitary. See Pituitary hormone(s); specific hormones
  posterior pituitary, 297–298
  releasing, 294–295. See also specific hormones
  sex. See Sex hormone(s); specific hormones
  sweat glands and, 442
  thyroid. See Thyroid hormone(s)
  thyroid stimulating, 298
  triglycerides and, 213
Human chorionic gonadotropin, adverse effects of, 310
  clinical indications for, 309–310
  function of, 301
Human immunodeficiency virus, 226
Human menopausal gonadotropin(s), 309–310
Hydantoin(s), as anticonvulsant agents, 39–40
  structure of, 37, 37
  See also specific agents
Hydatidiform mole, treatment of, 432
Hydralazine, as antihypertensive agent, 195, 195
  interaction of, with propranolol, 195
    with thiazide diuretics, 204–205
Hydrochloric acid, antacids and, 390–391
  in digestion, 378–379
  in gastrointestinal ulcers, 383–384
Hydrochlorothiazide, clinical indications for, 277, 280
Hydrocodone, 50
Hydrocortisone, adverse effects of, 320
  clinical indications for, 318–320
  interaction of, with cholestyramine, 328

lithium carbonate and, 66
  mechanism of action of, 318
Hydromorphone, 49
Hydroxyamphetamine, 135
Hydroxychloroquine sulfate, 455
p-Hydroxynorephedrine, dextroamphetamine and, 54
Hydroxyperoxyeicosatetraenaic acid(s), in prostaglandin synthesis, 430, 431
5-HT,5-Hydroxytryptamine pathway(s), 11–12, 12
Hydroxyurea, as antineoplastic agent, hematologic, 251
Hydroxyzine, 75–76
Hymen, anatomy of, 416
l-Hyoscine, 121
l-Hyoscyamine, 121
Hyoscyamus niger, 119, 121
Hyperactivity, in attention deficit disorder, 23
Hypercalcemia, treatment of, 317
Hyperchloremia, from diuretics, 282
Hypercholesterolemia, treatment of, 241–243
Hyperchylomicroanemia, 227t, 227–228
Hyperglycemia, adrenergic receptors and, 105
  from epinephrine, 131
  from thiazide diuretics, 278
  in diabetes mellitus, 307–308
Hyperinsulinemia, 309
Hyperkalemia, from diuretics, 280, 282
Hyperlipidemia(s), adrenergic receptors and, 105
  treatment of, 241–244, 241t
Hyperlipoproteinemia(s), 227–228
  treatment of, 243–244
  types of, 227t
Hyperparathyroidism, 306
Hypersensitivity, to amobarbital, 34
  to antihemophilic agents, 236
  to asparaginase, 252
  to cephalosporins, 359
  to iron dextran, 230
  to loperamide, 403
  to penicillin, 357–358
  to pentobarbital, 3
  to phenobarbital, 35
  to sulfonamides, 424
  to tocainide, 174
  to vitamin B_{12}, 231
  to vitamin K, 233
  treatment of, epinephrine in, 131
  types of, 340
Hypertension, 167–168
  defined, 167
  essential, 168
  from oxytocin, 314
  in congestive heart failure, 166
  in polycythemia vera, 223
  incidence of, 168
  influences on, 167–168
  perioperative, 187
  rebound, 192
  treatment of, 190–199
    alpha-adrenergic blocking agents in, 137–139
    beta-adrenergic blocking agents in, 140–143
    diuretics in, 273–274
    nicotinic blocking agents in, 125–126
    regimen for, 199, 199
Hypertensive crisis, treatment of, 196
Hyperthermia, malignant, 27, 128

Hyperthyroidism, 305
    treatment of, 316–317
Hyperuricemia, from chlorambucil, 246
    treatment of, 274
        uricosuric agents in, 280–281
Hypervitaminosis A, 451–452
Hypodermis, anatomy of, 440, 441
Hypoglycemia, from insulin, 325
    treatment of, 326
    from sulfonylureas, 327
Hypoglycemic agent(s). See Antidiabetic agent(s)
Hypogonadism, female, 321
    male, 324
Hypokalemia, from diuretics, 278–279, 281–282
Hyponatremia, from diuretics, 282
Hypoparathyroidism, 305–306
Hypophyseal portal system, 296, 297
Hypophysis. See Pituitary gland
Hypopituitarism, female, 321
    male, 324
Hypopituitary dwarfism, 304
Hypoprothrombinemia, vitamin K in, 232–233
Hypotension, from antihypertensive agents, 193–197
    from antiparkinsonism agents, 78
    from bretylium tosylate, 176
    from isoflurane, 27
Hypothalamus, anatomy and physiology of, 7–8, 8
    in autonomic nervous system, 94
    in schizophrenia, 22
    levodopa and, 78
    pituitary gland and, 294–296, 296–297
Hypothyroidism, 30
    treatment of, 315–316
Hypoxia, cardiac arrhythmias in, 161
    in congestive heart failure, 165

Ileum, in digestion, 381
Ileus, adynamic, 107–108
Ilopan, 404
Imbalance hypothesis of depression, 21
Imipramine, adverse effects of, 63
    clinical indications for, 63
    history of, 59
    structure of, 59, 59
Immune system, in acquired immune deficiency syndrome, 226
    in asthma, 109
    lymphocytes in, 210, 212, 214–215
    thymus gland in, 214–215
    tonsils in, 214
Immunization, against acquired immune deficiency syndrome, 226
    agents in, 464t
Immunoglobulin E, in hypersensitivity reactions, 340
Immunologic agent(s), 464t
Immunosuppression, from mechlorethamine, 246
Immunosuppressive agent(s), 465t
Impetigo, 442–443
Indanedione(s), anticoagulant, 239
Indoleamine hypothesis of depression and mania, 20
Indomethacin, interaction of, with anticoagulants, 457
    with bumetanide, 456–457
    with captopril, 203, 457
    with corticosteroids, 329, 457
    with furosemide, 457
    with lithium carbonate, 457
    with loop diuretics, 284
    with prazosin, 204
    with triamterene, 457
Infection(s), cardiac, 168
    treatment of, 199
    central nervous system, 24
    chlamydial, 419
    cholangitis from, 389
    diarrhea from, 385–386
    ear, 342–343
    fungal. See Fungal infection(s); specific disorders
    gastrointestinal, treatment of, 406–408
    genitourinary, 419–420
    glaucoma from, 107
    hepatitis from, 389
    herpes virus, 419, 427, 443
    in acquired immune deficiency syndrome, 226
    in diabetes mellitus, 308
    in leukocyte disorders, 224–225
    laryngotracheal, 342
    leukocytes in, 212–213
    nasal, 342
    parasitic, 376, 444
    respiratory. See Respiratory infection(s)
    skin, 442–443
    stomatitis from, 382
    treatment of, glucocorticoids in, 319
    urinary tract, 420–421, 423–426
    vascular fragility from, 226
    venereal, 419–420
    See also Viral infection(s); specific disorders
Infectious mononucleosis, 342
Infertility, treatment of, 309–310
Inflammatory disorder(s), treatment of, 318–320
    See also specific disorders
Inhalation anesthetic agent(s), 25t, 26–28
    interaction of, with neuromuscular blocking agents, 145
Injury(ies), in organic brain psychosis, 21
    vascular, 217
Inotropism, defined, 153
    from digitalis, 179
Insomnia, 18–19
    causes of, 19
    from central nervous system stimulants, 55–56
    incidence of, 16
    treatment of, antihistamines in, 347
        ethchlorvynol in, 36
        ethinamate in, 36
        flurazepam in, 31
        glutethimide in, 36
        methyprylon in, 36
        pentobarbital in, 33
        phenobarbital in, 35
        talbutal in, 34
        temazepam in, 31
        triazolam in, 31
Insulin, adverse effects of, 325–326
    clinical indications for, 325
    dosages of, 326t
    drug interactions with, miscellaneous, 329
    epinephrine and, 308
    function of, 302
    in treatment, of diabetes mellitus, 308, 325, 326t
    interaction of, with beta-adrenergic blocking agents, 329
        with bronchodilators, 145
        with cardiac glycosides, 329

with metoprolol, 143
with other hormones, 329
with propranolol, 140
with thiazide diuretics, 329
mechanism of action of, 325
secretion of, 302
in diabetes mellitus, 308
smoking and, 330
types of, 325, 326t
Insulin receptor(s), hormones and, 290–291
Integumentary/connective tissue system, 439–457
anatomy and physiology of, 441–442, 441
disorders of, 442–446
See also specific disorders
drugs in, 446–457
introduction to, 440
summary of, 457
Intermittent claudication, treatment of, 241
Interstitial cell-stimulating hormone, 300–301, 309
Intestine, large. See Colon
small, 379–381, 380
Intestine(s), disorders of, 384–389
Intestino-intestinal reflex, in adynamic ileus, 107–108
Intracranial pressure, morphine and, 48
pentazocine and, 52
Intravenous anesthetic agent(s), 25t, 28–29
See also specific agents
Iodide, interaction of, with gallamine, 127
with metocurine, 127
thiazide diuretics and, 277
See also Iodine
Iodination reaction, defined, 298
Iodine, adverse effects of, 369
hypothyroidism and, 305
Lugol's solution of, 316
mucolytic preparations of, 367t, 369
thyroid gland and, 298, 303
topical, 450
See also Iodide
Ion flux(es), cardiac, 156–158, 157
Ipratropium bromide, 368
Iproniazid, history of, 57
Iron, deficiency of, 215–217, 221
treatment of, 228t–229t, 228–230
dietary requirements of, 215, 221
in treatment, of anemia, 228–230, 228t
interaction of, with allopurinol, 457
with antacids, 253, 410
with chloramphenicol, 253
with penicillamine, 253
with tetracycline, 253
metabolism of, 215–216, 216
overdose of, 229
Iron dextran, in anemia treatment, 228t, 229–230
Islets of Langerhans, anatomy of, 301–302
Isocarboxazid, 64
Isoetharine, 136
Isofluorophate, 118
Isoflurane, 27
Isoniazid, adverse effects of, 360
clinical indications for, 57, 360
interaction of, with phenytoin, 81
Isoproterenol, adrenergic receptors and, 104, 104
adverse effects of, 135–136
as beta-adrenergic receptor, 95, 104, 104
clinical indications for, 135

in digitalis toxicity, 184
interaction of, with decongestants, 146
mechanism of action of, 135
Isoquinoline, structure of, 45
Isosorbide, dosage of, 275t
Isosorbide dinitrate, 186–187
Isotretinoin, 450–451

Jacksonian seizure(s), defined, 19
Jaundice, digestion and, 389
Jejunum, anatomy of, 380–381, 380
Jock itch, 443
Joint(s), anatomy and physiology of, 441–442
disorders of, 445–446, 446t, 445, 447
treatment of, 453–456
See also Arthritis entries
Juvenile onset diabetes, 308

Kabikinase, 240
Kanamycin, 362
Kaolin, as antidiarrheal, 401
interaction of, with pseudoephedrine, 410
Kaolin-pectin, interaction of, with digitalis, 202
with lincomycin, 371
Keratolytic agent(s), 451
Ketamine, 28–29
interaction of, with thyroid preparations, 328
Ketoacidosis, causes of, 325
in diabetes mellitus, 307–308
Ketoconazole, 428
in respiratory infections, 366
Ketone body(ies), in diabetes mellitus, 325
Kidney, anatomy and physiology of, 263–271, 262–263, 265–267, 269, 271
disorders of. See Renal disorder(s)
See also Renal entries

Labetalol, 143
as antihypertensive agent, 197
Labor, induction of, 314, 431–432
Labyrinth, ear, 339–340, 339
Lactation, androgens and, 324
oxytocin and, 314
Lactic dehydrogenase, valproic acid and, 42
Lactobacillus(i), antidiarrheal, 402
Lactulose, as stool softener, 399
Langerhans, islets of, 301–302
Larva migrans, cutaneous, 388
Laryngotracheobronchitis, acute, 342
Larynx, benign lesions of, 347
cancer of, 347
Laughing gas, 27–28
Laxative(s), 394–399, 396t
bulk, 398
drug interactions with, 410
fecal softeners as, 399
interaction of, with vitamin A, 410
lubricant, 397–398
saline, 398–399
stimulant, 395–397
synthetic cellulose, 398
Laxative/antidiarrheal agent(s), 403
Legionella pneumophila, 344
Legionnaire's disease, 344
treatment of, 363
Lennox-Gastaut syndrome, treatment of, 43
Leucovorin, 222

Leukemia, 224–225
　from melphalan, 247
　in polycythemia vera, 223–224
　treatment of, 246–252
Leukocyte(s), anatomy of, 212–213
　disorders of, 224–226
　formation of, 215
　in leukemia, 225
　types of, 212
Leukoplakia, oral cancer and, 382–383, 445
Leukotriene(s), in prostaglandin synthesis, 430
　rheumatoid arthritis and, 446
Leuprolide, 435
Levodopa, adverse effects of, 78
　clinical indications for, 78
　interaction of, with benzodiazepines, 83
　　with methionine, 83
　　with methyldopa, 204
　　with monoamine oxidase inhibitors, 82
　　with pyridoxine, 83
　mechanism of action of, 78
Levorphanol, 50
Levothyroxine, preparations of, 314–315
Leydig cell(s), 301
Lidocaine, as antiarrhythmic agent, 173
　electrophysiologic effects of, 173, *173*
　in digitalis toxicity, 184
　interaction of, with beta-adrenergic blocking agents, 200
　　with cimetidine, 200
　　with disopyramide, 200
　　with neuromuscular blocking agents, 200
　　with phenytoin, 200
　tocainide and, 174
Limbic system, anatomy and physiology of, 7, *7*
　in autonomic nervous system, 94
　meprobamate and, 76
　opiate receptors and, 46
Lincomycin, 364
　interaction of, with kaolin-pectin, 371
Lindane, 451
Liothyronine, preparations of, 314–315
Liotrix, 315–316
Lipid pneumonia, mineral oil and, 398
Lipid(s), bacterial, 351
　plasma, 213
Lipid solubility, of barbiturates, 32
Lipodystrophy, intestinal, 388
Lipogenase pathway, in prostaglandin synthesis, 430, *431*
Lipoprotein(s), function of, 213
　types of, 213, *214*
Lithium carbonate, adverse effects of, 66–67
　clinical indications for, 66
　interaction of, with haloperidol, 82
　　with indomethacin, 457
　　with methyldopa, 204
　　with neuromuscular blocking agents, 83
　　with phenothiazines, 82
　　with piroxicam, 83, 457
　　with thiazide diuretics, 283–284
　mechanism of action of, 66
Liver, anatomy of, 381–382
　disorders of. *See* Hepatic disorder(s); specific disorders
　in digestion, 381–382
　iron metabolism and, 215
Lobar pneumonia, defined, 344
Lobeline, 125

Local anesthetic agent(s), 29
　topical, 447
　See also specific agent(s)
Loewi, acetylcholine studies of, 96–97
Lomustine, in cancer treatment, 247
Loop diuretic(s), 278–279, 278*t*
　adverse effects of, 279
　clinical indications for, 278–279
　interaction of, with aminoglycoside antibiotics, 284
　　with cephaloridine, 284
　　with chloral hydrate, 284
　　with clofibrate, 284
　　with corticosteroids, 284
　　with digitalis, 284
　　with indomethacin, 284
　　with lithium carbonate, 284
　mechanism of action of, 278
Loperamide, as antidiarrheal, 403
Lorazepam, 74–75
Louse(lice), infestation with, 444
Lovastatin, as cholesterol-lowering agent, 243
Lown-Ganong-Levine syndrome, 163
Loxapine, 72
Lugol's solution, 316
Lumbago, defined, 441
Lumpy jaw, defined, 346
Lung(s), anatomy of, 336–338, *337–338*
　disorders of. *See* Pulmonary disorder(s); Respiratory disorder(s); specific disorders
　in circulatory system, 210–211, *211*
Lupron, 435
Lupus erythematosus, discoid, 445
　systemic, 446
　treatment of, 455
Lupus vulgaris, 443
Luteinizing hormone, function of, 300, 301
　mechanism of action of, 309
Lymphoma, Burkitt's, 224
Lymph node(s), sites of, 210
Lymphatic system, anatomy of, 213–215
　function of, 210, 213–214
Lymphocyte(s), in immune system, 210, 212, 214–215
　types of, 212
Lymphocytic leukemia, 224
Lymphoma(s), 224
　treatment of, 246–252
Lypressin, 313–314

Macroglobulinemia, Waldenstrom's, 225
Macrolide antibiotic(s), 363–364
Macrophage(s), anatomy of, 212
Magaldrate, as antacid, 392
Magnesium aluminum hydroxide, 410
Magnesium aluminum silicate, 402
Magnesium hydroxide, 391
Magnesium sulfate, as laxative, 398–399
　in obstetrics, 433
Magnesium trisilicate, 391–392
Malabsorption syndrome(s), celiac sprue as, 387
Malathion, 451
Malignancy(ies). *See* Cancer; specific tumors
Malignant hyperthermia, from halothane, 27
　from succinylcholine, 128
Malignant melanoma, 445
Malpighi, vascular anatomy and, 158

Mammary gland(s), cancer of, 324, 422, 433–435
  oxytocin and, 297
Mania, 21
Manic depression, treatment of, 66–67
  chlorpromazine in, 68
Mannitol, clinical indications for, 275, 282–283
Maprotiline, 65
Marey's law, defined, 159
Marijuana derivative(s), 435
Marinol, 435
Masculinization, from androgens, 324–325
Mastoiditis, 343
Mature onset diabetes, 308
Mecamylamine, 125
  as antihypertensive agent, 193
  interaction of, with decongestants, 146
    with ganglionic blocking agents, 145
Mechanoreceptor(s), pain and, 14
Mechlorethamine, in cancer treatment, 246
Mecillinam, 428–429
Meclizine, 350
Medial forebrain bundle, anatomy and physiology of, 8
Medulla oblongata, in autonomic nervous system, 91, 93–94
  in cardiac anatomy, 153–155, 153–155
Medullary depression, in anesthesia, 26
Megaloblast(s), defined, 222
Melanocyte-stimulating hormone(s), origin of, 294
Melanoma, malignant, 445
Melanosis coli, from cascara segrada, 397
Melphalan, in cancer treatment, 246
Menadione. See Vitamin K
Meningitis, 24
  treatment of, 423
Meninx(meninges), anatomy of, 5
Menopausal syndrome, 307
Menotropin(s), 309–310
Menstrual cycle, hormonal influences on, 300–301
  in gonadal hypofunction, 307
Meperidine, adverse effects of, 50
  clinical indications for, 50
  interaction of, with monoamine oxidase inhibitors, 82
  mechanism of action of, 50
Mephenteramine, 134–135
Mephenytoin, as anticonvulsant agent, 40
Mephobarbital, 35
  adverse effects of, 35
  as anticonvulsant agent, 39
  mechanism of action of, 35, 39
Meprobamate, 76
Mercaptopurine, in cancer treatment, 249
  interaction of, with allopurinol, 255, 457
Mersalyl, theophylline and, 280
Mesentery, anatomy of, 380
Mesolimbic pathway, in neurotransmission, 11
Metaproterenol, 136
Metaraminol, 134
Methacholine, 112
Methadone, 51
Methamine, as urinary tract antiseptic, 425
Methandrostenolone, interaction of, with corticosteroids, 329
  with oxyphenbutazone, 329
Metharbital, as anticonvulsant agent, 39
Methemoglobinemia, from bismuth, 406

Methenamine, interaction of, with acetazolamide, 435
  with carbonic anhydrase inhibitors, 283
  with sodium bicarbonate, 435
  with sulfonamides, 435
Methicillin, adverse effects of, 358
Methimazole, 317
Methionine, interaction of, with levodopa, 83
Methohexital, clinical indications for, 29
Methotrexate, clinical indications for, genitourinary, 434
  hematologic, 248–249
  in psoriasis, 451
  interaction of, with salicylates, 255
    with vaccinations, 255
Methoxamine, 135
Methoxyflurane, adverse effects of, 27
  clinical indications for, 27
  interaction of, with tetracyclines, 372
  mechanism of action of, 27
Methscopolamine, 122
Methsuximide, as anticonvulsant agent, 40–41
Methylcellulose, as laxative, 398
Methyldopa, as adrenergic inhibitor, 143
  as antihypertensive agent, 192–193
  interaction of, with decongestants, 146
    with levodopa, 204
    with lithium, 204
Methyldopate, as antihypertensive agent, 193
Methylergonovine maleate, 433
Methylhistamine, 341, 341
alpha-Methylnorepinephrine, 192–193
Methylphenidate, adverse effects of, 56
  clinical indications for, 56
  interaction of, with tricyclic antidepressants, 82
  mechanism of action of, 55
N-Methylphenobarbital, 3, 39
Methylprednisone, in rhinitis treatment, 369
Methyltetrahydrofolate, in anemia, 230–231, 230
Methylxanthine(s), as bronchodilators, 367–368, 367t
  clinical indications for, 55
  structure of, 55
Methyprylon, adverse effects of, 36
  clinical indications for, 36
  interaction of, with alcohol and depressants, 79
  mechanism of action of, 36
Methysergide, 139
Metoclopramide, adverse effects of, 114
  clinical indications for, 114
    gastrointestinal, 404
    in cancer therapy, 435
  interaction of, with digitalis, 202
  mechanism of action of, 114
Metocurine, 127
Metoprolol, 142–143
  as antihypertensive agent, 197–198
  interaction of, with insulin, 143
  postmyocardial infarction, 190
Metronidazole, clinical indications for, 408
  urinary tract, 426–427
  interaction of, with alcohol, 408, 435
    with disulfiram, 435
Metyrosine, 144
Mevalonic acid, clofibrate and, 243
Mevinolin, 243
Mexiletine, 174
Miconazole, 428
  in respiratory infections, 366

Microangiopathy, in diabetes mellitus, 308
Microfibrillar collagen hemostat, 235
Microvillus(i), anatomy of, 380–381, *381*
Midbrain, anatomy of, 4
Migraine, 110–111
 caffeine in, 55
 ergot alkaloids in, 139
Milk, interaction of, with tetracylcines, 372
Milk anemia, 221
Milk of magnesia, 391
Milk-alkali syndrome, 391
Mineral oil, as lubricant laxative, 397–398
 interaction of, with vitamin A, 410
Mineralocorticoid(s), function of, 299
 preparations of, 320
  dosages of, 319*t*
Minocycline, 362–363
Minoxidil, as antihypertensive agent, 195–196
Miotic agent(s), cholinergic agents as, 112–113, 116, 118
 drug interactions with, 144
 in treatment, of glaucoma, 107
Mite(s), scabies from, 444
Mitochondrion(mitochondria), in neurotransmission, 9
Mitomycin, 409
Mitosis, cancer therapy and, 244, *245*
Mole(s), in malignant melanoma, 445
Molindone, 71–72
Monday disease, defined, 187
Moniliasis. *See* Candidiasis
Monoamine oxidase, in catecholamine catabolism, 101–102
Monoamine oxidase inhibitor(s), 57*t*, 64–65
 adrenergic effects of, 144
 interaction of, with alcohol, 82
  with amitriptyline, 61
  with amphetamines, 81–82
  with anticholinergics, 145
  with antihistamines, 371
  with barbiturates, 80
  with bronchodilators, 145
  with decongestants, 145–146
  with ephedrine, 82
  with levodopa, 82
  with meperidine, 82
  with phenothiazines, 82
  with phenylpropanolamine, 82
  with reserpine, 204
  with tricyclic antidepressants, 82
 mechanism of action of, 57, 59
 See also specific agents
Monoamine(s), antidepressants and, 57, 59–61
 in neurotransmission, 9
Monocyte(s), anatomy of, 212
Monoethylglycinexylidide, 173
Mononucleosis, infectious, 342
Morphine, adverse effects of, 48
 clinical indications for, 48
 codeine versus, 49
 hydromorphone versus, 49
 interaction of, with scopolamine, 121
 mechanism of action of, 47–48
 methadone versus, 51
 opiate receptors and, 45–46, *46*
 opium composition and, 44–45
 oxymorphone versus, 49
 structure of, 45–46, *45*

Motion sickness, treatment of, 349–350
 scopolamine in, 121
Mouth, anatomy of, 376, *377–378*
 disorders of, 382–383
Moxalactam, 359
Mucolytic agent(s), 367*t*, 368–369
Mucormycosis, 342
Mucosal block phenomenon, iron metabolism and, 215, *216*
Mucus, expectorants and, 368–369
Multiple myeloma, 225
 treatment of, 246
Mumps, 383
Muscarinic acetylcholine receptor, 98–100, *100*
Muscarinic blocking agent(s), 118–123, 119*t*
 dosages of, 119*t*
 drug interactions with, 144–145
 naturally occurring, 118–123, 119*t*
 synthetic, 119*t*, 123
Muscle relaxant(s). *See* Neuromuscular blocking agent(s)
Muscle(s), arterial, 159
 calcium channels and, 188–189, *188–189*
 bronchial, 336
 gastrointestinal, 404
 in anesthesia, 26
 in congestive heart failure, 165–166
 skeletal, blood flow and, 160
  functions of, 441
 uterine, 429–433
 vascular, antianginal agents and, 186
Muscular disorder(s), from diuretics, 281
 from hyperparathyroidism, 306
 from hypoparathyroidism, 306
 in myasthenia gravis, 107
 in parkinsonism, 24
Muscular effect(s), autonomic, 92, 92*t*
 of adrenergic receptors, 103–104
 of androgens, 324
 of atropine, 119–120
 of etomidate, 29
 of neuromuscular blocking agents, 126–128
Myasthenia gravis, 107
 disopyramide and, 172
 streptomycin and, 361
 treatment of, 116–117
Mycobacterium tuberculosis, 345
 endometritis from, 420
Mycoplasma, antibiotics against, 363
Mycoplasma pneumonia, 345
Myelogenous leukemia, 224
Myocardial depression, from disopyramide, 172
Myocardial infarction, aspirin and, 240
 course of, 189
 drugs given after, 189–190
 in hyperlipoproteinemia, 228
 propranolol and, 140
 symptoms of, 167
 See also Cardiac disorder(s)
Myocardium, anatomy of, 152
 in congestive heart failure, 165–166
 in coronary artery disease, 166–167
Myoclonic seizure(s), defined, 19
Myxedema, 305
 treatment of, 315–316

Nadolol, 141
 as antianginal agent, 187–188
 as antihypertensive agent, 198

Nalbuphine, 52
Nalidixic acid, as urinary tract antiseptic, 425–426
Nalmefene, clinical indications for, 53
Naloxone, 52–53
Naltrexone, clinical indications for, 53
Narcolepsy, 18
   treatment of, dextroamphetamine in, 54
      methylphenidate in, 56
Narcotic analgesic antagonist(s), 52–53, 53t
   dosages of, 44t
   See also specific agents
Narcotic analgesic(s), 43–52, 44t, 45–46
   interaction of, with cimetidine, 410
      with neuromuscular blocking agents, 83
      with other agents, 83
   naturally occurring, 47–49
   semisynthetic opiate-like, 49–50
   synthetic, 50–52
   types of, 44
   See also specific agents
Narrow-angle glaucoma, 107
Nasal decongestant(s). See Decongestant(s)
National Center for Health Statistics, diuretics and, 260
Negatol, in hemostasis, 235
Neisseria gonorrheae, 419
   antibiotics against, 428–429
Nematode infestation, 388
Neomycin, 406
Neoplasm(s), malignant. See Cancer; specific tumors
Neostigmine, interaction of, with acetylcholinesterase, 115–116, 115
   with neuromuscular blocking agents, 116
Neostriatum, components of, 6
Nephron, anatomy and physiology of, 261, 263, 264–266, 265
Nephrotic syndrome, treatment of, 272
Nerve action potential, 94–95
Nerve(s), cardiac, 153, 153
   cranial, 5
   in anemia, 222
   in autonomic nervous system, 91, 93–95, 93
   in central nervous system, 2
   of skin, 442
   pain and, 14, 15
   vitamin B_{12} and, 222
   See also Neuron(s); Neurotransmission
Nerve terminal(s), in neurotransmission, 9, 10
Netilmicin, 362
Neuralgia, migraine, 111
Neuraxon(s), in median forebrain bundle, 8
   neurotransmission by, 5–6
   opiate receptors and, 46
Neuroeffector junction(s), in autonomic nervous system, 94
Neuroendocrine system, 290, 290
   See also Endocrine system
Neuroendocrine transducer(s), defined, 294
Neurohypophysis. See Pituitary gland, posterior
Neurokinin, migraine and, 110–111
Neuroleptanalgesia, from fentanyl and droperidol, 29
Neuroleptic malignant syndrome, from chlorpromazine, 69
Neurologic disorder(s), from digitalis, 184
   from paraldehyde, 5
   from syphilis, 420
   in acquired immune deficiency syndrome, 226
   in diabetes mellitus, 308
   in pernicious anemia, 231

Neuromuscular blocking agent(s), 126–129
   interaction of, with aminoglycosides, 361, 371
      with antibiotics, 145
      with diazepam, 145
      with digitalis, 145
      with diuretics, 145
      with edrophonium, 117
      with furosemide, 145
      with inhalation anesthetics, 145
      with lithium carbonate, 83
      with narcotic analgesics, 83
      with neostigmine, 116
      with quinidine, 201
      with thiazide diuretics, 284
   See also specific agents
Neuromuscular junction, acetylcholine receptor in, 98–99, 99
Neuron(s), adrenergic neurotransmission and, 101–102, 101
   autonomic ganglia and, receptors in, 124, 124
   central nervous system, anatomy and physiology of, 9–10, 10
   cholinergic, 12, 13
   dopaminergic, 11, 12
   GABA-ergic, 13
   in Alzheimer's disease, 23
   in autonomic nervous system, 93, 93–94
   in enkephalin-induced pain suppression, 16
   in neuroendocrine system, 294, 297
   noradrenergic, 10, 11
   normal loss of, 3
   seizures and, 19
   sensory, 5
   serotonergic, 11–12, 12
   volatile anesthetics and, 26
Neurosis. See Psychoneurosis
Neurotoxin(s), acetylcholine receptor and, 97
Neurotransmission, adrenergic, 100–105, 100–105
   cholinergic, 96–100, 96–100
   in Alzheimer's disease, 23
   in autonomic nervous system, 94–105, 96–105
      drugs in, 95–105
   in central nervous system, 9–13, 10–13
   in cerebral cortex, 5
   in depression, 20–21
   in mania, 21
   in parkinsonism, 24
   in schizophrenia, 23
   narcotics and, 47
   pain and, 14, 15, 16
Neurotransmitter(s), criteria for, 95
   dextroamphetamine and, 54
   monoamine oxidase inhibitors and, 64–65
   synthesis of, 95
Neutrophil(s), anatomy of, 212
Nicotine, adverse effects of, 125
   Buerger's disease and, 110
   clinical indications for, 125
   mechanism of action of, 124–125
Nicotinic acetylcholine receptor, 98–99, 98–99
Nicotinic acid, as antihyperlipidemic agent, 243
Nicotinic blocking agent(s), 123–128, 123t–124t
   drug interactions with, 145
Nifedipine, as antianginal agent, 188–189
Night sweats, in tuberculosis, 345
Nigrostriatal tract, in neurotransmission, 11

Nikethamide, 56–57
Nitrate(s), adverse effects of, 187
　clinical indications for, 186–187
　interaction of, with alcohol, 203
　　with ergot alkaloids, 203
　mechanism of action of, 186
Nitrofurantoin, as urinary tract antiseptic, 426
Nitrogen, in acetylcholine receptor, 98, *99*
Nitrogen mustard, 246
Nitroglycerin, as antianginal agent, 185–187, 186*t*
　tolerance to, 187
Nitroprusside, as antihypertensive agent, 196
Nitrous oxide, 27–28
Nocardiosis, pulmonary, 346
Nociceptor(s), pain and, 14
Nocturnal enuresis, 18
Nonmetaplastic gestational trophoblastic disease, 432
Nonsteroidal anti-inflammatory agent(s), 453–455, 454*t*
Noradrenaline. See Norepinephrine
Noradrenergic pathway(s), central nervous system, 10, *11*
Norepinephrine, adrenergic receptors and, 103
　adverse effects of, 131
　clinical indications for, 131
　depression and, 20
　dextroamphetamine and, 54
　function of, 299–300
　in autonomic nervous system, 94–96, 100–104, *101*, *103*
　in central nervous system, 10, *11*
　interaction of, with bretylium tosylate, 176
　　with tyramine, 102
　lithium carbonate and, 66
　migraine and, 110
　monoamine oxidase inhibitors and, 64–65
　narcotics and, 47
　re-uptake of, 102
　storage of, 101, *101*
　synthesis of, 100–102, *100–101*
　tricyclic antidepressants and, 60–64
Norfloxacin, as urinary tract antiseptic, 426
　interaction of, with theophylline, 426
　　with warfarin, 426
Nortriptyline, 63
Nose, anatomy of, *337*, *339*
　disorders of, 341–342
Nose brain, defined, 7
Nutrient(s), digestion of, 376–382
　replenishers of, 462*t*
Nutritional deficiency(ies), treatment of, 462*t*
Nystatin, 427–428
　topical, 450

Oat cell carcinoma, bronchogenic, 347
Obesity, diabetes mellitus and, 308
　hypertension and, 168
Obstetric(s), agents in, 429–433, 430*t*
　oxytocin as, 314
　See also Pregnancy
Ocular agent(s), anti-infective, 461*t*
　anti-inflammatory, 461*t*
Ocular disorder(s), from amiodarone, 176
　from chlorpromazine, 68–69
　from ethambutol, 365
　from glucocorticoids, 320
　from hydroxychloroquine sulfate, 455
　from isotretinoin, 451

　glaucoma as, 106–107
　in diabetes mellitus, 308
　treatment of, atropine in, 120
　　cholinergic agents in, 112–118, 120
　　muscarinic blocking agents in, 122
Ocular effect(s), of atropine, 120–121
Open-angle glaucoma, 106–107
Ophthalmia neonatorum, 419
Opiate receptor(s), 45–46, *46*
Opiate(s). See Narcotic analgesic(s); specific agents
Opisthotonus, in seizures, 19
Opium, composition of, 44–45
　history of, 45
Oral cancer, 382–383
　treatment of, 409
Oral contraceptive(s), adverse effects of, 323
　clinical indications for, 323
　estrogen in, 321–323
　interaction of, with aminocaproic acid, 253
　　with anticoagulants, 329
　　with barbiturates, 329
　　with benzodiazepines, 329
　　with phenytoin, 81
　　with tetracyclines, 372
　mechanism of action of, 322–323
　progestins in, 322–323
Organic brain psychosis, 21
Organomercurial agent(s), 280
Organophosphate(s), 144
Orgasm, defined, 418
Osmolarity, hypothalamus and, 8
　in renal physiology, 264–268, *266*
Osmoreceptor(s), in renal physiology, 268
　vasopressin and, 298
Osmosis, in renal physiology, 264–268, *266*
Osmostat, hypothalamus and, 8
Osmotic diuretic(s), 274–275, 275*t*
　drug interactions with, 283
　See also specific agents; Diuretic(s)
Osmotic laxative(s), 399
Osteitis, calcium and, 306
Osteitis deformans, 306, 317
Osteoarthritis, 446, 447
　treatment of, 453
Osteomalacia, from aluminum hydroxide, 391
　from glutethimide, 36
　from phenolphthalein, 395
Osteoporosis, from glucocorticoids, 320
　treatment of, 317, 321
　　diuretics in, 261
　　estrogens in, 321
Otitis media, 342–343
　treatment of, 357–358, 362–363
Ototoxicity, of cisplatin, 434
　of gentamicin, 362
　of streptomycin, 361
Ovary(ies), anatomy and physiology of, 300–301
　cancer of, 421–422
　　treatment of, 434
　gonorrhea of, 419
Oviduct(s), anatomy of, 300
Ovulation, 417
　disorders of, treatment of, 309–310, 322
　hormones in, 300
Oxazepam, 75
Oxazolidinedione(s), structure of, 37, *37*

Oxazolidinedione(s), as anticonvulsant agents, 41–42
  fetal malformations from, 41
Oxidized cellulose, in hemostasis, 236
Oxitriphylline, clinical indications for, 368
Oxycodone, 50
Oxygen, in circulatory system, 210–212, *211*
  in respiratory physiology, 336–338
Oxymorphone, 49–50
Oxyphenbutazone, in arthritis treatment, 454
  interaction of, with anticoagulants, 254
    with methandrostenolone, 329
Oxyprenolol, as antihypertensive agent, 198
Oxytetracycline, 362–363
Oxytocin, adverse effects of, 314
  clinical indications for, 314, 432
  ergonovine versus, 433
  function of, 297
  in posterior pituitary preparation, 312–313
  interaction of, with sympathomimetic agents, 328
  mechanism of action of, 314
  origin of, 294

Paget's disease, 306, 317
Pain, acute, 13–14
  chronic, 14
  from etomidate, 29
  function of, 13–14
  gate theory of, *15*, *16*
  in gastrointestinal ulcers, 384–385
  musculoskeletal receptors for, 441
  perception of, *15*, *16*
  relief of, aspirin in, 453
    by presynaptic inhibition, 16
    codeine in, 48–49
    morphine in, 47–48
    narcotics in, 44–52
    phenytoin in, 39
    semisynthetic narcotic analgesics in, 49–50
    synthetic narcotic analgesics in, 50–52
Pain disorder(s), 13–16, *15–16*
Pain fiber(s), 14, *15*, *16*
Pain threshold, 16
  morphine and, 47
  narcotics and, 44
Paleostriatum, anatomy of, 6
Pamabrom, 273
Panacinar emphysema, 343
Pancreas, anatomy and physiology of, 301–302
  cancer of, 389
  disorders of
    digestive, 389
    from asparaginase, 252
    hyperfunctional, 309
    hypofunctional, 307–309
    treatment of, 400
    See also Diabetes mellitus
  in digestion, 382
Pancreatic enzyme(s), as digestive aids, 400
Pancreatic hormone(s), preparations of, 325–328, 326t–327t
  drug interactions with, 329–330
Pancreatin, as digestive aid, 400
Pancreatitis, 389
Pancrelipase, as digestive aid, 400
Pancuronium, 127
  structure of, 98

Panhypopituitary abnormality(ies), 304
Panol, 404
Panthotenic acid, as gastrointestinal stimulant, 404
Pap smear, clinical indications for, 421
Papaver somniferum, 44–45
Papilloma(s), laryngeal, 347
  oral, 382
Para-aminobenzoic acid, as sunscreen, 453
  interaction of, with sulfonamides, 371, 408, 423, *424*
Para-aminophenol derivative, 456
Para-aminosalicylic acid, clinical indications for, 365
Parafollicular C cell thyroid hormone, 317–318
Paraldehyde, 35–36
Paralysis agitans, 24
Paralytic ileus, 107–108
Paramethadione, as anticonvulsant agent, 41–42
Paranoid schizophrenia, defined, 22
Parasitic infestation(s), dermatologic, 444
  gastrointestinal, 376
Parasomnia(s), 18
Parathormone, function of, 299
  in hypoparathyroidism, 305–306
  preparations of, 318
Parathyroid gland(s), anatomy and physiology of, 299
  hyperfunction of, 306
  hypofunction of, 305–306
  preparations of, 318
Paregoric, in diarrhea treatment, 47
Parkinsonism, as basal ganglia abnormality, 6
  symptoms of, 24
  treatment of, 77–79
    See also Antiparkinsonism agent(s); specific agents
Paroidin, 318
Parotitis, infectious, 383
Paroxysmal atrial tachycardia, 162, *162*
Paroxysmal supraventricular tachyardia, 163, *163*
Partial seizure(s), defined, 19
Pectin, as antidiarrheal, 401–402
Pediculosis, 444
  treatment of, 451
Pelvic inflammatory disease, treatment of, 429
Pemoline, 56
Penicillamine, 253
Penicillin, 355–359
  clinical indications for, genitourinary, 428–429
    in endocarditis, 199
  extended spectrum, 358–359
    clinical indications for, 428
  history of, 355
  interaction of, with chloramphenicol, 371
    with tetracyclines, 371
  natural, 356–357
  penicillinase-resistant, 357–358
    development of, 356
  structure of, 355–356
  types of, 355, 356t
Penicillin G, 356–357
Penicillin V, 357
Penicillinase, penicillin and, 355
Penicillinase-resistant penicillin, 357–358
Penis, anatomy and physiology of, 418, *418*
Pentaerythritol tetranitrate, 187
Pentazocine, 51–52
  adverse effects of, 52
  clinical indications for, 52
  interaction of, with naloxone, 52–53

Pentobarbital, 33
Pentolinium, 125
Pentoxifylline, as hemorrheologic agent, 240–241
Pepsin, antacids and, 393
  in digestion, 378–379
  in peptic ulcers, 383–384
Pepsinogen, in digestion, 378–379
Peptic ulcer(s), 108, 383–385
  treatment of, antacids in, 390–393, 390t
    antispasmodics/anticholinergics in, 394, 395t
    histamine receptor blocking agents in, 393–394, 393t
Peptide(s), in protein synthesis, 360–361
Peptidoglycans, antibiotics and, 354–355, 354–355
Pericarditis, 168
Peristalsis, in digestion, 377
Periventricular system, anatomy and physiology of, 8–9
Pernicious anemia, 216–217, 221–222
  folic acid and, 223, 232
  treatment of, 230–232, 230
Pertussis, treatment of, 363
Petechia(ae), in hemorrhagic disorders, 226–227
Petit mal seizure(s), defined, 19
  treatment of, 38–43
Peyer's patches, in typhoid fever, 385
pH, of skin, 442
  renal system in, 268–269
Phagocytosis, leukocytes in, 212–213
Pharmacist(s), in heart disease treatment, 204–205
Pharyngitis, 342
  streptococcal, 357, 359
Phenacemide, as anticonvulsant agent, 38, 43
Phenanthrene, 45–46
  structure of, 45
Phenelzine, 64–65
Phenethanolamine-N-methyltransferase, 303
Phenindione, 239
Phenobarbital, 34–35
  adverse effects of, 35, 38
  as anticonvulsant agent, 38
  clinical indications for, 35, 38
  interaction of, with corticosteroids, 328
    with digitalis, 202
    with quinidine, 201
  mechanism of action of, 34–35, 38
Phenolphthalein, as stimulant laxative, 395
Phenothiazine(s), 68–70
  as adrenergic blocking agents, 140
  as antihistamines, 349–350
  classes of, 67–68
  drug interactions with, 82
  interaction of, with amphetamines, 82
    with anticholinergic agents, 82
    with bronchodilators, 145
    with lithium carbonate, 82
    with monoamine oxidase inhibitors, 82
    with tricyclic antidepressants, 82
  receptor sites in, 60, 60
  structure of, 59–60, 59
  See also specific agents
Phenoxybenzamine, 137–138
  interaction of, with epinephrine, 138
Phenoxymethylpenicillin, 357
Phenprocoumon, 238
Phentolamine, 138
  interaction of, with bronchodilators, 145

Phenyl blanket, phenobarbital and, 38
Phenylalanine mustard, 246
Phenylbutazone, in arthritis treatment, 454
  interaction of, with anticoagulants, 254
    with corticosteroids, 329
    with phenytoin, 81
Phenylephrine, 133
Phenylethanolamine-N-methyltransferase, 101
Phenylpropanolamine, 133–134
  interaction of, with digoxin, 205
    with monoamine oxidase inhibitors, 82
Phenytoin, as antiarrhythmic agent, 174
  as anticonvulsant agent, 39–40
  in treatment, of digitalis toxicity, 184
  interaction of, with alcohol and depressants, 81
    with antacids, 81
    with anticoagulants, 81
    with barbiturates, 81
    with carbamazepine, 81
    with chloramphenicol, 81
    with cimetidine, 81
    with corticosteroids, 81
    with coumarin, 81
    with dexamethasone, 81
    with dicumarol, 81
    with digitalis, 174, 180, 184
    with disopyramide, 81, 200
    with disulfiram, 81
    with folic acid, 81, 253
    with furosemide, 81
    with isoniazid, 81
    with oral contraceptives, 81
    with phenylbutazone, 81
    with quinidine, 81, 201
    with salicylates, 81
    with sulfonamides, 81
Pheochromocytoma, treatment of, metyrosine in, 144
  phenoxybenzamine in, 137
  phentolamine in, 138
Phlebitis, defined, 220
Phosphate, in hyperparathyroidism, 306
  parathormone and, 299
  parathyroid preparations and, 318
Phosphodiesterase, prazosin and, 197
Phospholipase A_2, pain and, 14
Phospholipid(s), function of, 213
Phosphorylated carbohydrate solution, 405–406
Photosensitivity, from chlorpromazine, 69–70
  from tetracyclines, 363
Physostigmine, clinical indications for, 116
  history of, 115
  interaction of, with acetylcholine, 97
    with acetylcholinesterase, 115–116
  mechanism of action of, 116
Phytonadione. See Vitamin K
Pia mater, defined, 5
Pica, defined, 221
Pilocarpine, adverse effects of, 114
Pimozide, 71
Pindolol, 141
  as antihypertensive agent, 198
Pinworm infestation, 388
Pipbroman, in cancer treatment, 248
Piperazine antihistamine(s), 350
Piperazine phenothiazine(s), 68, 70

Piperidine antihistamine(s), 350
Piperidine phenothiazine(s), 68, 70
Piroxicam, interaction of, with lithium carbonate, 83, 457
Pituitary gland, anatomy and physiology of, 293-298, 296-297, 298t
　anterior, anatomy of, 293, 297
　　hormones of, 296-297, 298t
　　hyperfunction of, 304
　　hypofunction of, 304
　　hypothalamus and, 294-296, 297
　dysfunction of, 304-305
　embryology of, 302
　hypothalamus and, 8
　posterior, anatomy of, 294, 296
　　hormones of, 297-298
　　hypofunction of, 304-305
　preparations of, drug interactions with, 328
Pituitary hormone(s), anterior, 309-312, 309t
　in pregnancy, 302
　mechanism of action of, 290, 294
　origin of, 293-294
　posterior, 312-314, 312t
　　preparation of, 312-313
Placenta, hormones in, 301
Plantago seed, 398
Plaquenil, 455
Plasma cell dyscrasia(s), 225
Plasma cell leukemia, 225
Plasma lipid(s), function of, 213
Plasma membrane, antibiotics and, 354, 365-366
Plasmacytoma, 225
Platelet factor(s), anticoagulants and, 237-239
Platelet(s). *See* Thrombocyte(s)
Pneumonia, lipid, 398
　lobar, 344
　mycoplasma, 345
　pneumonococcal, 344
　primary atypical, 344-345
　treatment of, 357-359, 362-364
　viral, 344-345
Pneumonococcal pneumonia, 344
Poloxamer, 188, 399
Polycarbophil, 403
Polycythemia vera, 223-224
　treatment of, 248
Polymyxin B, 365
Polymyxin E, 406-407
Polyphagia, in diabetes mellitus, 308
Porphyria, phensuximide and, 41
　thiopental and, 28
　trimethadione and, 41
Portal system, hypophyseal, 296, 297
Posterior pituitary preparation, 312-313
　drug interactions with, 328
Postmenopausal syndrome, 307
Postpartum hemorrhage, treatment of, 433
Potassium, digitalis and, 179, 18
　diuretics and, 261-262, 281-282
　glucocorticoids and, 320
　in cardiac electrophysiology, 157-158, 157
　in renal physiology, 266-267, 266-267, 269-270, 275-276
　in treatment, of digitalis toxicity, 184
　quinidine and, 171
　thiazide diuretics and, 277-278

Potassium iodide, as antithyroid agent, 316
　as mucolytic agent, 367t, 369
Potassium-sparing diuretic(s), 279-280, 279t
　interaction of, with potassium, 284
Pralidoxime, 129
Pramoxine, 447
Prazepam, 75
Prazosin, 138-139
　as antihypertensive agent, 196-197
　interaction of, with beta-adrenergic blocking agents, 146
　　with indomethacin, 204
Preanesthetic medication, barbiturates as, 34-35
　morphine as, 48
　pentazocine as, 52
Prednisolone, sodium and, 319-320
Prednisone, clinical indications for, 319
　　genitourinary, 435
　　hematologic, 252
　　in allergic rhinitis, 369
　sodium and, 319-320
Preganglionic neuron(s), in autonomic nervous system, 93, 93-94
Pregnancy, breast cancer and, 422
　estrogens and, 321
　hormones in, 301
　hypothyroidism in, 305
　in diabetes mellitus, 308-309
　isotretinoin and, 451
　oxytocin and, 314, 432
　pituitary hormones in, 302
　prevention of, oral contraceptives in, 322-323
　progestins and, 322
　prostaglandins and, 431-432
　ritodrine and, 433
　toxemia of, 273
Premature atrial contraction(s), 161-162, 162
　treatment of, 171
Premature junctional contraction(s), 164, 164
Premature ventricular contraction(s), 164, 165
　treatment of, 171-173, 175
Premenstrual edema, treatment of, 273
Primary atypical pneumonia, 344-345
Primidone, as anticonvulsant agent, 43
Probenecid, as uricosuric agent, 280t, 280-281
　clinical indications for, 274
　drug interactions with, 284-285
Probucol, as cholesterol-lowering agent, 242
Procainamide, adverse effects of, 172
　clinical indications for, 172
　interaction of, with cholinergics, 200
　　with cimetidine, 200-201
　mechanism of action of, 171-172
Procaine penicillin G, clinical indications for, 428
Procarbazine, in cancer treatment, 251-252
　interaction of, with alcohol, 255
　　with sympathomimetics, 255
Procyclidine, 77-78
Progesterone, 322, 322t
　function of, 300
Progestin(s), 322, 322t
　clinical indications for, 435
Proinsulin, function of, 302
Prolactin, dopaminergic receptors and, 295
Promethazine, 349-350

Propantheline, 123
  interaction of, with digitalis, 202
Propoxyphene, 51
Propranolol, adverse effects of, 140–141
  as antianginal agent, 187–188
  as antianxiety agent, 76
  as antiarrhythmic agent, 175–176
    adverse effects of, 176
    clinical indications for, 175–176
    mechanism of action of, 175, *175*
  as antihypertensive agent, 198
  clinical indications for, 140
  in digitalis toxicity, 184
  interaction of, with bronchodilators, 145
    with digitalis, 175
    with hydralazine, 195
    with insulin, 140
  mechanism of action of, 140
  postmyocardial infarction, 190
Propylthiouracil, 317
Prostaglandin(s), acetaminophen and, 456
  aspirin and, 453
  defined, 14
  in obstetrics, 430–432, 430*t*, 430–431
  pain from, 14
  rheumatoid arthritis and, 446
  synthesis of, 430, *431*
  triglycerides and, 213
  types of, *430*
Prostate, cancer of, 422
    treatment of, 434–435
  urinary tract infections and, 419
Protamine, as heparin antagonist, 239–240
Protein kinase, adrenergic receptors and, 105, *105*
Protein synthesis, antibiotics affecting, 360–364, *361*
  bacterial, 360–361, *361*
  glucocorticoids and, 318
  in diabetes mellitus, 308
  in digestion, 381
  mineralocorticoids and, 320
Proteus, urinary tract infection from, 419
    treatment of, 424–426, 428
Prothrombin, in hemostasis, 217, 218*t*
Prothrombin time, dicumarol dosage and, 238
Protirelin, 312
Protriptyline, 63
Pseudoephedrine, 133
  interaction of, with kaolin, 410
Pseudomonas, antibiotics against, 358, 362, 365
Pseudoparkinsonism, from chlorpromazine, 69
Pseudotumor cerebri, drug-related, 451–452
Psoralen-ultraviolet light A, 451
Psoriasis, 444
  treatment of, 451–452
Psychologic depression, 20–21
  catecholamines and, 60–64
  treatment of, monoamine oxidase inhibitors in, 64–65
    tricyclic antidepressants in, 59–64
Psychologic disorder(s), from antiparkinsonism agents, 78
  from phenacemide, 43
  in acquired immune deficiency syndrome, 226
  in Alzheimer's disease, 23–24
  See also specific disorders
Psychologic effect(s), of chronic pain, 14
  of ethchlorvynol, 36
  of ketamine, 28–29
  of methyprylon, 36
  of pentobarbital, 33
Psychomotor seizure(s), defined, 19
Psychoneurosis, 21
  symptoms of, 21
Psychosis, attention deficit disorder and, 23
  from amphetamines, 54
  median forebrain bundle and, 8
  organic brain, 21
  schizophrenia as, 21–23
    See also Schizophrenia
Psychotherapeutic agent(s), 57–76, 57*t*–58*t*, 59–60
  See also specific agents and types
    of agents
Psychotogen(s), schizophrenia and, 23
Psychotropic agent(s), interaction of, with triazolam, 80
  See also specific agents and types of agents
Psyllium, 398
Pteroylglutamic acid. *See* Folic acid
Puberty, hormone release during, 303–304
Pulmonary cancer, 346–347, 370
Pulmonary disorder(s), antibiotics in, 352*t*
  chronic obstructive, 56, 343–344
  doxapram in, 56
  from bleomycin, 250, 409
  in congestive heart failure, 166
  neoplastic, 346–347
  See also Respiratory disorder(s); specific disorders
Pulmonary membrane, anatomy of, 336
Pupilloconstriction, from morphine, 48
Purine nucleotide(s), folic acid and, 231
Purkinje system, digitalis and, 180–182
  in cardiac electrophysiology, 155, *156*
Pyloric sphincter, anatomy of, 378, *379*
Pyrazolone(s), in arthritis treatment, 454
Pyridostigmine, 117
Pyridoxine, deficiency of, 223
  interaction of, with levodopa, 83
  isoniazid and, 360
Pyridoxine-responsive anemia, 223
Pyrimethamine, 253

Quaternary ammonium compound(s), atropine-like, 123
Quinidine, adverse effects of, 171
  clinical indications for, 171
  interaction of, with antacids, 201
    with anticoagulants, 201
    with barbiturates, 80–81, 201
    with cimetidine, 201
    with digitalis, 171, 201
    with disopyramide, 200
    with neuromuscular blocking agents, 201
    with phenytoin, 81, 201
    with rifampin, 201
  mechanism of action of, 170–171
  sources of, 170
Quinine, quinidine from, 170
Quinolone(s), as urinary tract antiseptics, 426

Radioactive isotope(s), antineoplastic, 252
Radiographic adjunct(s), 464*t*
Radiopaque agent(s), 464*t*
Ranitidine, in peptic ulcer treatment, 393–394
  interaction of, with antacids, 410
Rapid eye movement(s), in sleep, 17–18, *17*

Rauwolfia derivative(s), as antihypertensive agents, 194
Raynaud's disease, 110
Reagin(s), in hypersensitivity reactions, 340
Rebound hypertension, drug-induced, 192
Receptor(s), acetylcholine. *See* Acetylcholine receptor(s)
    adrenergic. *See* Adrenergic receptor(s)
    histamine. *See* Histamine receptor(s)
    insulin, 290–291
    opiate, 45–46, 46
Rectum, anatomy of, 381
Red blood cell(s). *See* Erythrocyte(s)
Red neck syndrome, from vancomycin, 360
Reed-Sternberg cell(s), 225
Reflex(es), cardiac, 153–155, *154–155*
Reflux, gastroesophageal, 377
Reflux esophagitis, 383
Reglan, 404
Renal blood flow, 261, *261*, 263–264, *263*, *265*
Renal calculus(i), in hyperparathyroidism, 306
Renal disorder(s), diabetes insipidus from, 305
    from amphotericin B, 366
    from bacitracin, 360
    from cisplatin, 434
    from gentamicin, 362
    from methoxyflurane, 27
    from polymyxin B, 365
    from streptomycin, 361
    from streptozocin, 408
    in diabetes mellitus, 308
    loop diuretics in, 279
    thiazide diuretics and, 278
    treatment of, diuretics in, 272–273
Renal failure, prevention of, diuretics in, 273
Renal system, 259–286
    anatomy and physiology of, 263–271, *262–263*, *265–267*, *269*, *271*
    disorders of, 271–274
        See also Renal disorder(s)
    drugs affecting, 274–281, 275t, 277t–280t
    introduction to, 260–263, *261*
    kidney function in, 268–271, *269*, *271*
    parathormone and, 299
    summary of, 285–286
    vasopressin and, 297–298
    See also Kidney; Renal entries
Renal waste excretion, 268
Renin, blood pressure and, 190, *190*
    prazosin and, 197
    renal secretion of, 270–271, *271*
    timolol and, 198
Renin-angiotensin-aldosterone system, 270–271, *271*
Repolarization, in neurotransmission, 95
Reproductive/genitourinary system, 415–436
    anatomy and physiology of, female, 416–417, *417*
        male, 417–418, *418*
    disorders of, 419–423
        treatment of, 423–435
        See also Genital disorder(s); specific disorders
    female, oxytocin and, 297
    introduction to, 416
    summary of, 435–436
Reserpine, as antihypertensive agent, 194
    interaction of, with anticholinergics, 144
        with decongestants, 146
        with monoamine oxidase inhibitors, 204
Respiration, 336–339

Respiratory depression, from codeine, 49
    from enflurane, 27
    from isoflurane, 27
    from morphine, 47–48
    from pentazocine, 52
    from phenobarbital, 5
    treatment of, 56
    infectious. *See* Respiratory infection(s)
    obstructive, 366–370
    See also Pulmonary disorder(s); specific disorders
Respiratory infection(s), 341–346
    fungal, 345–346
    lower, 343–346
        antibiotics in, 352t
    symptoms of, 336
    treatment of, 357–366
    upper, 341–343
Respiratory system, 335–372
    anatomy and physiology of, 336–340, *337–339*
    disorders of, 340–347, *341*
        treatment of, 336, 347–370
    introduction to, 336
    obstruction of, 366–370
    summary of, 272
Reticular core, function of, 6
Reticuloendothelial system, 209–256
    See also Circulatory/reticuloendothelial system
Retinoic acid, in acne treatment, 450–451
Retinopathy, in diabetes mellitus, 308
Rhabdomyolysis, from diuretics, 281
Rheumatoid arthritis, 445–446, *445*
    treatment of, 453–456
Rheumatoid factor, in rheumatoid arthritis, 446
Rhinencephalon, defined, 7
Rhinitis, allergic, 340, 342
    treatment of, 369
Rhinosinusitis, acute, 342
Ribonucleic acid, in protein synthesis, 360–361, *361*
Rice water stools, in cholera, 386
Ricinolic acid, castor oil and, 397
Rickets, from phenytoin, 40
Kidaura, 455
Rifampin, adverse effects of, 364
    clinical indications for, 364
    interaction of, with beta-adrenergic blocking agents, 203
        with anticoagulants, 254
        with digitalis, 371
        with disopyramide, 200
        with quinidine, 201
        with sulfonylureas, 330
    mechanism of action of, 364
Rifamycin(s), 364
Ringworm, 443
    treatment of, 450
Ritodrine, 137, 433
Rodenticide(s), warfarin as, 237
Roundworm infestation, 388

Saccharin, bladder cancer and, 423
Salbutamol, 136
Salicylate(s), interaction of, with anticoagulants, 254
    with corticosteroids, 329
    with methotrexate, 255
    with phenytoin, 81
Salicylic acid, topical, 451
Salicylism, 453

Saline laxative(s), 398–399
Salivary gland(s), anatomy of, 376, *378*
  disorders of, 382–383
Salmonella typhi, 385
Salmonellosis, 386
Salpingitis, 420
  gonorrheal, 419
San Joaquin fever, 346
Saponin(s), cardiac glycoside, 179
Scabies, 444
  treatment of, 451
Schizophrenia, 21–23
  age of onset of, 21
  biochemical theories of, 22–23
  symptoms of, 21–22
  treatment of, chlorpromazine in, 68
    molindone in, 72
    thioxanthines in, 70
Schofield, dicumarol and, 220
Scopolamine, 121
Scurvy, 226
Seborrhea, treatment of, 449, 451
Sebum, defined, 440
  function of, 442
Secobarbital, 33–34
Sedation, from nalbuphine, 52
  from phenobarbital, 35
Sedative and hypnotic agent(s), 30–37, 30t, 32–33
  drug interactions with, 79–81
  lorazepam as, 75
  See also specific agents and types of agents
Seg(s), defined, 212
Seizure(s), 19–20
  absence, treatment of, 38–43
  causes of, 19
  chemically induced, 41
  from barbiturate withdrawal, 33
  from chlorpromazine, 69
  from enflurane, 27
  gamma-aminobutyric acid and, 20
  grand mal, 38
  tonic-clonic, 38–40, 43
  treatment of, 37–43
    See also Anticonvulsant agent(s); specific agents
    phenobarbital in, 35
  types of, 19
Sella turcica, pituitary and, 293
Semen, 417–418
Seminoma(s), 422
Senile dementia, 23–24, 70–72
Senna preparation(s), as stimulant laxatives, 396–397
Sensory nerve fiber(s), in central nervous system, 2
Sensory neuron(s), in cerebral cortex, 5
Serotonergic pathway(s), central nervous system, 11–12, *12*
Serotonin, depression and, 20
  mania and, 21
  migraine and, 110
  narcotics and, 47
  schizophrenia and, 23
  tricyclic antidepressants and, 60–64
Serous otitis media, 343
Serturner, morphine isolation by, 45
Sex hormone(s), drug interactions with, 329
  function of, 299–301
  preparations of, 320–325, 321t–324t

Sexual intercourse, anatomic factors in, 416–418
Sexually transmitted disorder(s), 419–420
  acquired immune deficiency syndrome as, 226
Shigellosis, 385
Shingles, 443
Shock, 109–110
  thiopental and, 29
Shoulder(s), disorders of, 441
  See also Arthritis
Sick sinus syndrome, 161
Sickle cell anemia, 216–217
Sideroblast(s), defined, 223
Silicon dioxide, in antacids, 392
Simethicone, 404
Singer's node(s), laryngeal, 347
Single peak insulin, defined, 325
Sinoatrial disorder(s), 160–161, *160–161*
Sinus arrhythmia(s), 160–161, *160–161*
Skeletal effect(s), parathyroid, 299
Skeleton, components of, 441
Skin, anatomy and physiology of, 440–442, *441*
  disorders of. *See* Dermatologic disorder(s); specific disorder(s)
  pH of, 442
Sleep, ascending reticular activating system in, 6–7
  disturbances of, 16–19, *17*
    in depression, 20
    incidence of, 18
  in analgesia, 44
  rapid eye movement, glutethimide and, 36
    methyprylon and, 36
  stages of, 17–18, *17*
Sleep apnea, 18
Sleep wave(s), 17–18, *17*
Sleep-wake disorder(s), 18
Sleepwalking, 18
Slow reacting substance of anaphylaxis, in allergy, 340
Small intestine, anatomy of, 379–381, *380*
Smell, emotions and, 7
Sodium, blood pressure and, 190, *190*
  carbenicillin and, 358–359
  dietary restriction of, diuretics and, 285
  digitalis and, 179–180, *179–181*
  diuretics and, 282
  glucocorticoids and, 319–320
  histamine and, 341
  in cardiac electrophysiology, 157–158, *157*
  in renal physiology, 264–267, *266–267*, 275–276
  lithium carbonate and, 66
  mineralocorticoids and, 320
  phenytoin and, 39
Sodium bicarbonate, as antacid, 390–391
  interaction of, with methenamine, 435
Sodium chloride, in renal physiology, 260, 264–269, *266–267*
Sodium iodide, injection of, 316
Sodium iodide[131], 316–317
Sodium phosphate P32, in cancer treatment, 252
Sodium polystyrene sulfonate resin, 410
Somatostatin, function of, 302
Somatotropin. *See* Growth hormone
Somatrem, 312
Somnambulism, 18
Somnolence, from pentobarbital, 33
  from secobarbital, 34
Sore throat, 342, 357, 359

Spectinomycin, 429
Sperm cell(s), anatomy of, 417–418
Spermatogenesis, androgens and, 324–325
   hormonally induced, 310
   hormones in, 301, 324
Sperry, brain hemisphere research of, 3
Spinal anesthesia, 29. *See also* Local anesthetic agent(s); specific agents
Spinal cord, anatomy and physiology of, 3, 9
   in cardiac anatomy, 153–154, *153–154*
   in pernicious anemia, 231
   pain impulse transmission in, 15, 16
   volatile anesthetics and, 26
Spironolactone, clinical indications for, 279–280
   in cirrhosis, 272
   interaction of, with digitalis, 202
   mechanism of action of, 279
Sprue, celiac, 387
Squamous cell carcinoma, bronchogenic, 346
   defined, 445
   genital, 421
   oral, 382–383
Stab(s), defined, 21
Staphylococcus(i), antibiotics against, 358–360, 364
   food poisoning from, 386
   in endocarditis, 168
   skin infection with, 442
Starling's law, in congestive heart failure, 166
Sternum, anatomy of, 337
Steroid(s), adrenal, 303
   anabolic, 253, 329
   etomidate and, 29
   mechanism of action of, 291, *292*
   See also Corticosteroid(s); specific agents
Stevens-Johnson syndrome, from glucagon, 328
Stimulant(s), central nervous system. *See* Central nervous system stimulant(s); specific agents
   epithelial, 450
   uterine, 429–433
Stokes-Adams syndrome, treatment of, 135
Stomach, anatomy of, 377, *378*
   disorders of, 383–384
   motility of, 379
   secretion of, 378–379
Stomatitis, 382
Stool softener(s), 399
Streptococcus(i), antibiotics against, 357–359, 364
   in endocarditis, 168
   treatment of, 199
   skin infection with, 442–443
Streptococcus pneumoniae, 344
Streptokinase, as thrombolytic agent, 240
Streptomycin, adverse effects of, 361–362
   clinical indications for, 361
   interaction of, with neuromuscular blocking agents, 361, 371
   mechanism of action of, 361
Streptozocin, clinical indications for, gastrointestinal, 408
Stress, autonomic nervous system in, 92–93
   disease and, 7
   tachycardia from, 160
   ulcers and, 384
Striatum, components of, 6
Strong iodine solution, 316
Strongyloidiasis, 388
Substance P, narcotics and, 47

Succinimide(s), as anticonvulsant agents, 38, 40–41
   structure of, 37, *37*
Succinylcholine, 128
   interaction of, with cholinesterase inhibitors, 144
Sucralfate, as antacid, 393
Sulfacetamide sodium, 449
Sulfamethoxazole, clinical indications for, gastrointestinal, 407–408
   urinary tract, 424–425
Sulfasalazine, clinical indications for, 408
Sulfinpyrazone, as antithrombotic agent, 240
   clinical indications for, 274
      uricosuric, 280*t*, 281
   interaction of, with anticoagulants, 254
Sulfonamide(s), adverse effects of, 423–424
   clinical indications for, 423
      respiratory, 365
   dosages of, 423*t*
   interaction of, with anticoagulants, 254
      with methenamine, 435
      with para-aminobenzoic acid, 371
      with phenytoin, 81
      with sulfinpyrazone, 285
   mechanism of action of, 423, *424*
Sulfonylurea(s), 326–327, 327*t*
   dosages of, 327*t*
   drug interactions with, miscellaneous, 330
   interaction of, with beta-adrenergic blocking agents, 330
      with alcohol, 330
      with diazoxide, 330
      with digitoxin, 330
      with rifampin, 330
Sulindac, interaction of, with anticoagulants, 457
Sunlight, skin cancer and, 445
   sunscreens and, 452–453
Sunscreen(s), 452–453
Superinfection(s), antibiotics and, 354, 363
Surgical anesthesia, defined, 25–26
Sutilain(s), topical preparations of, 451
Sweat, function of, 442
   volume of, 442
Sweat gland(s), 442
Sympathomimetic agent(s), adrenergic receptors and, 103
   as nasal decongestants, 369
   interaction of, with anticholinergics, 145
      with digitalis, 202
      with oxytocin, 328
      with procarbazine, 255
Sympathomimetic amine(s), indirect acting, 131, *132*
Syncope, first dose, 139
   from prazosin, 197
Syndrome(s). *See* specific syndromes
Syphilis, 419–420
Systemic lupus erythematosus, 446
Systemic lupus erythematosus-like syndrome, from hydralazine, 195
   from procainamide, 172
Systole, defined, 152
Systolic pressure, defined, 159

T lymphocyte(s), anatomy of, 212
Tachyarrhythmia, sinus, 161
Tachy-brady arrhythmia, 161
Tachycardia, atrioventricular, 174
   defined, 153

Tachycardia, *(continued)*
  from hydralazine, 195
  paroxysmal atrial, 162, *162*
    treatment of, 172
  paroxysmal supraventricular, 163, *163*
  sinus, 160, *160*
  supraventricular, 178
  treatment of, methacholine in, 112
  ventricular, 164–165
    treatment of, 172–173, 175–176
Talbutal, 34
Tamoxifen, 435
T's and blues, abuse of, 349
Tapeworm infestation, 388–389
Tardive dyskinesia, from chlorpromazine, 69
Tartrazine, in ethchlorvynol preparations, 36
Tegison, 451–452
Telencephalon, anatomy of, 4–6
Temazepam, 31
  adverse effects of, 31
  clinical indications for, 31
  interaction of, with alcohol and depressants, 80
Tendinitis, defined, 441
Teratogenicity, of antineoplastic agents, 246–247
  of etretinate, 452
  of isotretinoin, 451
  of progestins, 322
  of trimethadione, 41
Teratoma(s), 422
Terbutaline, 136
Terfenadine, 350
Terpin hydrate, as mucolytic agent, 369
Testis(es), anatomy of, 301, 417, *418*
  cancer of, 422, 434–435
Testosterone, 323–325, 324*t*
  adverse effects of, 324–325
  clinical indications for, 324
  function of, 301
Tetany, in hypoparathyroidism, 306
Tetracycline(s), adverse effects of, 363
  candidiasis following, 354
  clinical indications for, 363
    gastrointestinal, 407
    genitourinary, 429
  interaction of, with antacids, 371–372
    with iron, 253
    with methoxyflurane, 372
    with milk, 372
    with oral contraceptives, 372
    with penicillin, 371
  mechanism of action of, 362–363
  topical, 448
Tetrahydrofolate, 222, 223
  in anemia, 230–231
Thalamus, anatomy of, 7
  emotional stimuli and, 7
  in brain stem formation, 4
  meprobamate and, 76
  opiates and, 46
T-helper cell(s), in acquired immune deficiency syndrome, 226
Theobromine, as diuretic, 280
Theophylline, adverse effects of, 368
  clinical indications for, 368
  interaction of, with beta-adrenergic blocking agents, 203
    with cimetidine, 410
    with erythromycin, 371
    with norfloxacin, 426
  mechanism of action of, 367–368
  mersalyl and, 280
Thermoreceptor(s), pain and, 14
Thermostat, hypothalamus and, 8
Thiamylal, clinical indications for, 29
Thiazide diuretic(s), 276–278, 277*t*
  adverse effects of, 278
  analogs of, 277
  clinical indications for, 277
    antihypertensive, 196, *196*, 199
  dosage of, 277, 277*t*
  drug interactions with, 283–284
  interaction of, with anticoagulants, 283
    with antidiabetics, 283
    with colestipol, 255, 284
    with corticosteroids, 284
    with diazoxide, 204
    with digitalis, 283
    with hydralazine, 204–205
    with insulin, 329
    with lithium carbonate, 283
    with neuromuscular blocking agents, 145, 284
    with trimethoprim-sulfamethoxazole, 283
  mechanism of action of, 276–277
  See also specific agents; Diuretic(s)
Thiobarbiturate(s), synthesis of, 32, *32*
Thioguanine, in cancer treatment, 249
Thiopental, 28
Thioridazine, 70
Thiothixene, 70–71
Thioxanthine derivative(s), 70–71
Thioxanthine derivative(s)
  See also specific agents
Thorax, anatomy of, 336–338, *337*
Threadworm infestation, 388
Throat, disorders of, 342
Thrombin, in hemostasis, 217, 235
Thromboangiitis obliterans, 110
Thrombocyte(s), anatomy of, 213
  aspirin and, 240
  formation of, 215
  in hemostasis, 217, 217*t*–218*t*
Thrombocytopenia, hemorrhage from, 226
Thromboembolism, from oral contraceptives, 323
Thrombolytic agent(s), 240
Thromboplastin, in hemostasis, 217, 218*t*
Thrombosis, from antihemophilic agents, 237
  from estramustine phosphate sodium, 434
  from thrombin, 235
  of hemorrhoids, 387
  prevention of, 240
  treatment of, 238–240
Thrombus(i), formation of, 217–218, 220
Thrush, 382
Thymidylate, in anemia, 230–231, *230*
Thymine synthesis, 230, *230*
Thymus, in immune system, 214–215
Thyroglobulin, function of, 298
  preparations of, 315
Thyroid disorder(s), from mucolytic iodides, 369
Thyroid gland, anatomy and physiology of, 298–299
  antithyroid drugs and, 316–317
  cancer of, 317

hyperfunction of, 305
hypofunction of, 305
iodine and, 303
preparations of, 314–316, 315t
  drug interactions with, 254, 328
Thyroid hormone(s), drug interactions with, 254, 328
  function of, 298–299
  iodine and, 303
  parafollicular C cell, 317–318
  preparations of, 314–316, 315t
Thyroid stimulating hormone, function of, 298
Thyroid storm, defined, 305
Thyrotoxicosis, 305
  treatment of, 316–317
Thyrotropin, 312
Thyroxine, function of, 298
Ticarcillin, clinical indications for, 358
Timolol, 141–142
  as antihypertensive agent, 198
  postmyocardial infarction, 190
Tinea infection(s), 443
  treatment of, 450
Tobacco, nicotine in, 124
Tobramycin, 362
Tocainide, 173–174
Toenail(s), growth of, 442
Tolazoline, 138
  interaction of, with beta-adrenergic blocking agents, 146
Tolbutamide, clinical indications for, 326–327
  interaction of, with alcohol, 330
    with anticoagulants, 253
    with rifampin, 330
Tonic-clonic seizure(s), treatment of, 38–40, 43
Tonsil(s), in immune system, 214
Tonsillectomy, controversy over, 342
Torus lesion(s), 382
Tourette's disorder, treatment of, 71
Tourniquet test, in hemorrhagic disorders, 226
Toxemia of pregnancy, 273
Tranquilizer(s), dosages of, 58t
  See also specific agents
Transaminase(s), valproic acid and, 42
Tranylcypromine, 65
Trauma. See Injury(ies)
Traveler's diarrhea, 386
Trazodone, 65–66
Tremor(s), from chlorpromazine, 69
  in parkinsonism, 24
Trental, 240–241
Treponema pallidum, 419
  antibiotics against, 428–429
Tretinoin, 450
Trexan, 53
Triamcinolone, clinical indications for, 320
Triamterene, 279–280
  interaction of, with indomethacin, 457
Triazolam, 31
  drug interactions of, 80
Trichinosis, 388
Trichloroethanol, effects of, 35
Trichomoniasis, treatment of, 426–427
  vaginal, 420
Trichuriasis, 388
Tricyclic antidepressant(s), 57t, 59–64, 59–60
  interaction of, with amphetamines, 82
    with anticholinergic agents, 82, 144

with barbiturates, 80, 82
with bronchodilators, 145
with cimetidine, 82
with clonidine, 203–204
with ethchlorvynol, 80
with guanethidine, 204
with methylphenidate, 82
with phenothiazines, 82
receptor sites in, 60, 60
structure of, 59
See also specific agents
Triethylenethlophosphoramide, 433–434
Triglyceride(s), drugs lowering levels of, 241t, 243–244
  function of, 213
  guanabenz and, 192
Triiodothyronine, function of, 298
Trimethadione, as anticonvulsant agent, 41
Trimethaphan, 125–126
  as antihypertensive agent, 193
Trimethoprim, clinical indications for, gastrointestinal, 407
  urinary tract, 424–425
Trimethoprim-sulfamethoxazole, interaction of, with thiazide diuretics, 283
1,3,7-Trimethylxanthine. See Caffeine
Trimipramine, 63–64
Tripelennamine, 349
Triple reaction of Lewis, 444
Troleandomycin, 364
Trophoblast, in choriocarcinoma, 421
Tropicamide, 122
Troponin-tropomyosin, digitalis and, 180, 181
Tuberculosis, 345
  of skin, 443
  treatment of. See Antituberculosis agent(s)
Tubocurarine, 126–127
d-Tubocurarine, structure of, 98
Tumor(s), esophageal, 383
  germ cell, 422
  in hyperparathyroidism, 306
  malignant. See Cancer; specific tumors
  oral, 382–383
  pulmonary, 346–347
Tunnel vision, in glaucoma, 107
Tympanic membrane, 339–340, 339
Typhoid fever, 385
  treatment of, 406
Tyramine, interaction of, with norepinephrine, 102
  neurotransmission and, 95
Tyrosine, in catecholamine synthesis, 100–101, 100–101
Tyrosine hydroxylase, parkinsonism and, 24

Ulcer(s), dermal, 451
  duodenal, 384–385
  esophageal, 383
  gastric, 383–384
  gastrointestinal, 108–109
    See also Peptic ulcer(s)
  herpetic, 419
  peptic. See Peptic ulcer(s)
Ulcerative colitis, 387
  loperamide in, 403
Ultraviolet light, sunscreens and, 452–453
Undifferentiated schizophrenia, defined, 22
Unipolar depression, defined, 20
Uracil mustard, in cancer treatment, 247
Urea, adverse effects of, 275

Urethra, anatomy of, 417, *418*
Urethritis, from sexually transmitted disorders, 419
Uric acid, in gout, 274
    thiazide diuretics and, 277–278
    uricosuric agents and, 274, 281
Uricosuric agent(s), 280–281, 280*t*
    defined, 263
    drug interactions with, 284–285
    in treatment, of gout, 274
Urinary bladder atony, 108
Urinary tract, anatomy and physiology of, 262, 264–267
    female, 416–417, *417*
    infections of, 420–421
        treatment of, 423–426
    male, 417–418, *418*
    See also Renal system
Urokinase, as thrombolytic agent, 240
Urticaria, 444
Uterus, agents affecting muscles of, 429–433, 430*t*
    anatomy of, 416, *417*
    cancer of, 421
        estrogens and, 321
        treatment of, 434–435
    disorders of, 420–421
    estrogens and, 321
    oxytocin and, 297
    progestins and, 322–323

Vaccination(s), interaction of, with methotrexate, 255
Vaccine(s), 464*t*
Vagina, anatomy of, 416, *417*
    cancer of, 421
Vaginitis, 420
    treatment of, 424
Vagus nerve(s), digitalis and, 182
    heart rate and, 153, *153*
    in digestion, 378–379
    quinidine and, 170–171
Vagusstoff, 97
Valproic acid, as anticonvulsant agent, 42
    interaction of, with barbiturates, 80
Van der Waals force(s), adrenergic receptors and, 103–104
    cholinergic receptors and, 98
Vancomycin, 359–360
Vas deferens, anatomy of, 417, *418*
Vascular anatomy and physiology, 158–160, *159*
Vascular collapse, in cirrhosis, 272
Vascular disorder(s), Buerger's, 110
    from oral contraceptives, 323
    in diabetes mellitus, 308
    migraine as, 110–111
    Raynaud's, 110
    treatment of, alpha-adrenergic blocking agents in, 137–139
    vasopressin and, 313
Vascular injury(ies), clotting and, 217
Vasoconstriction, from adrenergic agents, 130–135
    from caffeine, 55
    from ergot alkaloids, 139
Vasodilator(s), as antihypertensive agents, 194–196, *195*, 199
    diuretics and, 273–274
Vasopressin, drug interactions with, 328
    function of, 297–298

in diabetes insipidus, 304–305
in posterior pituitary preparation, 312–313
in renal physiology, 266, 267–268
injection of, 313
origin of, 294
vincristine and, 250
Vasopressin tannate, 313
Vecuronium, 128
Vein(s), anatomy of, 159–160
    antianginal agents and, 186
    in congestive heart failure, 165–166
Venereal disease(s), 226, 419–420
Venous pain, from etomidate, 29
Venous thrombosis, treatment of, 238–239
Ventricle(s), anatomy of, 150, *151–152*, 152
Ventricular arrhythmia(s), 164–165, *165*
Venule(s), anatomy of, 159
Verapamil, as antianginal agent, 188–189
    as antiarrhythmic agent, 177, *177*
    interaction of, with beta-adrenergic blocking agents, 203
        with digitalis, 202–203
Vibrio cholerae, 386
Vinblastine, in cancer treatment, 250
Vincent's infection, treatment of, 357
Vincristine, in cancer treatment, 250
Viral infection(s), hepatitis as, 389
    of skin, 443
    respiratory, 342–343, 344–345
Viral pneumonia, 344–345
Virus(es), herpes. *See* Herpes entries
    human immunodeficiency, 226
Visceral brain, defined, 7
Visual disturbance(s), from digitalis, 184
    from trimethadione, 41
    in glaucoma, 106–107
Vitamin A, in acne treatment, 450–451
    interaction of, with corticosteroids, 329
        with mineral oil, 410
Vitamin B_{12}, deficiency of, from nitrous oxide, 28
    treatment of, 230–231
    function of, 216, 222
    interaction of, with aminoglycosides, 23
        with aminosalicylic acid, 253
        with chloramphenicol, 253
    pernicious anemia and, 216, 221, 230–231
Vitamin C, deficiency of, 226
    capillaries and, 217
    urine pH and, 425
Vitamin D, in hypoparathyroidism, 306, 318
    phenytoin and, 40
Vitamin K, adverse effects of, 233
    anticoagulants and, 237–238
    clinical indications for, 232–233
    coagulation and, 220
    mechanism of action of, 232
Vitamin(s), 463*t*. *See also* specific vitamins
Volatile anesthetic agent(s), 26–28. *See also* specific agents
Vomiting, from ethchlorvynol, 36
    treatment of, 405–406, 405*t*
Von Willebrand's disease, desmopressin in, 314
Vulva, anatomy of, 416–417, *417*
    cancer of, 421

Waksman, streptomycin and, 361
Waldenstrom's macroglobulinemia, 225

Warfarin, adverse effects of, 239
  clinical indications for, 238
  drug interactions with, 253–254
  history of, 237
  interaction of, with danazol, 328
    with norfloxacin, 426
    with quinidine, 201
  mechanism of action of, 238
Wart(s), 443
Water balance, renal system in, 269
  skin in, 440, 442
Water purification system, renal system versus, 260, *261*
Water/electrolyte balance, renal system in, 260, *261*, 264–267, *266–267*, 269–270
Wheal and flare reaction, 444
Whipple's disease, 388
Whipworm infestation, 388

White blood cell(s). *See* Leukocyte(s)
Wolff-Parkinson-White synrome, 163, *164*

Xanthine oxidase, allopurinol and, 456
Xanthine(s), as bronchodilators, 367–368, 367t
  as diuretics, 280
  structure of, *55*
Xanthoma(ta), in hyperlipoproteinemia, 228
Xerostomia, from atropine, 120–121
  from isotretinoin, 451

Yeast cell preparation(s), antihemorrhoidal, 404

Zinc oxide, as sunscreen, 453
Zollinger-Ellison syndrome, treatment of, 394
Zovirax, 427